Nutrition and Diet Therapy

Carroll A. Lutz, MA, RN

Associate Professor
Jackson Community College
Jackson, Michigan

Karen Rutherford Przytulski, MS, RD

Director of Dietary and Registered Dietitian
Doctors Hospital of Jackson
Supplemental Instructor
Allied Health
Jackson Community College
Jackson, Michigan

F. A. Davis Company

F. A. DAVIS COMPANY • Philadelphia

F. A. Davis Company
1915 Arch Street
Philadelphia, PA 19103

Printed in the United States of America

Last digit indicates print number: 10 9 8 7 6 5 4 3

Publisher, Nursing: Robert G. Martone
Nursing Development Editor: Melanie Freely
Production Editor: Gail Shapiro
Cover Design By: Steven Morrone

As new scientific information becomes available through basic and clinical research, recommended treatments and drug therapies undergo changes. The author(s) and publisher have done everything possible to make this book accurate, up to date, and in accord with accepted standards at the time of publication. The authors, editors, and publisher are not responsible for errors or omissions or for consequences from application of the book, and make no warranty, expressed or implied, in regard to the contents of the book. Any practice described in this book should be applied by the reader in accordance with professional standards of care used in regard to the unique circumstances that may apply in each situation. The reader is advised always to check product information (package inserts) for changes and new information regarding dose and contraindications before administering any drug. Caution is especially urged when using new or infrequently ordered drugs.

Library of Congress Cataloging–in–Publication Data

Lutz, Carroll A.
  Nutrition and diet therapy / Carroll A. Lutz, Karen Rutherford Przytulski
    p.   cm.
  Includes bibliography references and index.
  ISBN 0-8036-5681-5
  1. Dietetics.   2. Diet Therapy.   3. Nutrition.   4. Nursing.
  I. Przytulski, Karen Rutherford.   II. Title.
  [DNLM: 1. Nutrition.   2. Diet Therapy.   WB 400 L975n 1994]
  RM217.L88 1994
  613.2—dc20
  DNLM/DLC
  for Library of Congress   94–17986
                                                                 CIP

To my parents with gratitude for teaching me by their example that a commitment to your chosen profession brings satisfaction that is difficult to derive elsewhere. To my children with hope that I have taught them that a commitment to one's work is an important part of emotional well-being.

Karen Rutherford Przytulski

To all my students who ever asked something I could not answer:
Thanks for the stimulus to learn; and
To all my teachers, including family, friends, and colleagues:
Thanks for your ongoing support over the years.

Carroll A. Lutz

Preface

This first edition of *Nutrition and Diet Therapy* is designed to provide the beginning student with an understanding of the fundamentals of nutrition and how these fundamentals relate to the promotion and maintenance of optimal health. It emphasizes the practical applications of the current principles of nutrition and diet therapy in the prevention and treatment of nutrition-related pathologies.

This book was written to meet the educational needs of nursing students, dietetic assistants, diet technicians, and others. Support materials for the nursing student (and instructor) include charting tips and case studies with examples of care plans presented throughout the text. In addition, when the role of the healthcare professional is discussed, the specific role of the nurse is accentuated, if deemed appropriate.

This text can be used to teach a complete course in nutrition and supplement as a desk reference for practitioners. The student using this book needs no previous exposure to anatomy, physiology, or medical terminology. To enable students to more easily absorb the material, the foundation is carefully planned so that ideas are presented simply at first and then built up slowly in complexity until complete concepts emerge. More challenging subjects are fully supported by diagrams, illustrations, figures, or tables.

The content of *Nutrition and Diet Therapy* is organized into three units.

Unit I, **The Role of Nutrients in the Human Body,** consists of Chapters 1 through 9. This unit covers all the essential nutrients including definitions, functions, effects of excesses and deficiencies, and food sources. Chapter 5 clearly and concisely discusses how the body uses food to obtain energy for continued growth and/or maintenance. How the body maintains energy balance is discussed in detail in Chapter 8.

Unit II, **Family and Community Nutrition,** consists of Chapters 10 through 12. This unit provides an overview of topics such as nutrition in the life cycle, food and preparation, storage, and safety.

Unit III, **Clinical Nutrition,** consists of Chapters 13 through 22. This unit focuses on the care of patients with pathologies either caused by or causing nutritional impairments. Pathological conditions include diabetes mellitus and hypoglycemia, cardiovascular disease, renal disease, gastrointestinal disease, cancer, and AIDS. Other topics discussed in this unit include food, nutrient, and drug interactions, weight control, and nutrition during stress and surgery.

There are several special features used throughout the text that facilitate the teaching and learning process. All of the chapters include the following learning aids:

Chapter Outline—Quickly identifies chapter contents.

Key Terms—List important terms in the chapter. Following each key term in the list, a page number reference appears in parentheses so that the student can easily locate the terms in the chapter text. In addition, key terms are identified in the text as either **bold face** or *italic*, and all can be found in the extensive glossary.

Learning Objectives—Identify student outcomes.

Introductory Paragraph—Provides an overview of the chapter's key topic.

Chapter Summary—Briefly summarizes of contents of the chapter.

Marginal Notes—Highlight definitions of key terminology.

Study Aids—Include **Chapter Review Questions** and an **NCLEX Style Quiz.** These help the student to review chapter contents and to prepare for the kinds of questions that may appear on the NCLEX examination. *Answers to the Study Aids are Located in the Appendix.*

Bibliography—Lists publication sources of information; can be used by the student for further reading.

Tables, graphs, and illustrations—Aid the student and instructor in conceptualizing the material.

Additional special features appearing in most chapters that assist the student in the integration of information and the application of this information in clinical decision making include the following:

Case Study with a proposed **Nursing Care Plan**—Allows the student to see how the nutrition principles described in the chapter are applied in a specific clinical situation.

Charting Tips—Include documentation advice for charting.

Clinical Applications—Cover a variety of topics that emphasize text material as applied to clinical practice or current use in the health-care professions.

Clinical Calculations—Isolate and explain in detail many of the mathematical calculations that are used in nutritional science.

This text also includes the following aids:

Appendices—Include a Food Composition Table, Height and Weight Tables, Growth Charts, a sample Food Frequency Questionnaire, Recommended Dietary Allowance Table, Estimated Safe and Adequate Daily Dietary Intakes of Selected Vitamins and Minerals, Estimated Minimum Requirements of Sodium, Chloride, and Potassium, Food Exchange List of the American Dietetic and Diabetic Association, Body Fat and Skinfold Tables, An Outline of Subjective Data for Nutritional Screening, Guide to Evaluate Dietary Status, Selected Religious Dietary Restrictions, Characteristic Eating Patterns of Selected Cultural Groups, New Food Labels, Calculation Aids and Conversion Factors, and Answers to Study Aids.

Glossary—Includes over 700 entries, which eliminates the need for a medical dictionary.

Index—Provides a quick reference to the main contents of the book. An instructor's MAT Test Bank is available for this book.

The text is comprehensive, clearly written, and fully supported by the many learning aids described above. We feel that *Nutrition and Diet*

Therapy provides the clinical information necessary for a fuller understanding of the relationship between knowledge and its clinical application. This text balances the simple direct explanations of the underlying basic sciences and the actual clinical responsibilities of the healthcare professional.

Acknowledgments

A project as massive as the writing of a textbook requires the assistance of many people. We would first like to thank all the organizations and publishers that gave permission for the use of their material. We would also like to thank Russell Tobe, J.D., D.O., B.S.E.E. for the multiple hours he spent reviewing selected portions of the manuscript. This textbook would have been much less without his unselfish devotion to this project

Many of our peers contributed to this project. In particular we would like to thank Janice Wohlgemuth B.S., P.T., Gayle Easton P.A., Ruby Mann, B.A., and Stephanie Huffman, R.N. for their review of selected chapters. We would also like to thank all the talented people at F. A. Davis for their assistance and ongoing encouragement. A special thanks to Bob Martone, Ruth DeGeorge, Melanie Freely, Bob Butler, and Gail Shapiro for taking a chance on two unknown writers. We would also like to thank our students for their challenging questions and continuing inspiration. Lastly, we would like to thank our husbands, Bob and Paul, for understanding our compulsion to write. We know it has been difficult to live with us during the past five years.

Consultants

Cheryl Brown, RN
Erwin Vocational School
Tampa, FL

Phyllis Campbell, MS
LPN Program
Lee County Voc Tech
Ft. Myers, FL

LaDeena Cantrell, RN, BSN
Ivy Tech
Indiana Vocational Technical College
Terre Haute, IN

Eileen Monahan Chopnick, MBA, RD
Adjunct Faculty
Widener University
School of Nursing
Chester, PA

Marcia Costello, MS, RD
Assistant Professor
College of Nursing
Villanova University
Villanova, PA

Sandra Freeman, RN, BS, Ed
Practical Nursing Coordinator
Hinds Community College
Jackson, MS

Mary Bridget Jordan, BS
Practical Nursing Instructor
St. Louis Board of Education
St. Louis, MO

Glenda Lindseth, PhD, RN, LRD
Associate Professor
Eastern Michigan University
Ypsilanti, MI

Mary Mirch, RN, MS
Associate Professor
Glendale Community College
Glendale, CA

Mary Courtney Moore, PhD, RN, RD
Research Associate
Vanderbilt University
Nashville, TN

Carol Nelson, RN, BSN, MSN
Instructor
Spokane Community College
Spokane, WA

Rose Rash, RN, BSN
Corsicanna, TX

Laura Waddle
Mesquite, TX

Contents

Unit One
The Role of Nutrients in the Human Body

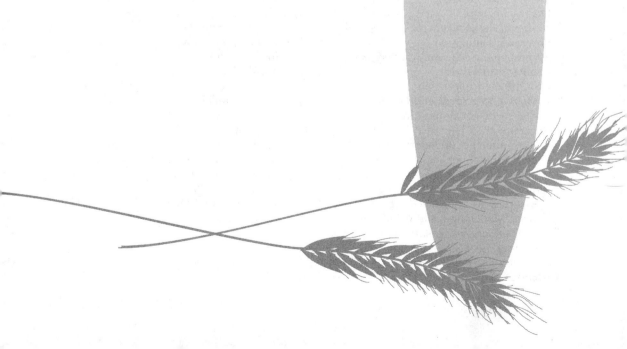

Chapter Outline

Evolution of the Human Body and Emergence of Health Issues
Effect of Agriculture
Adaptation to Feast and Famine
Conditions
Food Safety Issues
Our Ancestors' View of Health
Current Attitudes toward Health and
Health Care
The Emerging Role of the Healthcare Professional
Physician
Registered Dietitian
Dietetic Technician
Registered Nurse
Licensed Practical Nurse
Other Healthcare Personnel
Patient or Client as the Focus of the
Healthcare Provider
Nutrition Is a Science
Nutrients
Functions of Nutrients
Nutrient Deficiencies and Excesses
Undernutrition
Overnutrition
Nutrition and Health
Physical Growth and Development
Body Composition
Mental Development
Diet as Therapy
Nutritional Assessment
Physical Examination
Anthropometric Measurements
Laboratory Tests
Food Intake Information
Nutritional Standards and Guides
Tables of Food Composition
Recommended Dietary Allowances
US Recommended Dietary Allowances
Dietary Guidelines
The Food Pyramid
American Dietetic and Diabetic
Associations Exchange Lists
Variety, Moderation, and Balance
The Delivery of Nutritional Care
Screening
Referring
Summary

Study Aids
Chapter Review Questions
NCLEX-Style Quiz
Clinical Application 1–1: Dietary Guidelines
Clinical Calculation 1–1: Percent Healthy Body Weight
Clinical Calculation 1–2: Determination of Body Frame Type

Key Terms

As a study aid, each term is followed by the page number where the term is defined in the chapter. Terms that appear **boldface** or <u>underscored</u> in the chapter text are located in the glossary.

anthropometry (12)
anthropometric measurements (12)
ash (9)
balanced diet (24)
cyclical variation (4)
dementia (11)
dietary recall, 24-hour (15)
dietary status (11)
energy (7)
energy nutrients (8)
essential nutrient (7)
exchange (22)
food frequency (15)
Food Pyramid (20)
food record (15)
health (5)
malnutrition (8)
metabolism (7)
nonessential (7)
nutrient (7)
nutrition (6)
nutritional assessment (11)
nutritional status (11)
overnutrition (9)
Recommended Dietary Allowance (17)
undernutrition (8)

Chapter One
Evolution, Nutrition, and the Nurse

Learning Objectives

After completing this chapter, the student should be able to:

1. Discuss the relationship between the biological evolution of the human body and present nutritional concerns.
2. State the three functions of nutrients.
3. Identify the six classes of nutrients.
4. Discuss the effects of malnutrition on health and provide examples.
5. Describe the relationship between nutrition and health.
6. List three standards or guides used by healthcare workers to either evaluate or educate patients about nutrition.

*W*hy does the body need fat? What are the effects of eating more (or less) food than we should? How does nutrition impact health?

The answer to the first of these questions requires an inquiry into human evolution. In this chapter, we compare our ancestors' food habits and their effect on health with those of modern people. The world and basic concepts about health and nutrition have changed considerably in the intervening 5 to 8 million years. We will discuss past and present views about health and health care and how these views affect the role of the healthcare professional. We will consider the effects of nutrition and health and the importance of nutrients in the diet.

EVOLUTION OF THE HUMAN BODY AND EMERGENCE OF HEALTH ISSUES

Throughout history our ancestors survived on a number of different diets. What early humans ate in any particular geographic area depended on the climate, their hunting and gathering skills, the state of their food-processing technology, and what foods were available. The human body evolved the capability to subsist on a wide variety of foodstuffs of both plant and animal origin.

Effect of Agriculture

The emergence of agriculture led to population expansion. Individuals learned to work together to grow crops and began to live together in larger groups to protect the cultivated fields and harvested food stores, leading to the development of villages and towns. Food distribution systems evolved for the rationing of the harvest from one growing season to the next. This helped assure a food supply in the event of a poor harvest or natural disaster.

However, agriculture, especially single-crop agriculture, limited the variety of foods eaten in a given community. Today we understand that growth deficiencies can result from diets based on single-crop agriculture, because no single food can furnish all the raw materials necessary for human growth and healthful maintenance. Variety, moderation, and balance in the diet are all necessary for health.

Adaptation to Feast and Famine Conditions

When archaeologists study fossils and draw conclusions about the diet of early humans, other relationships between human beings, food, and the environment become evident. Seasonal and cyclical variations in food availability affected our ancestors. An example of a seasonal variation is the abundance of food during summer and fall compared with the scarcity of food late in winter. A **cyclical variation** refers to a recurring series of events such as a period of drought and famine followed by a period of plentiful rainfall.

Cyclical variation—A recurring series of events during a specified time period

Biologically, the human body adapted to these feast-or-famine conditions by developing the capacity to store energy as fat. While this adaptation enabled human beings to survive famine, individuals did not always receive optimal nourishment. The situation is much the same today. Famine still exists in many Third World countries, and even in the developed countries there are population groups—notably, the poor, the young, and the elderly—that suffer from malnutrition.

Food Safety Issues

Frequently, we paint a picture of the so-called natural man or woman, imagining a time when healthy, happy people subsisted on unprocessed foods. Though free from pesticides and additives, the food our ancestors ate was not always safe. Meat, for example, was often rancid and contained parasites; fungal infestations contaminated not only stored grain but also grain in the fields; and heavy metals leached out of utensils into food, often with fatal effects. Notwithstanding these and other hazards, humans still managed to survive as a species.

Our Ancestors' View of Health

In the past, attitudes about health were often linked to following or not following the laws of a supernatural being. For example, the recurrent epidemics of bubonic plague that swept Europe during the Middle Ages were thought to be the result of witchcraft and the work of the devil. With the discovery of bacteria in the late 1880s and the subsequent discovery and use of antibiotics in the 1940s, many diseases were better understood and treatable. Until recent decades, the primary focus of health care was on curing an existing disease. Slowly, in part as a result of scientific progress, the thrust of healthcare delivery has shifted from curing an existing disease to preventing disease. The use of vaccines is one form of prevention. The consumption of substances in food, which can help to prevent certain diseases, is another example of prevention.

Health—A state of complete physical, mental, and social well-being, not just the absence of disease or infirmity

Current Attitudes toward Health and Health Care

Today many diseases are linked to lifestyle behaviors such as smoking, lack of adequate physical activity, and poor nutritional habits. Healthcare providers, in their role as educators, emphasize the relationship between lifestyle and risk of contracting disease. People are increasingly managing their health problems and making personal commitments to lead healthier lives. Nutrition is, in part, a preventive science. How and what one eats is a lifestyle choice.

The ability to detect disease early with the help of highly sophisticated technology is another major focus of healthcare delivery. Not only can it sometimes reduce suffering and mortality, but early disease detection also enables people to alter behaviors, including food habits, which can help to retard disease progression. Although early identification of disease frequently results in a cost saving to the patient, educating and screening patients for disease is expensive to society. Can we afford to pay for disease detection and health education? The answer depends largely on the willingness of healthcare providers to educate patients during each patient encounter.

THE EMERGING ROLE OF THE HEALTHCARE PROFESSIONAL

Changing attitudes about health have altered the role of the healthcare professional. No longer is the patient totally reliant on the physician; his or her care is now in the hands of a number of allied health personnel. Indeed, a hospital patient's healthcare team may include more than 15 members.

The respective titles and responsibilities of the major members of the healthcare team are outlined below.

Physician

The physician is responsible for the diagnosis and treatment of the medical condition. He or she manages all care, orders laboratory tests, prescribes medications and diet, and explains the treatment plan to the patient.

Registered Dietitian

The registered dietitian (RD), together with the physician, has the responsibility to meet the patient's nutritional needs. This includes interpreting the physician's diet order in terms of the patient's food habits and food choices; evaluating the patient's response to the therapeutic diet; and providing nutrition education and counseling for patients.

Dietetic Technician

The dietetic technician (DT) assists the dietitian by taking nutrition histories and body measurements, reviewing records, and monitoring patients' food intake.

Registered Nurse

The registered nurse (RN) is responsible for the patient's daily health care, including his or her nutritional care. The RN communicates with the physician and the dietitian regarding the patient's response to food, including intake and tolerance; provides nutrition education, if needed, and records information on the patient's chart.

Licensed Practical Nurse

The licensed practical nurse (LPN), supervised by an RN, feeds clients, monitors food consumption, measures intake and output, and records data.

Other Healthcare Personnel

Other healthcare personnel who may be involved in patient care include the clinical pharmacist, the licensed social worker, the medical technologist, the nurse practitioner, and the physical therapist.

Patient or Client as the Focus of the Healthcare Provider

The patient is the focus of the healthcare team, and both the patient and the family members should be involved in the care plan. Patients who participate in their own care are more likely to achieve the goals or objectives set.

NUTRITION IS A SCIENCE

Nutrition—The science of food and its relation to humans

Stated simply, **nutrition** is the relationship of humans to food. Our study of nutrition will include a discussion of the following topics:

- The chemical content of food
- The use of food by the body
- The relationship of food to health
- The selection of food
- Techniques to change food behavior
- The diet as treatment for disease
- The relationship between medications and food intake

As this list shows, the science of nutrition encompasses ideas from many other sciences: biology, chemistry, economics, educational theory, medicine, pharmacology, physiology, psychology, and sociology. This connection with other disciplines suggests far-reaching implications of good nutrition.

Nutrients

The science of nutrition is based on the nutrients found in food. **Nutrients** are chemical substances supplied by food that the body needs for growth, maintenance, and repair. Nutrients can be divided into six groups:

1. Carbohydrates (often abbreviated as CHO)
2. Fats (lipids)
3. Proteins
4. Minerals
5. Vitamins
6. Water

Nutrient—A chemical substance supplied by food that the body needs for growth, maintenance, and repair

Each group will be discussed in a separate chapter.

Nutrients may be either essential or nonessential, depending on whether the body can or cannot manufacture them. When the body requires a nutrient for growth or maintenance but lacks the ability to manufacture it in amounts sufficient to meet bodily needs, the nutrient is called essential and must be supplied by foods in the diet. Vitamin C, vitamin A, and calcium are just three examples of the more than 40 essential nutrients. However, if the nutrient is not needed in the diet because the body can make its own, the nutrient is called nonessential.

Food—Any material that provides the nutrients necessary to maintain growth and physical well-being

Functions of Nutrients

All nutrients perform one or more of the following functions: they serve as a source of energy or heat, support the growth and maintenance of tissue, and/or aid the regulation of basic body processes. These three life-sustaining functions collectively fall under the term metabolism. *Metabolism* is the sum of all physical and chemical changes that take place in the body. Nutrients have specific metabolic functions and interact with one another to maintain the human organism.

Essential nutrient—One which must be present in the diet because the body lacks the ability to manufacture it in sufficient amounts for optimal health

Source of Energy or Heat

Energy is defined in the physical sciences as the capacity to do work. Energy can take several forms: electrical, thermal (heat), and mechanical. All food enters the body as potential chemical energy. The body processes the chemical energy stored in food and converts it into other energy forms. For example, chemical energy can be transformed into electrical signals in nerves, which is changed to mechanical energy in muscles. Carbohydrates,

Energy—The capacity to do work

Energy nutrients—The chemical substances in food that are able to supply fuel; refers collectively to carbohydrates, fat, and protein

fats, and proteins are the nutrients that supply energy, and for this reason they are referred to as the **energy nutrients.**

Growth and Maintenance of Tissues

Some nutrients provide the raw materials for building the body's structure and participate in the continued growth and maintenance of the necessary tissues. Water, proteins, fats, and minerals are the nutrient classes that contribute in a major way to building the body's structure.

Regulation of Body Processes

Some nutrients control or regulate the chemical processes in the body. For example, certain minerals and protein help regulate how water is distributed in the body. Vitamins participate in the series of reactions needed to generate energy. Even though vitamins themselves are not energy sources, if the body lacks a particular vitamin, the body will not be an efficient producer of energy.

NUTRIENT DEFICIENCIES AND EXCESSES

Malnutrition—Poor nutrition; results when the body's cells receive either an excess or a deficiency of one or more nutrients

Too much or too little of a nutrient can interfere with health and well-being. There is a beneficial range of intake for any nutrient; to go below or above that range is incompatible with optimal health. If there is inadequate nutrient intake, the result will be malnutrition. If there is an excessive intake of a nutrient, the result will be malnutrition. Thus, **malnutrition** (poor nutrition) occurs when body cells receive too much or too little of one or more nutrients.

Undernutrition

Malnutrition includes <u>undernutrition,</u> which is the result of a deficiency of one or more nutrients. Undernutrition can be related to:

- The inability to obtain foods that contain the essential nutrients
- Failure to consume essential nutrients
- The poor use of nutrients by the body
- Disease conditions that increase the body's need for nutrients
- A too-rapid excretion of nutrients from the body

Undernutrition can result from many different circumstances. For example, stress caused by trauma, surgery, or burns is frequently a cause of malnutrition. Some persons exposed to severe and prolonged stressors of these kinds may be malnourished even though they are eating a "normal diet." Prolonged stress causes the body to break down internal protein stores, resulting in larger than usual amounts of nutrients being lost in the urine. Mental and emotional stress has not been as clearly linked to malnutrition.

Although not widespread, undernutrition in the United States does exist. It generally occurs as a result of poverty, illness, neglect, poor dietary planning, environmental hazards, and prolonged hospitalization. Especially vulnerable groups are children, pregnant women, and the elderly. For example, malnourished children grow at a slower rate, are prone to infections, and are more likely to have mental and developmental problems.

Overnutrition

Malnutrition includes overnutrition, which is the excessive intake of nutrients. For example, when ingested in very high doses once or habitually, preformed vitamin A can cause a headache, vomiting, bone abnormalities, and liver damage. Vitamin D toxicity can lead to the deposit of calcium in soft tissues, with consequent irreversible kidney and cardiovascular damage. Overnutrition is often associated with the use of self-prescribed over-the-counter vitamin and mineral supplements. Overnutrition is also often associated with eating too much food and hence an excessive intake of many nutrients.

NUTRITION AND HEALTH

Good nutrition is essential for good health. Nutrition is related to physical growth and development, body composition, and mental development. Research has shown that certain dietary substances can either protect persons from chronic diseases or predispose them toward chronic diseases. Medical treatment for many diseases includes diet therapy. Nutrition is thus both a preventive and therapeutic science.

Physical Growth and Development

Heredity determines much of the growth pattern and genetic potential of each individual. Malnutrition can slow down or prevent an individual from achieving his or her genetic potential. For example, without calcium, phosphorus, and protein, bones cannot grow properly; children who are malnourished may never reach their genetic potential for height. Slowed growth may be one of the first clinically measurable indicators of inadequate dietary intake in children. This is one reason why an infant's height and weight are measured and plotted on growth charts by diligent physicians and nurse practitioners on each visit. Examples of growth charts commonly used to plot the height and weight of infants and children can be found in Appendix C.

Body Composition

Nutrient intake can affect body composition, which in turn can affect health. The composition of the human body can be divided into four main substances: water, fat, ash, and protein and one minor substance, carbohydrate (see Figure 1–1). One half to three quarters of the body is made up of water. A normally active female has a body fat content of between 18 and 22 percent. A normally active male has a body fat content of between 15 and 19 percent. Body ash comprises about 6 percent of body weight. Ash is the leftover portion or residue that remains after something is burned, as in a charcoal fire. Body ash is the body's mineral content. For example, the human skeleton is partly composed of the minerals calcium and phosphorus.

About 15 percent of body weight consists of protein. The male body contains more protein than the female body. With age, the typical person's

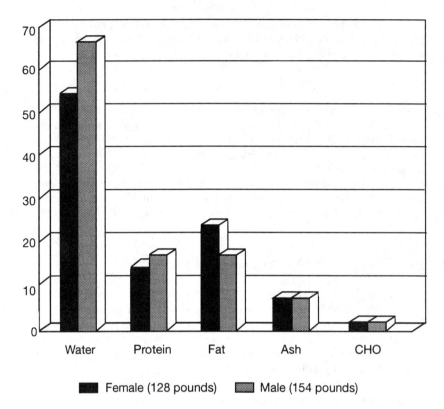

FIGURE 1–1. Approximate body composition of a sample 25-year-old man (154 pounds) and woman (128 pounds). Note that the typical woman has a higher percentage of body fat than does the typical man. The man has a higher percentage of lean body mass. The percentage of ash content is equal in both sexes. The human body has a minimal carbohydrate content.

body composition becomes higher in fat and lower in protein. Protein is stored primarily in muscle tissue, organs, and certain body chemicals. When a person loses body protein, he or she is losing muscle tissue, organ mass, and/or the protein stored in body chemicals. Preservation of body protein and optimal health go hand-in-hand. Common sense dictates that a loss of structural body content (heart muscle, kidney, liver, blood proteins, etc.) is undesirable.

A person's body fat and protein content can be modified by food intake and/or exercise. For example, exercise increases body protein content by increasing muscle content. Eating too much food or the wrong kind of food increases the fat content of the body, since fat is stored for future use.

Mental Development

The relationship between undernutrition and the development of a child's brain in structure, size, and function is being researched. It has been found that undernourished babies have smaller and fewer brain cells. However, the relationship between intelligence and the size and number of brain cells is not clear. There is some evidence that infants less than 6 months of age are particularly vulnerable to the effects of malnutrition on their mental development. Some nutritional deficiencies may cause permanent impairment of the central nervous system (CNS) in young infants.

Some conditions that affect the CNS may be reversible through diet. For example, nutrition plays an important role in the prevention and management of some forms of dementia. **Dementia** is defined as the impairment of intellectual function that is usually progressive and interferes with normal social and occupational activities. "Impairment" means any condition that causes one to deteriorate; "progressive" means to become more severe or to spread to other parts. Excessive alcohol intake or nutritional deficiencies may result in dementia. Correction of the deficiency or the removal of alcohol from the diet may improve intellectual function. Not all forms of dementia are directly related to poor nutrition. Alzheimer's disease may not be.

Dementia— Impairment of intellectual function that usually is progressive and interferes with normal social and occupational activities

Diet as Therapy

A special or modified diet is often an important component of a patient's total medical care. For example, diet is an important part of the treatment for patients with metabolic diseases such as diabetes and hypoglycemia. Special dietary measures are often required to maintain the lives of patients who have chronic heart, kidney, liver, and gastrointestinal diseases. These diets must also take into consideration the effects of medications on nutrients. Adjustments in the diet are also necessary for other situations, such as highly stressful or traumatic events. Persons suffering from severe burns, broken bones, or surgery may require dietary adjustment.

Although rare, some patients have a single-nutrient deficiency. Often, just adding foods to the diet that contain the missing nutrient is sufficient. The last section of this book is devoted to describing various diets for specific clinical situations.

NUTRITIONAL ASSESSMENT

How do healthcare practitioners determine whether a patient is well nourished or suffering from malnutrition? Before this question can be answered, two terms need to be defined. **Nutritional status** refers to the condition of the body as it relates to the intake and use of nutrients. All members of the healthcare team have a role to play in the effective evaluation of a patient's nutritional status. **Dietary status** tells us what a patient is eating. A patient's dietary status can be adequate, but his or her nutritional status may nevertheless be poor. An evaluation of a patient's dietary status can help to determine the reason for his or her poor nutritional status or to rule out poor diet as the source of the patient's problem.

When a physician attempts to diagnosis a potential nutritional problem, a complete **nutritional assessment** is frequently prescribed. A thorough, reliable, and concise nutritional assessment includes a physical examination, anthropometric measurements, laboratory data, and food intake information.

Nutritional status—The condition of the body as related to the intake and use of nutrients

Dietary status— Description of what a person has been eating

Nutritional assessment— The evaluation of a patient's nutritional status based on a physical examination, anthropometric measurements, laboratory data, and food intake information

Physical Examination

Well-nourished persons appear alert and responsive, and generally have a more positive outlook on life. Weight is reasonable for the person's height, age, and body build; skin is smooth and firm; eyes are bright and clear; hair is glossy and full; and posture is erect. Appetite is normal, as are digestion, elimination, and sleeping habits. The person has not recently experienced unintentional weight loss or frequent infections.

Anthropometric Measurements

Anthropometric measurement—
Physical measurements of the human body such as height, weight, skinfold thickness, and so forth; used to determine body composition and growth

For clinical purposes, body size, weight, and proportions are determined by what are called **anthropometric measurements.** *Anthropometry* is the science of measuring the human body. Such measurements are used to determine body composition and growth. Anthropometric measurements are also frequently used to assess a person's nutritional status. Specifically, the body's kilocalorie and protein stores can be determined by these measurements. These measurements are usually compared with standard measurements for persons of the same sex and age. Our discussion will focus on height-weight tables, triceps skinfold, midarm circumference, and abdominal circumferences.

Height-Weight Tables

A reliable height-weight table includes information on shoe heel height; it should also indicate the amount of weight attributable to clothing. The information from height-weight tables is used to calculate a patient's percent healthy body weight (HBW). (To assess percent HBW, see Clinical Calculation 1–1 at the end of this chapter.)

Using percent HBW helps members of the healthcare team to interpret height-weight relationships more readily. If a range of body weights is given on the table, the weight that is midpoint for the patient's frame size is used for the calculation. Please see Clinical Calculation 1–2 to determine an individual's body frame type. See Appendix B for an example of a height-weight table.

Skinfold Thickness Index

This measurement, which involves the triceps muscle in the upper arm, provides an estimate of the amount of body fat. Such a measure can be used to differentiate between a person who is heavy because of muscle mass and one who is heavy because of excess fat. Athletes, for example, are frequently much heavier than the weight given on height-weight tables. However, these individuals are not overly fat. Instead, they have a much higher body protein content than the average person because exercise increases body protein content. Figure 1–2 demonstrates measurement of a person's triceps skinfold using an instrument called a skin caliper.

The technique used to take a skinfold measurement determines how accurate it is. Much practice is needed to take accurate measurements; the interpretation of the value requires special training. Although nurses usually do not take skinfold measurements, they do need to be able to answer patient's questions.

Midarm Circumference

The circumference of a circle describes the distance around the area enclosed by the circle. This number is usually expressed in inches or cen-

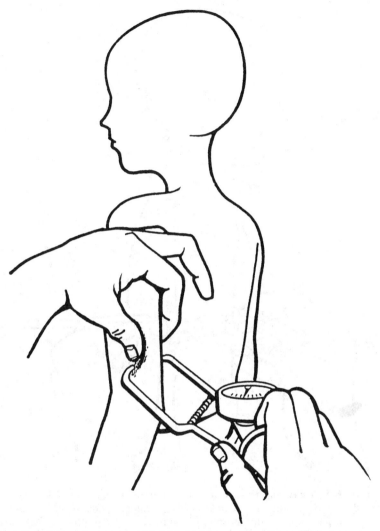

FIGURE 1–2. Measuring triceps skinfold thickness with calipers. This measurement can be used to help determine the percentage of body fat present. (Reprinted from *Nutrition Assessment: A Comprehensive Guide for Planning Intervention* by M. Simko, C. Cowell, and J. Gilbride [eds], © 1984 with permission.)

timeters (1 inch equals 2.54 centimeters). The circumference of the midarm is used to provide information about body protein stores. Since 50 percent of the body's protein stores are located in muscle tissue, measuring a person's midarm can provide an estimate of soft tissue in the arm. Figure 1–3 illustrates the measurement of a child's midarm circumference.

Abdominal Circumference

This measurement provides information on water retention. It is frequently made when an individual is accumulating fluid in his or her abdomen. How-

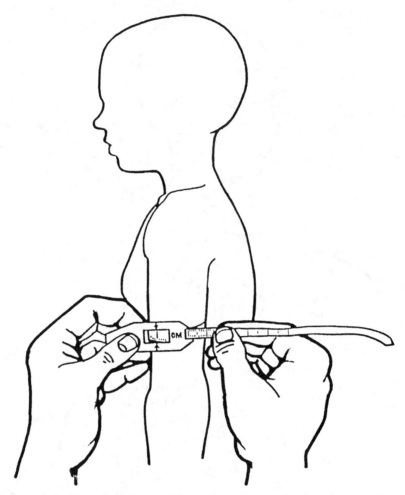

FIGURE 1–3. Measuring triceps midarm circumference. An insertion tape is one method used to measure the circumference of the upper midarm. This measurement can be used to help determine body protein content. (Reprinted from *Nutrition Assessment: A Comprehensive Guide for Planning Intervention* by M. Simko, C. Cowell, and J. Gilbride [eds], © 1984 with permission.)

ever, it is also done for other reasons—for example, to monitor the growth of abnormal tissue within the abdomen.

Laboratory Tests

Laboratory data include results from blood, urine, and stool tests. The results of these tests reveal much of what a person has eaten, what his or her body has stored, and how nutrients are being used by the body. Laboratory tests are not infallible, however, and good clinical judgment must be used in selecting tests and interpreting test results. Some studies have shown that a thorough physical assessment and nutritional history (Table 1–1) are as effective in identifying malnutrition as are a battery of laboratory analyses

TABLE 1–1 *Commonly Used Techniques to Obtain Food Intake Information*

Technique	Comments
Comparison with the Food Pyramid Model Healthcare worker asks patient what he or she eats and compares this reported food intake with the Food Pyramid model.	Can be used to screen many patients quickly Does not require a trained interviewer Not comprehensive May overlook some patients who would benefit from nutritional care
Food Frequency Healthcare worker requests patient to fill out a questionnaire asking about usual food intake during specified times such as "What do you usually eat for breakfast?"	Questionnaire can be tailored to particular nutrients of interest (e.g., lactose, gluten). May assess food usage for any length of time: day, week, month, weekends versus weekdays, summer versus winter, etc. Initial patient contact does not require a trained interviewer. May require special resources (e.g., computer database) to evaluate the information collected Provides limited information on a patient's food behaviors such as meal spacing, length of usual mealtime, etc.
Food Records Healthcare worker asks patient to record his or her food intake for a specified length of time (1 or 3 or 7 days).	A motivated patient will provide reasonably accurate information. A less highly motivated patient will "forget to keep" part or all of the food record. Research shows some patients will change their food habits while keeping a food record; therefore, this technique works poorly to assist in determining a patient's dietary and/or nutritional status. This technique works well when a behavior change is desired. May require special resources (e.g., a computer database) to evaluate the information obtained Patient needs to be available for a follow-up visit to review the evaluated food records. Analysis of results is time-consuming.
24-Hour Dietary Recall Healthcare worker asks patient what he or she has eaten during the previous 24 hours.	Fairly simple technique Interviewer should be trained not to ask leading questions.

TABLE 1–1 *Commonly Used Techniques to Obtain Food Intake Information (Continued)*

Technique	Comments
	Yields limited information only about the kinds of foods and beverages consumed within the previous 24 hours
	The previous 24 hours may not have been usual for the patient.
	Frequently patients may not remember what they ate and the amounts consumed.
Diet History	
A diet history is an in-depth interview which yields information about the usual food intake, drug and medication usage, alcohol and tobacco use, financial ability to obtain food, special dietary needs, food allergies and intolerances, weight history, cultural and religious preferences which may influence food selection, ability to chew and swallow foods, previous dietary instructions received, patient knowledge about nutrition, and elimination patterns.	Comprehensive
	Requires a trained interviewer who is usually a dietitian
	An analysis of the results obtained can usually be provided on the same day the information is collected.
	A good technique for high-risk patients when information is needed to evaluate the need for nutritional support.
	Highly dependent on the willingness of the patient to reveal information to the interviewer
	Patient must be a good historian
	Time consuming

SOURCE: Adapted from Moore,[1] p. 10, and from Mason, M, Wenberg, BG, and Welsch, PK: The Dynamics of Clinical Dietetics, p. 10. John Wiley & Sons, New York, 1982.

(Moore, 1993). Throughout this text you will be introduced to specific laboratory tests used in a variety of clinical situations.

Food Intake Information

Food intake information is used to determine a patient's dietary status or as one part of a nutritional assessment. Table 1–1 summarizes commonly used techniques to obtain food intake information from patients.

NUTRITIONAL STANDARDS AND GUIDES

All healthcare workers use specific standards and guides to deliver nutritional care. This section of the text introduces you to some of these tools. Tables of food composition are introduced first, followed by an explanation of Recommended Dietary Allowances, US Recommended Dietary Allowances, Dietary Guidelines, the Food Pyramid, and ADA Exchange Lists of the American Dietetic and Diabetic Associations.

Tables of Food Composition

Food composition tables list foods and the amounts of selected nutrients for a specified volume or weight of the food. The US Department of Agriculture (USDA) publishes a food composition table titled Nutritive Values of the Edible Part of Foods (see Appendix A). From a practical viewpoint, tables of food composition can be used as a reference to look up the nutritive content of a particular food.

Recommended Dietary Allowances

Recommended Dietary Allowances (RDAs) are defined as the levels of essential nutrients that, on the basis of scientific knowledge, are judged by the Food and Nutrition Board of the National Research Council as adequate to meet the known nutrient needs of practically all healthy persons (Subcommittee on the 10th edition of the RDAs, 1989). RDAs were designed to be used to plan and evaluate diets for groups of people. For example, RDAs are used to plan menus for prisoners, school lunch programs, and for institutionalized patients. Individual requirements for nutrients are highly variable, and therefore RDAs may not necessarily indicate if an individual has a deficiency. A copy of the 1989 RDA table can be found in Appendix E. Other governments have published standards similar to the US government's RDAs. For example, the Canadian Council on Nutrition has published its standards, which in some respects are different from the US standards.

Many computer software programs are available to compare an individual's nutritive intake with the RDA standard. It is important to remember that a person's diet is not necessarily deficient if he or she consumes less than the RDA. When comparing an individual's nutritive intake with the RDA standard, the only scientifically correct statement a healthcare worker can make is that the intake does or does not meet the RDA standard. It is inappropriate to make an evaluation of a patient's nutritional and/or dietary status based completely on a comparison with the RDA. A complete nutritional assessment is needed to evaluate an individual's nutritional status.

US Recommended Dietary Allowances

The US RDA are standards used for nutrition labeling prior to the Nutrition Labeling and Education Act of 1990. This law significantly changed labeling requirements. You may still see some food labels that use the US RDA, however. These standards are based on the 1968 Recommended Dietary Allowances of the National Academy of Sciences, National Research Council, which makes them about 20 years old. The highest needs in the RDA table for each age and sex were selected for use as the US RDA, so the values are quite generous. The information on food labels is presented as a percent of US RDA.

Dietary Guidelines

The US Departments of Agriculture and Health and Human Services jointly publish a pamphlet entitled "Nutrition and your Health: Dietary Guidelines for Americans" (Fig. 1–4). The seven guidelines for health promotion and the rationale for each can be found in Clinical Application 1–1. These guidelines are targeted to the healthy general population to assist in the prevention of chronic and degenerative diseases. They do not apply to individuals who need special diets because of disease or conditions that alter normal nutritional requirements.

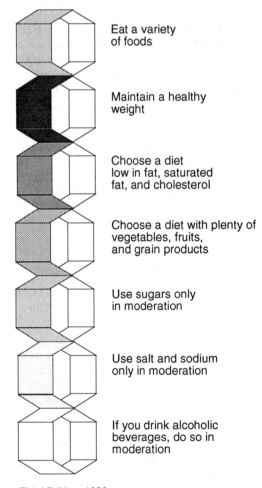

Nutrition and your Health:
Dietary Guidelines for Americans

Eat a variety of foods

Maintain a healthy weight

Choose a diet low in fat, saturated fat, and cholesterol

Choose a diet with plenty of vegetables, fruits, and grain products

Use sugars only in moderation

Use salt and sodium only in moderation

If you drink alcoholic beverages, do so in moderation

Third Edition, 1990
U.S. Department of Agriculture
U.S. Department of Health and Human Services

FIGURE 1–4. *Nutrition and Your Health: Dietary Guidelines for Americans.* This booklet was developed by the US Departments of Agriculture and Health and Human Services. Information on how to put guidelines into practice can be obtained by contacting the Human Nutrition Information Service, USDA, Room 325-A, 6505 Belcrest Road, Hyattsville, MD 20782.

CLINICAL APPLICATION 1–1
Dietary Guidelines

Guideline	Rationale
Eat a wide variety of foods.	Benefits of eating a wide variety of food food include increasing assurance of adequate nutrient intakes, avoiding deficiencies or excesses of any single nutrient, ensuring an appropriate balance of trace minerals, and reducing the likelihood of exposure to contaminants in any single food.
Maintain healthy weight.	The chances of developing health problems are increased when a person is overly fat. Excess body fat is connected with high blood pressure, stroke, heart disease, the most common form of diabetes, certain cancers, and other types of illness.
Choose a diet low in fat, saturated fat, and cholesterol.	Populations like ours with diets relatively high in fat tend to have more obesity and certain types of cancers. A high intake of saturated fat and cholesterol is linked to our increased risk of heart disease.
Choose a diet with plenty of vegetables, fruits, and grain products.	Healthy adults need at least three servings of vegetables, two servings of fruits, and six servings of starches (preferably whole-grain) each day. These foods contain complex carbohydrates, dietary fiber, and other components that are linked to good health.
Use sugars only in moderation.	A significant health problem from eating too much sugar is tooth decay. Contrary to widespread belief, too much sugar in the diet does not cause diabetes. Sugar provides kilocalories (fuel) but few other nutrients. Thus, diets with large amounts of sugar should be avoided because they often displace other, more healthful foods in the diet.
Use salt and sodium in moderation.	A high sodium intake may predispose a person to high blood pressure. In populations with low salt intakes, high blood pressure is less common than in populations with diets high in salt. Other factors besides salt intake affect blood pressure. At present there is no way to

Box continued on next page.

CLINICAL APPLICATION 1–1(Continued)

	predict who might develop high blood pressure and who will benefit from reducing dietary salt and sodium. However, most experts consider it wise for most people to eat less salt and sodium because they need much less than they now eat, and such reduction will benefit those people whose blood pressure rises with salt intake.
If you drink alcoholic beverages, do so in moderation.	Alcoholic beverages are high in calories and low in nutrients. Even moderate drinkers who are overweight should decrease their intake of alcohol. Heavy drinkers often develop nutritional deficiencies as well as more serious diseases, such as cirrhosis of the liver and certain forms of cancer. Consumption of alcohol by pregnant women may cause birth defects or other problems during pregnancy; there is no known "safe" level of alcohol intake in pregnancy.

The Food Pyramid

The Food Pyramid is a general guideline on how to choose a healthful diet and is based on the concept that foods within a group contain similar nutrients (Fig. 1–5). Foods are arranged in the following groups: (1) bread, cereal, rice, and pasta group; (2) vegetable group; (3) fruit group; (4) meat, poultry, fish, dry beans, eggs, and nuts group; (5) milk, yogurt, and cheese group; (6) fats, oils, and sweets group. Each group contains foods of similar nutrient content. For example, foods in the milk, yogurt, and cheese group are high in calcium, riboflavin, and protein. Each of the food groups supply some but not all of the essential nutrients, and some servings from each of the groups should be eaten daily. In terms of quantity, the group at the bottom of the pyramid—bread, cereal, rice, and pasta—should provide the foundation of the diet and supply the most servings eaten. The group at the top of the pyramid—fats, oils, and sweets—should provide the fewest daily servings.

American Dietetic and Diabetic Associations Exchange Lists

The American Dietetic Association and the American Diabetic Association jointly publish a food guide commonly called the ADA Exchange Lists.

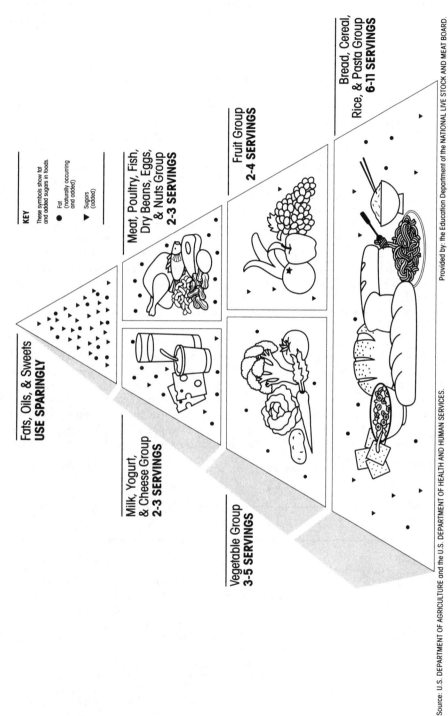

FIGURE 1–5. The food pyramid. This guide is commonly used to evaluate the dietary status of individuals and to educate patients about food choices.

These lists are used in clinical practice to aid in meal planning. Individuals with diabetes, hypoglycemia, and obesity are taught to plan their meals using exchange lists. The ADA Exchange Lists are revised and updated about every 10 years. The last revision was in 1986. It is possible to approximate a patient's carbohydrate, fat, protein, and kilocalorie intake with exchange lists. Exchange lists are used not only for calculating a patient's food intake but also for education, meal planning, and counseling.

Exchange list— A food guide developed by the American Dietetic and Diabetic Association; often used in clinical practice to aid in meal planning

There are six basic **exchange lists:** (1) starch; (2) meat in three subgroups (lean, medium fat, and high fat); (3) vegetable; (4) fruit; (5) milk subdivided into three groups (skimmed, low-fat, and whole); and (6) fat subdivided into two groups (unsaturated and saturated). Table 1–2 identifies typical foods in each exchange list. In addition, some foods are considered "free." Free foods are on a separate list. See the complete exchange lists in Appendix H.

Foods are placed on each list based on their energy nutrient composition and because foods within each list contain similar nutrient composition. For example, corn is on the starch list because it is closer in composition to a slice of bread than to green beans. Table 1–3 shows the amount of carbohydrate, protein, fat, and kilocalories in one exchange on each list. As you can see from the table, one exchange on the fruit list is not equal to one exchange on the starch list. To correctly use this method of meal planning, it is necessary for patients to choose the correct number of items from each appropriate list.

Learning to use exchange lists can be confusing for both patients and healthcare practitioners. Understanding the meaning of the term "exchange" is important. In this context, the term <u>exchange</u> means only and precisely a defined quantity of food within an exchange list. For example, one exchange of bread is one slice (a defined quantity). Individual food items within an exchange list are essentially equal to each other in nutrient composition and can thus be exchanged or "swapped" for each other. This is possible because portion sizes for various items were adjusted at the time the

---

TABLE 1–2 *Typical Foods in Each Exchange List*

Exchange List	Food Items
Starch	Cereals, grains, pasta, dried beans, peas, lentils, starchy vegetables, bread, crackers
Meat	Beef, pork, veal, poultry, fish, wild game, cheese, eggs, tofu, peanut butter
Fruit	Fresh, frozen, or unsweetened canned fruit; dried fruit; fruit juice
Vegetable	Raw or cooked vegetables, vegetable juices
Milk	Milk, yogurt, evaporated milk, powdered milk
Fat	Avocado, margarine, mayonnaise, nuts, seeds, oil, salad dressing, bacon, coconut, powdered coffee whitener, cream, sour cream, whipped cream, cream cheese, salt pork

TABLE 1–3 *Energy Nutrient Composition of the Six Exchange Lists*

Exchange Lists	CHO (grams)	Protein (grams)	Fat (grams)	Calories
Starch	15	3	Trace	80
Meat				
Lean	0	7	3	55
Medium fat	0	7	5	75
High fat	0	7	8	100
Vegetables	5	2	0	25
Fruit	15	0	0	60
Milk				
Skimmed	12	8	Trace	90
2 percent	12	8	5	120
Whole	12	8	8	150
Fat	0	0	5	45

SOURCE: The exchange lists are the basis of a meal planning system designed primarily for people with diabetes and others who must follow special diets. The exchange lists are based on principles of good nutrition that apply to everyone. © With permission 1986 American Diabetes Association and American Dietetic Association.

lists were created to make each exchange approximately equal. For example, Table 1–4 shows items equal to one starch exchange.

Patients at any prescribed kilocalorie, protein, fat, or carbohydrate level can use exchange lists. Exchange lists should always include a specific meal plan for the patient to follow. A meal plan is a food guide that shows the number of choices or exchanges the patient should eat at each meal or snack. Table 1–5 illustrates two different meal plans for two different kilocalorie levels. One example is provided for distributing the various exchanges among the meals.

It is also possible to calculate two different meal plans for the same kilocalorie level. Table 1–6 illustrates two 1200-kilocalorie meal plans.

Using exchange lists and following a meal plan allows the patient a variety of food choices. This method can also be used to control the distribution of nutrients throughout the day. For clinical reasons, many patients need to modify meal frequency.

TABLE 1–4 *Examples of One Starch Exchange*

Bread	1 slice
Corn	½ cup
Rice	⅓ cup

TABLE 1–5 *1500- and 1800-Calorie Meal Plan Using Exchanges for One Day*

	1500 Calories	1800 Calories
Starch	7	7
Meat, lean	1	3
Meat, medium	3	3
Vegetable	4	5
Fruit	3	5
Milk, skimmed	2	2
Fat	6	7

Distribution of Exchange throughout the Day			
	1500-Calorie Meal Plan		
	Breakfast	Lunch	Dinner	Snack
---	---	---	---	---
Starch	2	2	2	1
Meat, lean	0	1	0	0
Meat, medium	0	0	3	0
Vegetable	0	2	2	0
Fruit	1	1	1	0
Milk, skimmed	1	0	0	1
Fat	2	2	2	0

Variety, Moderation, and Balance

Balanced diet— One that contains all the essential nutrients in required amounts

The terms variety, moderation, and balance are frequently used to describe a healthful diet. Variety means choosing foods from each of the five food groups daily and eating many different foods within each food group. The five major food groups are all the food groups listed on the Food Pyramid, with the exception of fat, oils, and sweets. Moderation means avoiding too much or too little of any one food or food group. For example, even water is harmful if consumed in excess. Balance is the automatic result of eating a wide variety of foods in moderation. Variety, moderation, and balance are easy guidelines to follow when planning daily meals.

TABLE 1–6 *Two 1200-Calorie Meal Plans Using Exchanges for One Day*

Exchanges	Meal Plan 1	Meal Plan 2
Starch	5	6
Meat, lean	4	1
Meat, medium	1	3
Vegetable	2	4
Fruit	3	2
Milk, skimmed	2	1
Fat	4	4

THE DELIVERY OF NUTRITIONAL CARE

All healthcare providers have some responsibility for the nutritional care of patients. Nutritional care can be divided into three activities: screening patients for nutritional risk, referring at-risk patients to other healthcare providers, and directly treating the patient. Nurses use a systematic approach called the nursing process when treating problems directly. Every subsequent chapter contains a case study and a nursing care plan to aid in integrating nutrition knowledge into the practice of nursing. Let us now turn our attention to the process of screening for care and to the nature of referral systems.

Screening

The goal of a nutritional screening program is to identify those patients who need nutritional care. A screening system assumes that patients at greatest risk have first priority for nutritional care. A systematic approach to nutrition screening recognizes that healthcare resources are limited. In addition, information collected during the screening process is frequently used to evaluate the effectiveness of any nutritional care provided. For example, how much weight has the patient gained since admission?

Nutrition screening should be brief enough that the information can be gathered in 5 to 10 minutes. A broad-based screening form usually screens

---

TABLE 1–7 *Nutrition Screening Form*

Name _____ Date _____ Adm Date _____
Sex _____ Birthdate _____ Physician's Name _____
Adm Dx. _____

Diet Information	Diet order _____ Date Prescribed _____ Accepts all major groups _____ Feeds self _____ Type of assistance needed _____
Physical	Height _____ Weight _____ Healthy body weight % _____ Weight change in last 3 months _____ Chewing ability _____ Weight history _____ Swallowing ability _____ Hearing _____ Vision _____ Bowel function _____ Bladder function _____ Edema _____ Nausea _____ Pressure ulcer _____ Stage _____ Allergies _____
Laboratory	Blood glucose _____ Albumin _____ Potassium _____ Lymphocytes _____ Hemoglobin _____ Hematocrit _____ Cholesterol _____
Medications	Insulin _____ Diuretics _____ Laxatives _____ Vit/min supp ___ Antibiotics _____ Thyroid _____ Anticoagulants _____ Antidepressants (MAO) _____ Antabuse _____ Flagel _____ Lithium _____

If the above identifies a problem, continue with in-depth assessment.
_____ *(Signature)* _____ *(Date)*

for basic information such as height, weight, weight change, pertinent laboratory values, refusal of one of the basic food groups, routine elimination, chronic aliments, medications, and allergies. Table 1–7 is an example of a nutrition screening form.

Referring

After screening patients for nutritional risk, the healthcare worker may identify patients who have needs that he or she cannot address. Some of the reasons for not being able to address a particular patient's needs include lack of resources (including time), lack of adequate knowledge, and the wasteful practice of duplicating existing services and information. The referral system has two functions. First, it ensures that the patient gets comprehensive care. Second, it informs patients about the service of a nutrition program by making them aware of their need for and the benefits of that service. The nurse is in a unique position to assist patients in achieving optimal nutritional status by referring patients to the appropriate resource.

Summary

Nutrition has been defined as the science of food and its relation to people. Our bodies and our attitudes about health and nutrition have evolved over millions of years. Health is a state of complete physical, mental, and social well-being, not just the absence of disease or infirmity. Nutrition is vital to optimal health. The principles of nutrition are applied by a team of healthcare members to promote health and treat many diseases. The science of nutrition is based on chemicals in foods called nutrients, which function (1) as fuel sources, (2) to support tissue growth and maintenance, and/or (3) to regulate body processes. A nutrient is called essential if the body requires it and is unable to manufacturer it in sufficient amounts to meet bodily needs. A balanced nutrient intake is vital for physical growth and development, optimal body composition, mental development, and the prevention of disease.

The tools used by health professionals rendering nutritional care are accepted throughout the United States. Healthcare professionals estimate an individual's nutrient stores by completing a nutritional assessment. A physical examination, anthropometric measurements, laboratory tests, and food intake information are all necessary components of a nutritional assessment. Healthcare professionals use specific standards and guides to evaluate the food intake either of groups of people or of an individual. These standards or guides are the Food Pyramid, Recommended Dietary Allowances (RDAs), Dietary Guidelines, and ADA Exchange Lists. The nurse is in a position to help patients receive optimal nutritional care by screening patients for nutritional problems, referring patients to nutritional services, or providing care directly.

STUDY AIDS

Chapter Review Questions

1. An example of cyclical variation is:
    a. A period of drought and famine followed by a period of cloudy skies
    b. A period of rain followed by a period of plentiful sunshine
    c. A period of drought and famine followed by a period of plentiful rainfall
    d. A period of stormy weather followed by clear skies

2. Which of the following statements is true?
    a. The terms "nutrient" and "food" mean the same.
    b. Nonessential nutrients must be provided in the diet for health.
    c. Malnutrition can occur only during starvation.
    d. There are more than 40 essential nutrients.

3. A diet is adequate or _____ if it provides nutrients in proportions that best meet the body's needs.
    a. Balanced
    b. Correct
    c. Appropriate
    d. Organic

4. The following is *not* considered one of the six classes of nutrients as described in the text:
    a. Carbohydrate
    b. Water
    c. Fiber
    d. Minerals

5. The functions of a nutrient include all of the following items except:
    a. Serves as a fuel source
    b. Fosters a sense of well-being
    c. Builds and maintains the body's structure
    d. Regulates body processes

6. The food groups included as part of the Food Pyramid are:
    a. Meat, milk, fruits, and vegetables
    b. Fat, carbohydrate, protein, and fiber
    c. Milk, fiber, protein, and fat
    d. Breads, cereal, rice, and pasta; vegetables; fruits; milk, yogurt, and cheese; meat, poultry, fish, dry beans, eggs, and nuts

7. _____ percent of the human body is ash or mineral.
    a. 6
    b. 15
    c. 25
    d. 50

8. Which statement about the ADA Exchange Lists is true?
    a. One starch exchange is equal to two fruit exchanges.
    b. Exchange lists are used to calculate an individual's RDA.
    c. The word "exchange" means a defined quantity of a food on a particular exchange list.
    d. All 1000-calorie meal plans are the same.

9. Which of the following is *not* a dietary guideline?
    a. Eat foods with adequate starch and fiber.
    b. Avoid too much sugar.
    c. Everyone would benefit from drinking alcohol in moderation.
    d. Maintain a healthy body weight.

10. The following statement about the relationship between nutrition and health is true.
    a. Your physical and mental development depend on the nutrients obtained from a balanced diet.
    b. Any person with a heightened sense of well-being most likely eats a balanced diet.
    c. Nutrients in excess have a positive impact on health.
    d. The health benefits from a well-balanced diet are considered more important than other lifestyle behaviors.

NCLEX-Style Quiz

Situation One

1. Ms. A. has a body fat content of 15 percent and an HBW of 105 percent. The nurse might correctly conclude that:
   a. Ms. A. is overweight.
   b. Ms. A. is athletic.
   c. Ms. A. would benefit from an increase in her fat intake and a decrease in her kilocalorie intake.
   d. Ms. A. would benefit from a decrease in her fat and kilocalorie intake.

Situation Two

2. A nurse is developing a nutrition screening form to be used in a long-term nursing home. Each nurse will have approximately 5 minutes to evaluate each patient's dietary status. In this situation, the best technique to obtain food intake information would be to:
   a. Ask each patient how many servings of food he or she consumes each day from each group in the Food Pyramid
   b. Ask each patient to record his or her food intake for the previous 24 hours
   c. Ask each patient to record his or her food intake for 3 days
   d. Ask each patient to fill out a three-page food frequency questionnaire

Situation Three

3. Mr. B. has a body fat content of 30 percent and his weight is 97 percent HBW. This patient would benefit from (by):
   a. Increasing his water intake to increase his body water content
   b. A nutritional assessment
   c. Decreasing his fat intake to decrease his percent body fat
   d. Increasing his protein intake to increase his muscle mass

Situation Four

4. Ms. C. refuses to eat fruits and vegetables. As her nurse, you should:
   a. Notify the doctor
   b. Drop the issue because the patient is upset
   c. Refer the patient to another healthcare provider or address the problem yourself
   d. Document urinary output

Situation Five

5. Ms. D. has just completed a health risk assessment. She learned that high-fat diets are related to colon and breast cancer. Her father died from colon cancer, and her mother has had surgery for breast cancer. Ms. D. expressed inter-

est in modifying her fat intake. Which of the following Food Groups should Ms. D. eat less of?

a. Fruit and grain
b. Fat and meat
c. Meat and starch
d. Milk and cereal

CLINICAL CALCULATION 1–1

Percent Healthy Body Weight

The formula for calculating percent healthy body weight is:

$$\frac{\text{Patient's weight}}{\text{Weight from table}} \times 100 = \% \text{ healthy body weight}$$

For example, according to the height-weight table in Appendix B, a 5-foot 8-inch woman who is 30 to 39 years old would have a healthy body weight of 145 pounds. This assumes the woman was weighed wearing light indoor clothing and 1-inch heels, and has a medium frame. If she weighed 145 pounds, her healthy body weight would be 100 percent. If she weighed 100 pounds, her healthy body weight would be 69 percent, calculated as follows:

$$\frac{100 \text{ pounds}}{145 \text{ pounds}} \times 100 = 69\%$$

CLINICAL CALCULATION 1–2

Determining Body Frame Type

Measure the smallest part of the wrist between the wrist bones and the hand. For the system we are using, use inches. If the person's height is not known, measure him or her, in feet and inches, without shoes. Taking that information, look at the chart below. Find the person's height on the left and his or her wrist size at the bottom, and compare the shaded area with the boxes at the bottom. As an example, find the frame size of a person who is 5 feet 4 inches and has a wrist circumference of 6¼ inches. (The person has a medium frame.)

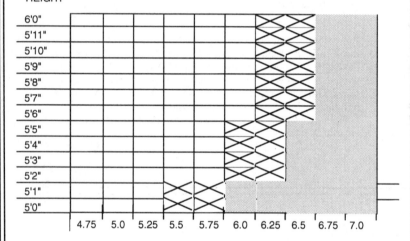

HEIGHT

WRIST MEASUREMENT IN INCHES
(Distance around smallest part of wrist, between wrist bones and hand)

☐ = Small frame

✕ = Medium frame

▨ = Large frame

BIBLIOGRAPHY

Feldman, EB: Essentials of Clinical Nutrition. FA Davis, Philadelphia, 1988.

Food and Nutrition Board of the National Research Council: What Is America Eating? National Academy Press, Washington, DC, 1986.

Garn, SM and Leonard, WR: What did our ancestors eat? Nutr Rev 47:11, 1989.

Gray, GE: Nutrition and dementia: J Am Diet Assoc 12:1800, 1989.

Life Sciences Research Office: Nutrition Monitoring in the United States. US Department of Health and Human Services, DHHS Publication No. (PHS) 89-1255, Washington, DC, 1989.

Mason, M, Wenberg, BG, and Welsch, PK: The Dynamics of Clinical Dietetics. John Wiley & Sons, New York, 1982.

Moore, MC: Pocket Guide, Nutrition and Diet Therapy. Mosby Year Book, St. Louis, 1993.

National Research Council: Diet and Health: Implications for Reducing Chronic Disease Risk. Report of the Committee on Diet and Health, Food and Nutrition Board, Commission on Life Sciences. National Academy Press, Washington, DC, 1989.

Schmitz, A: Food News Blues. Hippocrates, Sausalito, CA, 1991.

Simko, MD, Cowell, C, and Judith, JA: Nutrition Assessment. Aspen Publications, Rockville, MD, 1984.

Subcommittee on the Tenth Edition of the RDAs. Food and Nutrition Board. Commission on Life Sciences. National Research Council: Recommended Dietary Allowances. National Academy Press, Washington, DC, 1989.

US Department of Agriculture and US Department of Health and Human Services: Nutrition and Your Health: Dietary Guidelines for Americans, ed 3. Human Nutrition Information Service, USDA, Hyattsville, MD, 1990.

Chapter Outline

Key Terms

As a study aid, the key terms are followed by the page number where the term is defined in the chapter. Terms that appear **boldface** or <u>underscored</u> in the chapter text are located in the glossary.

acetone (39)
bacteria (40)
chlorophyll (34)
complex carbohydrate (34)
dental caries (39)
dextrose (35)
diacetic acid (39)
disaccharide (34)
element (34)
enrichment (43)
fiber, dietary (37)
fructose (35)
galactose (35)
genetic susceptibility (40)
glucose (35)
glycogen (37)
high-fructose corn syrup (HFCS) (35)
insoluble (37)
intravenous (35)
ketone bodies (39)
ketosis (39)
lactose (35)
maltose (35)
milling (43)
molecule (34)
monosaccharide (34)
nursing-bottle syndrome (42)
photosynthesis (34)
polysaccharide (36)
satiety (38)
simple carbohydrate (34)
solubility (37)
soluble (37)
sucrose (35)

Carbohydrates

Learning Objectives

After completing this chapter, the student should be able to:

1. Describe the types of carbohydrates and identify food sources and individual needs.
2. List the major functions and storage methods in the human body for carbohydrates.
3. Discuss dietary fiber and list its functions and food sources.
4. Describe the relationship between carbohydrates and dental health.
5. List the carbohydrate content (in grams) of each appropriate exchange list.
6. List two dietary recommendations relating to carbohydrates.

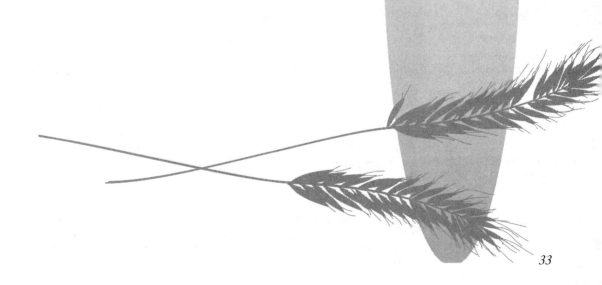

Photosynthesis —Process by which plants containing chlorophyll are able to manufacture carbohydrates from carbon dioxide and water using the sun's energy

Molecule—The smallest quantity into which a substance may be divided without loss of its characteristics

Element—A substance that cannot be separated into simpler parts by ordinary means

Atom—Smallest particle of an element that has all the properties of the element. An atom consists of the nucleus, which contains protons (positively charged particles), neutrons (no-charge particles), and surrounding electrons (positively charged particles).

Monosaccharide —A simple sugar composed of one unit of $C_6H_{12}O_6$; examples include glucose, fructose, and galactose

Disaccharide—A simple sugar composed of two units of $C_6H_{12}O_6$ joined together; examples include sucrose, lactose, and maltose

NATURE OF CARBOHYDRATES

Carbohydrates, along with fats and proteins, provide the body's basic fuel or energy needs. Carbohydrates, however, are the recommended major source of energy; they break down rapidly and are therefore readily available for use by the body. In this chapter we discuss the role of carbohydrates in the body and their relationship with the other energy nutrients. We also consider carbohydrates in the diet and health issues related to carbohydrate intake.

Carbohydrates are manufactured by green plants during a complex process known as **photosynthesis.** In this process, sugars and starches are formed in the plant by the combination of carbon dioxide from the air and water from the soil. Sunlight and the green plant pigment called chlorophyll are necessary for this conversion to occur. Through photosynthesis the sun's energy is transformed into food energy in the form of carbohydrates.

Carbohydrates may be divided into two major groups: sugars and starches. The chemical structure of each carbohydrate determines whether it is classified as a sugar or starch. Sugars have the simplest chemical structure, while starches are more *complex.* Thus sugars are frequently referred to as simple carbohydrates and starches as complex carbohydrates. The terms sugar, starch, simple, and complex all refer to the intricacy of the chemical structure of the carbohydrate.

COMPOSITION OF CARBOHYDRATES

To understand the composition of carbohydrates, three terms need to be defined: molecule, element, and atom. A **molecule** is the smallest quantity into which a substance may be divided without loss of its characteristics. For example, water's formula is H_2O. If the hydrogen atoms are pulled apart from the oxygen atom, the resulting products are the two gases hydrogen and oxygen, which bear no resemblance to water. Molecules are made of elements. In the case of water, H_2O, the elements are hydrogen and oxygen. An **element** is a substance that cannot be separated into simpler parts by ordinary means. An **atom** is any of the smallest parts of an element.

CLASSIFICATION OF CARBOHYDRATES

Carbohydrates are composed of the elements carbon, hydrogen, and oxygen. The ratio of hydrogen to oxygen is the same as that for water, two parts of hydrogen to one part of oxygen. The simplest carbohydrates have the formula $C_6H_{12}O_6$, or six molecules each of carbon and oxygen and twelve molecules of hydrogen. Carbohydrate is frequently abbreviated CHO.

Carbohydrates are classified as either simple or complex. Simple carbohydrates include monosaccharides and disaccharides. Complex carbohydrates are called polysaccharides.

Simple Carbohydrates

Simple sugars can be either monosaccharides or disaccharides. Mono- means one, di- means two, and saccharide means sweet. A **monosaccharide** contains one molecule of $C_6H_{12}O_6$. A **disaccharide** is composed of two molecules of $C_6H_{12}O_6$ joined together (minus one unit of H_2O). When the body joins two molecules of monosaccharides together, a molecule of water is released at the same time.

Monosaccharides

The monosaccharides are the building blocks of all other carbohydrates. The three monosaccharides of importance in human nutrition are glucose, fructose, and galactose. Note the *-ose* ending for each of these sugars. All monosaccharides and disaccharides end with the letters "o-s-e."

GLUCOSE   The monosaccharide glucose is commonly called the "blood sugar" because it is the major form of sugar in the blood. No matter what form of sugar is consumed, the body readily converts it to glucose, which it obtains mostly from the breakdown of more complex carbohydrates. Glucose is present in only small amounts in some fruits and vegetables and is moderately sweet.

Another name for glucose is **dextrose.** A common practice in almost all healthcare facilities is to place patients on intravenous feedings. Intravenous simply means within or into a vein. The most common intravenous feeding is D_5W, used primarily to deliver fluids to the patient. The abbreviation D_5W means that the solution contains 5 percent dextrose (glucose) and water. For now, it is sufficient to remember that dextrose is the same sugar as glucose. More will be said about D_5W and fluid balance in the chapter on water.

Dextrose—Another name for the simple sugar glucose

FRUCTOSE   Found in fruits and honey, fructose is commonly referred to as the honey sugar. It is the sweetest of all the monosaccharides. Relatively new on the list of sweeteners is **high-fructose corn syrup (HFCS),** commercially introduced in the 1970s. Because it is cheaper than table sugar, high-fructose corn syrup is now used extensively in soft drinks, canned foods, and a number of other processed foods. (Tufts University Diet and Nutrition Letter, 1985). The human body readily converts fructose to glucose after ingestion.

High-fructose corn syrup (HFCS)—A common food additive used as a sweetener; made from fructose

Dietary treatment for certain chronic diseases includes restricting many forms of concentrated sugars from the diet. Because fructose is now so prevalent in our food supply, nurses need to teach patients that fructose is a form of concentrated sugar.

GALACTOSE   The monosaccharide galactose comes mainly from the breakdown of the milk sugar lactose. Yogurt and unaged cheese may contain free galactose. It is the least sweet of all the monosaccharides. The body converts galactose into glucose after ingestion.

Disaccharides

When two monosaccharides are linked together, a disaccharide is formed. The three disaccharides of importance are sucrose, lactose, and maltose.

SUCROSE   The most prevalent disaccharide, sucrose, is ordinary white table sugar made commercially from sugar beets and sugar cane. Brown, granulated, and powdered sugar are all forms of sucrose. Sucrose is also found in molasses, maple syrup, and fruits. The two monosaccharides joined together to form sucrose are glucose and fructose. The total average daily intake of both sucrose and fructose is considered excessive and has been approximated to be 80 grams a day or 18 percent of energy intake. (National Research Council, 1989). See Clinical Calculation 2–1 for an explanation of how to convert grams of simple sugars to teaspoons of sugar. This calculation is designed to help you learn to read and interpret food labels.

LACTOSE   Because it occurs naturally only in milk, lactose is commonly referred to as the milk sugar. However, during lactation the body forms lactose from glucose to supply the needed sugar component of breast milk; hence the name lactose. Lactose is the least sweet of the disaccharides. The two monosaccharides that make up lactose are glucose and galactose.

MALTOSE   The disaccharide maltose is produced when starches are broken down by the body into simpler units. This disaccharide is present in malt, malt products, beer, some infant formulas, and sprouting seeds. Maltose consists of two units of glucose joined together.

Complex Carbohydrates

Polysaccharide
—Complex carbohydrates composed of many units of $C_6H_{12}O_6$ joined together; examples important in nutrition include starch, glycogen, and fiber

Complex carbohydrates are called **polysaccharides.** Poly- means "many," and polysaccharides are many molecules of $C_6H_{12}O_6$ joined together, with many molecules of water produced (released). Polysaccharides can be composed of various numbers of monosaccharides and disaccharides. The three types of complex carbohydrates of nutritional importance are starch, glycogen, and fiber. See Table 2–1 for a summary of the composition of carbohydrates.

Starch

Starch is the major source of carbohydrate in the diet. Starch is found primarily in grains, cereals, breads, pasta, starchy vegetables, and legumes. Legumes include dried peas and beans such as black beans, pinto beans, kidney beans, navy beans, soybeans, black-eyed peas, split green or yellow peas, chick peas (garbanzo beans), and lentils. Many consumers erroneously believe that complex carbohydrate foods are fattening. In fact, as you will learn in later chapters, gram for gram, fat has more than twice the kilocalories as carbohydrate. Strictly speaking, all starches yield simple sugars on digestion; starchy foods are mostly low in fat and high in carbohydrates and some starchy foods contain much fiber (see below).

TABLE 2–1 *Composition of Carbohydrates*

Elements	C (carbon)
	H (hydrogen)
	O (oxygen)
Molecule	$C_6H_{12}O_6$
Monosaccharide (simple)	One unit of $C_6H_{12}O_6$
Disaccharide (simple)	Two units of $C_6H_{12}O_6$ minus one unit of H_2O
Polysaccharide (complex)	Many units of $C_6H_{12}O_6$ minus many units of H_2O

Glycogen

The polysaccharide **glycogen** is commonly called the animal starch. It is a starch-like substance in the liver and muscle tissues that is changed to glucose as needed for muscular work and for liberating heat. Glycogen represents the body's carbohydrate stores. Liver glycogen helps sustain blood glucose levels during sleep.

The typical human body has an available store of glucose in the form of glycogen for about one day's energy needs. The body's ability to store carbohydrate in the form of glycogen is limited, so adequate intake of dietary carbohydrates is essential. When a person stores glycogen, water is also stored. Each glycogen molecule attracts many molecules of water because of the way the elements are arranged. The average person after eating, that is, with glycogen stores completely filled, will also store about 4 pounds of water.

Glycogen—A polysaccharide commonly called the animal starch; the form in which carbohydrate is stored in liver and muscle tissue; formed in the body from glucose

Dietary Fiber

Dietary fiber refers to that portion of foods, mostly from plants, that the human body cannot break down or digest. It is eliminated from the body in the form of fecal material. Sometimes called roughage or bulk, fiber adds almost no fuel or energy value to the diet, but it does add volume.

In the United States, approximately one half of the population eats more than 12 grams of fiber per day, while one half eats less. (Food and Nutrition Board, 1986). Experts recommend that a healthy adult eat 20 to 35 grams of dietary fiber a day, twice what the average American consumes.

Can eating too much fiber cause problems? The answer is unquestionably yes. There is much evidence to suggest that eating more than 50 grams of fiber a day can interfere with mineral absorption, which can lead to problems like anemia and osteoporosis. The current recommendation is that a desirable fiber intake be achieved *not* by adding fiber concentrates to the diet, but by the consumption of fruits, vegetables, legumes, and whole-grain cereals, because they are excellent sources of fiber that also provide minerals and vitamins.

Fiber is classified as either **soluble** or **insoluble.** Solubility is defined as the ability of one substance to dissolve into another. For example, oil does not dissolve in water, so oil is insoluble in water. Insoluble fiber does not dissolve in water, whereas soluble fiber does. Both types of fiber react differently in the body and are needed for different reasons.

Dietary fiber— Material in foods, mostly from plants, that the human body cannot break down or digest

Soluble—Able to be dissolved

Insoluble—Incapable of being dissolved

SOLUBLE FIBER   Examples of sources of soluble fibers include beans, oatmeal, barley, broccoli, and citrus fruits. Oat bran is a good source of soluble fiber. Soluble fibers dissolve in water and thicken to form gels. The reported health benefits of soluble fibers include reduced cholesterol levels, regulated blood sugar levels, and weight loss (by helping dieters control their appetites).

INSOLUBLE FIBER   Examples of sources of insoluble fibers include the woody or structural parts of plants, such as fruit and vegetable skins, and the outer coating (bran) of wheat kernels. Insoluble fibers have been reported to promote regularity of bowel movements, reduce the risk of diverticular disease, and reduce the risk of some forms of cancer. Table 2–2 relates the solubility of each type of fiber to food sources and lists the reported health benefits attributed to each.

TABLE 2–2 *Food Sources and Reported Benefits of Fiber*

	Insoluble Fiber	Soluble Fiber
Solubility	Does not dissolve in water	Dissolves in water
Food Sources	Wheat bran	Oatmeal
	Corn bran	Oat bran, barley
	Vegetables	Some fruits such as
	Nuts	apples, oranges
	Fruit skins	Broccoli
	Some dry beans	Some dry beans*
Reported Benefit	Promotes regularity	May help reduce
	May help reduce risk of	cholesterol levels
	some forms of cancer	May assist in regulating
	May reduce risk of	blood sugar levels
	diverticular disease	May promote weight loss
		by increasing satiety†

*Current laboratory methods to assay soluble fiber content of individual foods are imprecise. This is the subject of much research.
†Satiety is defined as the sensation of fullness after eating.

FUNCTIONS OF CARBOHYDRATES

Carbohydrates play the following roles in the body: they provide fuel, spare body protein, and help prevent ketosis.

Provide Fuel

Carbohydrates, fats, and proteins provide the body's basic fuel or energy needs. Perhaps no other concept in science is more difficult to understand than the concept of energy, which is defined as the capacity to do work. You cannot see, feel, hear, or smell energy. To understand the concept of energy, it may be helpful to think of the human body as a machine. Just as gasoline is a car's fuel, so carbohydrate, protein, and fat are the human machine's fuel. Without fuel, of course, a car will not operate; without a fuel source over an extended period of time, death by starvation is the result for the human machine. Just as you cannot substitute something other than gasoline for your car (if you have a gasoline engine), you cannot substitute something other than carbohydrate, protein, and fat for fuel in your body.

The brain, other nervous tissue, and the lungs use carbohydrate as a primary source of fuel. In addition, the brain cannot store carbohydrate. This means that the brain must have an uninterrupted source of carbohydrate on an ongoing basis. This has a multitude of clinical implications, which will be discussed throughout this book.

Spare Body Protein

When we eat inadequate carbohydrate, our bodies suffer. We must have a continuous supply of glucose for all cells to function, particularly those of the central nervous system. Remember, our glycogen stores are limited. But the body can convert protein to glucose. An adequate supply of dietary carbohydrates spares body protein stores from being partially converted into glucose and allows protein to be used for growth and repair of body tissue. This principle has important ramifications for human nutrition, which will be discussed repeatedly throughout the text.

Help Prevent Ketosis

A balanced intake of the energy nutrients is vital. If a person's carbohydrate intake is too low, the body will break down stored fat to meet its fuel needs. The human machine cannot handle the excessive breakdown of stored body fat because the body lacks the necessary equipment. As a result, partially broken-down fats accumulate in the blood in the form of ketones and the person is said to be in a state of **ketosis.** Fatigue, nausea, and a lack of appetite are some of the undesirable consequences of ketosis. Coma and death have occurred in severe cases. The presence of ketosis is easily determined by testing for the presence of <u>acetone</u> or <u>diacetic acid</u> in the urine. Acetone and diacetic acid are **ketone bodies.** A minimum of 50 to 100 grams of carbohydrate each day is usually enough to prevent ketosis.

Ketosis—The physical state of the human body when ketones are elevated in the blood and present in the urine; as, for example, in diabetic ketoacidosis

Ketone bodies—Compounds such as acetone and diacetic acid that are formed when fat is metabolized incompletely

CONSUMPTION PATTERNS

Most of the world's population subsist primarily on carbohydrates. Foods rich in carbohydrates are easily grown in most climates, are low in cost, and are easily stored. They do not require refrigeration or electricity, and their shelf life may stretch to years. In Asia, where rice is a dietary staple, carbohydrates provide as much as 80 percent of the fuel in the diet.

Several trends reveal important information about the consumption of carbohydrates. For example, the percentage of fuel available from carbohydrates has decreased from 57 percent from the period covering 1909 to 1913 to 46 percent in 1985. Americans are eating less carbohydrate and more fat and protein as a percentage of total kilocaloric intake. In addition, back in 1909 Americans obtained about 66 percent of their total carbohydrate from starches such as corn, potatoes, wheat, and beans, and about 33 percent of their carbohydrate from sugars such as table sugar, maple sugar, molasses, jelly, and jam. By 1980, sugars furnished more than 50 percent of the carbohydrate in the food supply.[2]

RELATIONSHIP TO DENTAL HEALTH

Several studies have shown a relationship between carbohydrate consumption and dental caries. *Dental caries* is defined as the gradual decay of the teeth. A dental cavity is a hole in a tooth caused by dental caries. Dental caries results from four interactions: a genetically susceptible tooth, bacteria, carbohydrate, and time. All four of these factors must occur simultaneously for a cavity to form, as Figure 2–1 illustrates.

Genetic Susceptibility

Diet is not the sole contributor to health. Considerable genetic variability exists in the population. Even dental caries or a cavity is subject to genetic

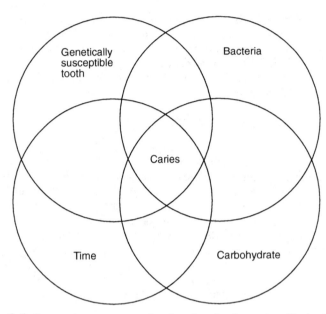

FIGURE 2–1. Interactions necessary for dental caries formation. Each of these four variables are necessary for a cavity to form. We cannot control our genetic susceptibility for cavities, and bacteria is always present in our mouths and is difficult to eliminate. However, we can control the length of time carbohydrate-containing foods are in our mouths and the kinds and amounts of carbohydrates we eat.

influences. Although the subject of genetics is beyond the scope of this text, the reader should be aware that studies have demonstrated remarkable genetic diversity among humans. Thus, for example, one individual's teeth may be more genetically susceptible or prone than another's to caries. **Genetic susceptibility** is the likelihood of an individual developing a given trait as determined by heredity. This is one reason why each patient must be evaluated as a unique individual.

Genetic suscep- tibility—The like- lihood of an indi- vidual developing a given trait as determined by heredity

Bacteria—Sin- gle-celled microorganisms that lack a true nucleus; may be either harmless to humans or dis- ease-producing

Other Factors Related to Cavity Formation

Bacteria, carbohydrate-containing foods, and the length of time that teeth are exposed to sugars influence cavity formation. Bacteria normally present in the mouth interact with dietary carbohydrate and produce acids. It is the acids, not the sugar itself, that cause decay (see Fig. 2–2) (Thomas, 1993). All types of sugars can promote cavity formation, including fructose, glucose, maltose, lactose, and sucrose. A strong relationship exists between the length of time sugars are actually present in the mouth and the development of caries. For example, sticky foods like caramels and raisins, which adhere to the tooth surface for longer periods, can lead to tooth decay in susceptible people. Sipping sweetened beverages continually throughout the day can also lead to tooth decay. Clinical Application 2–1 discusses a common healthcare problem known as nursing-bottle syndrome.

DENTAL CARIES

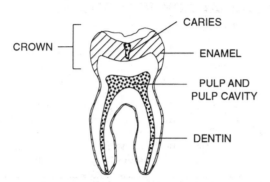

CROWN

CARIES

ENAMEL

PULP AND
PULP CAVITY

DENTIN

ACID BREAKS DOWN THE ENAMEL
THAT COVERS THE CROWN
OF THE TOOTH

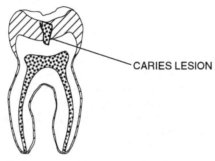

CARIES LESION

DECAY PENETRATES THE DENTIN,
THE LAYER UNDER THE ENAMEL,
CAUSING THE CAVITY

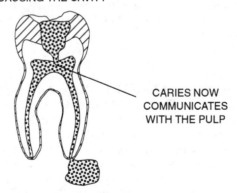

CARIES NOW
COMMUNICATES
WITH THE PULP

THE CAVITY, IF NOT REPAIRED,
SPREADS INTO THE PULP OF THE
TOOTH. THIS MAY CAUSE INFLAMMATION
AND AN ABSCESS. THEN THE TOOTH
MAY HAVE TO BE EXTRACTED.

FIGURE 2–2. The process of cavity formation. (From Thomas, CL [ed]: Taber's Cyclopedic Medical Dictionary, ed 16. FA Davis, Philadelphia, 1989, p 297, with permission.)

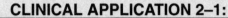

CLINICAL APPLICATION 2–1:
Nursing-Bottle Syndrome

Nursing-bottle syndrome is a dental condition caused by the frequent and prolonged exposure of an infant or young child to liquids containing sugars. Milk, formula, fruit juice, or other sweetened drinks can all cause rampant dental caries.

Typically, nursing-bottle syndrome occurs when a caretaker habitually puts a baby to bed with a bottle of milk, juice, or other sweetened liquid. During sleep the flow of saliva decreases, which allows the liquids from the nursing bottle to pool around the teeth, undiluted, for extended periods. Mothers need to be cautioned against this practice.

Certain foods may help counteract the effects of the acids produced by oral bacteria. Chewing fibrous foods such as apples or celery stimulates the production of generous amounts of saliva. Saliva helps clear the mouth of food and counteracts acid production. Because saliva production is increased during a meal, sugars eaten with a meal are less likely to cause decay than those eaten between meals.

FOOD SOURCES

As indicated earlier, carbohydrates consist of two groups: sugars and starches. All starches contain fiber; however, all starches do not provide equal amounts of fiber.

Sugars

Sugar, as mentioned in Clinical Calculation 2–1, contains 4 grams of carbohydrate per teaspoon. When determining a person's sugar consumption, you need to consider not only the simple sugars such as honey, jam, and jelly but also the sugars present in carbonated beverages, ice cream, sherbet, cakes, pies, cookies, and donuts. Tables of Food Composition may be used to approximate the actual intake a person may have from combination foods (See Appendix A). Simple sugar intake can be estimated using the value of 4 grams of carbohydrates per teaspoon (see Table 2–7).

Starches

Starches provide complex carbohydrate and are important sources of fiber and other nutrients. Fig. 2–3 illustrates a typical cereal grain. Its main parts, the germ, bran, and endosperm, are labeled. Most of the nutrients in cereal are in the bran and germ.

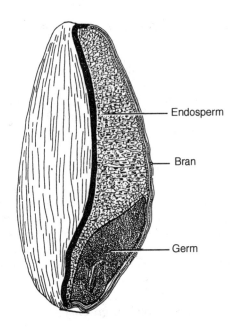

Endosperm

Bran

Germ

FIGURE 2–3. A grain of wheat. The most nutritious part of a grain of wheat is the bran and germ, which are removed during the milling of grain. For this reason, the use of whole-grain products should be encouraged.

Emphasis on Whole Grain

During the **milling** of grain, the germ and bran from the grain kernel are removed. Products made from the milling process are said to be refined. White flour results from the milling of wheat, white rice from the milling of rice. Oat products are not normally milled. Refined cereals and bread products are not as nutritious as their whole-grain counterparts since the bran and germ contain appreciable vitamins, minerals, and fiber. The nutritive value of cereal depends on the amount of bran and germ retained during the milling process. For this reason, you should encourage the use of whole grains whenever possible.

Milling—the process of grinding grain into flour

Enrichment

The addition of nutrients previously present in a food but removed during food processing or lost during storage is called **enrichment.** Enrichment of bread and white flour is mandatory in about two thirds of the United States, but in fact nearly all white bread in the United States is enriched with certain B vitamins and iron (National Research Council, 1989). Other enriched products include macaroni, noodles, spaghetti, and ready-to-eat cereals. Enriched products are not nutritionally equal to their whole-grain counterparts because not all of the nutrients lost during the milling process are replaced under government-mandated enrichment laws. The fiber lost during the milling of whole-grain products, for example, is not replaced by enrichment. The nutritive value of refined enriched food depends on the nutrients retained during milling and those added by enrichment. If a person will not eat whole grains, encourage him or her to select enriched grain products.

Enrichment— The addition of nutrients previously present in a food but removed during food processing or lost during storage

EXCHANGE LIST VALUES

The concept of exchange lists was introduced in the first chapter. In this section we will focus on those exchange lists that contain carbohydrates. A complete copy of the exchange lists is located in Appendix H. Exchanges that include carbohydrate are the starch/bread, vegetable, fruit, and milk lists. Learning the carbohydrate content of each of these exchange lists will assist in your understanding of food composition.

Starch/Bread Exchange List

One American Dietetic Association/American Diabetic Association (ADA) exchange of starch contains approximately 15 grams of carbohydrate. For example, each of the food items in Figure 2–4 is equal to one starch exchange. Whole-grain products average about 2 grams of fiber per serving. Some foods are higher in fiber (Table 2–3). A general rule to follow is ½ cup of cooked cereal, grain, or pasta or 1 ounce of a bread product is equal to one starch exchange.

Vegetable Exchange List

Vegetables eaten raw or cooked are also good sources of carbohydrates. Vegetables contain between 2 and 3 grams of fiber per serving. One vegetable exchange contains approximately 5 grams of carbohydrate. Table 2–4 defines one vegetable exchange. Vegetables, like fruits, are also good sources of vitamins and minerals.

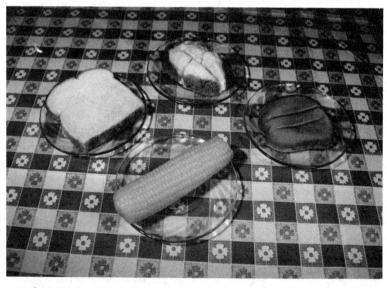

FIGURE 2–4. Each of these foods is equal to one starch exchange. An exchange is a defined quantity of a food item. One slice of bread, one small potato, one half of a hamburger bun, and one medium ear of corn are all defined quantities (amounts) of a food. (Courtesy of Mike Anderson, 808 S. Durand, Jackson, MI 49303.)

TABLE 2–3 *Selected Starch Exchanges*

Bran cereals, concentrated*	⅓ cup
Cooked cereal	½ cup
Ready-to-eat, unsweetened cereals	¾ cup
Beans and peas (cooked)*	⅓ cup
Corn*	½ cup
Potato, baked	1 small (3 ounces)
Whole wheat bread	1 slice (1 ounce)

General rule: ½ cup of cereal, grain, or pasta or 1 ounce of a bread product is equal to one starch exchange.

*Higher in fiber.

TABLE 2–4 *Vegetable Exchanges*

½ cup of cooked vegetables
½ cup of vegetable juice
1 cup of raw vegetables

TABLE 2–5 *Selected Fruit Exchanges*

Apple (raw, 2 inches across)	1 apple
Banana (9 inches long)	½ banana
Blueberries*	¾ cup
Grapefruit (medium)	½ grapefruit
Nectarine (1 ½ inches across)*	1 nectarine
Strawberries (raw, whole)*	1 ¼ cup
Prunes (dried)*	3 medium
Orange (2 ½ inches across)	1 orange
Orange juice	½ cup

*Contain 3 or more grams of fiber.

TABLE 2–6 *Carbohydrate and Fiber Content of ADA Exchanges*

	Carbohydrate (grams)	Fiber (grams)
Milk	12	0
Fruit	15	2*
Starch	15	2*
Vegetable	5	2–3

*Unless identified as a food with 3 or more grams of fiber per serving.

Fruit Exchange List

Fruits are another source of carbohydrate. One ADA exchange of fruit contains approximately 15 grams of carbohydrate. Many fruits are excellent sources of fiber (Table 2–5) and contain vitamins and minerals.

Milk Exchange List

Milk, with its lactose content, is an important source of carbohydrate. One cup of milk contains 12 grams of carbohydrate. Skim, whole, and 2 percent milk all contain approximately equal amounts of carbohydrate. Eight ounces of plain low-fat yogurt (with added nonfat milk solids), ⅓ cup dry nonfat milk, ½ cup evaporated milk, and 1 cup of buttermilk are all equal to 1 cup of milk—they also contain 12 grams of carbohydrate.

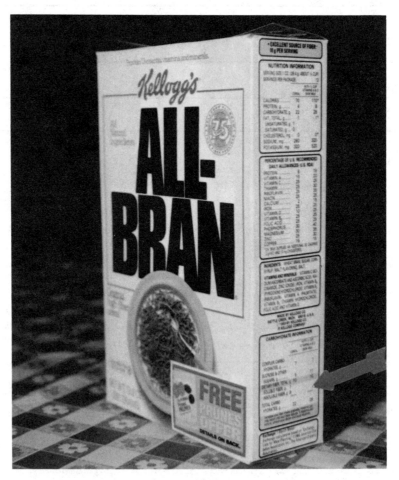

FIGURE 2–5. One half cup of All-Bran cereal contains 10 grams of fiber. Bran products are high in insoluble fiber. (Courtesy of Mike Anderson, 808 S. Durand, Jackson, MI 49303.)

Estimating the Fiber Content of Foods

Table 2–6 lists the carbohydrate and approximate fiber content in one serving from each of the carbohydrate-containing exchange lists. Because the fiber content of starches, fruits, and vegetables is highly variable, using the exchange list to approximate a patient's fiber intake provides only an estimate. For example, Figure 2–5 shows that ⅓ cup of All-Bran cereal contains 10 grams of fiber. This is several more grams than would have been approximated if the exchange list value of 2 grams had been used.

The fiber values given in Table 2–7 may be useful to screen large numbers of patients to locate individuals with a potential fiber deficiency. If a more accurate intake of a patient's fiber intake is necessary, you may need to use another technique to calculate this value. Other techniques include a computerized nutritional analysis or looking up individual food items in a Table of Food Composition. Both of these techniques are time-consuming.

DIETARY RECOMMENDATIONS

There is no recommended dietary allowance for carbohydrate. According to the 1989 edition of *Diet and Health*, the following minimal recommendations relating to carbohydrate-containing food groups were published:

1. Every day, eat five or more servings of a combination of vegetables and fruits, especially green and yellow vegetables and citrus fruits. (One serving equals ½ cup.)
2. Increase intake of starches and other complex carbohydrates by eating six or more daily servings of a combination of breads, cereals, and legumes. (One serving equals one slice of bread or ½ cup cooked cereal, grain, or pasta.)

If individuals consume the recommended number of servings of fruits, vegetables, and starches, they will most likely be taking in the recommended amount of dietary fiber.

Summary

Carbohydrates are divided into groups: sugars and starches. All carbohydrates are composed of one or more units of $C_6H_{12}O_6$ singly or joined together. The average American's intake of sugars is considered excessive, while the intake of starches is considered low. Many Americans would also benefit by increasing their fiber intake with the consumption of more starches, fruits, and vegetables. The use of whole-grain starches should be encouraged. It has been established that dietary carbohydrate promotes tooth decay in susceptible individuals. The ADA Exchange Lists that contain carbohydrate are the starch, vegetable, fruit, and milk lists.

There are adverse consequences to inadequate carbohydrate consumption. The human body can make glucose from either protein or carbohydrate in the diet. The human body must find a continuous source of glucose for proper central nervous system function. Remember that the body's glycogen stores are limited. Therefore, when there is no carbohydrate in the diet and the body uses protein or fat for a fuel source, the body in effect cannibalizes itself for glucose. Muscle and organ mass are lost in the process. A minimum of 50 to 100 grams of carbohydrate a day is usually adequate to prevent these consequences.

A case study and a sample plan of care appear below. Both are designed to show you how the information you have studied in this chapter can be used in nursing practice.

CASE STUDY 2–1

The nurse was in Ms. D.'s room when her tray and menu for the following day arrived. Ms. D., a 22-year-old, 5-foot 6-inch, 142-pound patient, was having some trouble manipulating her pencil because she had a cast on her right arm. Ms. D. was on a general diet, and the nurse offered to assist her in marking her menu. As the nurse read the menu, Ms. D. indicated her selections. The patient selected eggs and bacon for breakfast, a double order of chicken for lunch, and a double order of roast beef for dinner. Ms. D. refused all milk, fruit, vegetables, and starches. When the nurse questioned Ms. D. as to why she refused these items, she stated, "I am following a high-protein diet to lose weight." Upon further questioning, the nurse learned that the patient has been following this diet for about 2 weeks. In addition, laboratory analysis of her urine was positive for ketones.

Applying the principles learned on the nursing process, a nurse might construct a nursing care plan similar to the one illustrated below. Remember, however, that real patients may have far more complex needs and problems and that other nurses may devise other equally valid and effective interventions.

NURSING CARE PLAN FOR MS. D.

Assessment
Subjective: Refuses foods containing CHO
Objective: Ketone bodies in urine
Height: 5 feet 6 inches
Weight: 142 pounds

Nursing Diagnosis
Nutrition, altered: Less than body requirements, related to knowledge deficit as evidenced by refusal to select CHO-containing foods on menu and urine positive for ketones

Desired Outcome/Evaluation Criteria
1. Patient will state at least one reason why she needs CHO by midnight tonight (date).
2. Patient will select at least 100 grams of CHO on menu each day beginning tomorrow (date).
3. Patient will consume at least 100 grams of CHO each day beginning the day after tomorrow (date).

Nursing Actions
1. Encourage patient to consume milk, vegetables, fruits, and starches. Refer to dietitian for instruction on normal nutrition and possible appropriate weight reduction strategies. Request order from physician for a low-kilocalorie diet.
2. Assist with daily menu selections.
3. Document food intake (may be called a calorie count).

Rationale

1. Explaining the reason carbohydrates are necessary in the diet may motivate the patient to eat carbohydrates. Milk, vegetables, fruits, and starches are all good sources of carbohydrates. The nurse may need to educate the patient about dietary sources of carbohydrates.
2. The minimum daily recommended intake to prevent ketosis is 50 to 100 grams of carbohydrate. Helping the patient fill out his or her menu is a good method to determine if the patient understands the dietary sources of carbohydrate.
3. Directly observing a patient's food intake and documenting the observations made are necessary to evaluate if the approach taken by nursing was successful.

If objectives are met, continue interventions. If objectives are not met, reassess.

STUDY AIDS

Chapter Review Questions

1. The following are all monosaccharides except:
   a. Glucose
   b. Lactose
   c. Fructose
   d. Galactose

2. _____ is (are) the body's carbohydrate stores.
   a. Polymers
   b. Glycogen
   c. Soluble fiber
   d. Ketones

3. Eight grams of simple carbohydrate is equal to _____ teaspoon(s) of sugar.
   a. 1
   b. 2
   c. 3
   d. 8

4. The following are all good sources of fiber except:
   a. Honey
   b. Whole-grain bread
   c. Beans
   d. Nectarines

5. Reported benefits of insoluble fiber include:
   a. May help reduce cholesterol levels
   b. May assist in regulating blood sugar levels
   c. May help reduce the risk of some forms of cancer
   d. May promote weight loss by increasing satiety

6. Beans, oatmeal, barley, broccoli, and citrus fruits are foods that contain much _____.
   a. Lactose
   b. Maltose
   c. Soluble fiber
   d. Insoluble fiber

7. The following statement is true:
   a. Sugar is harmful to the human body.
   b. A person should consume a minimum of 50 to 100 grams of carbohydrate per day to prevent ketosis.
   c. The human body has the capacity to store about 3 days' worth of carbohydrate.
   d. If a person consumes some oat bran daily, he or she need not worry about including other sources of fiber in the diet.

8. Choose the *incorrect* statement:
   a. Ketosis can occur when a person avoids carbohydrate.
   b. Acetone and diacetic acid are ketone bodies that can be measured in the urine.
   c. A minimum of 50 to 100 grams of CHO is needed each day to prevent ketosis.
   d. A person can always tell when he or she is in a state of ketosis because he or she becomes faint.

9. One cup of milk contains approximately _____ grams of carbohydrates:
   a. 5
   b. 8
   c. 10
   d. 12

10. The following practice is the most likely to promote cavity formation:
    a. Eating apples between meals
    b. Skipping meals
    c. Slowly sipping a soft drink continually throughout the day
    d. Eating a piece of cake as part of a meal

NCLEX-Style Quiz

Situation One

1. Mrs. D. is trying to lose weight and complains of hunger. She asks the nurse to recommend fruit exchanges that "have a large volume." Which of the following would you recommend?
   a. Orange juice
   b. Prunes
   c. Strawberries
   d. Raisins

Situation Two

2. Ms. B. takes Dolores, who is 18 months old, to the clinic for a routine checkup. The nurse notices that Dolores has rampant dental caries. This can usually be attributed to:
   a. Feeding the child only liquids and not enough solids
   b. Feeding the child all solids and not enough liquids
   c. The occasional ingestion of candy
   d. Dolores's caretaker putting her to bed for a nap or a night's sleep with a bottle of milk or juice

Situation Three

3. Mrs. A. has read about the health benefits of fiber. She is considering adding fiber concentrates to her diet. Which of the following statements would be the nurse's best response?
   a. Fiber is best obtained from starches, fruits, and vegetables because these foods provide other necessary nutrients. In addition, too much fiber interferes with the absorption of some vitamins and minerals.
   b. Fiber concentrates are best taken before meals.
   c. Fiber concentrates are best taken with meals.
   d. It is difficult to obtain adequate fiber from foods, so the use of fiber concentrates is a recommended practice.

Situation Four

4. Mr. P. has a high-fiber diet order. The nurse should encourage the intake of:
   a. Milk, yogurt, and ice cream
   b. Eggs, cheese, and chicken
   c. Fruits, vegetables, and starches
   d. Margarine, salad dressings, and oils

CLINICAL CALCULATION 2–1

Converting Grams of Sugar into Teaspoons of Sugar

The expression "eighty grams of sugar" does not mean much to the average American consumer, since most Americans are unfamiliar with the metric system. Unfortunately, many food labels use the metric system to list the nutritional content of a product. To help acquaint you with the metric system, we will demonstrate how to convert 80 grams of sugar to its equivalent in teaspoons. The number you need to remember to make this conversion is four. One teaspoon of sugar contains 4 grams of carbohydrate.

$$\frac{80 \text{ grams of sugar}}{4 \text{ grams of sugar per teaspoon}} = 20 \text{ teaspoons of sugar}$$

Eighty grams of sugar is equal to 20 teaspoons. Table 2–7 lists sweeteners that also contain 4 grams of carbohydrate.

TABLE 2–7 *Sweeteners that Contain 4 Grams of Carbohydrates per Teaspoon*

Molasses
Granulated sugar
Powdered sugar
Syrup
Brown sugar
Jam
Marmalade
Honey
Jelly

Now that you know how to convert grams of sucrose into common measures, compare the following two cereal labels in Figure 2–6. One label contains 3 grams of sucrose and the other contains 14 grams. This converts to ¾ teaspoon and 3½ teaspoons of sugar, respectively. If you remember the number 4, you can easily convert grams of sucrose into teaspoons of sugar. Divide grams by 4 to obtain teaspoons.

First label:

$$\frac{3 \text{ grams of sugar}}{4 \text{ grams per teaspoon}} = \frac{3}{4} \text{ teaspoon}$$

Second label:

$$\frac{14 \text{ grams of sugar}}{4 \text{ grams per tsp}} = 3\frac{1}{2} \text{ teaspoons}$$

Box continued on next page.

CLINICAL CALCULATION 2–1 *(Continued)*

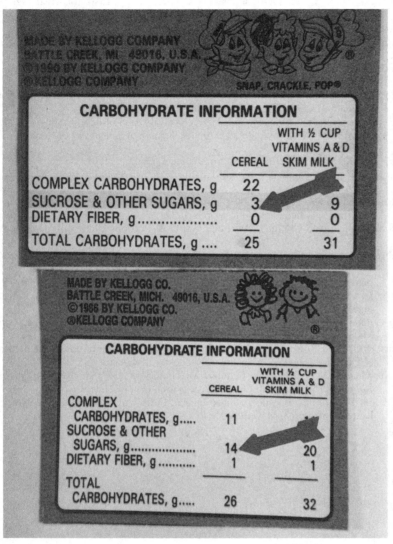

FIGURE 2–6. A comparison of two cereal labels. Use this photograph as you read Clinical Calculation 2–1. (Courtesy of Mike Anderson, 808 S. Durand, Jackson, MI 49303.)

BIBLIOGRAPHY

American Dental Association: Diet and Dental Health (Publication No. W159). American Dental Association, Chicago, 1986.

American Dietetic and Diabetic Associations: Exchange Lists for Meal Planning. The American Dietetic Association, Chicago, 1986.

American Institute for Cancer Research: Newsletter 23, Spring, 1989.

Cady, B: Cancer Manual, ed 7. American Cancer Society, Massachusetts Division, Boston, 1986.

Feldman, EB: Essentials of Clinical Nutrition. FA Davis, Philadelphia, 1988.

Finn, SC: Rough Stuff. Ross Laboratories, Columbus, OH, 1989.

Food and Nutrition Board: Proceedings of a Symposium. What Is America Eating? National Academy Press, Washington, DC, 1986.

Glinsmann, WH, Irausquin, H, and Park, YK: Evaluation of health aspects of sugars contained in carbohydrate sweeteners: Report of Sugars Task Force, 1986. J Nutr (Suppl) 116:1, 1986.

Hughes, MS: All eyes on the potato. Smithsonian, October, 1991.

National Research Council: Diet and Health. National Academy Press, Washington, DC, 1989.

Owen, AL: Fiber in Your Diet. Nutrition Counselor. Health Team Interactive Communications, Inc., New York, March, 1989.

Pennington, JA and Church, HW: Food Values of Portions Commonly Used, ed 14. Harper & Row, New York, 1985.

Subcommittee on the Tenth Edition of the Recommended Dietary Allowances: National Research Council: Recommended Dietary Allowances, ed 10. National Academy Press, Washington, DC, 1989.

Thomas, CL (ed): Tabers Cyclopedic Medical Dictionary, ed 17, FA Davis, Philadelphia, 1993.

Tri-County Health Department: Market to Market. American Heart Association of Michigan, Lathrop Village, 1989.

Watson, GE and Bowen, WH: The influence of sugar on dental caries. Department of Dental Research, University of Rochester, Rochester, NY, 1989.

White-Graves, MV and Rosita Schuler, M: History of foods in the caries process. Journal of the American Dietetic Association (Suppl 2) 86:916, 1986.

Why sugar continues to concern nutritionists. Tufts University Diet and Nutrition Letter. Vol 3, no 3, May 1985.

Chapter Three
Fats

Chapter Outline

Key Terms

As a study aid, each key term is followed by the page number where the term is defined in the chapter. Terms that appear in **boldface** or <u>underscored</u> in the chapter text are located in the glossary.

Fats

Learning Objectives

After completing this chapter, the student should be able to:

1. Describe the different types of fats and identify food sources for each.
2. Identify how fats are classified and discuss their physical properties.
3. List the major functions of fats both in the diet and in the body.
4. Discuss the relationship of cholesterol, saturated fat, polyunsaturated fat, and monounsaturated fat to health.
5. List three current recommendations of the Food and Nutrition Board of the National Research Council that pertain to fats.
6. Correctly interpret a food label for a margarine or salad dressing.

Lipid—Any one of a group of fats or fat-like substances that are insoluble in water; includes true fats (fatty acids and glycerol), lipoids, and sterols

*T*he descriptive name for fats of all kinds is **lipids.** You will see the term lipid used in patients' medical records. The group of lipids includes true fats and oils, and related fat-like compounds such as lipoids and sterols. Fats and oils are both present in the body and also found in foods. Fats are typically thought of as solids, while oils are regarded as liquids. For example, your body produces oil adjacent to your hair. Not as readily apparent to some people is the layer of fat beneath the skin, which is solid. At room temperature, dietary fats such as lard and butter are solid, whereas corn and olive oils are liquid.

Lipids exhibit the physical property of insolubility in water, and are greasy to the touch. When two insoluble substances are mixed together, they separate readily, the classic example being that of vinegar and oil. You can shake the vinegar and oil combination repeatedly, and it will still separate after the agitation stops.

COMPOSITION

Glycerol—The backbone of a fat molecule

Lipids are composed of the elements carbon, hydrogen, and oxygen. These are the same three elements that make up carbohydrates, but the proportion of oxygen to carbon and hydrogen is lower in fats. The implications of this will be discussed later in the chapter. The basic structural unit of a true fat is one molecule of **glycerol** joined to one, two, or three **fatty acid** molecules. Glycerol is thus the backbone of a fat molecule.

Fatty acid—Part of the structure of a true fat

A fatty acid is composed of a chain of carbon atoms with hydrogen and a few oxygen atoms attached. The fatty acid chains joined to the glycerol molecule vary in length (depending on the number of carbon atoms present) and composition. The different taste, smell, and physical appearance of each fat results from the variety of fatty acids and their physical arrangement in the fat molecules. Beef fat tastes, smells, and looks different from chicken fat or corn oil. All fats contain fatty acids.

Number of Fatty Acids

A fat can have from one to three fatty aids. As you will see, the number of fatty acids a fat contains has important implications for both diet and health.

Monoglycerides and Diglycerides

When a single fatty acid is joined to a glycerol molecule, the resulting fat is called a monoglyceride. When two fatty acids are joined to a glycerol molecule, the fat is called a diglyceride. The terms monoglyceride and diglyceride are commonly seen on food labels.

Triglyceride—Three fatty acids joined to a glycerol molecule

Triglycerides

When three fatty acids are joined to a glycerol molecule, a **triglyceride** is formed. Most of the fat found in our diets and in the body is in the form of triglycerides. Excess triglycerides are stored in the specialized adipose cells that make up **adipose tissue.** The human body has a virtually unlimited capacity to store fat. Figure 3-1 illustrates the structure of monoglycerides, diglycerides, and triglycerides.

Adipose tissue—Tissue containing masses of fat cells

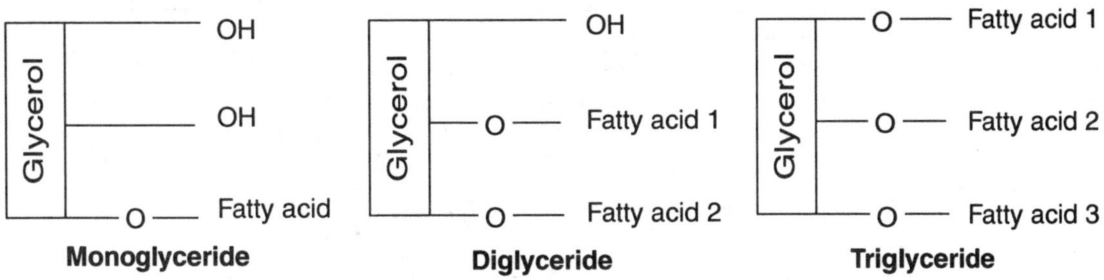

FIGURE 3–1. Monoglycerides, diglycerides, and triglycerides. A monoglyceride has one fatty acid attached to the glycerol molecule, a diglyceride has two fatty acids attached to the glycerol molecule, and a triglyceride has three fatty acids attached to the glycerol molecule.

Length of Fatty Acid Chain

As mentioned earlier, fatty acids vary in the length of their fatty acid chains. The length of each fatty acid chain is determined by the number of carbon atoms present, and can vary from 2 to 24 carbons. The length of the fatty acid chain determines how the body transports the fat in the body, since fatty acid chains of short length (< 6 carbon atoms) and medium length (8 to 12 carbon atoms) are processed differently than fats with longer chains.

Degree of Saturation

The terms saturated, unsaturated, monounsaturated, and polyunsaturated have become household words. Both news and feature stories about health issues revolve around these terms. Whether you get your information from newspapers, magazines, television, or radio, you know that degree of fat saturation is important. Consumers and patients ask sophisticated questions about fats and turn to all healthcare professionals to define and explain the terminology. Technically, all of these terms refer to the chemical structure of fatty acids, based on the degree of hydrogen atom saturation.

The degree of saturation of a fatty acid depends on the extent to which hydrogen is joined to the carbon atoms that are present. A saturated fatty acid is filled with as many hydrogen atoms as the carbon atoms can bond with, and has no double bonds between carbons. In this case, a **double bond** describes the type of chemical connection between two neighboring carbon atoms, each lacking one hydrogen atom. In an unsaturated fatty acid, the carbon atoms are joined together by one or more of such double bonds.

Wherever a double bond occurs, another hydrogen atom could potentially "join" the chain. In other words, the fatty acid chain is lacking hydrogen atoms and is thus less saturated than a chain that is completely filled. A fatty acid with only one carbon-to-carbon double bond is monounsaturated. A fatty acid with more than one carbon-to-carbon bond is polyunsaturated. See Figure 3–2 for a structural comparison of saturated, monounsaturated, and polyunsaturated fatty acids.

Double bond—A type of chemical connection in which a fatty acid has only two neighboring carbon atoms, each lacking one hydrogen atom

Saturated

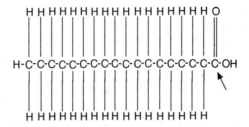

Saturated (no carbon–to–carbon double bonds)

Unsaturated

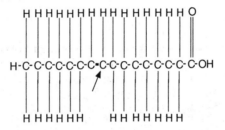

Monounsaturated (one carbon–to–carbon double bond)

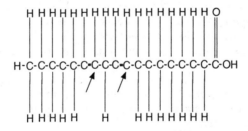

Polyunsaturated (more than one carbon–to–carbon double bond)

FIGURE 3–2. Saturated, monounsaturated, and polyunsaturated fatty acids. A saturated fatty acid has no carbon-to-carbon double bonds. A monounsaturated fatty acid has one carbon-to-carbon double bond. A polyunsaturated fatty acid has more than one carbon-to-carbon double bond.

In addition to the fats in the body, the fats found in foods are combinations of saturated and unsaturated fatty acids. They are designated as follows:

> *Saturated fat*—Composed mostly of saturated fatty acids
> *Unsaturated fat*—Composed mostly of unsaturated fatty acids
> *Monounsaturated fat*—Composed mostly of monounsaturated fatty acids
> *Polyunsaturated fat*—Composed mostly of polyunsaturated fatty acids

PHYSICAL PROPERTIES AND FOOD SOURCES

Saturated Fats

Saturated fats are likely to be solid at room temperature and usually occur in products of animal origin such as meat, poultry, and whole milk. The exceptions are the tropical coconut and palm-kernel oils, and cocoa butter, which are of vegetable origin. See Table 3–1 and 3–2 for a more complete list of foods containing saturated fat. Saturated fats become <u>rancid</u> very slowly because the chemical bond between carbon and hydrogen is very stable. A rancid fat has an offensive odor and taste caused by the partial chemical breakdown of the fat's molecular structure. Products made with saturated fats have a long **shelf life** because the fat in the product is stable. Saturated fats have been targeted for reduction in the average American's diet by the Committee on Diet and Health of the National Research Council. You will learn more about this in the chapter on cardiovascular disease.

Shelf life—The time a product can remain in storage without deterioration

Unsaturated Fats

Unsaturated fats are likely to be liquid at room temperature, to be of plant origin, and to become rancid more quickly than saturated fats. The double carbon bonds in unsaturated fatty acids are very unstable and therefore easily broken. For this reason, many convenience products have been made with saturated fats to lengthen their shelf life. The food industry is slowly changing this practice; increasingly, more convenience products are being made with unsaturated fats. Examples of unsaturated fats are corn, cottonseed, safflower, soybean, and sunflower oils. See Table 3–3 for a more complete list of unsaturated fats.

TABLE 3–1 *Food Sources of Saturated Fats*

Meat products	Visible fat and marbling in beef, pork, and lamb, especially in prime-grade and ground meats, lard
Processed meats	Frankfurters
	Luncheon meats such as bologna, corned beef, liverwurst, pastrami, and salami
	Bacon, sausage, lard, suet, salt pork
Poultry and fowl	Chicken and turkey (mostly beneath the skin) cornish hens, duck, and goose
Whole milk and whole-milk products	Butter
	Cheeses made with whole milk or cream, condensed milk, ice cream, whole-milk yogurt, all creams (sour, half-and-half, whipped)
Plant products	Coconut oil, palm-kernel oil, cocoa butter
Miscellaneous	Fully hydrogenated shortening and margarine, many cakes, pies, cookies, and mixes

TABLE 3–2 *Selected Foods High in Cholesterol and/or Saturated Fat*

Foods	Amount	Cholesterol (mg)	Saturated Fat (mg)
Caviar	3 ½ ounces	580	4.0
Oysters, Eastern	3 ½ ounces	530	0.5
Liver	3 ounces	410	2.4
Cream puff	1	228	10.0
Baked custard	1 cup	213	7.0
Egg, hard cooked	1	215	5.0
Waffles, homemade	2	204	8.0
Coconut custard pie	1 piece	183	8.0
Cheesecake	3.25 ounces	170	10.0
Shrimp, boiled	6 large	167	0.2
Eggnog, commercial	1 cup	149	11.0
Bread pudding/raisins	1 cup	142	4.5
Whole milk	1 cup	124	5.0
Ground beef, 21% fat	3 ounces	76	7.0

Hydrogenation

Hydrogenation
—The process of adding hydrogen to a fat to make it more highly saturated

Commercial food processing frequently involves taking a fat of vegetable origin (unsaturated) and adding hydrogen to either extend the fat's shelf life or make the fat harder. This process of adding hydrogen to a fat is called **hydrogenation.** If only some of the fat's double bonds have been broken by hydrogenation, the product becomes "partially hydrogenated." If all of the double bonds are broken, the product becomes "completely hydrogenated." Completely hydrogenated fats are highly saturated fats. That is, they have no carbon-to-carbon double bonds. For example, a completely hydrogenated corn oil is closer to lard in saturation than a partially hydrogenated corn oil. All vegetable spreads such as corn oil margarine have been hydrogenated to some extent. If these spreads had not been hydrogenated, they would be liquids (except for the saturated tropical oils). Patients are usually advised to avoid products that contain completely hydrogenated fats when the therapeutic goal is to decrease saturated fat intake.

TABLE 3–3 *Food Sources of Unsaturated Fats*

Monounsaturated oils	Canola, olive, peanut
Foods	Avocados, olives, peanuts; nuts such as almonds, cashews, and filberts
Polyunsaturated oils	Corn, cottonseed, safflower, sunflower, sesame, soybean, and mustard seed
Fish	Halibut, herring, mackerel, salmon, sardines, fresh tuna, trout, and whitefish

CLASSIFICATION

Lipids can be classified according to three criteria: whether the fat is emulsified or nonemulsified, whether the fat is visible or invisible, and/or whether the fat is simple or compound.

Emulsified or Nonemulsified Fats

Fats can be classified as emulsified or nonemulsified. The term <u>emulsion</u> is applied to a liquid dispersed in another liquid with which it does not usually mix. The body emulsifies dietary fat so that it can be transported throughout the body by the blood, which is water-based. Emulsification takes place in the small intestine through the action of bile salts during the digestive process (see Chapter 5).

Visible or Invisible Fats

Dietary fat can be classified as either **visible fat** or **invisible fat,** according to whether it can or cannot be seen. More than 40 percent of dietary fat is ingested as visible fat (Feldman, 1988). This 40 percent includes vegetable oils, butter, margarine, lard, mayonnaise, salad dressings, visible fat on meats, and shortening. If a person is trying to decrease the fat content of his or her diet, it is prudent to eliminate visible fats first. Invisible fats cannot be identified as readily. These fats are present in grains, egg yolks, poultry, emulsified milk and milk products, the marbling in meat, and in many baked goods and snacks. Invisible fat accounts for the remaining 60 percent of fat in the American diet. Even if patients eliminate all visible forms of fat from their diet, large amounts of invisible fat may be present. Patients should be taught to identify invisible forms of fat.

Visible fat— Dietary fat that can be easily seen, such as the fat on meat or in oil

Invisible fat— Dietary fats that cannot be seen easily; hidden fats in foods such as baked goods, peanut butter, emulsified milk, and so forth

Simple or Compound Fats

Fats are also classified as simple or compound. *Simple fats* are lipids that have only fatty acids or a hydroxyl molecule joined to glycerol. Think of the hydroxyl molecule as being just a simple chemical "filler." Monoglycerides, diglycerides, and triglycerides are all simple fats.

When one of the fatty acid chains joined to the glycerol molecule is replaced by a protein, the result is a *compound fat*. This structure is then called a **lipoprotein.** Lipoproteins are composed of fat, protein, and fat-related components. They transport fat in the blood stream. The human body makes four types of lipoproteins: chylomicrons, very low-density lipoproteins (VLDL), low-density lipoproteins (LDL), and high-density lipoproteins (HDL). As is evident by their names, the lipoproteins vary in density. The higher the protein content of the lipoprotein, the greater the density. Lipoproteins also vary in the proportional amounts of fat and protein each contains. The type and amounts of lipoproteins in a person's blood can either protect them from, or predispose them to, heart disease.

Lipoprotein—A fat and protein complex in which one of the fatty acids joined to the glycerol molecule is replaced by a protein; may combine with cholesterol, phospholipids, and triglycerides

FUNCTIONS OF FATS

Lipids are important in the diet and serve many functions in the human body. Fats in food serve as a fuel source, carry the essential fatty acids, act as a vehicle for fat-soluble vitamins, and help add satiety to the diet. Fats in the body supply fuel to most tissues, function as an energy reserve, insulate the body, support and protect vital organs, lubricate body tissues, insulate nerve fibers, and form an integral part of cell membranes.

Fats in Food

Fuel Source

Fats are the major dietary source of fuel. Because fats have proportionately more carbon and hydrogen and less oxygen than carbohydrates, they have a greater potential for the release of energy. In practical terms, this means that fats are a concentrated source of fuel or kilocalories. Fats furnish more than twice the kilocalories, gram for gram, as carbohydrates. Each gram of fat yields 9 kilocalories, so one teaspoon of fat, which is equivalent to 5 grams of fat, will yield 45 kilocalories. Compare this with carbohydrates, each gram of which yields only 4 kilocalories. A teaspoon of sugar contains 4 grams of carbohydrate and will therefore yield only 16 kilocalories.

Vehicle for Fat-Soluble Vitamins

In foods, fats act as a vehicle for vitamins A, D, E, and K; in the body, fats assist in the absorption of these fat-soluble vitamins.

Satiety Value

Satiety—The feeling of satisfaction after eating

Fats also contribute flavor, **satiety,** and palatability to the diet. They supply texture to food, trap and intensify its flavor, and enhance its odor. Consider for a moment the different sensations felt when eating 2 cups of ice cream versus eating six apples.

Sources of Essential Fatty Acids

Linoleic acid— An essential fatty acid

As you learned in Chapter 1, an essential nutrient is one that must be supplied by the diet because the body requires it but cannot manufacture the nutrient. Fat contains the essential fatty acid **linoleic acid.** Linoleic acid strengthens cell membranes and has a major role in the transport and metabolism of cholesterol. Two necessary fatty acids, gamma-linolenic (γ-linolenic) acid and arachidonic acid, can be synthesized by the body from linoleic acid. These fatty acids taken together help prolong blood clotting time, hasten fibrolytic activity, and are involved in the development of the brain.

Prostaglandins —Long-chain, unsaturated fatty acids mostly synthesized in the body from arachidonic acid; has hormone-like effects

Prostaglandins, compounds with extensive hormone-like actions, require arachidonic acid for synthesis. Recent evidence has shown that a group of fatty acids such as alpha-linolenic (α-linolenic) may also be essential. (Neuringer and Conner, 1986)

A deficiency of linoleic acid can occur in infants and hospitalized patients under certain conditions. Linoleic acid deficiency was first observed in infants fed formulas deficient in linoleic acid. Drying and flaking of the skin has been observed (Wiese, Hansen, and Adam, 1958). This deficiency was again observed in the early 1970s in hospitalized patients fed exclusively with intravenous fluids containing no fat. The symptoms included scaly skin, hair loss, and impaired wound healing. Linoleic acid deficiency is still being diagnosed today.

Fats in the Body

Fuel Supply

Fat needs to be available in the body as fuel to supply needed energy for all tissues except in the central nervous system and the brain, which rely on glucose for their energy needs.

Fuel Reserve

Fat also functions as the body's main fuel or energy reserve. Excess kilocalories consumed are stored in specialized cells called <u>adipose cells.</u> When an individual does not eat enough food to meet the energy demands of the body, the adipose cells release fat for fuel.

Organ Protection

Fatty tissue cushions and protects vital organs by providing a supportive fat pad that absorbs mechanical shocks. Examples of organs supported by fat are the eyes and kidneys.

Lubrication

Fats also lubricate body tissue. The human body manufactures oil in structures called <u>sebaceous glands.</u> Secretions from the sebaceous glands lubricate the skin to retard loss of body water to the outside environment.

Insulation

The subcutaneous layer of fat beneath the skin helps to insulate the body by protecting it from excessive heat or cold. A sheath of fatty tissue surrounding nerve fibers provides insulation to help relay nerve impulses.

Cell Membrane Structure

Fat serves as an integral part of cell membranes, helps transport nutrient materials and metabolites, and provides a barrier against water-soluble substances.

CHOLESTEROL

Cholesterol is not a true fat, but belongs to a group called sterols. Cholesterol is a component of many of the foods in our diet. In addition, the human body manufactures about 1000 milligrams of cholesterol a day, mainly in the liver. The liver also filters out excess cholesterol and helps to eliminate it from the body.

Cholesterol—A fat-like substance made in the human body and found in foods of animal origin.

Functions

Cholesterol has several important functions. It is an essential component of all cell membranes and is found in brain and nerve tissue and in the blood. Cholesterol is necessary for the production of several hormones, including cortisone, adrenalin, estrogen, and testosterone. A <u>hormone</u> is a substance produced by the endocrine glands and secreted directly into the bloodstream. By this route, hormones are carried to target areas of the body, where they act to stimulate increased functional activity or the secretion of another hormone. In this way hormones regulate the functions of many organs and cells. (More information on hormones will be presented in later chapters.) Cholesterol is also a component of bile salts, which aid in digestion.

Blood Cholesterol Levels

An elevated level of cholesterol in the blood is a major cause of coronary artery disease. Lowering blood cholesterol levels reduces the risk of heart attacks due to coronary disease. Individuals with cholesterol levels below 200 milligrams per deciliter have the least risk. Individuals with cholesterol levels between 200 and 239 milligrams per deciliter have a borderline to high risk. A cholesterol level in excess of 240 milligrams per deciliter places the individual in the high-risk category. The consumption of cholesterol is considered to be less of a risk factor for coronary heart disease than the consumption of saturated fats (National Research Council A, 1989).

Food Sources

Cholesterol is present in the foods we eat. In fact, many of the products now sold in supermarkets are targeted to shoppers interested in controlling their blood cholesterol level through diet. Cholesterol occurs naturally in all animal foods and is produced only in liver tissue. When we ingest animal products, we also ingest the cholesterol the animal made. For this reason, The American Heart Association recommends that a healthy woman eat no more than 6 ounces of lean meat per day and a healthy man no more than 7 ounces of lean meat per day. Cholesterol is not present in foods of plant origin.

Table 3–2 lists selected foods high in cholesterol. Note that one egg supplies about 215 milligrams of cholesterol. Eggs are the major contributor of cholesterol in the average American's diet. The American Heart Association recommends that consumers limit egg yolks to no more than four per week.

FATS IN THE AMERICAN DIET

Fat available in the food supply increased from an average of 124 grams per day per person in 1909 to 172 grams per day per person in 1985. There are approximately 5 grams of fat in a teaspoon; therefore, 124 grams converts to 25 teaspoons of fat and 172 grams to 34½ teaspoons. Thus, as of 1985, American were eating about 9½ more teaspoons of fat per day than they did in 1909. The relative contribution of fat from saturated versus polyunsaturated sources has changed since that time. The intake of animal fat from red meat has declined while that of vegetable fat has risen. Americans are also consuming less whole milk and more low-fat milk.[5] Notwithstanding, fat intake in the American diet is still considered excessive. Recent estimates indicate that Americans derive approximately 37 percent of their total caloric intake from fat, whereas most experts agree that less than 30 percent of total caloric intake should be derived from fat.

Calculating the amount of fat as a percentage of total kilocalories is a convenient way of evaluating the level of fat in a food item. Clinical Calculation 3–1 demonstrates how to calculate the percent of kilocalories from fat in a food item. If a food item contains more than 30 percent fat, it should be balanced with other items that contain less fat, such as fruits and vegetables. What is important is *balance*. The main objective is to reduce overall fat intake during the course of a day or a week.

DIETARY RECOMMENDATIONS CONCERNING FAT

There is no RDA for fat. The Food and Nutrition Board's Committee on Diet and Health recommends that the fat content of the US diet not exceed 30 percent of kilocaloric intake. They also recommend that less than 10 percent of kilocalories should be provided from saturated fatty acids and that dietary cholesterol should be less than 300 milligrams per day. Some fat is needed to provide linoleic acid, an essential fatty acid. The Food and Nutrition Board of the National Research Council recommends a minimum adequate intake of linoleic acid as opposed to a set amount. The minimum adequate amount of linoleic acid is 1 to 2 percent of total dietary kilocalories. The healthy adult can obtain this amount from about 1 teaspoon of oil per day. For infants consuming 100 k calories per kilogram, this would correspond to a daily intake of 0.2 grams per kilogram.

FAT INTAKE AND HEALTH

Dietary Fat

Excess dietary fat has been associated with an increased risk of cardiovascular disease, the development of obesity, and an increased risk of certain cancers, especially cancers of the colon and prostate. Although it is difficult to predict exactly which conditions will lead to a disease in a particular individual, scientists have been able to develop a list of factors closely associated with particular diseases in large population groups. These factors are called risks. Saturated fat increases the risk of coronary heart disease independent of other factors. High dietary cholesterol also contributes to the development of atherosclerosis and increased coronary heart disease risk in the population, but to a lesser extent. Table 3–4 shows the maximum recommended grams of fat an individual should consume at selected kilocalorie levels.

Monounsaturated Fats

Recently, the health benefits of monounsaturated fatty acids have been much in the news. The Committee on Diet and Health of the National Research Council recommends that the average American *increase* his or her intake of monounsaturated fats. There is some evidence that individuals with a high intake of monounsaturated fats, a low intake of saturated fats, and a low total fat intake may have a decreased risk of colorectal cancer (National Research Council B, 1989).

Polyunsaturated Fats

The Committee on Diet and Health of the National Research Council does *not* recommend that the average American increase his or her intake of

TABLE 3-4 *Recommended Maximum Fat Intake at Selected Kilocalorie Levels*

Kilocalorie Level	Total Fat (grams)
1200	40
1500	50
1600	53
1800	60
2000	67
2200	73
2400	80
2500	83

polyunsaturated fat. At very high levels of polyunsaturated fat intake, animal studies consistently show an increase in colon and mammary cancers. Observations in humans have shown that a polyunsaturated fat intake of less than 10 percent of kilocalories does not increase the population's risk of cancer.

Body Fat

Both the amount of body fat and its location are related to health risk. Many experts feel that the ratio of body fat to total weight is more important than total weight. Healthy ranges for body fat are between 15 and 19 percent for men and between 18 and 22 percent for women. A high percentage of body fat has been associated with increased risk of disease, even when total body weight is normal. The location of excess body fat is also important. Excessive fat on the lower body, specifically on the hips and thighs, appears to be less dangerous than excessive fat on the abdomen and upper body, which is associated with a much higher risk of diseases such as cancer, heart disease, and diabetes. To assist in planning meals low in fat, the exchange lists in the next section may be used.

EXCHANGE LISTS

Exchange categories that include fat are the milk, meat, and fat lists. The amount of fat in one exchange of either meat or milk varies within the list. Some foods not on any of the exchange lists are also high in fat. Many of such foods may be found in tables like the Nutritive Values of Edible Parts of Food (see Appendix A).

Milk Exchange List

The fat content of milk varies according to which type is consumed. Table 3-5 shows the grams of fat in one milk exchange for each kind of milk. Whole milk and 2 percent milk contain saturated fat and cholesterol. Whole milk contains 48 percent fat, 2 percent milk contains 38 percent fat, and skimmed milk contains less than 1 percent fat. The protein, carbohydrate, vitamin, and mineral content of whole, 2 percent, and skimmed milk are comparable. Skimmed milk is thus a nutritional bargain.

TABLE 3–5 *Grams of Fat in One Milk Exchange*

Type	Fat (grams)
Whole milk	8
2% (low-fat)	5
Skimmed milk	Trace

Meat Exchange List

The meat exchange list is divided into three subgroups: one lean meat exchange contains 3 grams of fat; one medium-fat meat exchange contains 5 grams of fat; and one high-fat meat exchange contains 8 grams of fat. Table 3–6 lists selected food examples from each of these meat exchanges.

Many patients have misconceptions about meat. Some patients avoid all red meat because they believe that all red meat contains excessive fat. Many beef and pork products are not excessively high in fat. Figure 3–3 compares

TABLE 3–6 *Examples of Lean, Medium-Fat, and High-Fat Meat Exchanges*

Each of the following is one lean meat exchange and contains 3 grams of fat:		
Beef	USDA good or choice; round	1 ounce
Veal	Chop or roast	1 ounce
Poultry	Chicken (no skin)	1 ounce
Pork	Tenderloin	1 ounce
Fish	All fresh or frozen	1 ounce
	Tuna (water packed)	¼ cup
Cheese	Any cottage cheese	¼ cup
Other	Egg whites	3 whites
	95% fat-free lunch meat	1 ounce
	Egg substitute	¼ cup
Each of the following is one medium-fat meat exchange and contains 5 grams of fat:		
Beef	All ground beef	1 ounce
Pork	Chops	1 ounce
Poultry	Chicken (with skin)	1 ounce
Fish	Salmon (canned)	¼ cup
Cheese	Mozzarella, part skim	1 ounce
Other	86% fat-free lunch meat	1 ounce
	Egg (high in cholesterol)	1
Each of the following is one high-fat meat exchange and contains 8 grams of fat:		
Beef	USDA prime cuts; corned beef	1 ounce
Pork	Spare ribs, pork sausage	1 ounce
Fish	Any fried fish product	1 ounce
Cheese	American, cheddar	1 ounce
Other	Bologna	1 ounce

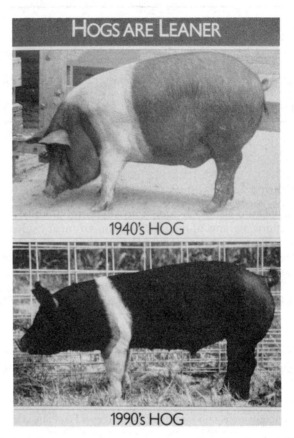

FIGURE 3–3. The fat content of hogs has decreased during the last 50 years. Consumers are increasingly demanding leaner red-meat products, and farmers are responding. (From the National Live Stock and Meat Board, 444 North Michigan Ave, Chicago, IL 60611, with permission.)

prized 1940 hogs with 1990 hogs, and Figure 3–4 compares 1940 steers with 1990 steers. In both figures, note how much leaner the 1990 animals appear than the 1940 animals. Many consumers are not aware of the lean cuts of beef or pork. On the other hand, not all fish and poultry items are lean meat exchanges.

Different methods of food preparation can greatly influence the fat content of these foods. Some patients are also under the misconception that if they eat only lean meats, they can eat as much as they like. This is not true because all meat contains fat. The total amount of meat any healthy individual should eat each day is between 6 and 7 ounces.

Meat exchanges are usually eaten in multiples of one. Table 3–7 totals the fat content of three meat exchanges. Three meat exchanges equals 3 ounces of cooked meat. In each example, the grams of fat in one meat exchange was multiplied by three. Typically, meats such as prime rib are eaten in large amounts (from 6-ounce to 16-ounce servings). Teaching patients meat portion sizes is usually indicated when the goal is to decrease a patient's fat intake.

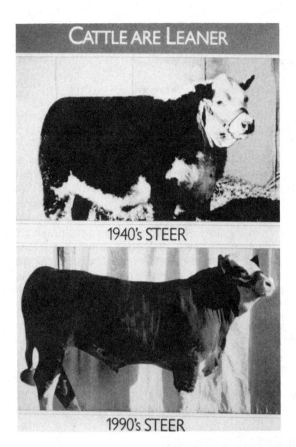

FIGURE 3–4. For beef, the ideal 1940 market animal was short-legged, short and deep in the body, and exhibited good evidence of body fat. By the 1980s and 1990s, improved breeding techniques and animal nutrition had resulted in a dramatic change in the characteristics of the typical beef animal. Muscle now replaces much of the fat in today's beef animal. (From the National Live Stock and Meat Board, 444 North Michigan Ave, Chicago, IL 60611, with permission.)

TABLE 3–7 *Total Fat in Three Meat Exchanges*

Meat (cut/kind)	Subgroup	Grams of Fat per Exchange	Grams of Fat per 3-Ounce Serving
Tuna, water pack	Lean	3	9
Hamburger patty, broiled*	Medium fat	5	15
Prime rib*	High fat	8	24

*About 4 ounces of raw meat.

Regardless of whether the meat is classified as a lean, medium-fat, or high-fat meat exchange, the grams of fat in each exchange was calculated based on the following assumptions:

- Visible fat on meat is not consumed.
- Meat is weighed after cooking.
- Meat is baked, boiled, broiled, grilled, or roasted (unless indicated otherwise).

New food labeling regulations became effective as of May, 1994. Regarding the fat content of meat, poultry, seafood, and game meats, two terms now have legal definitions: "lean" and "extra lean." The term "lean" can only be used on a meat, poultry, seafood, or game meat product if the product contains less than 10 grams of fat, less than 4 grams of saturated fat, and less than 95 milligrams of cholesterol per serving and 100 grams (3½ ounces). The legal term "lean" will thus equal the ADA exchange list definition for a lean meat exchange. The term "extra lean" can only be used if the product contains less than 5 grams of fat, less than 2 grams of saturated fat, and less than 95 milligrams of cholesterol per serving and per 100 grams (3½ ounces) (US Food and Drug Administration, 1992).

Fat Exchange List

Each fat exchange provides 5 grams of fat. The fat list is subdivided into two groups: unsaturated fats and saturated fats. Table 3–8 lists selected exchanges from each group. You probably would have classified butter and margarine as fats. Would you have thought of cream cheese, olives, or nuts as fat?

Additional Food Sources of Fat

As mentioned earlier, snack foods including crackers, cakes, pies, donuts, and cookies may be high in fat. When making food choices, you might check

---

TABLE 3–8 *Examples of Saturated and Monounsaturated or Polyunsaturated Fat Exchanges*

Each of the following is one fat exchange high in saturated fat and contains 5 grams of total fat:

Butter	1 teaspoon
Bacon	1 slice
Cream cheese	1 tablespoon

Each of the following is one fat exchange high in monounsaturated or polyunsaturated fat and contains 5 grams of fat:

Margarine	1 teaspoon
(Tub or stick listing safflower, corn, or sunflower oil as the first ingredient)	
Olives	5 small
Cashews	1 tablespoon
Peanuts	20 small or 10 large

the fat content in potato chips, gravies, cream sauces, and soups, and in combination foods such as pizza with sausage, tacos, and spaghetti. They may be high in fat. You may not be aware of this, but microwave popcorn is higher in fat than hot-air popped popcorn (without added fat).

You can select a low-fat meal at a fast-food restaurant. However, many of the specialty fast-food hamburgers are high in fat. A small hamburger is the best "burger" choice. A small side salad with low-fat dressing is a better low-fat choice than french fries. Skimmed milk is lower in fat than either a milk shake or whole milk. Consumers who desire low-fat foods need not avoid eating out, but they do need to make wise food choices.

Food labeling regulations spell out what terms may be used to describe the level of fat in a food and how they can be used. "Fat-free" on a food label means that the food contains no more than 0.5 grams of fat per serving. Synonyms for "free" include "without," "no," and "zero." All of these terms can legally be used on a food label only if the product contains no amount of—or only trivial or "physiologically inconsequential" amounts of—fat, saturated fat, and cholesterol.

"Low-fat" is legally defined as a food that contains no more than 3 grams of fat in a serving. "Low saturated fat" is legally defined as a food that contains no more than 1 gram of saturated fat per serving. "Low cholesterol" is defined as a food that contains less than 20 milligrams per serving. Synonyms for low include "little," "few," and "low source of." Additionally, serving sizes listed on food labels are standardized to make nutritional comparisons of similar products easier.

Summary

The group name for all fats is lipids. Lipids include true fats and oils and related fat-like compounds such as lipoids and sterols. Lipids are insoluble in water and greasy to the touch.

Hydrogen, oxygen, and carbon are the primary elements in fats. Gram for gram, fats contain over twice the kilocalories as carbohydrates because they contain less oxygen than carbohydrates. All fats contain fatty acids. The number of fatty acids in a fat determines whether it is a monoglyceride, a diglyceride, or a triglyceride. Most food fats and fat stored in the body are triglycerides. The length of a fatty acid chain determines how the body transports fat. The degree of hydrogen atom saturation, or the presence or lack of carbon-to-carbon double bonds in a fatty acid, make it either saturated or unsaturated.

Fats are labeled according to the amount and type of fatty acids they contain as saturated, unsaturated, monounsaturated, or polyunsaturated. Fats can also be classified as emulsified or nonemulsified, visible or invisible, and simple or compound. Fats serve many important functions both in our diets and in the human body.

Americans currently derive about 37 percent of their kilocalories from fat. Many experts feel this is excessive. Excess fats in our diets are related to cardiovascular disease, obesity, and some types of cancer. Cholesterol is a fat-like substance that is both present in food and produced by the human body. Many Americans would receive a health benefit by decreasing their cholesterol and saturated fat intake. The ADA exchanges that contain fat are the milk, meat, and fat lists. The current recommendation is that the fat content of the diet should not exceed 30 percent of kilocaloric intake, that less than 10 percent of kilocalories should be provided from saturated fats, and that dietary cholesterol should be less than 300 milligrams per day.

A case study and a sample plan of care appear below. Both are designed to show you how the information you have studied in this chapter can be used in nursing practice.

CASE STUDY 3–1

Mr. D. had his cholesterol level analyzed during a community screening program. Results from this program were mailed to his family physician. The nurse employed in the office of Mr. D.'s doctor is responsible for the following:

1. Scheduling the patient for follow-up with the physician.
2. Developing a nursing care plan that addresses the patient's nursing problem to complement the medical diagnosis.

Mike Rod, the nurse, scheduled the appointment. Mr. D. was instructed by the nurse to write down all food he consumed for 1 day prior to the appointment. The patient was advised to choose a typical day to record his food intake, so as to provide a more accurate analysis of his usual diet. Mr. D. arrived as scheduled on the appropriate day and handed his food record to the nurse for review. Mike calculated the grams of fat in Mr. D.'s food record, based on a combination of ADA exchanges and a table of food composition similar to the table in the appendix of this text (see Appendix A). Mr. D.'s food record and Mike's calculations follow:

11:00 AM Restaurant

Food	*Fat* (grams)
Salad bar:	
Assorted vegetables and lettuce	0
4 teaspoons blue cheese dressing	10 (2 fats)
1 ounce shredded cheese	7 (1 high-fat meat)
1 ounce diced ham	3 (1 lean meat)
½ cup potato salad	10*
Dinner roll	0
1 tsp butter	5 (1 fat)
1 cup clam chowder	7*

7:00 PM Restaurant

4 ounce hamburger, cooked weight	20 (4 medium-fat meats)
1 ounce cheese	8 (1 high-fat meat)
1 tablespoon mayonnaise	15 (3 fat)
Bun	0
6 onion rings	15*
Tossed salad	0
4 teaspoons blue cheese dressing	10 (2 fats)

*Values obtained from a table of food composition.

11:00 PM Home

1 cup 2% milk	5 (1 2% milk)
1 orange	0
	115 grams of fat

The physician has just seen the patient, reviewed Mr. D.'s food record and Mike's calculations, and determined that the patient's elevated cholesterol level is secondary to his dietary habits. Mr. D.'s cholesterol level was 225 milligrams per deciliter, he weighed 135 pounds, and is 5 feet 6 inches tall. Mr. D. stated, "I cannot understand why my cholesterol is elevated. My weight is stable. I always select the salad bar for lunch, avoid sweets, and drink low-fat milk." See Charting Tip 3–1.

NURSING CARE PLAN FOR MR. D.

Assessment
Subjective:
  Admitted knowledge deficit
  Food record for 1 day contained 115 grams of fat
Objective:
  Cholesterol level: 225 milligrams per deciliter
  Height: 5 feet 6 inches
  Weight: 135 pounds

Nursing Diagnosis
  Nutrition, altered: more than body requirements related to knowledge deficit as evidenced by admitted lack of understanding and a cholesterol level of 225 milligrams per deciliter.

Desired Outcome/Evaluation Criteria:
  1. Cholesterol level of < 200 milligrams per deciliter in 3 months (*date*).
  2. Patient will decrease his total fat intake by at least 35 grams per day as evidenced by repeated food record data over the next 3 months (*date*).
  3. Patient will decrease his visible fat intake.

Nursing Actions:
  1. Remind the patient to have his serum cholesterol level checked in 6 weeks per standing physician's order (*date*) and complete a 1-day food diary just prior to having the blood sample drawn.
  2. Remind the patient to complete a 3-day* food record just prior to having his blood sample drawn. Review patient's food records with him at 6-week intervals.
  _____ (*date*) _____ (*date*) _____ (*date*)
  3. Review visible dietary sources of fat with the patient; concentrate on blue cheese dressing, butter, and mayonnaise. Suggest alternatives to using visible fats. Review the diet selected by the physician with the patient. Completed _____ (*date*). Specific diets used to treat elevated cholesterol can be found in the chapter on cardiovascular disease.
  4. Tell patient to call the nurse if he is having trouble interpeting dietary instructions at home.

Rationale

1. Individuals with a cholesterol level <200 milligrams per deciliter are at a lower risk of cardiovascular disease.
2. The keeping of food records will remind the patient of the importance of decreasing his fat intake.
3. It is prudent to eliminate visible fats first from an individual's diet as they are easily identifiable.
4. Offer the patient support between visits.

STUDY AIDS

Chapter Review Questions

1. When _____ and fatty acids are joined, a fat is formed.
   a. Glycerol
   b. Glycogen
   c. Linoleic acid
   d. Triglyceride

2. The body is able to store _____ in unlimited amounts.
   a. Dextrose
   b. Glycogen
   c. Fat
   d. Protein

3. The most common from of fat found in both the body and food is:
   a. Monoglycerides
   b. Diglycerides
   c. Triglycerides
   d. Cholesterol

4. The manufacturing process that makes unsaturated fats more stable is called:
   a. Hydrogenation
   b. Emulsification
   c. Modification
   d. Saturation

5. Polyunsaturated fats are:
   a. Solid at room temperature
   b. Unlikely to become rancid
   c. Primarily of animal origin
   d. Composed of many double bonds

6. According to the Committee on Diet and Health, the average American would benefit by increasing his or her intake of which of the following fats?
   a. Corn oil
   b. Olive oil
   c. Safflower oil
   d. Lard

7. Recent estimates are that Americans derive _____ percent of their kilocaloric intake from fat.
   a. 25
   b. 30
   c. 37
   d. 46

8. One ounce of cheddar cheese contains 9 grams of fat and 115 kilocalories. What percent of kilocalories come from fat?
   a. 9
   b. 18
   c. 40
   d. 70

9. Please identify the following current recommendation of the Food and Nutrition Board of the National Research Council:
   a. Cholesterol intake should not exceed 500 milligrams per day.

    b. The fat content of the diet should not exceed 10 percent total kilocalories.

    c. All forms of dietary fat should be avoided.

    d. Ten percent or less of total kilocalories should be provided from saturated fat.

10. Which of the following exchange group(s) contain(s) significant amounts of fat?
    a. Skimmed milk
    b. Starch
    c. Meat
    d. Fruits

NCLEX-Style Quiz

Situation One

Mrs. S., 50 years old, has a cholesterol level of 233 milligrams per deciliter. She weighs 125 pounds and is 5 feet 5 inches tall. The dietitian has approximated her body fat content to be 35 percent.

1. When taking a nursing history, the nurse asks Mrs. S. if she eats any foods which may be related to her elevated cholesterol level. Which of the following groups of foods are most related to an elevated cholesterol level?
    a. Vegetable oils such as corn, cottonseed, and soybean
    b. Fruits and vegetables
    c. Starches such as bread, potatoes, rice, and pasta
    d. Animal fats such as butter, meats, lard, and bacon

2. Mrs. S.'s body fat content:
    a. Is not a problem because her weight is within the healthy body weight range
    b. Places her at a health risk
    c. Is within normal limits
    d. Indicates she is eating too much fat

Situation Two

3. Mr. B. is a new patient whose cholesterol level is 215 milligrams per deciliter. Mr. B.'s cholesterol level:
    a. Places him in the low-risk category
    b. Places him in the borderline to high-risk category
    c. Places him in the high-risk category
    d. Is sufficiently elevated enough for him to be a good candidate for drug therapy.

Situation Three

4. When Mrs. L. describes her regular intake of foods, you observe that her diet is especially low in monounsaturated fats. Which of the following oils would you recommend be used in place of corn oil?
    a. Safflower
    b. Soybean
    c. Canola
    d. Cottonseed

CHARTING TIPS 3–1

The following information should be charted:

✓ Specific fatty foods the patient is having trouble avoiding
✓ Statements the patient makes about knowledge deficits
✓ Height, weight, cholesterol levels, and percent body fat (if known)
✓ Recent behavioral changes the patient has made toward decreasing the fat content of his or her diet (to provide positive reinforcement)

CLINICAL CALCULATION 3-1:

Percent of Kilocalories from Fat

The following formula can be used to determine the percentage of kilocalories from fat in many packaged foods:

$$\frac{\text{Kilocalories from fat per serving}}{\text{Kilocalories per serving}} \times 100 = \%\ \text{kilocalories from fat}$$

Example: kilocalories from fat = 30
kilocalories per serving = 90

$$\frac{30}{90} = 0.33 \times 100 = 33\% \text{ kilocalories from fat}$$

---

*Food labeling regulations will require manufacturers to list both the number of kilocalories in a serving and the number of kilocalories from fat.

BIBLIOGRAPHY

American Dietetic and Diabetic Associations: Exchange Lists for Meal Planning, American Dietetic Association, Chicago, 1986.

American Institute for Cancer Research: Dietary Guidelines to Lower Cancer Risk. American Cancer Society, Washington, DC, 1990.

American Heart Association: Kitchen Cuisine. 1992.

Bennion, M: Introductory Foods, ed 7. Macmillan, New York, 1980.

Collins, FD, et al: Plasma lipids in human linoleic acid deficiency. Nutrition and Metabolism 13:150, 1971.

Consensus Conference: Lowering blood cholesterol to prevent disease. JAMA 253:2080, 1985.

Feldman, CB: Essentials of Clinical Nutrition. FA Davis, Philadelphia, 1988.

National Research Council: Diet and Health. National Academy Press, Washington, DC, 1989.

National Research Council: Recommended Dietary Allowances, National Academy Press, Washington, DC, 1989.

Neuringer, M and Connor, WE: n-3 Fatty acids in the brain and retina: Evidence for their essentiality. Nutr Rev 44:285, 1986

Report of the Expert Panel on Detection, Evaluation, and Treatment of High Blood Cholesterol in Adults: Cholesterol Education Program. National Heart, Lung, and Blood Institute, National Institutes of Health, Bethesda, 1987.

Scheve, LG: Elements of Biochemistry. Allyn & Bacon, Boston 1984.

Schmitz, D: Food News Blues. Hippocrates, Sausalito, CA, 1991.

Schrott, HG: Clinical considerations in managing hyperlipidemia. Journal of Osteopathic Medicine (Suppl 3) 3:16, 1989.

Tri-County Health Department: Market to Market. The American Heart Association of Michigan, Lathrop Village, 1989.

US Department of Health and Human Services: The Surgeon General's Report on Nutrition and Health. DHHS Publication No. (PHS) 88–55 210, Washington, DC, 1988.

US Food and Drug Administration (FDA): Backgrounder. BG 92-4. December 10, 1992.

Wiese, HF, Hansen, AE, and Adam, DJD: Essential fatty acids in infant nutrition. J Nutr 58:345, 1958.

Chapter Four

Protein

Chapter Outline

Key Terms

As a study aid, each key term is followed by the page number where the term is defined in the chapter. Terms that appear in **boldface** or <u>underscored</u> in the chapter text are located in the glossary.

Protein

Learning Objectives

After completing this chapter the student should be able to:

1. Discuss the functions of protein in the human body in health and in illness.
2. Explain the difference between complete and incomplete proteins and give examples of food sources of each.
3. Define anabolism and catabolism, and list possible anabolic and catabolic conditions.
4. List the grams of protein in each exchange list containing significant amounts of protein.
5. Calculate the protein allowance for a healthy adult when given the person's healthy body weight.
6. Design a daily meal plan containing adequate protein intake for a healthy adult.

*T*he importance of protein in nutrition and health was first emphasized by an ancient Greek who called this nutrient "proteos," meaning primary, or taking first place. Protein is essential for body growth and maintenance. If kilocalorie need is inadequate to support fuel requirements, dietary protein may be used for energy rather than for tissue growth and maintenance. If protein is eaten in excess it can contribute to body fat stores.

Proteins are the building blocks of blood and bone and all other tissues. Protein is a structural part of every cell. In fact, almost half the dry weight of the cells is protein. It is second only to water in amounts present in the body. A description of some of the tissues comprised of protein appears in Clinical Application 4–1.

COMPOSITION OF PROTEINS

Proteins, composed of carbon, hydrogen, oxygen, and nitrogen, make up the greater part of plant and animal tissue. Phosphorus, sulfur, iron, and iodine often form part of the protein molecule, but nitrogen is the element that distinguishes proteins from carbohydrates and fats. Proteins are made up of smaller building blocks called amino acids.

CLINICAL APPLICATION 4–1
Examples of Protein in the Human Body

Most of the cells of the body require periodic maintenance or replacement. Even bone tissue, which you might think of as fixed, undergoes change in the healthy adult. However, the body cannot repair tooth decay; hence the need for dental fillings.

Scar Tissue. The healing of even the simplest wound requires proteins. Many blood clotting factors, such as the protein prothrombin, quickly go into action to form a blood clot. The fibrin threads that form the mesh to hold the scar tissue in place are composed of protein. The white blood cells which dispose of the waste products of the injury and the healing process are also proteins.

Hair Growth. Hair cells are dead. This is the reason haircuts do not hurt. The new growth of hair does require protein building blocks, however. One sign of malnutrition is hair that can be easily and painlessly plucked.

Blood Albumin. Albumin is a transport protein. A transport protein functions as a vehicle taking other nutrients or elements to where they are needed. Albumin plays a significant role in medication absorption and metabolism (see Chapter 14). In addition to transporting substances to all the cells of the body, albumin also has functions relating to water balance (see Chapter 9).

Hemoglobin. Another transport protein, hemoglobin, is the oxygen-carrying part of the red blood cell. The *globin* part of this molecule is a simple protein.

Amino Acids

The chemical elements carbon, hydrogen, oxygen, and nitrogen combine in a specific arrangement to form **amino acids.** The amino acids, in turn, are linked in an exact order to make a particular protein. Amino acids are linked together by **peptide bonds.** A chain of two or more amino acids joined together by peptide bonds is called a **polypeptide.** A single protein may consist of a polypeptide of fifty to thousands of amino acids. Scientists have estimated that the body contains up to 50,000 different proteins, of which only about 1000 have been identified. Thus, we begin to see that an enormous variety of combinations are possible.

To visualize these combinations, take a moment to examine Figure 4–1, a schematic representation of the beef insulin molecule. It might also help to think of the elements as the letters of the alphabet, and amino acids as words. There are countless ways to make words, or amino acids, from the 26 letters (the elements). Words put into a certain order make up sentences that have a specific and unique meaning. In this comparison, a sentence is a protein. Each protein has a specific and unique sequence of amino acids. To complete the analogy of language to anatomy, see Table 4–1.

Primitive people sometimes drank the blood of an admired animal or brave enemy in the hope of gaining the qualities of that particular creature. In a way we do become what we eat. This is not literally true, of course: We do not turn into a steer or a hog after eating beef or pork. Instead, the animal proteins are disassembled in the digestive process into the component amino acids and then reassembled to form human proteins (see Chapter 5).

Precision is necessary to manufacture proteins. A slight error in the construction of a protein, such as occurs in sickle cell disease, can have severe consequences. Sickle cell disease is detailed in Clinical Application 4–2.

Twenty-four amino acids have been identified as being important in the body's metabolism. These amino acids are classified as either essential or nonessential.

Essential Amino Acids

As with other nutrients, the body's inability to construct an amino acid is the basis for classifying an amino acid as essential. Over 30 years ago Rose identified the amino acids found in proteins as nutritionally essential or nutritionally nonessential (Rose, 1957; Hunt and Groff, 1990). Histidine has more recently been added to the list of essential amino acids for both children and adults.

Other amino acids are conditionally essential or can become acquired essential depending on biochemical needs of the body. Table 4–2 lists the amino acids that have been classified as essential, conditionally and/or acquired essential, and nonessential. Acquired essential amino acids become essential in premature infants, in states of genetic and acquired disorders, and/or during severe stress. A very high intake of amino acids can cause other amino acids to become essential.

All essential amino acids must be available in the body simultaneously and in sufficient quantity for synthesis of body proteins. These amino acids may come from food or from the body's own cells as they age and are broken down and replaced.

Amino acid— Organic compounds that are the building blocks of protein; and products of protein digestion.

Peptide bond— Chemical bond that links two amino acids in a protein molecule.

Polypeptide— Chain of amino acids linked by peptide bonds that form proteins.

Essential amino acid—Nine amino acids that cannot be manufactured by the human body; must be obtained from food or artificial feeding.

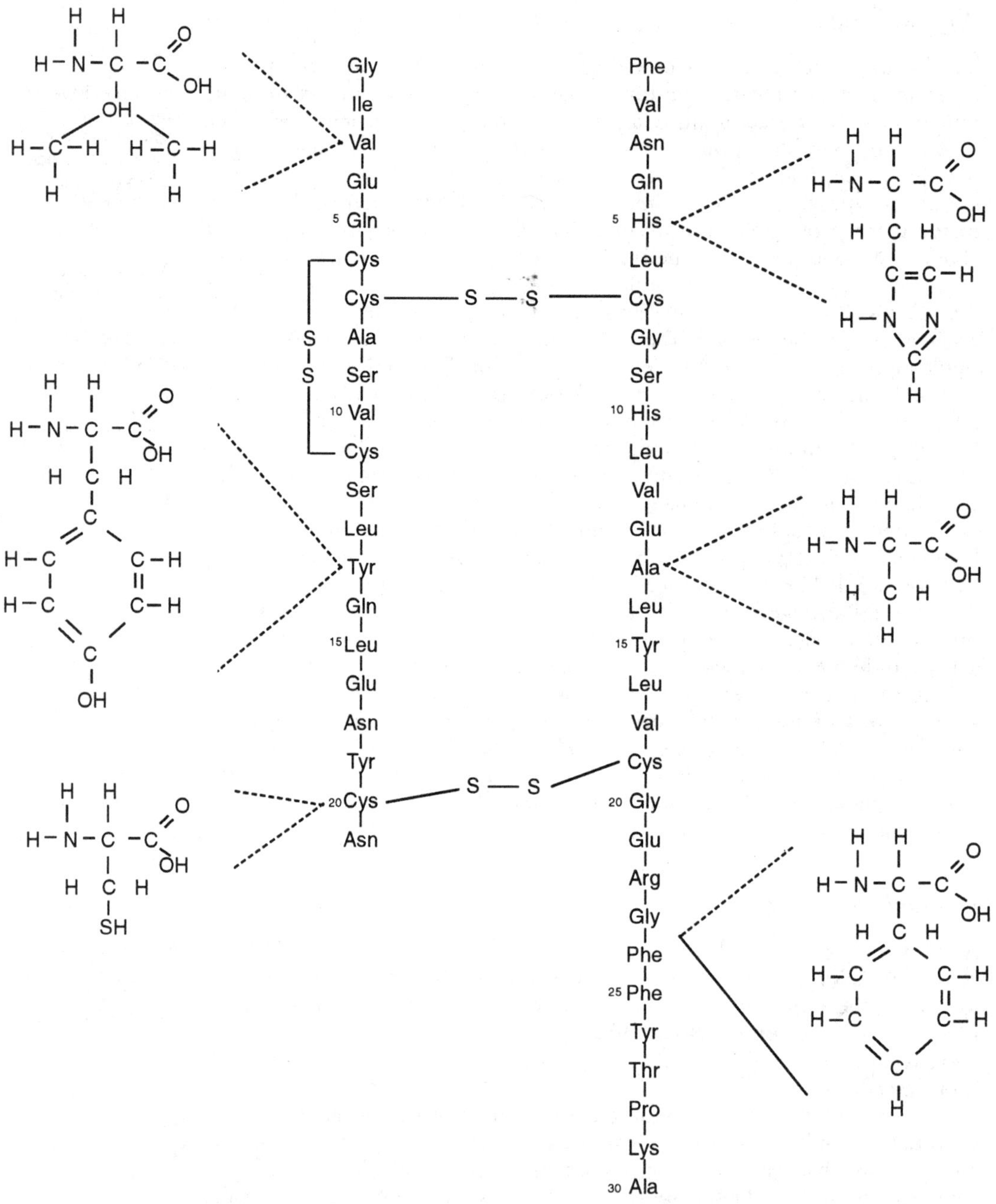

FIGURE 4–1. Beef insulin molecule. The long vertical chains represent the amino acids in the correct order for the beef insulin molecule. The boxes are enlargements of several amino acids showing the elements in their molecular structure. (From John W. Hole, Jr., HUMAN ANATOMY AND PHYSIOLOGY, 5th ed. Copyright © 1990 Wm. C. Brown Publishers, Dubuque, Iowa. All Rights Reserved. Reprinted by permission.)

TABLE 4–1 *Comparison of Language and Anatomy*

Component of Language	Component of Anatomy
Letters	Elements such as carbon, hydrogen, oxygen, nitrogen, sometimes sulfur
Word	Amino acid
Sentence	Protein
Paragraph	Cell
Chapter	Tissue
Book	Organ
Books on a given subject	System
Library	Human body

CLINICAL APPLICATION 4–2
Sickle Cell Disease

Normal hemoglobin is an important blood protein consisting of 146 amino acids combined in a specific order. In the hemoglobin of a person with sickle cell disease, one amino acid, glutamine, has been replaced by valine at one specific location on the protein chain.

Sickle cell disease is a hereditary condition in which the red blood cells become rigid and crescent-shaped. These abnormal cells tend to clump together and block small blood vessels in many different organs. In sickle cell disease the body is 99.3 percent correct in manufacturing the red blood cell. However, death results from the 0.7 percent error. No cure is known, and most patients die by the age of 50.

TABLE 4–2 *Essential, Conditionally and/or Acquired Essential, and Nonessential Amino Acids*

Essential	Conditionally Essential and/or Acquired Essential	Nonessential
Lysine	Cysteine*	Alanine
Threonine	Tyrosine	Glutamic acid
Histidine	Arginine	Aspartic acid
Isoleucine	Citrulline†	Glycine
Leucine	Taurine‡	Serine
Methionine	Carnitine§	Proline
Phenylalanine		Glutamine
Tryptophan		Asparagine
Valine		

*Also called cystine.

†Not used in protein synthesis but critical in the urea cycle.

‡Not used in protein synthesis but essential in retinal functioning, particularly in young children.

§In newborns, can enhance the use of fat as an energy source; can be made from lysine and methionine in adults.

Nonessential amino acid—Any amino acid that can be synthesized by the body.

Nonessential Amino Acids

Nonessential amino acids, according to the classic definition, are those which the body can build in suitable quantities to meet its needs. Often they are derived from other amino acids. Nonessential amino acids are necessary for good health but under normal conditions, adults do not have to eat them. One nonessential amino acid, aspartic acid, is combined with phenylalanine to make aspartame, a sugar substitute.

FUNCTIONS IN THE BODY

There are five major functions of protein in the body. Protein is required for maintenance and growth, for the regulation of body processes, for the development of immunity, for energy in some circumstances, and for proper water balance. Table 4–3 lists these functions and one example of each.

Maintenance and Growth

Because protein is a part of every cell (half the dry weight), adults as well as growing children require adequate protein intake. As cells of the body wear out, they must be replaced.

Anabolism versus Catabolism

Anabolism—The building up of body compounds or tissues by the synthesis of more complex substances from simpler ones; the constructive phase of metabolism.

Two terms that refer to the building up or the breaking down of body tissues are anabolism and catabolism. **Anabolism** is the building up of tissues as in growth or healing. **Catabolism** is the breaking down of tissues into simpler substances that the body can use or eliminate. Both of these processes are going on simultaneously in the body. For example, tissue proteins are constantly being broken down into amino acids, which are then reused for building new tissue and repairing old tissue. However, anabolism and catabolism are not always in balance. At times, one process may dominate the other.

Nitrogen Balance

Catabolism—The breaking down of body compounds or tissues into simpler substances; the destructive phase of metabolism.

Foods containing protein are the body's only external source of nitrogen. Nitrogen is excreted in the urine, feces, and sweat, and is sometimes lost

---

TABLE 4–3 *Functions of Protein in the Body, with Examples*

Function	Example
Maintenance and growth	Hair growth
Regulation of body processes	Glucagon (actions opposite those of insulin)
Immunity	Antibodies against measles
Energy source	If adequate carbohydrate and fat are lacking
Contribution to fluid balance	Albumin draws fluid back into capillaries from between the cells

through bleeding or vomiting. A person is in *nitrogen equilibrium* when the amount of nitrogen eaten is equal to the amount excreted. (See Clinical Calculation 4–1.) A healthy adult at a stable body weight is usually in nitrogen equilibrium. Under certain circumstances, however, nitrogen balance may be either positive or negative.

POSITIVE NITROGEN BALANCE   Positive nitrogen balance exists when a person consumes more nitrogen than is excreted. In other words, the body is building more tissue than it is breaking down. This finding is desirable during periods of growth such as infancy, childhood, adolescence, and pregnancy.

NEGATIVE NITROGEN BALANCE   Negative nitrogen balance exists when a person consumes less nitrogen than is excreted. Here, the person is receiving insufficient protein, and the body is breaking down more tissue than it is building. Situations marked by negative nitrogen balance include undernutrition, illness, and trauma.

Although skipping food for one day will undoubtedly create negative nitrogen balance, noticeable physical signs are not likely to occur. However, prolonged negative nitrogen balance can adversely affect the growth rate in children (Fig. 4–2).

Regulation of Body Processes

Protein contributes to the regulation of body processes. It is necessary for the manufacture of hormones, enzymes, and the nucleus of every cell. Table 4–4 lists the three kinds of regulators and gives examples of each.

Hormones

Hormones are chemicals secreted by various organs to regulate body processes. Hormones are secreted directly into the bloodstream rather than within an organ. Insulin and glucagon are two important protein hormones that help to control glucose metabolism (see Chapter 16).

Enzymes

The body also makes specialized proteins called **enzymes.** Enzymes are crucial to many body processes, such as digestion. The breakdown of foods in the stomach and small intestine involves enzymes, which act as **catalysts.** Catalysts influence the speed at which a chemical reaction takes place, but do not actually enter into the reaction. Without the aid of enzymes, many of the processes in the body would proceed too slowly to be effective.

Think of an enzyme as a dating service. Just as a dating service provides an opportunity for two people to meet and react in some fashion with each other, an enzyme provides a place (its surface) for two substances to meet and react with each other. If it were not for enzymes, these two substances would be less likely to encounter one another, and basic body functioning would be impossible.

In no way are enzymes optional equipment. Lack of a specific enzyme can have devastating effects on health, even on life itself. As an example, a disease called phenylketonuria is discussed in Clinical Application 4–3.

Nitrogen balance—The difference between the amount of nitrogen ingested and that excreted each day; the intake of more protein than is used produces positive nitrogen balance, and the intake of less protein produces negative nitrogen balance.

Enzyme—Complex protein produced by living cells that acts as a catalyst.

Catalyst—Substance that speeds a chemical reaction without entering into, or being changed by, the reaction.

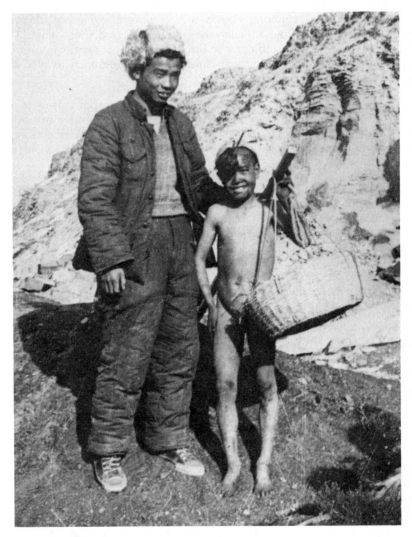

FIGURE 4–2. Two Asian boys of the same age. The boy on the right worked in a mine and ate protein-poor food. The boy on the left lived at a boarding school for 4 years where he received better food. (Courtesy of the Food and Agriculture Organization of the United Nations, Rome, Italy.)

TABLE 4–4 *Examples of Regulators of Body Processes*

Regulator	Examples
Hormones	Insulin, thyroid hormone
Enzymes	Lactase, Sucrase
Nucleoproteins	DNA, RNA

CLINICAL APPLICATION 4-3
Phenylketonuria

One of the enzymes necessary for the digestion of protein is phenylalanine hydroxylase. This enzyme is needed for the conversion of the essential amino acid phenylalanine to the amino acid tyrosine. If the enzyme is missing from the body or is defective, a disease called phenylketonuria (PKU) is the result. An infant with PKU cannot metabolize phenylalanine, which accumulates in the blood and eventually becomes toxic enough to cause mental retardation. As a preventive measure, infants are tested for phenylketonuria shortly after birth. Once diagnosed, the devastating effects of this enzyme deficiency can be avoided by strict regulation of the proteins the infant consumes.

Nucleoproteins

Nucleoproteins are the third example of regulatory proteins. The center or nucleus of every cell contains nucleoproteins. Their function is to direct the maintenance and reproduction of the cell. Two well-known nucleoproteins are DNA and RNA.

DNA **Deoxyribonucleic acid** (DNA) is present in all body cells of every species. It is the basic component of the **genes,** which serve as patterns to guide reproduction.

RNA **Ribonucleic acid** (RNA) is another nucleoprotein present in all living cells. It controls the manufacturing of cellular protein. Each of the common amino acids has its own RNA to transport it to the correct location in the protein chain.

Deoxyribonucleic acid (DNA)
Gene—Basic unit of heredity occupying specific locations on the chromosome.

Ribonucleic acid (RNA)—A substance which controls protein synthesis in all living cells.

Immunity

A specific protein called an **antibody** is produced in the body in response to the presence of a foreign substance or a substance that the body senses to be foreign. Antibodies provide **immunity** to certain diseases and other toxic conditions. A specific antibody is created for each foreign substance. Thus, if a person is exposed to a certain kind of disease-producing bacteria, the body creates an antibody that will only neutralize the harmful effects of that particular species or strain of bacteria. For some diseases, once the body has produced antibodies, it can respond quickly to another attack, making the individual immune. All antibodies belong to a group of blood proteins called immunoglobulins.

Antibody—A specific protein developed in the body in response to a substance that the body senses to be foreign.

Energy Source

Protein is a backup energy source. When the body has insufficient carbohydrate for energy, it will obtain energy from its own tissues. That is, the body converts its own muscle protein into energy. To spare protein for tissue building, adequate carbohydrate intake is necessary. The amount of energy obtained from a gram of protein is the same as the amount obtained from a gram of carbohydrate, 4 kilocalories.

CLASSIFICATION OF FOOD PROTEIN

Very few foods contain solely protein. Most foods embody various combinations of protein, fat, and carbohydrate. Nevertheless, some foods are better sources of protein than others.

Protein foods are classified according to the number and kinds of amino acids they contain. **Complete proteins** are foods that supply all eight essential amino acids in sufficient quantity to maintain tissue and support growth. **Incomplete proteins** lack one or more of the essential amino acids.

Complete protein—Protein containing all eight (nine for infants) essential amino acids that humans need; usually found in animal sources such as milk, meat, eggs, and fish.

Complete Protein

With few exceptions, single foods containing complete protein come from animal sources such as meat, poultry, fish, eggs, and cheese. Gelatin is an animal protein, but it is missing the essential amino acid tryptophan. Therefore gelatin is an incomplete protein.

Incomplete protein—Protein lacking one or more of the essential amino acids that humans need; usually found in plant sources such as grains and vegetables

Sources of Complete Protein

Both meat and milk products are good sources of complete protein. An adult following the Food Pyramid would consume two or three servings of meat, poultry, fish, or eggs daily. Two or three ounces of meat, poultry, or fish constitute a serving.

The recommendation from the Food Pyramid is that an adult consume two to three servings of milk, yogurt, or cheese every day. A serving of milk or yogurt is one cup. The amount of cheese constituting a serving varies with the type of cheese. Notice that the Food Pyramid categorizes cheese with milk, whereas the Exchange Group system places it with meat. (See Appendix H.)

Exchange Groups of Complete Protein

Foods in the milk and meat exchanges usually are comprised of complete protein. Each exchange of meat contains 7 grams of protein regardless of the amount of fat. (Review Table 3–6 or see the Exchange Lists in Appendix H.) Notice that not all beef is high in fat and not all fish or poultry is low in fat. To illustrate portion sizes, Figure 4–3 shows samples of two foods equal to 3 medium-fat meat exchanges.

Each milk exchange furnishes 8 grams of protein. Examples of one milk exchange are 1 cup of milk, buttermilk, or yogurt, ½ cup of canned evaporated milk, or ⅓ cup of dry skim milk. All of these milk products offer equal protein nutrition, but all are not nutritionally equivalent because of their fat content.

Incomplete Protein

Plant foods lack sufficient amounts of one or more of the essential amino acids. Thus, the protein they contain is incomplete.

Sources of Incomplete Protein

Grains, vegetables, legumes, nuts, and seeds are valuable sources of incomplete protein. These foods should not be avoided because of the term

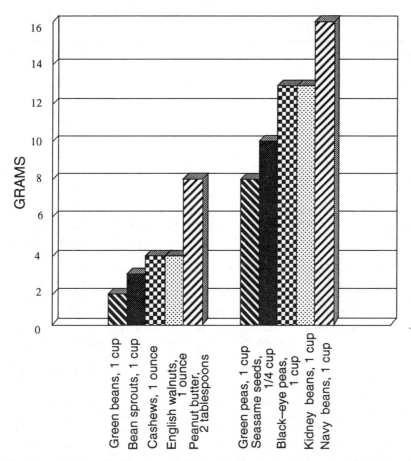

FIGURE 4–3. Protein content of selected food plants. Notice that all foods called peas or beans are not legumes. Green beans offer just 2 grams of protein compared to navy beans, which offer 16 grams. (Courtesy of Carroll A. Lutz.)

incomplete. First, they supplement the animal proteins in the diet. Second, a mixture of several different types of plant protein sources can yield all the essential amino acids. In this way, amino acids that are limited in one food will be supplied in one or more of the other foods.

Exchange Groups of Incomplete Protein

The vegetable and starch/bread exchanges are sources of incomplete protein. Some vegetables are closer in energy nutrient content to a slice of bread than to another vegetable. Vegetables such as corn, peas, and dried beans appear on the Starch/Bread Exchange List. Examples of one vegetable exchange are ½ cup of asparagus or ½ cup of chopped broccoli. A vegetable exchange contains 2 grams of protein. Examples of one exchange of starch/bread are ½ cup of corn, one small potato, ½ cup of winter squash, one slice of bread, a half a bagel or half an English muffin, or three square graham crackers. A starch/bread exchange contains 3 grams of protein. Table 4–5 lists the protein content of the exchanges that contain protein.

TABLE 4–5 *Grams of Protein per Exchange*

Exchange	Grams of Protein
Milk	8
Meat	7
Starch/Bread	3
Vegetable	2

Vegetarian Diets

For vegetarians or other individuals who limit their intake of animal foods, a group of plants classified as <u>legumes</u> are an important protein source. Legumes have roots containing nitrogen-fixing bacteria that "lock" nitrogen into the plant's structure, thus increasing its protein content. Legumes contain two to three times as much protein as most vegetables.

Commonly used legumes are peas, beans, lentils, and nuts. Not all peas and beans are legumes. Figure 4–4 compares the protein content of peas, beans, and nuts. Examples of one exchange of legumes are: ½ cup of peas, ⅓ cup of kidney beans, or ¼ cup of baked beans. On the exchange lists, these legumes are classified as starch/bread. Because many legumes are not only low in fat but also high in fiber, they are valued by health-conscious people.

Nuts appear on the fat exchange list. One tablespoon of cashews or 20 small peanuts is one exchange. Peanut butter is on the high-fat meat list; 1 tablespoon equals 1 exchange.

Because grains and legumes lack different amino acids, combining a grain with a legume will yield the equivalent of a complete protein. Some favorite combinations such as a peanut butter sandwich or baked beans with brown bread are grain-and-legume combinations. The Mexican burrito, a thin cornmeal bread filled with beans, is another example. Clinical Application 4–4 distinguishes various vegetarian diets.

Textured vegetable protein products from soybeans, peanuts, and cot-

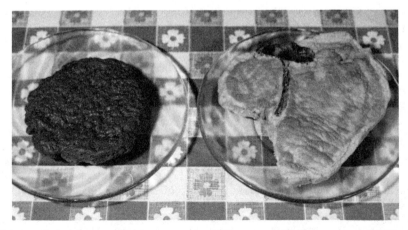

FIGURE 4–4. A 3-ounce hamburger patty or a 3-ounce pork chop each provide three medium-fat meat exchanges. (Courtesy of Mike Anderson, 808 S. Durand, Jackson, MI 49303.)

CLINICAL APPLICATION 4–4
Vegetarian Diets

Vegetarians practice different degrees of strictness. From most liberal to most restrictive, the vegetarian diets are ovolactovegetarian, lactovegetarian, ovovegetarian, and strict vegetarian or vegan. The prefixes ovo- and lacto- mean eggs and milk. So an ovovegetarian will consume eggs, a lactovegetarian milk, and an ovolactovegetarian both. A vegan eats no animal products.

FOODS PERMITTED IN THE VARIOUS VEGETARIAN DIETS

	Meat, Fish, Poultry	Dairy Products	Eggs
Ovolactovegetarian	No	Yes	Yes
Lactovegetarian	No	Yes	No
Ovovegetarian	No	No	Yes
Strict Vegetarian	No	No	No

The strict vegetarian diet requires careful planning. When foods are selected appropriately, often using vitamin and mineral supplements, adequate nutrition can be achieved.

tonseed can enhance the vegetarian diet. The protein is spun into fibers and flavored, colored, and shaped for use as a meat substitute.

Usually hospital dietitians can provide a balanced vegetarian diet. It is much better, when a nurse encounters a vegetarian patient, to inform the dietitian rather than expect the patient to select items from a general menu.

RECOMMENDED DIETARY ALLOWANCES

The RDA for adult protein is 0.8 grams of protein per kilogram of body weight. Clinical Calculation 4–2 shows you the procedure for calculating this amount based on a person's healthy body weight. Pregnancy and lactation increase the need for protein, as do periods of growth (Table 4–6).

During both pregnancy and breast-feeding the mother requires additional protein to build new tissue. The "eating for two" advice for pregnant women refers to the quality of foods eaten, not the quantity. Careful choices of foods will enhance the likelihood of a successful outcome. Infants up to the age of 6 months have the greatest protein requirement in proportion to their body size—2.2 grams per kilogram.

Overeating protein foods can adversely affect a person's health. Whole and 2 percent milk, medium- and high-fat meats derive more kilocalories from fat than from protein. High fat intake is associated with heart disease, certain cancers, and obesity, which itself is a risk factor for other pathology. The Committee on Diet and Health recommends that protein intake be no more than twice the RDA.

TABLE 4–6 *Protein RDA for Healthy Individuals of Various Ages*

Age in Years	Grams of Protein per Kilogram of Healthy Body Weight
0–½	2.2
½–1	1.6
1–3	1.2
4–6	1.1
7–14	1.0
15–18 (Males)	0.9
15–18 (Females)	0.8
19 and older	0.8
Pregnant	Nonpregnant RDA + 10 grams
Lactating	
First 6 months	Nonpregnant RDA + 15 grams
Remainder	Nonpregnant RDA + 12 grams

Wise selection and substitution of lower fat protein foods for medium- and high-fat ones would be prudent actions. Rinsing ground beef crumbles with warm water after cooking reduces fat content.

Aside from its association with fat, dietary protein itself taxes the body. Excreting excess nitrogen increases the kidneys' workload. Table 4–6 displays the protein RDA.

PROTEIN IN ANABOLISM AND CATABOLISM

Anabolism is the building of tissue; catabolism is the breaking down of tissue. Both processes are ongoing in everyone and usually balance one another. In certain conditions, some normal, some abnormal, either anabolism or catabolism becomes dominant.

Anabolism

The building of tissue occurs during pregnancy, lactation, childhood, and convalescence. Oftentimes during illness a person cannot eat a balanced diet. His or her body uses stored fat and sometimes protein for energy. After the acute phase of illness the body must replenish the protein stores, increasing the need for protein.

Catabolism

Tissue breakdown usually exceeds tissue build-up in severe illness. Persons who consume too little food, regardless of the reason, are likely to be breaking down more tissue than they are synthesizing.

Illness

There is an acute protein loss following surgery, burns, and fractures. An estimated 8 grams of protein is lost per day as a side effect of bed rest.

These patients may lose weight, become anemic, and be more susceptible to infections. The person who is well nourished before the surgery or injury is better prepared to weather the catabolism caused by surgery or injury.

Inadequate Energy Sources

Carbohydrate should be our chief source of energy, with fat as a readily available back-up source. Individuals who do not consume enough carbohydrates or fats for energy thereby force the body to use protein for energy.

Protein-Calorie Malnutrition (PCM)

Protein-calorie malnutrition (PCM)—Condition in which the person's diet lacks both protein and kilocalories.

Starvation in the classic sense means insufficient food due to famine. The term starvation is also used to describe individuals who receive inadequate food, sometimes for days, because of treatments or diagnostic tests. The alert nurse intervenes as patient advocate or coordinator of care in such cases to rearrange schedules or obtain food supplements.

Patients in institutions are susceptible to protein-calorie malnutrition (PCM) when they are unable to feed themselves. Individuals with wasting diseases may suffer from PCM. The following two conditions are types of PCM.

MARASMUS   In this condition the victim is not able to consume sufficient kilocalories or enough protein. Starvation is evident: the body is wasting away. Death occurs in 40 percent of the cases. Often the victim is a child in a developing country where food resources are scarce. Sometimes, however, a person with a debilitating disease, such as cancer or AIDS, develops marasmus.

KWASHIORKOR   This disorder occurs in a child shortly after weaning from breast milk, again frequently in a developing country. The victim lacks enough protein for growth. Clinically, he or she may appear chubby, but the reason is water retention related to protein deficiency. For this reason kwashiorkor is discussed in Chapter 9, which deals with water and bodily fluids.

CHOOSING PROTEIN FOODS WISELY

Producing meat is expensive. For every 5 pounds of vegetable or fish protein fed to livestock, only 1 pound of meat protein is produced.

For persons who wish to limit meat intake, Table 4–7 lists equivalent sources of protein. Prices of nationally advertised brands were employed, except for eggs, milk, and steak. Eggs, peanut butter, and tuna all provided 10 grams of protein for 12 cents. Water-packed tuna was the most nutrient dense, however, at 45 kilocalories. The most expensive source of protein was the frankfurter, both in dollars as well as kilocalories.

Knowledgeable shoppers read labels. Is the protein adequate? Is the fat excessive? Wise homemakers plan healthy meals, balancing high-fat foods with low-fat ones, offering a variety from all the food groups, and serving moderate portions of the foods closest to the top of the Food Pyramid.

TABLE 4–7 *Sources of 10 Grams of Protein with Kilocalories and Cost*

Food	Portion	Kilocalories	Cost/Amount	Cost/ Portion
Large eggs, poached	1.6 eggs	123	$0.89/dozen	$0.12
Peanut butter	2 tablespoons	190	$3.43/28 ounces	$0.12
Tuna, canned in water	1 ounce	45	$0.77/6.5 ounces	$0.12
Whole milk	1.25 cups	188	$2.35/gallon	$0.18
Whole wheat bread	3.3 slices	231	$1.39/20 ounces	$0.23
American cheese	1.6 oz.	168	$4.87/2 pounds	$0.24
Bean soup, condensed, prepared with water	1.25 cups	213	$0.52/11.5 ounces	$0.33
Boneless sirloin, broiled	1.2 oz.	72	$3.45/pound*	$0.35
Bologna, beef and pork, 1 ounce/ slice	2.9 slices	261	$2.49/pound	$0.45
Frankfurters, beef and pork, 8/ pound	1.6 franks	293	$2.39/pound	$0.48

*Shrinkage of 25% allowed for cooking

Summary

Protein is necessary for tissue maintenance and growth, for the regulation of body processes, for providing immunity, as a backup source of energy, and for water balance. Catabolism is the breaking down of tissues, and anabolism is the building up of tissues. These two processes go on in the body simultaneously. There are many situations in which the body may be in either a catabolic or anabolic state.

The element that distinguishes protein from carbohydrates and fats is nitrogen. The body combines carbon, hydrogen, oxygen, and nitrogen in certain ways to form amino acids, which then become the building blocks of various proteins. Eight essential amino acids must come from food.

Complete protein foods contain all eight essential amino acids in amounts sufficient to support growth. Complete protein foods usually come from animal sources, especially the meat and milk groups.

Incomplete protein foods are grains, vegetables, legumes, nuts, and seeds. If a person eats a grain product and a legume at the same meal, he or she is likely to receive all eight essential amino acids.

The normal healthy adult should consume 0.8 grams of protein per kilogram (2.2 pounds) of healthy body weight. A simple method of estimating protein intake uses the Exchange List system. Milk exchanges provide about 8 grams of protein, meat exchanges 7 grams, bread/starch exchanges 3 grams, and vegetable exchanges 2 grams.

A case study and a sample plan of care appear below. They are both designed to show you how the information you have studied in this chapter can be used in nursing practice.

CASE STUDY 4–1

Mrs. F. is a 72-year-old widow who eats independently in her family homestead. Her usual meals are tea and toast for breakfast, canned fruit and a muffin for lunch, and frozen potpie or canned hash for dinner. She complains that she has been having trouble chewing and has not been eating as much food as she usually does. She does not like milk.

NURSING CARE PLAN FOR MRS. F.

Assessment
Subjective
   Food deficit as evidenced by usual food intake information
   Has trouble chewing
   Does not like milk
Objective
   Height: 5 feet 4 inches
   Weight: 106 pounds
   Wrist circumference: 5.75 inches
   Examination of mouth: loose-fitting dentures

Nursing Diagnosis
Nutrition, altered: less than body requirements for protein and kilocalories, related to difficulty chewing, as evidenced by stated usual intake of 28–32 grams of protein per day and body weight 7 percent under minimum for weight and frame.

Desired Outcome/Evaluation Criteria
   1. Patient will gain 1 pound per week during next 2 weeks.
   2. Patient will increase her total protein intake by 9–13 grams per day.
   3. Patient will call for dental appointment within next 2 weeks.

Nursing Actions
   1. Encourage easily chewed sources of complete protein: cheese, eggs, ground meat, fish.
   2. Create a model meal plan with Mrs. F. using the Exchange System to count grams of protein.
   3. Explore sources of financial assistance for dental care if necessary.

Rationale
   1. Complete protein foods contain all eight essential amino acids necessary for tissue building.
   2. Mrs. F. requires 41 grams of protein for her healthy body weight. The meal plan she described in her history contains only 28 to 32 grams depending on dinner selection.
   3. Better fitting dentures would permit Mrs. F. a wider variety of foods.

STUDY AIDS

Chapter Review Questions

1. The special function of protein in the human body is to:
   a. Aid in the digestion and absorption of fats.
   b. Modify the passage time of selected medications.
   c. Provide energy.
   d. Serve as building materials for tissue repair.

2. The presence of which one of the following elements differentiates proteins from carbohydrates and fats?
   a. Carbon
   b. Hydrogen
   c. Nitrogen
   d. Oxygen

3. All proteins are composed of:
   a. Amino acids.
   b. Hormones.
   c. Immunoglobulins.
   d. Legumes.

4. Anabolism describes the process of:
   a. Building tissue.
   b. Destroying infected tissue.
   c. Losing weight due to disease.
   d. Providing immunity to specific diseases.

5. A catalyst is a substance that:
   a. Enters into a chemical reaction.
   b. Provides a safety value to prevent overreactions by certain chemicals.
   c. Serves as the clean-up crew for chemical reactions.
   d. Speeds up the rate at which a chemical reaction occurs.

6. Which of the following foods is a complete protein?
   a. Baked beans
   b. Broccoli
   c. Beef kabobs
   d. Bread sticks

7. If a person consumes ½ cup of orange juice, one banana, one English muffin, 2 teaspoons of margarine, and 1 cup of milk for breakfast, how many grams of protein does he or she receive?
   a. Nine
   b. Fourteen
   c. Nineteen
   d. Twenty-four

8. If a person had difficulty purchasing meat to serve every day, which of the following combinations of foods should the nurse suggest as offering the best source of protein?
   a. Applesauce and bran muffins
   b. Bean soup and rye bread
   c. Broccoli and French bread
   d. Carrot-and-raisin salad

9. How much protein should a normal healthy adult consume each day?
   a. 0.8 gram per kilogram of actual body weight
   b. 0.8 gram per kilogram of healthy body weight

c. 0.8 gram per pound of actual body weight

d. 0.8 gram per pound of healthy body weight

10. Which of the following persons would the nurse treat as being in a catabolic state?

a. Adolescent boy who is into body building

b. Lactating mother

c. Pregnant woman in the second trimester

d. Surgical patient, first day after a stomach resection

NCLEX-Style Quiz

Situation One

Mr. P., a 65-year-old widower of 6 months, has been referred to your home health agency for assistance in managing his nutritional intake. He has lost 10 pounds over the past 6 months, although a physical examination within the past month revealed no disease processes requiring treatment.

1. As the nurse assesses Mr. P., which of the following data would she gather first?

a. Availability of family members to assist Mr. P.

b. Blood protein levels analyzed during the recent physical examination

c. A description of the procedure Mr. P. uses to weigh himself

d. Twenty-four hour recall of Mr. P.'s food and fluid intake

2. In addition to a possible nursing diagnosis of dysfunctional grieving, which of the following nursing diagnoses is best supported by the data given above?

a. Nutrition, altered: less than body requirements

b. High risk for fluid volume deficit

c. Knowledge deficit related to nutritional needs

d. Self-care deficit in feeding

3. Which of the following plans would be most appropriate to increase Mr. P.'s protein consumption immediately?

a. Refer patient to nutrition education program.

b. Have Mr. P. apply for meals on wheels.

c. Recommend that Mr. P. supplement his meals with one of the milk-based instant breakfast products.

d. Suggest to Mr. P. that he sign up for cooking lessons at the local high school or community college.

4. Considering both the dysfunctional grieving and the nursing diagnosis you selected in item 2, which of the following actions should the nurse explore with Mr. P. in hopes of impacting both problems?

a. Becoming active in a church group which meets monthly

b. Moving into a daughter's home

c. Regularly obtaining a hot meal at a nearby senior nutrition site

d. Starting a walking program to serve as an appetite stimulant

5. Which of the following outcomes would indicate achievement of the nutritional objective for Mr. P.?

a. A gain in weight of 2 pounds in 2 weeks

b. An invitation to the nurse to join him for a dinner he has learned to cook

c. A report by Mr. P. that he is eating better

d. A visual inspection of Mr. P.'s refrigerator revealing fresh meat and milk products in abundance

CLINICAL CALCULATION 4–1

Nitrogen Balance Studies

To calculate an individual's nitrogen balance, the amount of nitrogen in the foods he or she consumes is compared with the amount of nitrogen excreted in the urine. (Other potential losses are estimated.) Protein is approximately 16 percent nitrogen, so to calculate the nitrogen content in the foods, the amount of protein consumed (in grams) is multiplied by 0.16. Thus, a person who ingests 50 grams of protein has a nitrogen intake of 8 grams. To be in nitrogen equilibrium, he or she would therefore be expected to excrete or lose 8 grams of nitrogen.

CLINICAL CALCULATION 4–2

RDA for Protein

To determine a person's daily protein allowance, first determine his or her healthy body weight, as explained in Chapter 1. Taking the body weight in pounds, convert the pounds to kilograms. There are 2.2 pounds per kilogram. Consider a 5-foot 4-inch woman, whose healthy body weight is 131 pounds.

$$\frac{\text{weight in pounds}}{2.2 \text{ pounds per kilogram}} = \text{weight in kilograms}$$

$$\frac{131 \text{ pounds}}{2.2 \text{ pounds per kilogram}} = 59.5 \text{ kilograms}$$

The adult RDA for protein is 0.8 gram of protein per kilogram of healthy body weight. So multiply the weight in kilograms by 0.8 gram per kilogram.

59.5 (weight in kilograms) × 0.8 (grams per kilogram) = 47.6 grams of protein daily

Thus the daily protein allowance for our sample woman is 47.6 grams.

BIBLIOGRAPHY

Brenner, BM, Meyer, TW, and Hostetter, TH: Dietary protein intake and the progressive nature of kidney disease: The role of hemodynamically mediated glomerular injury in the pathogenesis of progressive glomerular sclerosis in aging, renal ablation, and intrinsic renal disease. N Engl J Med 307:652, 1982.

Brown, JE: The Science of Human Nutrition. Harcourt Brace Jovanovich, San Diego, 1990.

Burtis, G, Davis, J, and Martin, S: Applied Nutrition and Diet Therapy. WB Saunders, Philadelphia, 1988.

Cella, JH and Watson, J.: Nurse's Manual of Laboratory Tests. FA Davis, Philadelphia, 1989.

Chandra, RK: Antibody formation in first and second generation offspring of nutritionally deprived rats. Science 190:289, 1975.

Chandra, RK, et al: Nutrition and immunocompetence of the elderly: Effects of short-term nutritional supplementation on cell-mediated immunity and lymphocyte subsets. Nutrition Research 2:223, 1982.

Eschleman, M: Introductory Nutrition and Diet Therapy, ed 2. JB Lippincott, Philadelphia, 1991.

Fischbach, FT: A Manual of Laboratory Diagnostic Tests, ed 3. JB Lippincott, Philadelphia, 1988.

Hamilton, EU, Whitney, EN and Segeo, FS: Nutrition Concepts and Controversies, ed 5. West Publishing, St Paul, 1991.

Hole, JW, Jr: Essentials of Human Anatomy and Physiology, ed 2. William C. Brown, Dubuque, IA, 1986.

Hui, YH: Human Nutrition and Diet Therapy. Wadsworth, Monterey, CA, 1983.

Hunt, TK: Nutritional requirements of repair. In Ballenger, WF, et al (eds): Manual of Surgical Nutrition. WB Saunders, Philadelphia, 1975.

Hunt, SM and Groff, JL: Advanced Nutrition and Human Metabolism. West Publishing Company, St Paul, 1990.

Krause, MV and Mahan, LK: Food, Nutrition, and Diet Therapy, ed 7. WB Saunders, Philadelphia, 1984.

Lehninger, AL: Biochemistry, ed 2. Worth, New York, 1981.

Love, JA and Pruska, KJ. Nutrient composition and sensory attributes of cooked ground beef: Effects of fat content cooking method and water rinsing. J Am Diet Assoc. 92(11):1367, 1992.

National Research Council: Recommended Dietary Allowances, ed 10. National Academy Press, Washington, DC, 1989.

National Research Council. Diet and Health. National Academy Press, Washington, DC, 1989.

Rose, WC: The amino acid requirement of adult man. Nutr Abst Rev 27:631–643, 1957.

Rosenfeld, A: The great protein hunt. Science 81:64, 1981.

Scanlon, VC and Sanders, T: Essentials of Anatomy and Physiology. FA Davis, Philadelphia, 1991.

Thomas, PR (ed): Improving Americans Diet & Health. National Academy Press, 1991.

Whitney, EB and Cataldo, CB: Understanding Normal and Clinical Nutrition, ed 3. West Publishing, St Paul, 1991.

Williams, SR: Nutrition and Diet Therapy, ed 6. CV Mosby, St Louis, 1989.

Chapter Outline

Overview of the Major Processes
Digestion
    Alimentary Canal
    Accessory Organs
    Digestive Action
    The Food Pathway
Absorption
    Small Intestine
    Large Intestine
    Elimination of Unabsorbed Material
    Factors Interfering with Absorption
    Food Allergies
Metabolism
    Catabolic Reactions
    Anabolic Reactions
Excretion of Waste Products
Summary
Case Study
Study Aids
    Chapter Review Questions
    NCLEX-Style Quiz
Clinical Application 5–1: Carbohydrate
Intolerances
Clinical Application 5–2: Surgical
Removal of All or Part of the Alimentary
Canal
Clinical Application 5–3: Inadequate
Absorption
Clinical Application 5–4: Lipid
Malabsorption

Key Terms

As a study aid, each key term is followed by the page number where the term is defined in the chapter. Terms that appear in **boldface** or <u>underscored</u> in the chapter text are located in the glossary.

How the Body Uses Food

Key Terms *(Continued)*

Learning Objectives

After completing this chapter, the student should be able to:

1. List the anatomical structures which make up the gastrointestinal tract.
2. Describe digestion, absorption, metabolism, and excretion.
3. Discuss how nutrients are used by the cells.
4. Describe appropriate dietary treatments for lactose intolerance, lipid malabsorption, food allergies, and gluten-sensitive enteropathy.
5. List the ways the body eliminates waste.

*E*very part of the human body requires nutrients for energy, maintenance, and growth. Food supplies the necessary nutrients. However, food is composed of complex substances that must be broken down to simpler forms that can be used by the cells. The underline{cell} is the ultimate destination for the nutrients found in food. Digestion, absorption, and metabolism are the three interrelated processes that act on food to prepare it for use by the body. A fourth process, excretion, is the elimination of undigestible or unusable substances. In this chapter we will discuss all the bodily activities, organs, and systems involved in these major processes.

OVERVIEW OF THE MAJOR PROCESSES

The first step in preparing food for use by the cells is digestion. Digestion is the process by which food is broken down mechanically and chemically in the gastrointestinal tract into forms small enough for absorption to occur. The end products of digestion move from the gastrointestinal tract into the blood or lymphatic system in a process called absorption. After absorption, the nutrients usually are transported to the liver where they may be adjusted to suit the needs of the body. Metabolism, the sum of all physical and chemical changes that take place in the body, determines the final use of the individual nutrients and medications. What the cells have no use for becomes waste that is eliminated through excretion.

DIGESTION

Digestion—The process by which food is broken down mechanically and chemically in the gastrointestinal tract into forms small enough for cells to use.

Digestion takes place in the alimentary canal and the accessory organs (see Fig. 5–1).

Alimentary Canal

The alimentary canal is a long, hollow, muscular tube passing through the body that extends from the mouth to the anus. It includes the oral cavity, pharynx, esophagus, stomach, small intestine, and large intestine.

Muscle rings, called sphincters, separate segments of the alimentary canal. They act as valves to control the passage of food. When the muscles contract, the passageway closes; when the muscles relax, the passageway opens.

Structure of the Alimentary Canal

Structurally, the alimentary canal has four layers: the mucosa, the submucosa, the external muscle layer, and the serosa. See Figure 5–2 for a cross-sectional diagram of the small intestine (a typical example). Each layer has a specific structure and use:

Mucus—A thick fluid secreted by the mucous membranes and glands.

1. Mucosa. The mucosa lines the alimentary canal. It secretes **mucus,** which lubricates the canal and helps facilitate the smooth passage of food. The mucosa secretes digestive enzymes of the stomach and small intestine. The mucosal muscle layer between the mucosa and the submucosa raises intestinal folds to increase the surface area for better absorption.

2. Submucosa. The submucosa layer contains many blood and lymphatic vessels.

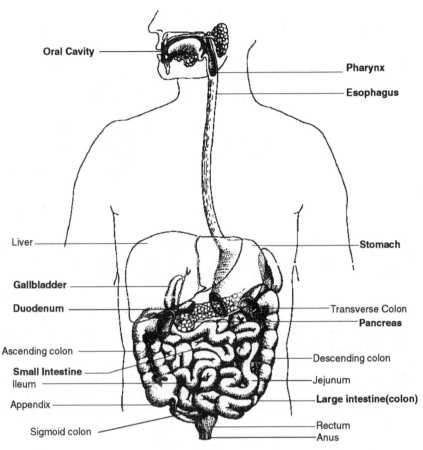

Oral Cavity

Pharynx

Esophagus

Liver

Stomach

Gallbladder

Duodenum

Transverse Colon

Pancreas

Ascending colon

Descending colon

Small Intestine
Ileum

Jejunum

Appendix

Large intestine(colon)

Sigmoid colon

Rectum
Anus

FIGURE 5–1. Alimentary canal and accessory organs. The alimentary canal is a hollow tube that runs through the body. The liver, gallbladder, and pancreas are part of the digestive system. Secretions from these organs enter the alimentary canal through ducts.

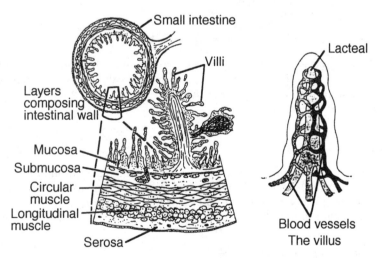

Small intestine

Lacteal

Villi

Layers
composing
intestinal wall

Mucosa

Submucosa

Circular
muscle

Longitudinal
muscle

Blood vessels

Serosa

The villus

FIGURE 5–2. A cross section of the small intestine. Structural layers typical of the alimentary canal (*left*); mucosal folds and villi that are covered with microvilli increase the surface area of the small intestine (*center*); Each villus has a capillary network and a lacteal (*right*).

3. <u>External Muscle Layer.</u> Typically, the external muscle layer consists of two layers of smooth muscle—the circular and longitudinal layers. The muscular actions of these two layers will be discussed later in the chapter.

4. <u>Serosa.</u> The serosa is usually a serous membrane that covers internal organs and lines body cavities. Serous fluid prevents friction between organs.

Variations on these layers of the alimentary canal do occur. For example, the stomach has a third smooth muscle layer in addition to the other two.

Accessory Organs

Three <u>organs</u> located outside of the alimentary canal are considered part of the digestive system. These are the liver, gallbladder, and pancreas. They make important contributions to the digestive process.

Liver

Liver—A digestive organ that aids in the metabolism of all the energy nutrients, screens toxic substances from the blood, manufacturers blood proteins, and performs many other important functions.

The **liver** is the second largest single organ in the body (skin is the largest). Many functions are performed by the liver, but the only digestive function is the production of **bile**. Bile is important in breaking down dietary fats. Bile is taken out of the liver by the hepatic duct. A <u>duct</u> is a narrow tube that permits the movement of fluid from one organ to another. Later in the chapter we will discuss some of the tasks the liver performs after the absorption of nutrients.

Gallbladder

Bile—Dark yellow secretion of the liver that alkalinizes the intestine and breaks large fat globules into smaller ones to facilitate enzyme digestive action.

The <u>gallbladder</u> is a 3-to-4-inch sac that concentrates and stores bile until it is needed in the small intestine. Bile is delivered to the small intestine through the common bile duct. About 2 to 3 cups of bile are secreted each day into the alimentary canal.

Pancreas

Mechanical digestion—The digestive process that involves the physical breaking down of food into smaller pieces.

The <u>pancreas</u> secretes enzymes that are involved in the digestion of all the energy nutrients. These secretions are collectively known as pancreatic juice. Pancreatic juice is carried to the small intestine via the pancreatic and common bile ducts.

Digestive Action

Chemical digestion—Digestive process that involves the splitting of complex molecules into simpler forms.

Mechanical and chemical digestion occur simultaneously throughout the alimentary canal. **Mechanical digestion** is the physical breaking down of food into smaller pieces. **Chemical digestion** involves the splitting of complex molecules into simpler forms.

Mechanical Digestion

Peristalsis—A wavelike movement that propels food along the alimentary canal.

Examples of mechanical digestion include chewing or <u>mastication,</u> swallowing, peristalsis, and emulsification. **Peristalsis** is a wavelike movement that propels food along the entire length of the alimentary canal. This one-way movement is caused by the alternate contraction and relaxation of the circular and longitudinal muscles that make up the external muscle layer of the alimentary canal. Other muscular activity churns the food, which reduces it to successively smaller particles and mixes it with digestive secretions. All of these muscular actions are regulated by a network of nerves within the wall of the alimentary canal. Emulsification is discussed later in the chapter.

Chemical Digestion

Many chemical reactions are involved in digestion. For example, the conversion of starch to maltose, of fat to glycerol and fatty acids, and of protein to amino acids all involve the process of **hydrolysis.** The hydrolysis of nutrients is achieved mostly through the action of digestive enzymes, which are present in saliva, gastric juice, pancreatic juice, and intestinal juice. Each enzyme is specific in its action; it will only act upon a certain substance and no other. Enzymes sometimes require the presence of additional substances such as activators, coenzymes, or hormones to make them active. There are more than 500 enzymes involved in the digestive process. However, only a few of the major ones will be discussed in this chapter.

Hydrolysis—A chemical reaction that splits a substance into simpler compounds by the addition of water.

In addition to enzymes, other secretions and chemicals are used in the chemical digestion of food. These include mucus, electrolytes, and water. As mentioned earlier, mucus lubricates passages and facilitates the movement of food. It also protects the inside walls of the alimentary canal from acidic solutions. Electrolytes are substances that conduct an electric current in solution (see Chapter 9). One example of an electrolyte is the hydrochloric acid (HCl) secreted by the stomach. It performs many functions necessary to the digestive process. The ways in which HCl aids digestion will be discussed later in the chapter. In addition to participating in chemical reactions (hydrolysis), water promotes peristalsis and the activities of digestive enzymes. The release of enzymes and other substances necessary for chemical digestion can be affected by many factors.

Control of Secretions

The amount of mucus, electrolytes, water, and enzymes released during the digestive process depends on several factors. Hormones frequently turn on or turn off a given secretion. For example, the acid content of the food causes a hormone called secretin to be released. The release of secretin in the small intestine causes the pancreas to send pancreatic juices into the small intestine.

How you feel about a food can affect the amount of a secretion released. There is a relationship between your nervous system and your digestive system. For example, the smell of a roasting turkey on Thanksgiving Day will cause the release of hydrochloric acid in the stomach. Stress and tension can also produce this effect sometimes with deleterious results.

The very presence of food in the gastrointestinal tract can influence the release of alimentary canal secretions. For example, coffee causes a hormone to be released into the stomach, which in turn causes the secretion of hydrochloric acid. Another example is the release of bile from the gallbladder caused by the presence of fat in the small intestine. This chain of reactions whereby one event causes another and then another is very common in all biological systems.

End Products of Digestion

Within about four hours after you have eaten a meal, your body has broken down the food into some two hundred million, million, million molecules. Each of the energy nutrients is broken down into simpler molecules. Carbohydrates are digested into monosaccharides. Fats are broken down into molecules of glycerol, fatty acids, and monoglycerides. The end products of protein digestion are amino acids and small peptides. Up to one third of dietary protein is believed to be absorbed into mucosal cells as di- and tri-peptides. Vitamins, minerals, and water are also released during digestion. In the next section we will follow the pathway of food as it goes through the digestive process. Then, the digestive activities that occur along this pathway (by location in the alimentary canal) will be discussed in detail.

The Food Pathway

Food passes through the mouth into the oral cavity, where it is chewed and exposed to chemicals in the saliva. The tongue voluntarily forces the mass of food, called a bolus, into the pharynx, which is responsible for the reflex action of swallowing. When swallowed, the bolus enters the esophagus, a muscular, mucus-lined tube, and is propelled downward by peristalsis to the stomach. Both mechanical and chemical digestion occur in the stomach, reducing the food to a semifluid mass that is then released into the small intestine. Further digestion takes place in the small intestine, and most of the absorption of nutrients occurs here as well. Any food remaining after digestion and absorption passes into the large intestine and is excreted as fecal matter.

Oral Cavity

The oral cavity is the hollow space in the skull directly behind the mouth. Its boundaries are the roof of the mouth, the cheeks, and the floor of the mouth. Within the oral cavity are the teeth, tongue, and the openings of the ducts of the salivary glands.

Salivary amylase—An enzyme that initiates the breakdown of starch in the mouth.

DIGESTIVE ACTION   Food entering the oral cavity is chewed and thus broken into smaller particles. This mechanical action increases the surface area of the food for exposure to saliva, a digestive secretion produced by the salivary glands. Saliva moistens and softens the food for swallowing and contains the digestive enzyme known as **salivary amylase.** Salivary amylase converts starch to maltose (a disaccharide) or to shorter chains of glucose. Because they require no digestion, some absorption of simple sugars (monosaccharides) may occur in the mouth. The chemical digestion of carbohydrates (starch) continues until the hydrochloric acid in the stomach halts the action of the salivary amylase. After being chewed, the bolus (food mass) is maneuvered backward by the tongue into the pharynx.

Pharynx

The pharynx is a muscular passage between the oral cavity and the esophagus. No digestive action occurs here. The pharynx continues the movement of the bolus by the reflexive action of swallowing. The bolus then enters the esophagus.

Esophagus

The esophagus is a muscular tube about 10 inches long that takes food from the pharynx to the stomach. No digestive action occurs here. Peristalsis forces the bolus into the stomach with the help of mucous secretions. At the end of the esophagus is the cardiac sphincter (closes the entrance to the stomach), which opens to receive the food. The sphincter closes after the passage of food to prevent the backup of stomach contents.

Stomach

The stomach is a J-shaped sac that extends from the esophagus to the small intestine. Folds in the mucous membrane, called rugae, smooth out when the stomach is full. They allow the stomach to expand. The need to eat constantly is prevented because the stomach serves as a reservoir for food, which takes from 2 to 6 hours to completely pass through to the small intestine. Gastric juice, the collective secretions of the stomach, consists of hydrochloric acid, mucus, and the enzymes pepsin, rennin, and gastric lipase.

DIGESTIVE ACTION   In the stomach, the chemical digestion of protein begins and further mechanical digestion takes place. Some water and minerals, certain drugs, and alcohol are absorbed in the stomach. Even before food enters the mouth, the sight or smell of food will cause the gastric mucosa to excrete the hormone **gastrin.** This hormone stimulates the secretion of gastric juice so that there is some present in the stomach when the food arrives. The stomach's lining is partially protected from the corrosive effects of gastric juice by mucus.

Gastrin—A hormone secreted by the gastric mucosa; stimulates the secretion of gastric juice.

The hydrolysis of protein is initiated when hydrochloric acid activates and then converts pepsinogen to its active form, **pepsin.** A protein molecule is made up of possibly hundreds of amino acids joined together by peptide bonds. Such chains of amino acids linked by peptide bonds are called polypeptides. What pepsin does is to break down large polypeptides into smaller polypeptides. In infants, the milk protein casein is broken down by the enzyme rennin. The action of rennin coagulates (curdles) the milk. In addition to activating pepsin, hydrochloric acid destroys harmful bacteria, makes certain minerals such as iron and calcium more absorbable, and maintains the pH (1 to 2) of the gastric juice.

Pepsin—An enzyme secreted in the stomach that begins protein digestion.

Some butterfat molecules of milk are also broken down into smaller molecules in the stomach. The enzyme that accomplishes this is gastric lipase. This enzyme is most active in infants because the more alkaline environment of the infant's stomach enables gastric lipase to work more effectively.

The mechanical digestion that occurs in the stomach is a result of the churning action of the muscular walls. This muscular activity agitates the contents of the stomach, thoroughly mixing the food with gastric juice. In this way, the food is reduced to a semifluid mass of partially digested material called **chyme.** Peristaltic waves push the chyme toward the pyloric sphincter, the valve separating the stomach from the small intestine. With each peristaltic wave, a small amount of chyme is forced through the pyloric sphincter into the small intestine.

Chyme—The mixture of partly digested food and digestive secretions found in the stomach and small intestine during digestion of a meal.

Small Intestine

The small intestine is the longest portion of the alimentary canal, approximately 20 feet in length. It extends from the pyloric sphincter of the stomach to the large intestine. The small intestine is looped and coiled in the central part of the abdominal cavity, surrounded by the large intestine. It consists of three parts: the duodenum is the first 10 inches, the jejunum is the middle 8 feet, and the ileum is the last 11 feet. Ninety percent of the digestive action in the alimentary canal and nearly all absorption of the end products of digestion occurs in the small intestine. Its anatomy will be discussed further in the section on absorption.

The entry of chyme into the duodenum stimulates the secretion of two hormones, secretion and cholecystokinin. Collectively, these hormones are responsible for the secretion and release of bile and the secretion of pancreatic juice. **Secretin** stimulates the production of bile by the liver and the secretion of sodium bicarbonate juice by the pancreas. The bile salts in bile emulsify fats, and sodium bicarbonate juice (which is alkaline) neutralizes the gastric juice that enters the duodenum. This neutralization is necessary to prevent damage to the lining of the duodenum. Mucus secreted by intestinal glands also provides some measure of protection against such damage. **Cholecystokinin** stimulates the contraction of the gallbladder, an action that forces stored bile into the duodenum. It also stimulates the secretion of pancreatic enzymes, which are essential for the breakdown of carbohydrates, fats, and proteins. Intestinal juice is also secreted in response to the presence of chyme in the duodenum. Peristaltic action of the small intestine mixes the bile, the pancreatic juice, and the intestinal juice together with the chyme as it moves toward the colon. It is the collective action of these juices that yields the final end products of the digestive process.

Secretin—A hormone that stimulates the production of bile by the liver and the secretion of sodium bicarbonate juice by the pancreas.

Cholecystokinin—A hormone secreted by the duodenum; stimulates contraction of the gallbladder (releases bile) and the secretion of pancreatic juice.

DIGESTION OF CARBOHYDRATES Carbohydrate digestion is completed through the action of pancreatic and intestinal enzymes. Pancreatic amylase breaks down any remaining starch into maltose. The disaccharides maltose, sucrose, and lactose are reduced to monosaccharides (simple sugars) by the action of three enzymes located in the walls of the small intestine. Each of these enzymes is specific for a given disaccharide: maltase breaks down maltose to glucose and glucose, sucrase breaks down sucrose to glucose and fructose, and lactase breaks down lactose to glucose and galactose. Often, low levels of these enzymes can lead to intolerances for the respective disaccharides.

In fact, approximately 70 percent of the world's population has some degree of lact*ose* intolerance. This intolerance is the result of a lack of the intestinal enzyme lact*ase*. Clinical Application 5–1 discusses carbohydrate intolerances, including lactose intolerance. Table 5–1 lists food items that are lactose-free, low in lactose, and high in lactose.

DIGESTION OF FATS Fats are emulsified by bile salts in the small intestine before they are digested further. Emulsification is the physical breaking up of fats into tiny droplets. Lingual lipase is an important enzyme in infants, although not in adults. In this way, more surface area of the fat is exposed to the chemical action of the pancreatic enzyme **pancreatic lipase.** Pancreatic lipase completes the digestion of fats by reducing triglycerides to diglycerides and monoglycerides, fatty acids and glycerol.

Pancreatic lipase—An enzyme that splits fats into fatty acids and glycerol; present in pancreatic juices; also known as pancreatic lipase.

DIGESTION OF PROTEIN Although hundreds of enzymes are involved in protein digestion, this text reviews only a few of the major ones.

CLINICAL APPLICATION 5–1
Carbohydrate Intolerances

Some individuals have a deficiency of one or more of the enzymes lactase, maltase, or sucrase. This means that they are unable to digest these disaccharides into monosaccharides. The resulting disease is called a lactose intolerance, maltose intolerance, or sucrose intolerance. Lactose intolerance is the most common of these diseases. Lactose intolerance may occur in 60 percent to 100 percent of Hispanics, blacks, and southeast Asians. The condition can be hereditary or can be secondary to other disease processes involving the small intestine.

A lactose intolerance results when the enzyme lactase is not produced in sufficient quantities to digest the lactose that is consumed. Dietary treatment of a lactose intolerance involves three steps: (1) identifying food items that contain lactose; (2) eliminating all sources of lactose from the diet; and (3) establishing an individual tolerance level for the patient on a trial-and-error basis. There is a broad range of tolerance levels for lactose in these patients.

Symptoms of a lactose intolerance include abdominal cramping and pain, loose stools, and flatulence (gas) after eating or drinking milk products. Lactose is the disaccharide found only in milk and milk products. The treatment for a lactase deficiency is dietary. The patient should be educated not to drink milk or to eat foods made from milk in excess of tolerated amounts.

Patients on a lactose-free diet should read all labels carefully to see if milk or milk solids, lactose, or whey have been added to the products. Whey is the thin watery portion of milk that separates from the thicker part, or curd, during cheese production. The whey contains the milk sugar or lactose. Many toothpastes or over-the-counter medications contain a small amount of lactose. Generally, the amount is very small and is tolerated well.

Because the lactose content of cheeses is a source of confusion for both nurses and patients, a brief discussion on cheese follows. One gallon of milk is required to produce 1 pound of cheese. During cheese making, the whey is separated from the curd. The whey is the liquid and the curd is the solid material (similar to the curd in cottage cheese). Most of the lactose in cheese is removed when the whey is separated from the curd. In ripened cheese, the small amount of lactose entrapped in the curd is transformed into lactic acid, which does not require lactase for absorption.

Generally, cheese must age for more than 90 days to be lactose free. The following cheeses are considered hard ripened (low in lactose): blue, brick, Brie, Camembert, Cheddar, Colby, Edam, Gouda, Monterey, Muenster, Parmesan, Provolone, and Swiss. The following cheeses are considered "soft cheeses" and thus contain more lactose: cream cheese, Neufchatel, ricotta, mozzarella, and cottage cheese.

Lactaid is an over-the-counter product specially designed for individuals with a lactose intolerance. Lactaid is a natural enzyme which is available in liquid or tablet form. The liquid form is typically added to milk, whereas the tablet form is chewed before consumption of a food product containing lactose. Some grocery stores also sell milk that has been pre-treated with Lactaid. This product will digest 70 percent of the lactose in a product into glucose and galactose. As a result, most lactose-intolerant persons can drink Lactaid-treated milk or eat foods

Box continued on next page.

CLINICAL APPLICATION 5–1 *(Continued)*

which contain lactose and digest it comfortably. Figure 5–3 pictures a person drinking lactose-treated milk.

A lactose-restricted diet may be low in calcium, riboflavin, and vitamin D. Patients should be instructed in alternate sources of these nutrients or advised to take supplements.

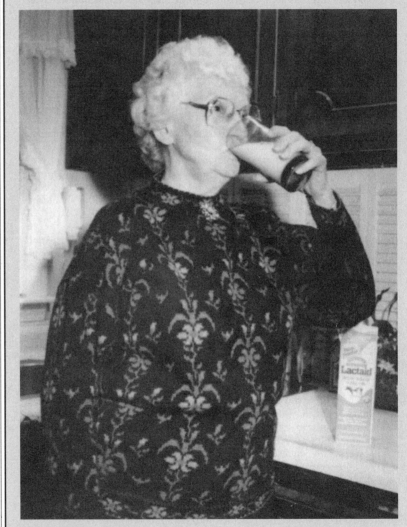

FIGURE 5–3. A person drinking Lactaid-treated milk. Milk treated with Lactaid is slightly sweeter than regular milk. The sweeter taste results naturally when lactose is broken down into its digestible form.

The shorter polypeptides resulting from the digestive action in the stomach are broken down even further by the action of pancreatic and intestinal enzymes. Two of the major enzymes produced by the pancreas that are responsible for this additional protein-splitting are <u>trypsin</u> and <u>chymotrypsin.</u>

TABLE 5–1 *Lactose Content of Foods*

Lactose-Free Foods	Low-Lactose Foods (0 to 2 grams/serving)	
Broth-based soups	½ cup	Milk treated with lactase enzyme
Plain meat, fish, poultry, peanut butter	½ cup	Sherbet
Breads that do not contain milk, dry milk solids, or whey	1–2 ounces	Aged cheese
Cereal, crackers	1 ounce	Processed cheese
Fruit, plain vegetables		Butter or margarine
Desserts made without milk, dry milk solids, or whey		Commercially prepared foods containing dry milk solids or whey
Tofu and tofu products, such as tofu-based ice cream substitute	Some medications and vitamin preparations may contain a small amount of lactose. Generally, the amount is very small and is tolerated well.	
Nondairy creamers		

High-Lactose Foods (5 to 8 Grams/Serving)

½ cup	Milk (whole, skim, 1%, 2%, buttermilk, sweet acidophilus)	½ cup	White sauce
⅛ cup	Powdered dry milk (whole, nonfat, buttermilk—before reconstituting)	½ cup	Party chip dip or potato topping
		¾ cup	Creamed or low-fat cottage cheese
¼ cup	Evaporated milk	1 cup	Dry cottage cheese
3 Tbsp	Sweetened condensed milk	¾ cup	Ricotta cheese
		2 oz	Cheese food or cheese spread*
¾ cup	Heavy cream	¾ cup	Ice cream or ice milk
½ cup	Half and half	½ cup	Yogurt†
½ cup	Sour cream		

*Lactose content is higher than that of aged cheese and of processed cheese because of the addition of whey powder and of dry milk solids.

†Yogurt may be tolerated better than foods with similar lactose content because of hydrolysis of lactose by bacterial lactase found in the culture. Tolerance may vary with the brand and the processing method.

Mayo Clinic Diet Manual, 1988, with permission.

Both trypsin and chymotrypsin have inactive precursors that are activated by other enzymes. The intestinal wall also secretes a group of enzymes known as **peptidases.** The peptidases act on the smaller molecules produced by the pancreatic enzymes, reducing them to single amino acids and small peptides, the final end products of protein digestion.

Peptidases— Enzymes that assist in the digestion of protein by reducing the smaller molecules to single amino acids.

Table 5–2 shows a summary of the digestion of carbohydrates, fats, and proteins by body organ (mouth, stomach, or small intestine). The subcategories in the table identify whether the digestive action is mechanical or chemical. This table includes only the material that is covered in the text. You may find it helpful to refer to an anatomy and physiology text.

TABLE 5–2 *Summary of Digestion*

Nutrient	Mouth and Esophagus	Stomach	Small Intestine
Carbohydrates yield	*Mechanical* Mastication Swallowing Peristalsis Mucus	*Mechanical* Peristalsis Mucus	*Mechanical* Peristalsis Mucus
	Chemical Salivary amylase	*Chemical* None	*Chemical* Pancreatic enzymes: Pancreatic amylase Intestinal enzymes: Maltase Sucrase Lactase
Monosaccharides			
Fats yield	*Mechanical* Mastication Swallowing Peristalsis Mucus	*Mechanical* Peristalsis Mucus	*Mechanical* Peristalsis Mucus Gallbladder: Bile
	Chemical None Lingual lipase in infants	*Chemical* Gastric lipase†	*Chemical* Pancreatic enzymes: Pancreatic lipase
Glycerol, fatty acids, and monoglycerides			
Proteins yield	*Mechanical* Mastication Swallowing Peristalsis Mucus	*Mechanical* Peristalsis Mucus	*Mechanical* Peristalsis Mucus
	Chemical None	*Chemical* Rennin Pepsin Hydrochloric acid	*Chemical* Pancreatic enzymes: Trypsin Chymotrypsin Intestinal enzymes: Peptidases
Amino acids and small peptides			

*Emulsifies fat.

†Digests butterfat only.

ABSORPTION

The end products of digestion move from the gastrointestinal tract into the blood or <u>lymphatic system</u> in a process called **absorption.** The lymphatic system transports <u>lymph</u> from the tissues to the bloodstream. This system is technically part of the circulatory or cardiovascular system. Eventually, all fluid in the lymphatic system enters the blood. It is only after nutrients have been absorbed into either the blood or lymphatic system that they can be utilized by the cells of the body.

The end products of digestion include the monosaccharides from carbohydrate digestion, the fatty acids and glycerol (and often monoglycerides) from fats, and small peptides and amino acids from protein digestion. Absorption occurs primarily in the small intestine.

Absorption—The movement of the end products of digestion from the gastrointestinal tract into the blood and/or lymphatic system.

Small Intestine

The inner surface of the small intestine has mucosal folds, villi, and microvilli to increase the surface area for maximum absorption (refer again to Fig. 5–2). The mucosal folds can be compared to pleats in fabric. On each fold (or pleat) are millions of fingerlike projections, called <u>villi</u> (plural of villus). Each villus has hundreds of microscopic, hairlike projections (resembling bristles on a brush), called <u>microvilli,</u> on its surface. The large surface area resulting from this arrangement fosters the movement of nutrients into the blood or lymphatic system. This is similar to the idea that four lanes of traffic move more quickly than two—the surface area of the highway is larger so more traffic can be accommodated. The structure of the mucosa serves as a unit that accomplishes the absorption of nutrients.

Within each villus is a network of blood **capillaries** and a central lymph vessel called a <u>lacteal.</u> The villi absorb nutrients from the chyme by way of these blood and lymph vessels. Monosaccharides, amino acids, glycerol (which is water soluble), minerals, and water-soluble vitamins are absorbed into the blood in the capillary network. Because short- and medium-chain fatty acids have fewer carbons in their chain length, they are more water soluble than long-chain fatty acids. Thus, they are absorbed directly into the blood as well. These water-soluble nutrients, including short- and medium-chain fatty acids, eventually enter into hepatic portal circulation (via the portal vein) and travel to the liver. **Hepatic portal circulation** is a subdivision of the vascular system by which blood from the digestive organs and spleen circulates through the liver before returning to the heart. In the liver, the nutrients are modified according to the needs of the body.

Capillary—A tiny tube (vessel) that brings the blood into contact with cells.

Hepatic portal circulation—A subdivision of the vascular system by which blood from the digestive organs and spleen circulates through the liver before returning to the heart.

Because long-chain fats are not soluble in water and the blood is chiefly water, the fat-soluble nutrients cannot be absorbed directly into the blood. Instead, fat-soluble nutrients—including long-chain fatty acids, any monoglycerides remaining from fat digestion, and fat-soluble vitamins—are first combined with bile salts as a carrier. Then, this complex of fat-soluble materials is absorbed into the cells lining the intestinal wall. Once absorbed, the bile separates from the fat and returns to recirculate. Within the intestinal cells, any remaining monoglycerides are reduced to fatty acids and glycerol by an enzyme. Glycerol, fatty acids, and absorbed long-chain fatty acids are recombined (within the intestinal cells) to form human triglycerides in a process called triglyceride synthesis.

TABLE 5-3 *Metabolic Modifications in the Liver*

Energy Nutrient	Modification
Carbohydrates	Fructose and galactose changed to glucose, excess glucose converted to glycogen
Lipids	Lipoproteins formed, cholesterol synthesized, triglycerides broken down and built
Amino acids	Nonessential amino acids manufactured, excess amino acids deaminated and then changed to carbohydrates or fats, ammonia removed from the blood, plasma proteins made
Other	Alcohol, drugs, and poisons detoxified

Chylomicron—A lipoprotein that carries triglycerides in the blood after meals.

After triglyceride synthesis, the newly formed triglycerides and any other fat materials present (such as cholesterol) are covered with special proteins, forming lipoproteins called **chylomicrons.** The chylomicrons are released into the lymphatic system via the lacteals. Remember that the lymphatic system is connected to the blood system. The protein "wrapping" these packages of fat enables the chylomicrons to move into the blood via the thoracic duct (and hence into portal blood). In the liver, lipids are also modified to suit the needs of the body before distribution to body cells. (Table 5–3) describes some of the nutrient modifications that are made in the liver.

After absorption of nutrients in the small intestine, the watery chyme moves into the large intestine, where final absorption and elimination take place. No digestion occurs in the large intestine.

Large Intestine

The large intestine, also called the colon, extends from the ileum (last part of the small intestine) to the anus. When any remaining chyme leaves the small intestine it enters the first portion of the large intestine, the cecum. The appendix, an organ with no known function, is attached to the cecum. Further passage of undigested food is controlled by the ileocecal valve, which relaxes and then closes with each peristaltic wave. This valve prevents backflow and ensures that chyme remains in the small intestine long enough for sufficient digestion and absorption. Chyme leaves the cecum and travels slowly through the remaining parts of the large intestine: the ascending colon, the transverse colon, the descending colon, the sigmoid colon, the rectum, and the anal canal.

Water is the main substance absorbed by the large intestine. However, the absorption of some minerals (as electrolytes—see Chapter 9) and vitamins also occurs in the colon. Most of the water, up to 80 percent, is extracted in the cecum and the ascending colon. Vitamins synthesized by intestinal bacteria, including vitamin K and some of the B-complexes (see Chapter 6), are absorbed from the colon. After absorption and digestion have taken place, the remaining waste products are eliminated in the feces by way of the rectum.

Elimination of Unabsorbed Materials

Absorption of water into the body reduces the water content of the material left inside the large intestine slowly, so in the end a solid consistency remains. This solid material is the feces. Mucus, the only secretion in the large intestine, provides lubrication for the smooth passage of the feces. By the time the feces reach the rectum they consist of 75 percent water and 25 percent solids. The solids include cellular wastes, undigested dietary fiber, undigested food, bile salts, cholesterol, mucus, and bacteria.

Indigestible Carbohydrates

The body cannot digest some forms of carbohydrate because it lacks the necessary enzyme to split the appropriate molecule. Some vegetables and legumes contain these indigestible sugars and fibers. Intestinal gas is formed in the colon by the decomposition of undigested materials. Examples of gas-forming foods are beans, onions, cabbage family vegetables, and radishes.

Factors Interfering with Absorption

Malabsorption is the inadequate movement of digested food from the small intestine into the blood or lymphatic system. Malnutrition can be caused by malabsorption. Table 5–4 lists factors that interfere with the absorption of nutrients. Note from the table that many diseases, medications, and some

Malabsorption— Inadequate movement of digested food from the small intestine into the blood or lymphatic system.

TABLE 5–4 *Factors Decreasing Absorption*

Medications	Antacids
	Laxatives
	Birth control pills
	Anticonvulsants
	Antibiotics
Parasites	Tapeworm
	Hookworm
Surgical procedures	Gastric resections
	Any surgery on the small intestine
	Some surgical procedures on the large intestine
Disease states	Infection
	Tropical sprue
	Gluten-sensitive enteropathy
	Hepatic disease
	Pancreatic insufficiency
	Lactase deficiency
	Sucrase deficiency
	Maltase deficiency
	Circulatory disorders
	Cancers involving the alimentary canal
Medical complications	Effects of radiation therapy

Note: Most of these conditions will be discussed in later chapters.

CLINICAL APPLICATION 5–2

Surgical Removal of All or Part of the Alimentary Canal

Patients may need to have a portion of their small intestine surgically removed for a variety of reasons. These patients are frequently at a nutritional risk because they are either permanently or temporarily unable to absorb essential nutrients. In such cases, a nutritional assessment is indicated. In the past, some patients elected to have a portion of their alimentary canal removed in order to lose weight. The surgical removal of the alimentary canal for weight reduction is discussed in Chapter 15.

---

medical treatments have a negative impact on the absorption of nutrients. Clinical Application 5–2 discusses surgical removal of all or part of the alimentary canal and the effect on absorption. Clinical Application 5–3 discusses inadequate absorption.

CLINICAL APPLICATION 5–3

Inadequate Absorption

The healthcare worker can often determine whether or not a patient's digestion and absorption of food are normal. A visual inspection of a patient's feces can confirm a suspicion of poor digestion or poor absorption. Large chunks of food indicate a problem with digestion. A large amount of liquid or near-liquid stools suggests poor absorption. A simple question directed to the patient, such as "Are your stools normal?" can provide some information. However, be advised that a patient's concept of normal may be different from your own.

Absorption may be affected by several factors (refer again to Table 5–4). Laboratory results are also used to identify problems with digestion and absorption. The physician's clinical evaluation of a patient may lead to a diagnosis of malabsorption, the inadequate absorption of nutrients from the intestinal tract. Patients with malabsorption usually suffer from malnutrition.

The cells lining the inside layer of the small intestine have a very short life. The smallest structures are replaced every 2 to 3 days. Although this rapid cell turnover helps to promote healing after injury, it also allows vulnerability to any nutritional deficiency or process that might interfere with cell reproduction.

"Gut failure" is a term used to describe a situation in which the small intestine fails to absorb nutrients properly. Symptoms include diarrhea, malabsorption, and a poor response to oral feedings. A vicious cycle starts when the cells lining the small intestine fail to reproduce because they do not have the necessary nutrients for cell replacement. This in turn leads to chronic diarrhea caused by malabsorption. In turn, the malabsorption leads to malnutrition which prevents cell reproduction. Figure 5–4 diagrams this cycle.

Box continued on next page.

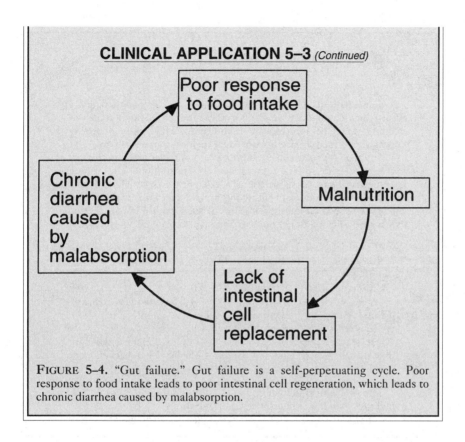

CLINICAL APPLICATION 5–3 *(Continued)*

FIGURE 5–4. "Gut failure." Gut failure is a self-perpetuating cycle. Poor response to food intake leads to poor intestinal cell regeneration, which leads to chronic diarrhea caused by malabsorption.

Steatorrhea

Some diseases and medications result in the malabsorption of fat. In these conditions, patients have <u>steatorrhea,</u> or fat in the stools. Frequently the condition is caused by the inhibition of pancreatic lipase, an enzyme necessary for the digestion of fats. Clinical Application 5–4 discusses lipid malabsorption and dietary treatment.

Nontropical Sprue

Nontropical <u>sprue</u> is a disorder of the small intestine. This disease is commonly referred to as **celiac disease** or <u>gluten-sensitive enteropathy.</u> Gluten-sensitive enteropathy results from the toxic effects that occur from the ingestion of <u>gluten,</u> a protein present in the following grains: wheat, rye, oats, and barley. Individuals with this disease suffer from a wide variety of nutritional problems.

The result of the toxic effect of gluten is the direct destruction of intestinal cells. This may be related to an allergic reaction and can be either severe or mild. In the severe form, the loss of the intestinal mucosa causes lactose intolerance.

Treatment in this situation would involve the use of medium-chain triglycerides to increase the kilocaloric content of the diet and a lactose-free, gluten-free diet. This is a complex diet for the healthcare professional to plan and for the patient to follow. Usually, frequent consultations with the physi-

Celiac disease (gluten-sensitive enteropathy)—An intolerance to dietary gluten, which damages the intestine and produces diarrhea and malabsorption.

CLINICAL APPLICATION 5–4
Lipid Malabsorption

Some patients for a variety of reasons are unable to digest and absorb long-chain fatty acids. For these patients, the use of MCT (medium-chain triglyceride) oil is indicated. MCT oil can provide a kilocalorie source for patients with a fat malabsorption problem.

Any food that contains fat must be carefully planned into the diet of any patient who suffers from a lipid malabsorption. The American Dietetic and Diabetic Associations' Exchange Lists for Menu Planning can be used as a guide in planning this type of diet. Usually the physician will order a specified number of grams of fat. A typical low-fat diet order may read: 40-gram fat diet. Such as diet may be planned as follows:

Exchange	Number of Exchanges/Day	Grams of Fat
Skimmed milk	Unlimited	0
Starches	8	4 (0.5 grams of fat/exchange)
Fruits	Unlimited	0
Vegetables	Unlimited	0
Meat, lean	7	21 (7 × 3 grams/exchange)
Fat	3	15 (3 × 5 grams/exchange)
		40 grams fat/day

The MCT oil is then added to the diet to bring the kilocalories up to meet the patient's kilocalorie requirement.

More information on fat-restricted diets appears in later chapters.

---

cian regarding the status of the patient's intestinal cells are necessary. These patients are often malnourished. As such, the patient benefits from being kept on this severe a diet only until intestinal cell regeneration is completed. Once the patient is able to tolerate both lactose and long-chain triglycerides they should be included in the diet. This will increase the patient's compliance in maintaining a high kilocalorie intake and assist in treating the malnutrition.

In milder forms, only a gluten-restricted diet is indicated (Table 5–5). Gluten is present in a number of prepared foods that contain thickened sauces. Extensive patient teaching is necessary for a positive patient outcome. Removal of all forms of wheat, rye, oats, and barley from the diet frequently results in remission or improvement within weeks.

Food Allergies

A <u>food allergy</u> is a sensitivity to a food that does not cause a negative reaction in most people. Individuals may be genetically predisposed to a food allergy. Almost any food can cause an allergic reaction, but milk, eggs, wheat, shellfish, chocolate, and oranges are frequent offenders. Some food allergies may be due to an alteration in absorption. The susceptible person absorbs a

TABLE 5–5 *Sources of Gluten*

Food Groups	Foods That Contain Gluten	Foods That May Contain Gluten	Foods That Do Not Contain Gluten
Beverage	Cereal beverages (e.g., Postum), malt, Ovaltine, beer and ale	Commercial* chocolate milk; cocoa mixes; other beverage mixes; dietary supplements	Coffee; tea; decaffeinated coffee; carbonated beverages; chocolate drinks made with pure cocoa powder; wine; distilled liquor
Meat and meat substitutes		Meat loaf and patties, cold cuts and prepared meats, stuffing, breaded meats, cheese foods and spreads; commercial souffles, omelets, and fondue; soy protein meat substitutes	Pure meat, fish, fowl, egg, cottage cheese, and peanut butter
Fat and oil		Commercial salad dressing and mayonnaise, gravy, white and cream sauces, nondairy creamer	Butter, margarine, vegetable oil
Milk	Milk beverages that contain malt	Commercial chocolate milk	Whole, low-fat, and skim milk; buttermilk
Grains and grain products	Bread, crackers, cereal, and pasta that contain wheat, oats, rye, malt, malt flavoring, graham flour, durham flour, pastry flour, bran, or wheat germ; barley; millet; pretzels; communion wafers	Commercial seasoned rice and potato mixes	Specially prepared breads made with wheat starch,† rice, potato, or soybean flour or cornmeal; pure corn or rice cereals; hominy grits; white, brown, and wild rice; popcorn; low protein pasta made from wheat starch
Vegetable		Commercial seasoned vegetable mixes; commercial vegetables with cream or cheese sauce; canned baked beans	All fresh vegetables; plain commercially frozen or canned vegetables
Fruit		Commercial pie fillings	All plain or sweetened fruits; fruit thickened with tapioca or cornstarch
Soup	Soup that contains wheat pasta; soup thickened with wheat flour or other gluten-containing grains	Commercial soup, broth, and soup mixes	Soup thickened with cornstarch, wheat starch, or potato, rice or soybean flour; pure broth

TABLE 5-5 *Sources of Gluten (Continued)*

Food Groups	Foods That Contain Gluten	Foods That May Contain Gluten	Foods That Do Not Contain Gluten
Desserts	Commercial cakes, cookies and pastries;	Commercial ice cream and sherbet	Gelatin; custard; fruit ice; specially prepared cakes, cookies, and pastries made with gluten-free flour or starch; pudding and fruit filling thickened with tapioca, cornstarch, or arrowroot flour
Sweets		Commercial candies, especially chocolates	
Miscellaneous‡		Ketchup; prepared mustard; soy sauce; commercially prepared meat sauces and pickles; vinegar; flavoring syrups (syrups for pancakes or ice cream)	Monosodium glutamate; salt; pepper; pure spices and herbs; yeast; pure baking chocolate or cocoa powder; carob; flavoring extracts; artificial flavoring

*The terms "commercially prepared" and "commercial" are used to refer to partially prepared foods purchased from a grocery or food market and to prepared foods purchased from a restaurant.

†Wheat starch may contain trace amounts of gluten. Avoid if not tolerated.

‡Medications may contain trace amounts of gluten. A pharmacist may be able to provide information on the gluten content of medications.

Mayo Clinic Diet Manual, 1988, with permission.

part of a food before it has been completely digested. The incomplete digestion of protein in particular is responsible for many allergic reactions. The body does not recognize the sequence of amino acids (because the protein was absorbed partly undigested) and therefore treats the protein as a foreign substance and tries to destroy it. This attempt produces the symptoms of food allergy, including skin rash, nausea, vomiting, diarrhea, intestinal cramps, swelling in various parts of the body, and spasm of the small intestine. The treatment for a food allergy is to avoid the offending food.

METABOLISM

Metabolism—The sum of all the physical and chemical changes that take place in the body; the two fundamental processes involved are anabolism and catabolism.

After digestion and absorption, nutrients are carried by the blood (usually after being modified in the liver cells) to all cells of the body. After entry into the cells, the nutrients from food undergo many chemical changes, which result in either the release of energy or the use of energy. **Metabolism** is the sum of all chemical and physical processes continuously going on in living organisms, comprising both anabolism and catabolism with the release of energy for vital body processes. Catabolic reactions usually result in the release of energy. The other main metabolic process, anabolism, is the building up of complex substances from simpler ones. Anabolic reactions require energy. In the next section we will describe how cells utilize the end products of digestion—the glucose from carbohydrates, the glycerol and fatty acids from fats, and the amino acids from proteins—to meet the energy needs of the body.

Catabolic Reactions

Glucose, glycerol, fatty acids, and amino acids can be broken down even further. These nutrients are held together by bonds that, when broken, release energy. The breakdown of the fuel-producing nutrients yields carbon dioxide, water, heat, and other forms of energy. The carbon dioxide is eventually exhaled and the water becomes part of the body fluids or is eliminated in the urine. Fifty percent or more of the total potential energy usually is lost as heat. The remaining available energy is temporarily stored in the cells as ATP, adenosine triphosphate.

ATP, a high-energy compound that has three phosphate groups in its structure, is thus available in all cells. Practically speaking, ATP is the storage form of energy for the cells since each cell has enzymes that can initiate the hydrolysis (breakdown through the addition of water) of ATP. In this reaction, one or more phosphate groups split off and subsequently release energy. If one phosphate group is removed, the result is ADP (adenosine diphosphate) plus phosphate.

Many steps are involved in the catabolic process responsible for the release of this energy. These steps require one or more of the following agents: enzymes, coenzymes, and/or hormones. Some vitamins and minerals act as coenzymes. Oxygen is also necessary for the full release of any potential energy. This addition of oxygen to the reaction is called <u>oxidation.</u> During the many steps that occur, the energy is released little by little and stored as ATP. The breakdown process includes the formation of intermediate chemical compounds such as <u>pyruvate</u> (pyruvic acid) and <u>acetyl CoA.</u> Acetyl CoA can be broken down further by entering a series of **chemical reactions** known as the *Kreb's cycle* or the TCA (tricarboxylic acid) cycle. See Figure 5–5 for a simplified schematic of the steps involved in the release of energy by the cells.

Chemical reaction—the process of combining or breaking down substances to obtain different substances.

Storage of Excess Nutrients

If the cells do not have immediate energy needs, the excess nutrients are stored. Glucose is stored as glycogen in liver and muscle tissue; surplus amounts are converted to fat. Glycerol and fatty acids are reassembled into triglycerides and stored in adipose tissue. Amino acids are used to make body proteins; any excess is deaminated (stripped of nitrogen) and ultimately used for glucose formation or stored as fat. If energy is not available from food, the cells will seek energy in body stores.

Anabolic Reactions

Once immediate energy needs have been met, the cells utilize the nutrients as needed for growth and repair of body tissue. The cellular supply of ATP is used first. When this instant energy source is exhausted, glycogen and fat stores are used. In addition to building up body protein, other anabolic reac-

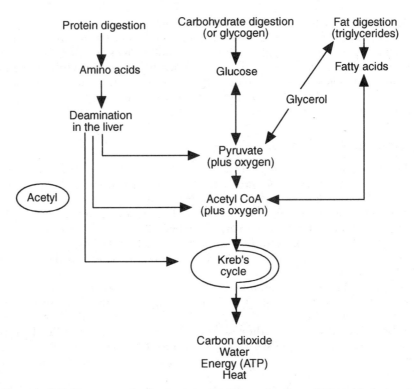

FIGURE 5–5. Energy production in the cells. Energy is released bit by bit during the further breakdown of amino acids, glucose, glycerol, and fatty acids.

tions include the recombination of glycerol and fatty acids to form triglycerides and the formation of glycogen from glucose.

EXCRETION OF WASTE PRODUCTS

Excretion—the elimination of waste products from the body in feces, urine, exhaled air, and perspiration.

What the cells have no use for becomes waste that is eliminated through **excretion.** Solid waste is disposed of in the feces. The digestive system needs assistance from other body systems in the disposal of nonsolid waste. The lungs dispose of gaseous waste. Most liquid waste is sent first to the kidneys and then to the <u>bladder</u> to be eliminated in the urine. Some liquid waste is disposed of by the skin through perspiration.

Carbon dioxide (CO_2) is a gas that is eliminated through the lungs each time you exhale. The amount of carbon dioxide exhaled depends on the type of fuel (lipid, protein, or carbohydrate) and/or the source of fuel that the body is currently burning for energy. For example, more CO_2 is produced when carbohydrate is being utilized than when the body is burning either protein or fat.

The skin removes some of the liquid waste in the form of perspiration or water and some is excreted in the feces. The kidneys eliminate most of the excess water, sodium, hydrogen, and urea. <u>Urea</u> is synthesized in the liver from the nitrogen resulting from the breakdown of amino acids. Some water is also removed from the body each time you exhale.

Summary

The cell is the ultimate destination for the nutrients in food. For food to be of use to the cells, it must first be broken down into many tiny particles and then absorbed into the body. Digestion is the process whereby food is broken down into a form usable by the cell: carbohydrates are broken down to monosaccharides, fats are reduced to glycerol and fatty acids, and proteins are split to yield amino acids. This is accomplished by both mechanical and chemical means. Secretions from the salivary glands, stomach, small intestine, liver, and pancreas assist in chemical digestion. Absorption refers to the movement of food from the gastrointestinal tract into the blood and lymphatic system. Metabolism involves the two processes of anabolism and catabolism. The liver plays a major role in metabolism.

After absorption, water-soluble nutrients go directly to the liver for further processing. The liver releases the nutrients into the bloodstream for delivery to the cells. Most of the fat-soluble nutrients are absorbed into the lymphatic system before entering the bloodstream. Short- and medium-chain triglycerides are absorbed differently than long-chain triglycerides. The cells remove the nutrients from the bloodstream as needed for energy and growth. Energy is released little by little from the end products of digestion in a series of chemical reactions. Energy nutrients not needed immediately by the cells are placed in storage as glycogen and adipose tissue.

The metabolism of food produces waste. Waste products are released from the body in the feces, urine, perspiration, and exhaled air.

Many ailments and diseases are related to the structure and function of the gastrointestinal system. Many forms of malabsorption, including disaccharide intolerances and gluten-sensitive enteropathy, are related to structural damage of the small intestine.

A case study and a sample plan of care appear below. Both are designed to show you how the information you have studied in this chapter can be used in nursing practice.

CASE STUDY 5–1

Mr. H. is a 25-year-old male who is 6 feet 0 inches tall and weighs 170 pounds (dressed without shoes). He has a medium frame, as determined by measuring his wrist circumference. Mr. H. has just been admitted to the hospital where you are employed for an elective arthroscopic (surgical procedure) on his right knee. During the nursing admission process, Mr. H. complained of gas pains and frequent loose stools. He stated that he does not avoid any particular foods and has a healthy appetite. He claims to drink about three cups of milk each day. The patient complained of a loss of 5 pounds during the prior month. Mr. H needed to use the restroom twice during the interview to "move his bowels." The second time the nurse inspected the stool. The patient's stool was loose and unformed.

The next day, upon reporting to work, you notice that a diagnosis of lactose intolerance had been made. A lactose-restricted diet was ordered.

The following nursing care plan originated on the day the patient was admitted. The physician used the information collected from the nurse in making his or her diagnosis. Please note that the patient has already met the first desired outcome and part of the second; they have been charted. The patient has not met the third desired outcome.

NURSING CARE PLAN FOR MR. H.

Assessment

Subjective: Patient complains of gas pains and loose stools. Patient stated that he does not avoid any particular foods.

Objective: Patient observed to use the restroom twice in 10 minutes to defecate. Visual inspection showed stool to be loose and unformed.

Nursing Diagnosis

Alteration in bowel elimination: diarrhea related to patient's complaints of loose stools as evidenced by the patient's need to use the restroom twice in a 10-minute period and by direct observation of one loose and unformed stool.

Desired Outcome/Evaluation Criteria

1. The patient will assist in ruling out causes for his loose stools and report his signs and symptoms to the nurse.
2. The patient will eliminate causative factors at once after these factors have been determined.
3. The patient will have formed stools within 24 hours after the causative factors have been eliminated.

Nursing Actions

1. a. Teach the patient to observe and record the pattern, onset, frequency, characteristics, amount, time of day, and precipitating events related to occurrence of diarrhea.
   b. Determine usual food intake and nutritional status, i.e., refer patient to the dietitian.
   c. Determine exposure to recent environmental contaminants, i.e., drinking water; food safety (see Chapter 12); illness of others
   d. Review drug intake for medications affecting absorption (refer to Table 5–4, Factors Decreasing Absorption).
2. a. Follow through with the elimination of causative factors—i.e., restrict intake if necessary, note change in drug therapy, if any.
3. a. Document the stool consistency.

Rationale

1. Observation and documentation of the patient's response to these factors will assist in determining the cause of his loose stools.
2. Elimination of the causative factors should decrease the frequency of loose, unformed stools.
   The patient needs to be instructed on the relationship of his diarrhea to causative factors.
3. Whenever possible an objective measure should be used to evaluate the success of any patient intervention.
   Stool consistency is an objective measure for treatment response to diarrhea and malabsorption.

STUDY AIDS

Chapter Review Questions

1. A patient on a gluten-free diet can usually tolerate which of the following (refer to Table 5–5)?
   a. Rice and granola
   b. Barley and wheat
   c. Oats and bulgur
   d. Corn and potatoes

2. Which of the following organs is not part of the digestive system?
   a. Kidney
   b. Gallbladder
   c. Liver
   d. Pancreas

3. After food leaves the stomach it enters the _____.
   a. Small intestine
   b. Esophagus
   c. Liver
   d. Large intestine

4. Most of the absorption of food takes place in the _____.
   a. Large intestine
   b. Gallbladder
   c. Small intestine
   d. Stomach

5. Metabolism is the _____.
   a. Breaking down of food into very small particles
   b. Movement of nutrients into the blood or lymphatic systems
   c. Excretion of body waste
   d. Sum of all chemical and physical processes continuously going on in living organisms, comprising both anabolism and catabolism with the release of energy for vital body processes

6. The body eliminates waste through all of the following except one. Identify the exception.
   a. Skin
   b. Hair
   c. Feces
   d. Lungs

7. The smallest functional unit of the human body is a _____.
   a. Molecule
   b. Cell
   c. Tissue
   d. Organ

8. Carbohydrates are absorbed as _____.
   a. A single monoglyceride
   b. Glycogen
   c. A single monosaccharide
   d. Glycerol

9. Which of the following elements is necessary for the *complete* release of energy from the end products of digestion?
   a. Nitrogen

    b. Chlorine
    c. Sodium
    d. Oxygen

10. Which of the following groups of food items should be restricted from a lactose-free diet? (Refer to Table 5-1.)
    a. Oranges, apples, bananas
    b. Green beans, peas, asparagus
    c. Sausage, nondairy creamers, some breads, canned soups
    d. Monosodium glutamate, angel food cake, pure cocoa powder, hard ripened cheeses such as cheddar and Swiss

NCLEX-Style Quiz

Situation One

1. Mrs. Hardy has been advised to follow a lactose-free diet. She can eat or drink:
    a. Any type of bread product, any type of cereal
    b. Fruit pies, angel food cake, parmesan cheese
    c. Frankfurters, ricotta cheese, caramels
    d. All fruit drinks, convenience desserts, any form of vegetable

Situation 2

2. Kathy, 24 months old, has been admitted to the pediatric unit you work on. She has a gluten-free diet ordered for celiac disease.
Which of the following meals would be permitted?
    a. Tuna noodle casserole, peas, milk, and fruit cocktail
    b. Swiss steak, mashed potatoes, corn, and chocolate pudding
    c. Tomato soup, grilled cheese sandwich, and french fries
    d. Roast turkey, baked potato, milk, green beans, and sour cream

3. When assessing Kathy's stools prior to dietary treatment, the nurse would expect the stool to be:
    a. Greasy, loose, and foul-smelling
    b. Brown and well-formed
    c. Odorless and yellow
    d. Frequent, seedy, and bulky

BIBLIOGRAPHY

Anatasio, P: Flatulence felled by gas-fighting enzyme. Environmental Nutrition 2:3, 1991.

Bozian, R. Nutrition and the gut: The concept of "gut failure." Clinical Consultations in Nutritional Support 4:2, 1984.

Christian, JL and Greger, JL: Nutrition for Living, ed 3. Benjamin and Cummings, Redwood City, CA, 1991.

Feldman, EB: Essentials of Clinical Nutrition. FA Davis, Philadelphia, 1988.

Guyton, AC: Textbook of Medical Physiology, ed. WB Sanders, Philadelphia, 1986.

Gylys, BA and Wedding, ME: Medical Terminology. FA Davis, Philadelphia, 1988.

Pecora, A A: Lactose Intolerance. Osteopathic Medical News 7:7, 1990.
Pemberton, CM et al: Mayo Clinic Diet Manual: A Handbook of Dietary Practice, ed 6. BC Decker, Philadelphia, 1988.
Robinson, CH and Weigley, ES: Basic Nutrition and Diet Therapy. Macmillan, New York, 1989.

Chapter Outline

Key Terms

As a study aid, each key term is followed by the page number where the term is defined in the chapter. Terms that appear in **boldface** or <u>underscored</u> in the chapter text are located in the glossary.

Key Terms (Continued)

Learning Objectives

After completing this chapter, the student should be able to:

1. Differentiate between fat-soluble and water-soluble vitamins.
2. State the functions of each of the vitamins discussed.
3. Identify three food sources for each of the vitamins discussed.
4. List diseases caused by specific vitamin deficiencies and identify associated signs and symptoms.
5. Identify the vitamins considered to be potential public health issues in the United States.
6. Discuss the wise use of vitamin supplements.

*V*itamins were first recognized by the effects of their absence. Some deficiency diseases have been known for centuries, but it is only in this century that vitamins have been completely identified and isolated in the laboratory. In this chapter we will consider the importance of vitamins in the body and in the diet, the general functions of vitamins, the classification of vitamins, and the use of vitamin supplements. Each of the vitamins will be discussed from absorption through excretion, including functions, sources, recommended dietary allowances, deficiencies and toxicities, and factors affecting stability.

THE NATURE OF VITAMINS

Vitamin—Organic substance needed by the body in very small amounts; yields no energy and does not become part of the body's structure.

Coenzyme—A substance that combines with an enzyme to activate it.

Vitamins are organic substances needed by the body in small amounts for normal metabolism, growth, and maintenance. Organic substances are derived from living matter and contain carbon. Vitamins themselves are not sources of energy nor do they become part of the structure of the body. Vitamins act as regulators of metabolic processes and as **coenzymes** in enzymatic systems.

Specific Functions

Vitamin functions are specific; the bodily processes do not permit substitutes. Thus, vitamins are similar to keys in a lock. All the notches in a key have to fit the lock, or the key will not turn. One vitamin cannot perform the functions of another. If a person does not take in enough vitamin C, for instance, taking vitamin D will not correct the deficiency. Vitamin D is the wrong key for the lock.

Classification

A major distinguishing characteristic among vitamins is their solubility in either fat or water. This characteristic allows vitamins to be classified as either fat soluble or water soluble. Vitamins A, E, D, and K are fat soluble. The eight B-complex vitamins and vitamin C are water soluble. See Table 6–1 for a list of the 13 known vitamins.

TABLE 6–1 *Classification of Vitamins*

Fat Soluble	Water Soluble
Vitamin A	B-Complex
Vitamin D	Thiamin
Vitamin E	Riboflavin
Vitamin K	Niacin
	Vitamin B_6
	Folic acid
	Vitamin B_{12}
	Biotin
	Pantothenic acid
	Vitamin C

FAT-SOLUBLE VITAMINS

Vitamins A, D, E, and K are generally more stable than the water-soluble vitamins. They are more resistant to the effects of oxidation, heat, light, and aging. However, the fat-soluble vitamins can be adversely affected by dehydration and the drying action of sunlight.

Fat-soluble vitamins are absorbed from the intestine in the same way as fats, and like fats, they can be stored in the body. Because of this storage capacity, excessive intake of fat-soluble vitamins, especially vitamins A and D, can be fatal. Another effect caused by the storage of these vitamins is the slow development of signs of deficiency. Of the fat-soluble vitamins, only vitamin A is considered to be a potential public health issue (US Department of Health and Human Services, 1989).

Vitamin A

Vitamin A comes in two forms: preformed vitamin A, underlineretinol, and provitamin A, carotene. A **preformed vitamin** is already in a complete state in ingested foods. A provitamin requires conversion in the body to be in a complete state. Carotene (provitamin A) is converted to vitamin A in the intestine. The term precursor is often used interchangeably with the term provitamin. A precursor is a substance from which another substance is derived.

Preformed vitamin—a vitamin already in a complete state in ingested foods, as opposed to a provitamin, which requires conversion in the body to be in a complete state.

Absorption, Metabolism, and Excretion

Of preformed vitamin A, 80 to 90 percent is absorbed, whereas only 33 percent of carotene is absorbed. Vitamin A is transported bound to a protein. This complex is too large for the kidney to filter, so it is retained in the body.

Up to a year's supply of vitamin A is stored in the body, 90 percent of it in the liver. Excessive carotene is stored in adipose tissue, giving fat a yellowish tint, but it is harmless.

Functions of Vitamin A

Several crucial body functions depend on vitamin A. It is necessary for vision, for healthy epithelial tissue, and for proper bone growth.

CHEMICAL NECESSARY FOR VISION   The eye is like a camera. It has a dark layer to keep out stray light, a lens to focus light, and a light-sensitive layer at the back of the eye, called the retina. In the retina, light rays are changed into electrical impulses that travel along the optic nerve to the back of the brain. Vitamin A is part of the molecules of a chemical in the retina that is responsible for this conversion. The body can synthesize this chemical, called **rhodopsin,** or visual purple, only if it has a supply of vitamin A.

When the eye is functioning in dim light, rhodopsin is broken down into a protein, called opsin, and vitamin A. In darkness or during sleep, opsin and vitamin A are reunited to become rhodopsin. Figure 6–1 diagrams this reaction. The body can keep reusing the vitamin A, but some of it is depleted during each visual cycle. This explains why a dietary deficiency produces night blindness. Clinical Application 6–1 discusses a practical method used to conserve a person's rhodopsin for night vision.

Rhodopsin—light-sensitive protein containing vitamin A in the retina; also called visual purple.

HEALTH OF EPITHELIAL TISSUE   Epithelial tissue covers the body and lines the organs and passageways that open to the outside of the

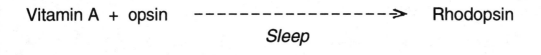

Vitamin A + opsin - - - - - - - - - - - - - - - -> Rhodopsin
Sleep

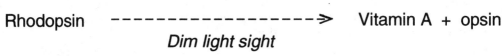

Rhodopsin - - - - - - - - - - - - - - - -> Vitamin A + opsin
Dim light sight

FIGURE 6–1. Vitamin A and the protein opsin combine while we sleep to form rhodopsin. When we need to see in dim light, the rhodopsin breaks down into vitamin A and opsin.

body. Skin is epithelial tissue, as is the surface of the eye and the lining of the alimentary canal. Epithelial tissue has a protective function, often producing mucus to wash out foreign materials. Vitamin A helps to keep epithelial tissue healthy by aiding the differentiation of specialty cells. This function has led some scientists to believe that vitamin A may play a role in cancer prevention. See Clinical Application 6–2 for more information on Vitamin A and cancer.

NORMAL BONE GROWTH   The mechanism by which vitamin A participates in bone growth and development is unclear. In children with vitamin A deficiency, some bones, such as those in the skull, stop growing, while other bones grow excessively.

Deficiency of Vitamin A

Even though vitamin A is stored in the body, deficiencies can occur. In some parts of the world vitamin A deficiency is widespread. Cases are common in India, south and east Asia, Africa, and Latin America. Vitamin A deficiency is second only to protein-calorie malnutrition as a nutritional problem affecting young people.

Vitamin A deficiency in the United States is due mostly to disease. For

---

CLINICAL APPLICATION 6–1

Red Light Conserves Rhodopsin

Red light breaks down rhodopsin more slowly than do other wavelengths of light. This is the reason aviators spend time in a red-lit room before flying at night. In the presence of red light, a buildup of rhodopsin occurs in the rods of the retina. Vision in dim light is thus enhanced. Red light is used on navigational instruments for the same reason.

CLINICAL APPLICATION 6–2
Vitamin A and Cancer

Fifty percent of fatal cancers begin with abnormal differentiation of epithelial cells. Vitamin A contributes to normal cell differentiation. It also functions as an antioxidant to neutralize free radicals. These highly reactive atoms or molecules can damage DNA, with resultant abnormal cell growth.

---

example, patients with long-lasting infectious disease, fat absorption problems, or liver disease are at risk of vitamin A deficiency.

SIGNS AND SYMPTOMS   Lack of vitamin A causes night blindness. In this condition the resynthesis of rhodopsin is too slow to allow quick adaptation to dim light.

All epithelial tissue suffers because of vitamin A deficiency. The person may have sinus trouble, a sore throat, and abscesses in the ears, mouth, and salivary glands. The most serious effect is the thickening of the epithelial tissue covering the eye. *Xerophthalmia* is an abnormal thickening and drying of the outer surface of the eye. It is a leading cause of blindness in some developing countries. An estimated 500,000 children are blinded each year by this deficiency. The unbelievable part of this tragedy is that a child's supplement of vitamin A would cost only 25 cents per year.

The other function of vitamin A is related to normal bone growth and development. In the person deficient in vitamin A, the cessation of bone growth produces brain and spinal cord injury.

Recommended Dietary Allowances

Vitamin A formerly was measured in <u>international units (IU).</u> You may have some patients who still think in those terms. Some supplements may be labeled in IU. The newer, more accurate measure of vitamin A activity is the **retinol equivalent (RE).** This measure encompasses both preformed vitamin A and carotene. One RE equals 3.3 IU from animal foods and 10 IU from plant foods; 1 RE corresponds to 1 **microgram** of retinol activity. Clinical Calculation 6–1 shows how IU are converted to RE.

The RDAs for vitamin A are: infants—375 micrograms RE; children—400 to 700 micrograms RE; male adolescents and adult men—1000 micrograms RE; female adolescents and adult and/or pregnant women—800 micrograms RE; lactating women: first 6 months—1300 micrograms RE, second 6 months—1200 micrograms RE.

Food Sources

Preformed vitamin A (retinol) is found in animal foods such as liver, kidney, egg yolk, butter, cream, milk, and fortified milk products. However, two thirds of the vitamin A in the American diet comes from carotene. Carotene is a yellow pigment found mostly in fruits and vegetables. Its presence can be readily seen in foods such as carrots, sweet potatoes, squash, apricots, and

Retinol equivalent (RE)—A measure of vitamin A activity which considers both preformed vitamin A (retinol) and its precursor (carotene); 1 RE equals 3.3 IU from animal foods and 10 IU from plant foods; 1 RE corresponds to 1 microgram of retinol.
Microgram—One millionth of a gram or one thousandth of a milligram; abbreviated mcg or μg.

cantaloupe. Although not as noticeable because chlorphyll masks the yellow color, carotene is also present in dark leafy green vegetables, including spinach, collards, broccoli, and cabbage.

Stability and Preservation

Vitamin A is fairly stable to heat, but sunlight, ultraviolet light, air, and oxidation easily destroy it. When you buy carrots, the ones that come packaged in plastic bags are better protected from light and air than the "bare" ones that have their tops secured by a rubber band.

Toxicity of Vitamin A

Because the liver can store large amounts of vitamin A, toxic effects may occur from the overconsumption of this fat-soluble vitamin.

Carotenemia— Excess carotene in body tissues, producing yellow skin but leaving whites of eyes white.

CAROTENEMIA   The condition resulting from ingesting too much carotene is called **carotenemia.** The person's skin becomes yellow, first on the palms of the hands and the soles of the feet. The whites of the eyes do not become yellow, however, as they do in jaundice caused by liver disease.

A person would have to eat 4 pounds of carrots per day or 1200 oranges in 6 weeks to develop this toxicity. Carotenemia has occurred in infants fed too many jars of carrots and squash. The skin returns to normal within 2 to 6 weeks after stopping the excessive intake. Carotenemia produces no adverse effects.

Hypervita-minosis—Condition caused by excessive intake of vitamins.

HYPERVITAMINOSIS A   Vitamin A toxicity is called **hypervitaminosis** A. Symptoms of vitamin A toxicity are similar to those of a brain tumor. Patients may complain of headaches and blurred vision and display signs of increased pressure within the skull. Other symptoms include pain in the bones and joints, dry skin, and poor appetite. Some patients developed symptoms after consuming beef liver once or twice a week.

One hazard is unique to the Arctic. Polar bear liver has made both men and dogs sick. It contains 390,000 IU per ounce or 354,545 micrograms RE per 3-ounce serving. This is 354 times the RDA for men. Other Arctic game poses similar hazards.

Vitamin D

Recently, vitamin D has come to be regarded as a hormone rather than a vitamin because of its functions. It may be many years before we stop calling it a vitamin, however.

Absorption, Metabolism, and Excretion

There are two metabolically active forms of vitamin D. Vitamin D_2, ergocalciferol, is formed when ergosterol (provitamin) in plants is irradiated by sunlight. Vitamin D_3 cholecalciferol, is formed when 7-dehydrocholesterol (another provitamin) in the skin is irradiated by ultraviolet or sunlight.

Both forms are absorbed into the blood. As with other fat-soluble vitamins, they are transported in the blood bound to protein. The liver alters the vitamin to calcidiol, an inactive form of vitamin D. By enzyme action, the kidney converts the calcidiol to calcitriol, the active form of vitamin D. Figure 6–2 diagrams the path of these processes.

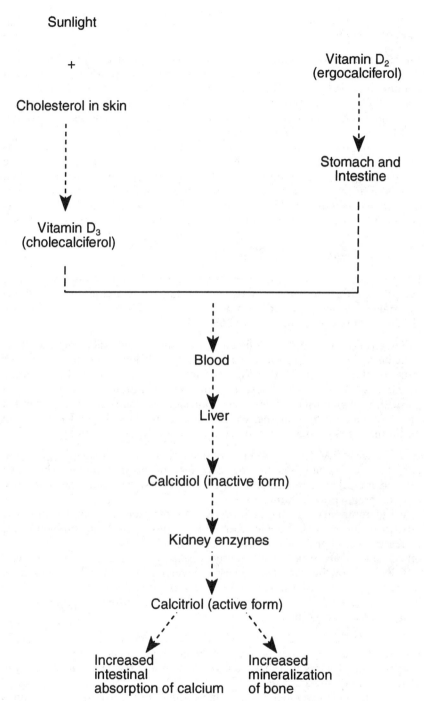

FIGURE 6–2. Vitamin D, whether from food or synthesis in the skin, is metabolized by the liver and the kidney to its most active form.

Functions of Vitamin D

Vitamin D functions to promote normal bone mineralization in three ways. (1) Vitamin D stimulates DNA to produce transport proteins, which bind calcium and phosphorus, thus increasing intestinal absorption of these minerals. (2) Once these minerals have been absorbed into the blood, vitamin D stimulates bone cells to use them to build and maintain bone tissue. (3) Vitamin D stimulates the kidneys to retain calcium.

Another control mechanism is also at work. Parathyroid hormone is secreted in response to a low serum calcium level. Parathyroid hormone causes the catabolism of bone to maintain a correct serum calcium level. The body's priority goal is maintenance of correct serum calcium for blood clotting, nerve function, and muscle contraction. Without this mechanism to sustain vital functions, a person would not live long enough to develop rickets.

Deficiency of Vitamin D

Lack of sunshine or vitamin D, chronic liver or kidney disease, or rare genetic disorders are causes of vitamin D deficiency. People in special circumstances are prone to developing deficiencies. Of particular concern are children whose bones are still growing.

RICKETS   Vitamin D deficiency in children is called rickets. This deficiency disease is seen in Canada and Great Britain, but there is almost none in the United States. Twenty-four cases occurred in Philadelphia between 1974 and 1978. These patients were children who belonged to a particular religious sect. They wore long hooded robes and ate vegetarian diets. At greatest risk in the United States are dark-skinned children in northern, smoggy cities or breast-fed infants not exposed to sunlight.

OSTEOMALACIA   Vitamin D deficiency in adults is called osteomalacia. This deficiency disease occurs most often in women who have insufficient calcium intake and little sunlight exposure, and who are frequently pregnant or lactating.

Environmental factors involved in osteomalacia are similar to those described for rickets. People with skin exposed to little sunlight have increased risk. Think of the probable sunlight exposure of cloistered nuns, office workers, institutionalized elderly persons, and residents of smoggy areas.

Because of the complex processes involved in vitamin D metabolism, liver or kidney disease can lead to bone deterioration. Chronic kidney failure has caused osteomalacia due to the inability of the kidneys to convert vitamin D to its active form.

SIGNS AND SYMPTOMS   Children with rickets have soft, fragile bones. Classic deformities occur, such as bowlegs, knock knees, and a misshapen skull. Infants may have **tetany** due to low levels of blood calcium. Calcium and tetany are discussed in Chapter 7.

Adults with osteomalacia also have increasing softness of the bones causing deformities due to loss of calcium. The bones most commonly affected are those of the spine, pelvis, and lower extremities.

Tetany—Muscle contractions, especially of the wrists and ankles, resulting from low levels of ionized calcium in the blood; causes include parathyroid deficiency, vitamin D deficiency, and alkalosis.

Recommended Dietary Allowances

Vitamin D is measured in micrograms of cholecalciferol. The RDAs for vitamin D are: infants—7.5 micrograms; children through adults age 24—10 micrograms; adult men and women—5 micrograms; pregnant and/or lactating women—10 micrograms.

As with vitamin A, vitamin D formerly was measured in International Units (IU). Some fortified foods or supplements still may be labeled this way. Four hundred IU of vitamin D is equal to 10 micrograms of cholecalciferol. Clinical Calculation 6–2 illustrates this conversion.

Sources of Vitamin D

Two sources of vitamin D are readily available to most people. Vitamin D is synthesized by the body, and it is added to most dairy products in the United States.

SUNLIGHT   A major source of vitamin D is the body itself. Vitamin D is manufactured in the skin. Children with low dietary intakes may escape rickets if they are exposed to sunlight.

Light-skinned adults can obtain the necessary 5 micrograms of cholecalciferol by exposing their hands, arms, and face to sunlight for 15 minutes twice a week. It is not possible to overdose on vitamin D by sunning yourself.

FOOD   If a person is not exposed to sunshine, food sources of vitamin D become important. Few natural foods contain enough vitamin D to meet recommended intakes. Our grandparents used cod liver oil. Although it does not taste very good, cod liver oil does contain 100 percent of the RDA in only 1 teaspoonful.

The major food source of vitamin D in the United States is fortified milk. One quart of fortified milk provides the RDA for children. Milk is the ideal food to link with vitamin D since it also contains calcium and phosphorus, which are necessary for bone anabolism. See Clinical Application 6–3 for a discussion of the fortification of foods.

Stability and Preservation

Vitamin D is stable to heat and not easily oxidized. Little special handling of foods is necessary.

 CLINICAL APPLICATION 6–3
Fortification of Foods

Fortification and enrichment of foods differ in meaning. Enrichment of grain products is done to replace some of the nutrients lost in milling. These vitamins and minerals are added to bring the grain closer to the original in amounts of thiamin, riboflavin, niacin, and iron.

Fortification is the process of adding nutrients to food products in amounts greater than those normally present. The original intent was to prevent deficiencies. Examples of fortification are the addition of vitamins A and D to milk and margarine. Also, many breakfast cereals are fortified with nutrients not naturally found in grains. Fluid milk must be fortified with vitamin D in the United States, but there are no mandates for other dairy products.

Interfering Factors

A high-fiber diet interferes with the absorption of vitamin D. Abnormalities of absorption such as diarrhea, fat malabsorption, and biliary obstruction also may lead to vitamin D deficiency.

Toxicity of Vitamin D

Since vitamin D is stored in the body, it is possible to ingest too much. Hypervitaminosis D is the term for toxicity from this vitamin.

MOST TOXIC OF VITAMINS   Vitamin D from supplements or even foods can be hazardous to your health. Vitamin D is the most toxic of all vitamins. Ten times the RDA for adults and two times the RDA for children, taken for a prolonged period, can be toxic. Infants face increased risk from multiple fortified foods. One quart of prepared commercial formula contains 10 micrograms of cholecalciferol, the same as a quart of fortified milk. Infants up to 6 months old require only 7.5 micrograms per day.

SIGNS AND SYMPTOMS   Early symptoms of hypervitaminosis D include loss of appetite, nausea, vomiting, diarrhea, bloody stools, polyuria, muscular weakness, and headaches. The more serious consequences of vitamin D overdose are related to the calcium that is deposited in soft tissue. The person develops calcium deposits in the heart, kidney, and brain. This will be discussed in greater detail in the chapter on kidney disease.

Vitamin E

The third fat-soluble vitamin is vitamin E. Much less is known about vitamin E than about vitamins A and D.

Absorption, Metabolism, and Excretion

Most vitamin E is stored in adipose tissue. Maximum transfer of vitamin E across the placenta occurs just before term delivery.

Functions of Vitamin E

Antioxidant— Substance that prevents or inhibits the uptake of oxygen; in the body, antioxidants prevent tissue damage from unstable molecules; in food, antioxidants prevent deterioration; vitamins A, C, and E and selenium are antioxidants.

The major function of vitamin E is as an **antioxidant.** Oxidation is the process of a substance combining with oxygen. Several substances can be destroyed by oxidation, including vitamin E, vitamin A, and vitamin C. Some molecules become very unstable when they are oxidized. Their accelerated movements can damage nearby molecules. Vitamin E accepts oxygen instead of allowing other molecules to become unstable. In this role, vitamin E protects vitamin A and unsaturated fatty acids from oxidation. One particular location where this is important is in the lungs. Vitamin E in lung cell membranes provides an important barrier against air pollution. It also protects the stability of the polyunsaturated fatty acids in the red-blood-cell membranes from oxidation in the lungs.

Deficiency of Vitamin E

In animals, vitamin E deficiency produces sterility. In several species of animals, a deficiency of vitamin E suppresses the immune system, whereas supplementation stimulates it.

Deficiency of vitamin E in humans is very rare. Muscle weakness and forms of muscular dystrophy are seen in cases of chronic fat malabsorption. Premature infants with inadequate reserves of vitamin E develop anemia. Without sufficient vitamin E the membranes of the red blood cells break down easily when exposed to oxygen or an oxidizing agent.

Recommended Dietary Allowances

Vitamin E is measured in milligrams of <u>alpha-tocopherol equivalents</u> (α-TE). As with vitamins A and D, the old measure of vitamin E was International Units. One milligram of alpha-tocopherol equivalents equals 1.5 International Units.

The RDAs for vitamin E are: infants—3 to 4 milligrams α-TE; children—6 to 7 milligrams α-TE; male adolescents and men—10 milligrams α-TE; female adolescents and women—8 milligrams α-TE; pregnant women—10 milligrams α-TE; lactating women: first 6 months—12 milligrams α-TE, second 6 months—11 milligrams α-TE.

Food Sources of Vitamin E

Vitamin E occurs with polyunsaturated fatty acids. The best source is vegetable oils, but whole grains and wheat germ also provide vitamin E. Other sources include milk, eggs, meats, fish, and leafy vegetables.

Stability and Preservation

Vitamin E is fairly stable to heat and acid. Normal cooking temperatures do not destroy it, but frying does. Vitamin E is unstable to light, alkalies, and oxygen.

Toxicity of Vitamin E

Very large supplemental doses of more than 600 milligrams of alpha-tocopherol daily (60 times the RDA) for a year or longer may cause excessive bleeding, impaired wound healing, and depression. Clinical Application 6–4 describes a patient with vitamin E toxicity.

Vitamin K

It is important for nurses to understand the functions of vitamin K because it is often prescribed as a medication. It also can interfere with a commonly prescribed anticoagulant.

Absorption, Metabolism, and Excretion

Three forms of vitamin K can meet the body's needs. Vitamin K_1, or <u>phylloquinone,</u> is the one found in foods. Vitamin K_2, or <u>menaquinone,</u> is synthesized by intestinal bacteria. Vitamin K_3, or <u>menadione,</u> is the synthetic, water-soluble pharmaceutical form of the vitamin. Vitamin K_3 is two to three times more potent than naturally occurring vitamin K.

CLINICAL APPLICATION 6–4
Vitamin E Toxicity

A patient was admitted to the hospital for narcolepsy. This is a disorder characterized by recurrent, uncontrollable, brief periods of sleep from which the individual is easily awakened. This patient would fall asleep while driving his car.

Narcolepsy can be a sign of uremia, hypoglycemia, diabetes, hypothyroidism, increased intracranial pressure, tumor of the brainstem or hypothalamus, or absence epilepsy. If all of these causes are ruled out, the medical diagnosis is either classical or independent narcolepsy.

During her assessment, the dietitian discovered only one unusual nutritional practice. She asked the patient if he was taking any vitamin or mineral supplements. Yes, he was. A clerk in a health foods store had recommended vitamin E. The patient had begun and continued this self-prescribed supplement.

The dietitian's investigation of vitamin E's adverse effects led her to suggest to the physician that the narcolepsy could be caused by excessive vitamin E. The patient discontinued the vitamin E and the narcolepsy disappeared.

In this case, a thorough nutritional assessment and an inquiring attitude saved the patient much discomfort (and his insurance company many dollars) by eliminating the need for extensive diagnostic tests. Often, patients do not think of dietary supplements as medications. The nurse should always ask specifically about what vitamin and mineral preparations, if any, the patient is taking.

Functions of Vitamin K

The role of vitamin K in blood clotting has been known for a long time. An additional function of vitamin K relates to bone metabolism.

BLOOD CLOTTING   At least 13 different proteins plus the mineral calcium are involved in blood clotting. Vitamin K is necessary for the liver to make factors II (**prothrombin**), VII, IX, and X. These factors are key links in the chain of events producing a blood clot.

BONE METABOLISM   In 1974, a protein was identified in bone which depends upon vitamin K. Vitamin K participates with vitamin D in synthesizing this bone protein which helps to regulate serum calcium.

Prothrombin—A protein essential to the blood clotting process; manufactured by the liver using vitamin K.

Deficiency of Vitamin K

The intestinal tract of the newborn infant is sterile. For this reason the baby is unable to produce vitamin K until the intestine picks up bacteria from the infant's environment, usually within 24 hours. To prevent bleeding problems, a dose of vitamin K_3 may be administered to the mother late in labor or to the infant immediately after birth.

Deficiencies have been associated with disease and drug therapy. Fat absorption problems may hinder vitamin K absorption, resulting in prolonged blood-clotting time. Antibiotics kill off the normal bacteria in the intestine as well as the organisms causing an infection. In one study, 31 percent of patients with gastrointestinal disorders given antibiotics for prolonged periods developed vitamin K deficiencies (Krasinski and Russell, 1985).

Recommended Dietary Allowances

The RDAs for vitamin K are: infants—5 to 10 micrograms; children—15 to 30 micrograms; boys and girls 11 to 14 years old—45 micrograms; male adolescents 45 to 65 micrograms; female adolescents 45 to 55 micrograms; men 19 to 24 years old—70 micrograms; women 19 to 24 years old—60 micrograms; adult men 25 years of age and older—80 micrograms; adult women 25 years of age and older and pregnant and lactating women—65 micrograms. The typical US diet supplies 300 to 500 micrograms.

Sources of Vitamin K

The body is capable of manufacturing some vitamin K. Many common foods contain adequate amounts also.

INTESTINAL SYNTHESIS Approximately half the body's needed vitamin K is manufactured by intestinal bacteria. This synthesis takes place in the large intestine.

FOOD SOURCES Liver, green leafy vegetables, vegetables of the cabbage family, and milk are the best sources of vitamin K. Examples of the vegetables include lettuce, spinach, asparagus, kale, cabbage, cauliflower, broccoli, and brussels sprouts.

Stability of Vitamin K

Vitamin K resists heat but is unstable in the presence of oxygen, light, alkalies, and strong acids.

Interfering Factors

Overconsumption of some vitamins can trigger a deficiency of others. Excessive intakes of vitamins A and E may interfere with vitamin K. The anticoagulant <u>warfarin sodium</u> interferes with the liver's use of vitamin K. However, this is the desired effect of the medication.

Toxicity of Vitamin K

The naturally occuring forms, vitamins K_1 and K_2, do not cause toxicity. Vitamin K_3, menadione, can cause liver damage, jaundice, excessive bleeding, hemolysis of red blood cells, and brain damage. As with all drugs, extra care must be taken when administering vitamin K to infants. Overdose in an infant may cause <u>hemolytic anemia,</u> hyperbilirubinemia, and irreversible brain damage.

Table 6–2 shows amounts of a variety of foods that would provide the

TABLE 6–2 *Amounts of Food Providing the Adult RDA for Fat-Soluble Vitamins*

Vitamin and Adult RDA	Amounts of Food Providing Adult RDA*	Number of Exchanges
Vitamin A	⅓ cup grated raw carrot	⅓ Vegetable
800–1000 micrograms	½ cup frozen or canned carrots	1 Vegetable
	3 pieces canned sweet potatoes, 3″ × 1 ″	1.5 Starch/Bread
		0.7 Medium-fat
	1 chicken liver	meat
Vitamin D	2 cups fortified milk	2 Milk
5 micrograms		
Vitamin E	2 tablespoons vegetable oil	6 Fat
8–10 milligrams	⅛ cup sunflower seeds	2 Fat
Vitamin K	¼ cup broccoli, cooked	½ Vegetable
65–80 micrograms	⅜ cup lettuce	Free
	⅜ cup cabbage, cooked	¾ Vegetable
	3 ounces liver	3 Medium-fat meat

*In cases with a range, food amounts were calculated to provide the higher RDA.

adult RDA for each of the fat-soluble vitamins; the table equates the amount of food to the Exchange System. Table 6–3 summarizes the stability of vitamins to environmental conditions. See Clinical Application 6–5 for a description of two conditions that mimic deficiencies of fat-soluble vitamins.

TABLE 6–3 *Factors Affecting Stability of Vitamins*

	Stable to				
Vitamin	Oxygen	Heat	Light	Acids	Alkalies
Fat Soluble					
A	No	Yes	No	No	*
D	Yes	Yes	Yes	*	*
E	No	Yes	No	Yes	No
K	No	Yes	No	No	No
Water Soluble					
C	No	No	No	Yes	No
Thiamin	No	No	*	*	No
Riboflavin	Yes	Yes	No	Yes	No
Niacin	Yes	Yes	Yes	Yes	Yes
B_6	*	Yes	No	Yes	No
Folic acid	No	No	No	No	Yes
B_{12}	No	Yes	No	No	No

*Data unavailable.

CLINICAL APPLICATION 6–5

CONDITIONS MIMICKING DEFICIENCIES OF FAT-SOLUBLE VITAMINS

PROTEIN DEFICIENCY

Water and fat do not mix. To circulate fats in the water-based blood, the liver attaches fat-soluble vitamins to protein carriers. Sometimes a protein deficiency hinders the use of the fat-soluble vitamins.

ZINC DEFICIENCY

Vitamin A is carried from storage in the liver to the tissues by a zinc-containing protein. For this reason zinc deficiency can mimic vitamin A deficiency.

WATER-SOLUBLE VITAMINS

Vitamins that dissolve in water are vitamin C, or ascorbic acid, and the B vitamins. Water-soluble vitamins cannot accumulate in the body in appreciable amounts. The B vitamins include thiamin, riboflavin, niacin, pyridoxine, folic acid, vitamin B_{12}, pantothenic acid, and biotin.

Water-soluble vitamins are easily destroyed by cooking. For example, one third to one half of the vitamin content is lost in the cooking water of boiled vegetables. However, in spite of the heavy losses of all water-soluble vitamins through cooking, only intakes of vitamin C, vitamin B_6, and folic acid are considered to be potential public health issues (US Department of Health and Human Services, 1989).

Vitamin C

A body deprived of vitamin C rapidly depletes its stores. The deficiency disease due to lack of vitamin C is **scurvy.** Most animals are not susceptible to scurvy; their livers manufacture vitamin C. Humans, along with other primates, guinea pigs, some birds, some fish, and fruit-eating bats, cannot synthesize vitamin C.

Scurvy—Disease due to deficiency of vitamin C, marked by bleeding problems and, later, by bony skeleton changes.

Absorption, Metabolism, and Excretion

Vitamin C is absorbed from the small intestine. A small amount of vitamin C is stored in the adrenal glands, liver, and spleen. As the amount of vitamin C consumed increases, the proportion of the vitamin that is absorbed decreases. So if 100 milligrams is ingested, 90 percent is absorbed. If 1,000 milligrams is ingested, less than 70 percent is absorbed. If 10,000 milligrams is taken, less than 20 percent is absorbed. Whatever is absorbed in excess of body needs is excreted in the urine.

Functions of Vitamin C

Vitamin C has diverse functions in the body. It contributes to wound and fracture healing, serves as an antioxidant, and is necessary for adrenal gland function. It enhances the absorption of iron and converts folic acid to an active form.

WOUND AND FRACTURE HEALING   Vitamin C contributes to the healing of wounds, burns, and fractures. It is necessary to the formation of **collagen,** the single most important protein of connective tissue. Both bone and scar tissue contain collagen.

Collagen—
Fibrous insoluble protein found in connective tissue.

ANTIOXIDANT   Vitamin C is a powerful antioxidant. By preventing the uptake of oxygen by other molecules, it deters the destruction of tissue by unstable molecules. Vitamin C is more susceptible to oxidation than either vitamin E or vitamin A; thus it is called the antioxidants' antioxidant.

ADRENAL GLAND FUNCTION   High concentrations of vitamin C are found in the adrenal glands. These are the organs that secrete adrenalin, the "fight or flight" hormone, in times of stress. Vitamin C aids in the release of adrenalin from the adrenal glands. Emotional and physical stress increase the body's need for vitamin C by three to four times.

IRON ABSORPTION   Vitamin C facilitates iron absorption. It acts with hydrochloric acid to keep iron in the more absorbable ferrous (2^+) form. Four ounces of orange juice nearly quadruples the iron absorbed from plant foods consumed with it.

FOLIC ACID CONVERSION   Vitamin C converts folic acid to an active form. For this reason deficiency of vitamin C can lead to **anemia** due to inefficient use of iron and folic acid.

Anemia—Condition of less than normal values for red blood cells or hemoglobin or both.

Deficiency of Vitamin C

Until the 17th century, sailors on long voyages often died of scurvy due to lack of vitamin C. The disease develops within 3 months after vitamin C is eliminated from the diet.

SIGNS AND SYMPTOMS   Early signs of scurvy are tender, sore gums that bleed easily and small skin hemorrhages due to weakened blood vessels. The later clinical picture of scurvy is related to the breakdown of collagen. Wound healing is delayed; even healed scars may separate. The ends of long bones soften, become malformed and painful, and fractures appear. The teeth loosen in their sockets and fall out. Hemorrhages occur about the joints, stomach, and heart. Untreated, scurvy progresses to often sudden death, probably from internal bleeding.

TREATMENT   Moderate doses of vitamin C will cure scurvy. A daily dose of 300 milligrams replenishes the body tissues in 5 days.

PREVALENCE OF VITAMIN C DEFICIENCY   As many as 25 percent of persons surveyed have a vitamin C intake well below the RDA. Intake may be less than half the RDA for infants, teens, and the elderly. At particular risk are elderly persons living alone, persons avoiding acidic foods, and patients receiving peritoneal or hemodialysis.

Recommended Dietary Allowances

The RDAs for vitamin C are: infants—30 to 35 milligrams; children—40 to 45 milligrams; boys and girls 11 to 14 years old—50 milligrams; men and women 15 years of age and older—60 milligrams; pregnant women—70 milligrams; lactating women: first 6 months—95 milligrams, second 6 months—90 milligrams.

As little as 10 milligrams per day *prevents* scurvy. A daily intake of 200 milligrams completely saturates the tissues. After major surgery or extensive burns, a patient may need up to 1000 milligrams of vitamin C per day.

Food Sources of Vitamin C

Many people automatically associate vitamin C with citrus fruits. They are excellent sources. Other good sources of vitamin C include tomatoes, white potatoes, cabbage, broccoli, chard, kale, turnip greens, asparagus, berries, melons, pineapple, and guavas. Figure 6–3 illustrates nutrient-dense produce that would meet the body's RDA for both vitamin A and vitamin C.

Stability and Preservation

Vitamin C is destroyed by air, light, heat, or alkalies. Oxygen or air destroys vitamin C. Boiling the cooking water for 1 minute before adding the food eliminates the dissolved oxygen that would oxidize the vitamin C. Because air destroys vitamin C, orange juice should be stored in a container which holds only an amount that can be consumed in a short time.

Vitamin C is destroyed by heat. Vegetables should be cooked as quickly

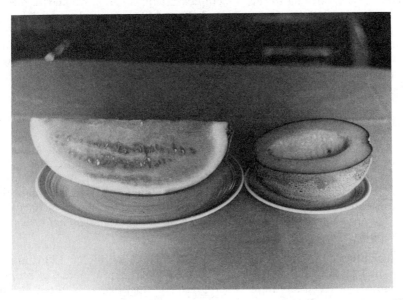

FIGURE 6–3. Both cantaloupe and watermelon are vitamin-dense fruits. One half of a cantaloupe or an 8 X 8 inch wedge of watermelon would each provide the adult RDA of both vitamin A and vitamin C.

as possible. Crisp-cooked is better than limp-cooked for retaining the vitamin C content.

Vitamin C is destroyed by alkalies. For example, adding baking soda to foods containing vitamin C destroys the vitamin C. In years past many food establishments routinely added baking soda to vegetables to enhance their color. Fortunately this is now illegal.

Interfering Factor

Smokers deplete vitamin C faster than nonsmokers. At least 140 milligrams per day are required by smokers to achieve the same tissue saturation as nonsmokers do with 60 milligrams. Unfortunately, many smokers do not consume even the RDA.

Toxicity of Vitamin C

Rebound scurvy—Vitamin C deficiency produced in a person following cessation of megadosing due to a habitually lessened rate of absorption.

Megadose—Dose ten times the RDA

The body's lackadaisical efforts at absorption in the presence of abundance explains **rebound scurvy**. If a person who is taking **megadoses** of vitamin C suddenly stops the supplement, the body cannot adjust quickly enough. It continues to absorb a meager proportion of the now smaller dose. A similar condition occurs in newborns whose mothers took megadoses of vitamin C during pregnancy. Scurvy can occur under these circumstances.

Excessive vitamin C causes false readings in two common laboratory tests. Some urine glucose tests will read falsely positive. Stool guaiac for occult blood will read falsely negative.

B-Complex Vitamins

Eight vitamins belong to the B-Complex group: thiamin, riboflavin, niacin, pyridoxine (B_6), folic acid, cyanocobalamin (B_{12}), pantothenic acid, and biotin. They all function as coenzymes. A coenzyme joins with an enzyme to activate it. If a person lacks the coenzyme, the effect is the same as lacking the enzyme itself. Many of the actions of the B-complex vitamins are interrelated. However, there are some diseases, including beriberi and pellegra, associated with single B-vitamin deficiencies.

Thiamin

Beriberi is the deficiency disease due to the lack of thiamin, a vitamin originally named B_1. The neurological symptoms of beriberi were recognized in China in 2600 BC, but it was not until 1937 that thiamin was chemically identified as the causative agent. The enrichment of food products has almost eliminated this disease, but it is still seen in alcoholics in the West and in persons in developing countries where enrichment may not be a standard practice.

ABSORPTION, METABOLISM, AND EXCRETION Thiamin is absorbed in the small intestine. The need for thiamin increases proportionately with carbohydrate intake. Excess thiamin is excreted in the urine.

FUNCTIONS OF THIAMIN Thiamin is a coenzyme in carbohydrate metabolism. It is involved in the production of energy from glucose and helps oxidize glucose to form a compound which stores energy. It is also used to metabolize alcohol to energy. Thiamin is required to convert tryptophan to niacin, another B-vitamin.

DEFICIENCY The deficiency disease beriberi is characterized by neurological, cerebral, and cardiovascular abnormalities. Initially, symptoms such as anorexia, indigestion, and constipation occur because the digestive process is disrupted due to interrupted glucose metabolism. Without a continual supply of glucose for the CNS, apathy, fatigue, and muscle weakness set in. The myelin sheaths covering peripheral nerves eventually degenerate, resulting in paralysis and muscle atrophy. If the thiamin deficiency continues, cardiac failure and then death is the result.

Wernicke-Korsakoff syndrome, a neurological disorder associated with chronic alcoholism, results from thiamin deficiency. Thiamin is used to convert alcohol to energy. Patients with Wernicke's encephalopathy display many motor and sensory deficits. The person with Korsakoff's psychosis has memory deficits.

RECOMMENDED DIETARY ALLOWANCES The RDAs for thiamine are: infants—0.3 to 0.4 milligram, children—0.7 to 1 milligram; boys 11 to 14 years old—1.3 milligrams; men 15 to 50 years old—1.5 milligrams; men 51 years of age and older—1.2 milligrams; girls 11 to 14 years old and women 15 to 50 years old—1.1 milligrams; women 51 years of age and older—1 milligram; pregnant women—1.5 milligrams; lactating women—1.6 milligrams.

The need for thiamin increases as kilocalorie consumption increases. An athlete consuming 4000 kilocalories needs twice as much as an office worker consuming 1800 kilocalories. Fasting does not decrease need for thiamin, however. The need is proportional to energy expenditure, not simply food intake.

FOOD SOURCES The table of the Nutritive Values of the Edible Part of Foods shows that few foods supply a day's allowance in a single serving for an adult (see Appendix (A). Pork, wheat germ, and brewer's yeast are the best sources. Many other commonly consumed foods—such as beef, liver, legumes, eggs, and fish—contain lesser amounts. A person who chooses enriched grains and eats a balanced diet should have no problems with lack of thiamin.

STABILITY Thiamin is destroyed by air and heat. The destruction is especially pronounced in the presence of alkalies.

INTERFERING FACTORS An enzyme in raw fish, thiaminase, destroys up to 50 percent of thiamin. A more commonly ingested substance in the United States is tea. Tea contains an **antagonist** to thiamin.

Antagonist—A substance that counteracts the action of another substance.

Riboflavin

Riboflavin, or B_2, was discovered when laboratory workers observed a yellow-green fluorescent pigment that formed crystals.

ABSORPTION, METABOLISM, AND EXCRETION Absorption of riboflavin occurs in the small intestine. Only small amounts are stored in the liver and kidneys, so daily needs must be supplied in the diet.

FUNCTIONS   Riboflavin is a coenzyme in the metabolism of protein. Thyroid and adrenal hormones control the conversion of riboflavin to the active coenzyme, which is involved in deamination and tissue building.

DEFICIENCY   Riboflavin deficiency often occurs with thiamine and niacin deficiencies. A person who avoids all dairy products, however, may be deficient in riboflavin alone, termed ariboflavinosis. Signs of this deficiency include lesions on the lips and in the oral cavity, seborrheic dermatitis, scrotal or vulval skin changes, and normocytic anemia.

RECOMMENDED DIETARY ALLOWANCES   The RDAs for riboflavin are: infants—0.4 to 0.5 milligram; children—0.8 to 1.2 milligrams; boys 11 to 14 years old—1.5 milligrams; male adolescents—1.8 milligrams; men 19 to 50 years old—1.7 milligrams; men 51 years of age and older—1.4 milligrams; girls 11 to 14 years old and women 15 to 50 years old—1.3 milligrams; women 51 years of age or older—1.2 milligrams; pregnant women—1.6 milligrams; lactating women: first 6 months—1.8 milligrams, second 6 months—1.7 milligrams.

Riboflavin needs increase as protein needs increase. Patients facing major healing processes, such as those with extensive burns, require more riboflavin than the average person.

FOOD SOURCES   Good sources are organ meats, milk, whole or enriched grains, legumes, and vegetables.

STABILITY   Riboflavin is relatively stable to heat but is sensitive to ultraviolet light. This is one reason to package milk in cardboard cartons. The other modern container, the plastic bottle, filters out more light than the old glass bottle.

Niacin

Niacin, or nicotinic acid, is also labeled as vitamin B_3. Lack of niacin causes a specific disease, pellagra.

ABSORPTION, METABOLISM, AND EXCRETION   Not all nutrients present in a food are available to the body. Niacin is a good example. Niacin is found in corn but in a bound form that cannot be absorbed. Treating the corn with lye, as is done in some Latin American cultures, frees the niacin for the body's use.

Not all the body's niacin has to come from preformed niacin in food. The body can convert the amino acid tryptophan to niacin. This is the only known vitamin with an amino acid for a provitamin.

FUNCTIONS OF NIACIN   Niacin is a coenzyme in the production of energy from glucose. Niacin also participates in the synthesis of fatty acids.

Pellagra—Deficiency disease due to lack of niacin and tryptophan; characterized by the 3 Ds: dermatitis, diarrhea, and dementia.

DEFICIENCY   **Pellagra** is the deficiency disease due to lack of niacin. To have a deficiency, a person must have a diet lacking in both niacin and tryptophan. Adults can get up to 67 percent of their niacin from foods containing complete proteins.

Pellagra has serious effects. The "three Ds" are its major symptoms: dermatitis, diarrhea, and dementia. The dermatitis is a red rash on the face, neck, hands, and feet. The rash is bilaterally symmetrical; on the hands and arms it sometimes resembles gloves.

RECOMMENDED DIETARY ALLOWANCES   Niacin is measured in niacin equivalents (NE). One milligram of niacin equivalent is the same as 1 milligram of preformed niacin or 60 milligrams of tryptophan.

The RDAs for niacin are: infants—5 to 6 milligrams NE; children—9 to 13 milligrams NE; boys 11 to 14 years old—17 milligrams NE; male adolescents—20 milligrams NE; men 19 to 50 years old—19 milligrams NE; men 51 years of age and older, girls 11 to 14 years old, and women 15 to 50 years old—15 milligrams NE; women 51 years of age and older—13 milligrams NE; pregnant women—17 milligrams NE; lactating women—20 milligrams NE.

FOOD SOURCES   Preformed niacin occurs in significant amounts of meat. Other sources include peanuts and other legumes. Coffee also contains niacin and prevents pellagra in cultures with low protein and high coffee intakes.

STABILITY   Niacin is a water-soluble vitamin. Small amounts are lost in cooking water. Niacin is stable to heat, light, air, acid, and alkalies. It is the most environmentally stable vitamin.

TOXICITY   Pharmacologic doses of niacin cause flushing. The large doses prescribed to lower blood lipid levels over the long term can cause liver damage (Committee on Diet and Health, 1989). A case of niacin toxicity from food is reported in Clinical Application 6–6. It explains how food poisoning epidemics are investigated and what the nurse's responsibilities are when assisting with the investigation.

CLINICAL APPLICATION 6–6
Niacin Toxicity

In late 1980, almost half the patients in a small nursing home in Illinois became ill after breakfast. Their faces became flushed, or they developed a rash 15 to 30 minutes after the meal. As in suspected food poisoning epidemics, the foods consumed were compared. Which food was eaten by all those who became ill, but by none of those who did not become ill? In this case, it was cornmeal mush.

Careful observation and documentation is important in food poisoning cases. The sequence of signs and symptoms may steer the investigators in the right direction. Often the signs and symptoms have disappeared by the time the physician arrives. In this nursing home, the signs and symptoms lasted only an average of 50 minutes.

If food poisoning is suspected, health authorities take samples of the food to examine in the laboratory. None of the leftover food should be discarded before health authorities arrive. The Food and Drug Administration tested the cornmeal from the nursing home's kitchen. It contained more than 1000 milligrams of niacin per pound. The recommended amount for cornmeal is 16 to 24 milligrams per pound.

Often a food poisoning epidemic has run its course by the time the source of the outbreak is known. In this case, the offending food was identified, but the method of contamination never was positively determined.

Vitamin B$_6$

This vitamin serves in many roles, but its lack is not described as a specific disease. The name for the pharmaceutical preparation of vitamin B$_6$ is <u>pyridoxine.</u>

ABSORPTION, METABOLISM, AND EXCRETION   Pyridoxine is absorbed in the small intestine and is found throughout the body (tissue saturation).

FUNCTIONS   Vitamin B$_6$ is a coenzyme in the synthesis and catabolism of amino acids. It is involved in the metabolism of more than 60 enzymes. Vitamin B$_6$ functions as a coenzyme in the conversion of tryptophan into niacin. It helps to manufacture antibodies. The hormone epinephrine and the neurotransmitters <u>dopamine</u> and <u>serotonin</u> all require vitamin B$_6$ as a coenzyme. It also participates in amino acid transport and the transfer of sulfur and nitrogen to form other compounds.

DEFICIENCY   A deficiency of B$_6$ is unlikely due to the large amounts present in the general diet. However, factors such as drug interactions or errors in food processing may cause a deficiency. In years past, improperly processed commercial infant formula produced vitamin B$_6$ deficiencies.
Vitamin B$_6$ deficiency risk is increased by the use of oral contraceptives. Women using oral contraceptives for more than 2 or 3 years require additional vitamin B$_6$ due to an abnormal tryptophan metabolism. Infants of mothers who took oral contraceptives for more than 30 months before pregnancy should also be monitored for deficiency.

RECOMMENDED DIETARY ALLOWANCES   The RDAs for vitamin B$_6$ are: infants—0.3 to 0.6 milligram; children—1 to 1.4 milligrams; boys 11 to 14 years old—1.7 milligrams; male adolescents and men—2 milligrams; girls 11 to 14 years old—1.4 milligrams; female adolescents—1.5 milligrams; women—1.6 milligrams; pregnant women—2.2 milligrams; lactating women—2.1 milligrams. An increase in protein metabolism increases the need for vitamin B$_6$.

FOOD SOURCES   Vitamin B$_6$ is widely distributed in foods. Pork and organ meats are the best animal sources. Whole grains and wheat germ are the best plant sources. Vitamin B$_6$ is not included in the enrichment of breads so whole wheat bread contains more of this vitamin than white bread. Other good sources include legumes, potatoes, oatmeal, and bananas.

STABILITY   As with other water-soluble vitamins, vitamin B$_6$ is preserved when vegetables are cooked as quickly as possible. Vitamin B$_6$ is relatively stable to heat and acids, but very sensitive to light and easily destroyed by alkalies.

TOXICITY   Pyridoxine toxicity has resulted from taking 2 to 6 grams per day for 2 to 40 months. These megadoses, 1000 to 2700 times the RDA, were self-prescribed. Signs and symptoms include sensory loss and numbness of the hands and feet, resulting in clumsiness and severe ataxia. Cessation of the drug permitted some, but not all, function to return.

Folic Acid

Also known as folate, <u>folic acid</u> affects many different tissues in the body. Inadequate supplies, understandably, produce extensive symptoms.

ABSORPTION, METABOLISM, AND EXCRETION The folic acid in food usually is bound to amino acids. The enzyme to split off the folic acid is called folate conjugase. It is found in salivary, gastric, pancreatic, and jejunal secretions. The unbound folate is absorbed through the intestinal wall and transported to the liver. In the liver some of the folate is processed for storage in the tissues and the liver. Some folate is secreted into bile. When the gallbladder releases bile into the duodenum, the folate may again be split off and absorbed. The recycling process is important because folate stores are adequate for only 2 to 4 months.

FUNCTIONS Folic acid is necessary for the formation of DNA. Thus, folate participates in the reproduction of every cell, not just the ovum and sperm. Folic acid is active in cell renewal and is necessary for rapidly growing cells, including those in the GI tract, blood, and fetal tissue. It also functions in the formation of **heme.**

Heme—The iron-containing portion of the hemoglobin molecule.

DEFICIENCY Folic acid deficiency is probably the most common vitamin deficiency due to inadequate food intake. At risk are poorly nourished children and the poverty-stricken. Pregnant women, growing infants, and young children are also at risk because increased folic acid is needed during periods of rapid growth.

A deficiency may also occur as a consequence of malabsorption disorders, or of conditions that increase the metabolic rate and hence the need for folic acid. Examples of such conditions include infections, cancer, and hyperthyroidism. For the same reason, serious burns, excessive blood loss, and gastrointestinal damage may lead to a deficiency.

Folic acid deficiency results in impaired cell division and protein synthesis (processes necessary to tissue growth) and the faulty synthesis of heme. Signs and symptoms include a red, smooth, and swollen tongue; heartburn, diarrhea, fainting, and fatigue. In addition, since folic acid functions in the production of heme, the person deficient in this vitamin develops **megaloblastic anemia.**

Megaloblastic anemia—anemia characterized by the formation of large, immature red cells that cannot carry oxygen properly; caused by folic acid deficiency.

RECOMMENDED DIETARY ALLOWANCES The RDAs for folic acid are: infants—25 to 35 micrograms; children—50 to 100 micrograms; boys 11 to 14 years old—150 micrograms; male adolescents and men—200 micrograms; girls 11 to 14 years old—150 micrograms; female adolescents and women—180 micrograms; pregnant women—400 micrograms, lactating women: first 6 months—280 micrograms, second 6 months—260 micrograms.

FOOD SOURCES From the meat group, liver is a good source of folic acid. Many common vegetables (such as spinach, asparagus, and broccoli) provide folic acid. Other vegetables containing appreciable folic acid are kidney beans, beets, and vegetables of the cabbage family. Fruits providing folic acid are oranges and cantaloupe.

STABILITY Folic acid is stable to alkalies but easily oxidized by light and acids. Some forms are easily destroyed by heat, so that cooking losses may be as high as 80 to 90 percent. To minimize losses, vegetables should be cooked as quickly as possible.

INTERFERING FACTORS Alcohol or oral contraceptives may interfere with the absorption of folic acid. Methotrexate, an anticancer drug, is a folic acid antagonist. Its purpose is to interfere with DNA in cancer cells, but at the same time it affects normal cells. Aspirin displaces folic acid from its carrier protein; the displaced folic acid is excreted.

TOXICITY   Folic acid toxicity is rare. Dose levels of over-the-counter vitamins are limited to 400 micrograms to make it inconvenient to overdose. This is done not to prevent toxicity from folic acid but to avoid masking signs of pernicious anemia, which will be discussed in the next section.

Vitamin B_{12}

Vitamin B_{12} is stored to a greater extent than the other B vitamins. Diverse causes can precipitate vitamin B_{12} deficiency, leading to serious consequences.

Intrinsic factor—specific protein-binding factor secreted by the stomach; necessary for the absorption of vitamin B_{12}.

ABSORPTION, METABOLISM, AND EXCRETION   Absorption of vitamin B_{12} requires a highly specific protein-binding factor called **intrinsic factor,** secreted by the gastric mucosal cells in the stomach. Vitamin B_{12}, also called **extrinsic factor,** and intrinsic factor combine in the stomach. The two factors form a complex that permits vitamin B_{12} to be absorbed in the only section of intestine possible, the ileum.

Vitamin B_{12} is not freely absorbed. The amount absorbed depends upon the body's storage levels. Vitamin B_{12} has a long half-life, so that a person's stores last from 3 to 5 years. The principal storage site is the liver.

Extrinsic factor—Vitamin B_{12}; necessary for proper red blood cell development.

FUNCTIONS   Vitamin B_{12} is required in a series of reactions that precede the use of folic acid in DNA replication. In fact, without vitamin B_{12}, folic acid is unable to assist in the manufacture of red blood cells. It is also essential for the synthesis and maintenance of myelin, the fatty insulation which speeds transmission of nervous impulses.

DEFICIENCY   Persons may be at increased risk of vitamin B_{12} deficiency because of stomach pathology, intestinal disease, or diet.

When a person lacks intrinsic factor, the result is a condition called **pernicious anemia.** It can also occur following the surgical removal of the stomach or a large portion of the stomach.

Pernicious anemia—Inadequate red blood cell formation due to lack of intrinsic factor from the stomach, which is required for the absorption of vitamin B_{12}.

In those cases vitamin B_{12} is not absorbed because intrinsic factor is missing. A person with Crohn's disease involving the ileum, or a patient whose ileum was removed, will not absorb vitamin B_{12}. Dietary treatment will be ineffective in these cases, so vitamin B_{12} must be given by injection. The pharmaceutical name for vitamin B_{12} is <u>cyanocobalamin.</u>

Symptoms of vitamin B_{12} deficiency are, in order of appearance, numbness and tingling in the hands and feet, red blood cell changes, moodiness, confusion, depression, delusions, and overt psychosis. Eventually, irreparable nerve damage occurs, and finally, death.

Diagnosis of vitamin B_{12} deficiency is difficult if the person consumes ample folic acid. The folic acid enables the body to continue manufacturing red blood cells in the correct size and number. In this way folic acid masks vitamin B_{12} deficiency. However, the neurological deterioration continues unabated. This is the reason the amount of folic acid in over-the-counter vitamins is limited to 400 micrograms.

Strict vegetarians are at risk of vitamin B_{12} deficiency because animal products are the best sources of vitamin B_{12}. In this case, additional vitamin B_{12}, from either food or supplements, is the treatment.

RECOMMENDED DIETARY ALLOWANCES   The RDAs for vitamin B_{12} are: infants—0.3 to 0.5 microgram; children—0.7 to 1.4 micrograms; male and female adolescents, men, and women—2.0 micrograms; pregnant women—2.2 micrograms; lactating women—2.6 micrograms.

FOOD SOURCES Vitamin B_{12} is synonymous with animal products. Healthy people who regularly eat meat, milk, cheese, or eggs are not at risk of vitamin B_{12} deficiency. Nutritional yeast and vitamin B_{12}-fortified soy milk are food sources available to strict vegetarians.

STABILITY Vitamin B_{12} is stable to heat. However, light, acids, and alkalies inactivate it.

INTERFERING FACTORS Megadoses of vitamin C interfere with vitamin B_{12} absorption and utilization. The body's use of vitamin B_{12} is also impaired by a deficiency of vitamin B_6 and gastritis.

Recently Emphasized Vitamins

Two B vitamins are so widely distributed in foods that only special circumstances have produced deficiencies. Long-term total parenteral nutrition is one such situation.

PANTOTHENIC ACID This vitamin plays a role in the metabolism of carbohydrates, fats, and proteins and in the synthesis of the neurotransmitter acetylcholine. No cases of deficiency of pantothenic acid have been docu-

TABLE 6–4 *Amounts of Food Providing the Adult RDA for Water-Soluble Vitamins*

Vitamin and Adult RDA	Amounts of Food Providing Adult RDA*	Number of Exchanges
Vitamin C 60 milligrams	1 orange or ½ cup orange juice	1 Fruit
	½ cantaloupe (5-inch diameter)	1.5 Fruit
	½ cup cooked broccoli or brussels sprouts	1 Vegetable
Thiamin	3 ounces pork roast	3 Medium-fat Meat
1.1–1.5 milligrams	13 tablespoons wheat germ	4.3 Starch/Bread
Riboflavin	1.4 ounces beef liver	1.4 Medium-fat Meat
1.3–1.7 milligrams	4 cups skim milk	4 milk
	4 cups cooked spinach	8 Vegetable
Niacin	0.9 cup light meat chicken	4 Lean Meat
15 milligrams	3.4 ounces water-packed tuna	1.7 Lean Meat
	¾ cup peanuts, oil-roasted, salted	14 Fat
B_6	5 ounces beef liver	5 Medium-Fat Meat
1.6–2 milligrams	1½ cups wheat germ	8 Starch/Bread
	1.9 cups instant oatmeal	4 Starch/Bread
	3 bananas, 9 inches long	6 Fruit
Folic acid	3 oz beef liver	3 Medium-fat Meat
180–200 micrograms	3.2 cups raw chopped broccoli	3.2 Vegetable
B_{12}	0.9 ounces beef liver	0.9 Medium-fat Meat
2 micrograms	2 cups skim milk	2 Milk

*In cases with a range, food amounts were calculated to provide the higher RDA.

mented in persons consuming a variety of foods, but deficiencies have been produced experimentally. There are no RDAs for pantothenic acid. Instead, an Estimated Safe and Adequate Daily Dietary Intake (ESADDI) of 4 to 7 milligrams has been set for adults. The average United States diet supplies 7 milligrams. Rich food sources include liver, egg yolk, milk, brussels sprouts, sweet potato, and dried beans. Intestinal bacteria are believed to synthesize small amounts of pantothenic acid.

BIOTIN Biotin, closely related to folic acid and vitamin B_{12}, is a coenzyme in the synthesis of fatty acids and amino acids. It is required to form purines, which are essential components of DNA and RNA. Deficiencies have been seen in children displaying the chief sign of skin rash. Deficiencies may occur in patients fed intravenously who also receive antibiotics. Antibiotics kill the intestinal bacteria that synthesize biotin. The ESADDI

TABLE 6–5 *Sources of Vitamins by Food Groups*

Vitamin	Synthesis/ Miscellaneous	Meats	Milk	Fruits/ Vegetables	Grains
A		Liver	Fortified	Deep yellow, dark green leafy	
D	In skin	Liver, eggs, some fish	Fortified		
E				Vegetable oil	Wheat germ, whole grains
K	In intestine	Liver, eggs	Milk	Green leafy	
C				Fresh, especially citrus	
Thiamin		Pork			Brewer's yeast
Riboflavin		Organ meats	Milk	Green vegetables	Brewer's yeast
Niacin	Coffee	Meat, tuna, eggs	Milk	Legumes	Brewer's yeast, whole grains
B_6		Pork, organ meats, chicken, fish		Potatoes, bananas, legumes	Whole grains, wheat germ, oatmeal
Folic acid		Liver		Cabbage family, dark green leafy, beets, kidney beans, cantaloupe, oranges	Whole grains
B_{12}		Meat, eggs	Milk		
Pantothenic acid	In intestine	Liver, kidney, egg yolk	Milk	Dried beans, brussels sprouts, sweet potato	
Biotin	In intestine	Meat, liver, kidney, egg yolk		Tomatoes	

for biotin is 30 to 100 micrograms. **Avidin,** a protein in raw egg white, binds with biotin. Humans given six raw egg whites per day developed dermatitis in 3 to 4 weeks. A week or two later they displayed mental changes, muscle pain, nausea, and loss of appetite. Five days of biotin therapy cured the symptoms. Good food sources of biotin include liver, kidney, meat, egg yolk, and tomatoes.

Avidin—Protein in raw egg white that inhibits the B-vitamin biotin.

Of the water-soluble vitamins, ascorbic acid is the most vulnerable to loss and niacin the most resistant. Table 6–4 shows amounts of a variety of foods that would provide the adult RDA for vitamin C and six of the B vitamins; the table also equates the amounts of food to the Exchange System. Table 6–5 summarizes sources of vitamins by food groups. A large percentage of Americans report consuming *no* fruit or fruit juice or vegetables on an average day. These choices indicate a high risk for vitamin deficiencies.

VITAMINS AS MEDICINE

Supplements

Healthy persons consuming normal foods in variety, balance, and moderation should not need vitamin supplements. If vitamins are taken as supplements, it is best not to exceed 100 percent of the RDA for each vitamin. This will prevent deficiency in the well individual and toxicity is unlikely.

The price of vitamin supplements varies widely. The average markup on vitamins is 43 percent. In some health food stores it is 500 percent.

Pharmacologic Uses

Vitamin supplements can be used to offset dietary deficiencies or to compensate for diseases causing malabsorption. They also have been given for some conditions unrelated to diet.

Treatment of Deficiencies

The obvious use of vitamins is to treat vitamin deficiencies. Vitamin C is the treatment for scurvy, vitamin D for rickets, and niacin for pellagra. Initially, the treatment of pernicious anemia involves frequent injections of vitamin B_{12}. Later, monthly doses are sufficient to control this condition.

Other Uses

MEGADOSES A dose ten times the RDA is called a megadose. Undoubtedly you have heard of individuals taking huge doses of vitamin C to prevent the common cold. Evidence of effectiveness has not been proved to the satisfaction of many scientists. Rebound scurvy is possible when megadoses of vitamin C are discontinued.

TREATING NONNUTRITIONAL DISORDERS Many vitamins have uses unrelated to prevention or treatment of deficiencies. Vitamins A, E, C, and niacin are examples. Vitamin A derivatives are often prescribed to control acne and the wrinkles of aging. Clinical Application 6–7 discusses

CLINICAL APPLICATION 6–7
Vitamin C and Smoked Meat

Vitamin C blocks the formation of nitrosamines from nitrates. Nitrates are chemicals added to smoked and cured meats to preserve them and enhance their flavor. In the small intestine, however, nitrates combine with amino acids to form nitrosamines. Nitrosamines have been linked to some cancers. For this reason meat packers have begun adding vitamin C to protect against nitrosamine formation.

Vitamin C as a food additive intended to reduce the formation of cancer-causing compounds. High doses of niacin, usually 3 to 6 grams per day have been used to lower serum cholesterol.

Summary

Vitamins are organic substances required in minute quantities that are necessary for many bodily processes. They do not become part of the structure of the body.

Vitamins were first recognized by the respective effects of their absence. Some deficiency diseases have been known for centuries. However, only in this century have each of the known vitamins been isolated in the laboratory. Even so, correct treatments prescribed were based on primitive and incomplete knowledge. Only low intakes of vitamins A, C, B_6, and folic acid are currently regarded as public health problems in the United States.

Vitamins A, D, E, and K are fat soluble and stable to heat. Sufficient dietary fat intake and adequate fat digestion and absorption are required for the proper utilization of these vitamins. Fat-soluble vitamins, especially A and D, can be stored by the body and hence can be sources of toxicity. Both vitamins A and D have clear-cut deficiency diseases: xerophthalmia and night blindness for vitamin A and rickets for vitamin D.

The water-soluble vitamins, C and the B-complexes, are not stored in the body in appreciable amounts. Vitamins C, B_{12}, thiamin, and niacin have specific diseases associated with deficiency: scurvy, pernicious anemia, beriberi, and pellagra, respectively.

Because of the interdependent functions of vitamins, we are well advised to rely on food for our vitamins. If a vitamin supplement is desired, it should be taken at the RDA levels only.

A case study and a sample plan of care appear below. They are both designed to show how the information in this chapter can be used in nursing practice.

CASE STUDY 6–1

Mr. J., a 79-year-old widower, prides himself on caring for himself in the past year since his wife died. His typical meal pattern is:

• Breakfast—egg, toast, jam, coffee

- Lunch—cheese or lunch meat sandwich, tea
- Dinner—canned stew or hash

Although Mr. J. has a refrigerator, he avoids buying fresh fruit or vegetables. He says he has difficulty consuming produce before it spoils. He seldom goes out to eat.

For the past few months Mr. J. has noticed that his gums are tender. He stopped wearing his dentures when his gums began to bleed.

The visiting nurse confirmed the inflammation of the gums. When the nurse took Mr. J.'s blood pressure, she noted a red, flat rash where the blood pressure cuff had been.

NURSING CARE PLAN FOR MR. J.

Assessment
Subjective
Sore gums
Diet lacks fresh fruits and vegetables
Objective
Erythematous petechiae under blood pressure cuff

Nursing Diagnosis

Nutrition, altered: possible vitamin C deficiency related to lack of fresh fruit and vegetables as evidenced by sore bleeding gums and pressure petechiae after minor pressure.

Desired Outcome/Evaluation Criteria

Will consume foods containing 60 milligrams of vitamin C every day within 3 days.

Nursing Actions

1. Teach importance of daily vitamin C.
2. Explore acceptability of good sources of vitamin C; list amounts necessary to obtain 60 mg.
3. If patient selects frozen vegetables, teach to boil water 1 minute before adding vegetables and to cook quickly till crisp-tender.

Rationale

1. Little vitamin C is stored in the body; must be consumed every day.
2. Foods would be better sources than vitamin supplements because other nutrients supplied also.
3. Heat and oxygen destroy vitamin C.

STUDY AIDS

Chapter Review Questions

1. Which of the following vitamins becomes part of the chemical in the eye necessary for vision?
   a. Vitamin A
   b. Vitamin B_6
   c. Vitamin C
   d. Vitamin D

2. Which of the following groups of foods would be the best sources of carotene?
   a. Bananas, cantaloupe, and pears
   b. Broccoli, lettuce, and lima beans
   c. Collards, spinach, and sweet potatoes
   d. Lemons, oranges, and strawberries

3. Which of the following combinations of foods would be the best sources of thiamin?
   a. Cabbage and cauliflower
   b. Eggs and milk
   c. Liver and onions
   d. Pork and whole wheat bread

4. Persons consuming ethnic foods emphasizing corn with limited protein should be assessed carefully for adequacy of _____ intake.
   a. Folic acid
   b. Niacin
   c. Riboflavin
   d. Thiamin

5. Which of the following persons run an increased risk of vitamin B_6 deficiency?
   a. Elderly residents of a home who seldom go outside
   b. Individuals with fat absorption problems
   c. Strict vegetarians
   d. Women taking oral contraceptives for more than 2 or 3 years

6. In the United States, over-the-counter vitamin supplements cannot contain more than 400 micrograms of:
   a. Biotin
   b. Folic acid
   c. Vitamin B_6
   d. Vitamin B_{12}

7. The need for which of the following vitamins increases whenever the need for protein increases?
   a. Riboflavin
   b. Vitamin A
   c. Vitamin C
   d. Vitamin K

8. The vitamin that is essential to the synthesis of several blood clotting factors is:
   a. Vitamin A
   b. Vitamin B_6
   c. Vitamin C
   d. Vitamin K

9. Which of the following precautions should be taken to minimize loss of vitamin C in foods?
   a. Adding baking soda to the cooking water
   b. Cooking thoroughly to kill any bacteria
   c. Eating good sources raw when possible
   d. Keeping food in a mesh bag to allow air to circulate

10. Which of the following groups of foods are the best sources of vitamin C?
    a. Cabbage, cantaloupe, and tomatoes
    b. Cheese, milk, and yogurt
    c. Liver, oysters, and shrimp
    d. Sweet potatoes, winter squash, and zucchini

NCLEX-Style Quiz

Situation One

Ms. C. is being seen in the well-baby clinic with her 3-month-old baby girl. Ms. C. states that the baby is taking 6 ounces of a commercial baby formula every 4 hours. Ms. C. has not added solid foods to the baby's diet. She was told to wait until the baby is 4 months old before adding cereal. Ms. C. is giving the baby the multivitamin preparation prescribed. She also has added cod liver oil to the infant's diet. "It's only a teaspoonful," she said. Ms. C.'s grandmother gave Ms. C. cod liver oil as a child. Ms. C. credits her grandmother's care during her own childhood for her strong bones and teeth. She admires her grandmother, who at age 75 still stands straight and tall.

1. Which of the following pieces of information should the nurse gather first to focus on the situation presented?
   a. The amount of vitamin C in the multivitamin supplement
   b. The conditions under which the vitamins are stored
   c. Ms. C.'s technique for measuring the vitamins
   d. The total amount of vitamin D the infant receives each day

2. Which of the following nursing diagnoses is likely to be correct in this situation?
   a. Nutrition, altered: less than body requirements
   b. Nutrition, altered: more than body requirements
   c. Altered growth and development
   d. High risk for infection

3. The nurse's action will be designed to:
   a. Educate Ms. C. as to safe amounts of vitamins for a child this age
   b. Measure the infant carefully for progress notes
   c. Obtain more formula for the infant from the community pantry
   d. Teach Ms. C. better hand washing and formula handling practices

4. Which of the following statements of possible rationale for the nurse's action is correct for this situation?
   a. The best protection against the spread of infection is good handwashing.
   b. Infants of 3 months should be taking 48 ounces of formula per day.
   c. An infant's growth and development are compared to standards to identify problems early.
   d. Too much of a vitamin is as undesirable as too little.

5. What would be a reasonable time frame to achieve the desired outcome in this situation?
   a. 1 day
   b. 1 week
   c. 1 month
   d. 3 months

CLINICAL CALCULATION 6–1

Converting International Units of Vitamin A to Retinol Equivalents

Since 1980, the vitamin A content of foods has been reported in retinol equivalents (RE). The previous unit of measure was international units (IU). Some tables report in both systems of measurement. When you have a choice, select the newer table. Not only will it be reported in RE, but the data will reflect the latest analyses.

Take for example, ½ cup of cooked, chopped broccoli. It contains 1090 IU of vitamin A. Since 1 microgram of RE equals 10 IU in plant foods, there will be fewer micrograms of RE than IUs in a given serving. Therefore, we divide 1090 by 10 to find that the broccoli contains 109 micrograms of REs.

To convert an animal food's vitamin A from IU to micrograms of RE consider the egg. One large egg contains 260 IUs. One microgram of RE from animal foods contains 3.3 IUs. Again there will be fewer REs than IUs. This time we divide 260 by 3.3 to get 78 micrograms of RE in one large egg.

CLINICAL CALCULATION 6–2

Converting International Units of Vitamin D to Micrograms of Cholecalciferol

If one quart of milk is fortified with 400 international units (IU) of vitamin D, what is the equivalent amount of cholecalciferol in the quart of milk?

We know that 5 micrograms of cholecalciferol is equal to 200 IU of vitamin D. Setting up a proportion gives us:

$$\frac{5 \text{ mcg}}{200 \text{ IU}} = \frac{x \text{ mcg}}{400 \text{ IU}}$$

$$200 \, X = 2000$$

$$X = 10 \text{ mcg}$$

Thus, 400 IU is equal to 10 micrograms of cholecalciferol.

BIBLIOGRAPHY

Angier, N. Chemists learn why vegetables are good for you. New York Times, April 13, 1993.

Brown, JE: The Science of Human Nutrition. Harcourt Brace Jovanovich, San Diego, 1990.

Committee on Diet and Health. Food and Nutrition Board. Commission on Life Sciences. National Research Council: Diet and Health: Implications for Reducing Chronic Disease Risk, National Academy Press, Washington, DC, 1989.

Deglin, JH, Vallerand, AH, and Russin, MM: Davis's Drug Guide For Nurses, ed 3. FA Davis, Philadelphia, 1993.

Feldman, EB: Essentials of Clinical Nutrition. FA Davis, Philadelphia, 1988.

Grimes, MR, Scardino, MA, and Martone, JF. Worldwide blindness. Nurs Clin North Am 27 (3): 807–816, 1992.

Hands, ES: Food Finder, ed 2. ESHS Research, Salem, OR, 1989.

Hui, YH: Human Nutrition and Diet Therapy. Wadsworth, Monterey, CA, 1983.

Krasinski, SD and Russell, RM: The prevalence of vitamin K deficiency in chronic gastrointestinal disorders. Am J Clin Nutr 41:639, 1985.

Medical Research Council Vitamin Study Research Group. Prevention of neural tube defects: Results of the Medical Research Council Vitamin Study. Lancet 338 (8760): 131–137, 1991.

Patient Care Flow Chart Manual, ed 3. Medical Economics, Oradell, NJ, 1982.

Scanlon, VT and Sanders, T: Essentials of Anatomy and Physiology. FA Davis, Philadelphia, 1991.

Shlafer, M and Marieb, E: The Nurse, Pharmacology, and Drug Therapy. Addison-Wesley, Redwood City, CA, 1989.

Townsend, CE: Nutrition and Diet Therapy, ed 5. Delmar Publishers, Albany, NY, 1989.

US Department of Health and Human Services: Nutrition Monitoring in the United States. US Government Printing Office, Washington, DC, 1989.

Whitney, EB, Cataldo, CB, and Rolfes, SR: Understanding Normal and Clinical Nutrition, ed 3. West Publishing Company, St Paul, MN, 1991.

Williams, SR: Essentials of Nutrition and Diet Therapy, ed 5. Times Mirror/Mosby, St Louis, 1990.

Williams, SR: Nutrition and Diet Therapy, ed 6. Times Mirror/Mosby, St Louis, 1989.

Chapter Outline

Key Terms

As a study aid, each key term is followed by the page number where the term is defined in the chapter. Terms that appear in **boldface** or <u>underscored</u> in the chapter text are located in the glossary.

Chapter Seven
Minerals

Key Terms *(Continued)*

Nonheme iron (185)
Osteoblasts (169)
Osteoclasts (169)
Osteoporosis (175)
Oxalates (172)
Parathyroid hormone (169)

Phytic acid (172)
Thyroxine—T_4 (190)
Total parenteral nutrition TPN (195)
Transferrin (185)
Triiodothyronine—T_3 (000)
Trousseau's sign (176)

Learning Objectives

After completing this chapter, the student should be able to:

1. Discuss the differences and similarities between minerals and vitamins.
2. Describe one or more functions of each mineral.
3. List at least two food sources for each mineral and identify any nonfood sources.
4. Describe individuals at increased risk for mineral deficiencies.
5. Identify the five minerals that are actual or potential public health problems in the United States due to low intake levels; identify the mineral that is a health risk because of overconsumption.

*I*n a broad sense, minerals are obtained for human use from the earth's crust. Through the effects of the weather, rocks that contain minerals are ground into smaller particles, which then become part of the soil. The mineral content in the soil is absorbed by growing plants. Animals eat the plants, and humans eat both the plants and the animals. In this way, minerals become part of the food chain.

MINERALS IN HUMAN NUTRITION

In nutrition, minerals make vital contributions toward promoting growth and maintaining health in the body. In this chapter we will discuss the minerals important in human nutrition and the role each plays in the body.

In this section we will first compare minerals with vitamins. Then we will discuss some of the general functions of minerals and explain how minerals are classified in nutrition.

Functions of Minerals

Minerals are similar to vitamins because they help regulate bodily functions without providing energy and are essential to good health. Minerals differ from vitamins not only because minerals are inorganic substances but also because minerals become part of the structure of the body. Minerals represent 4 percent of total body weight.

Structural Components of Body Systems

Minerals become part of the body's structure and part of the body's enzymes. For instance, calcium and phosphorus combine to give bones and teeth their hardness. Iron becomes attached to the protein globin to form hemoglobin. Iodine becomes part of the thyroid hormones.

Regulators of Bodily Functions

Most minerals serve a variety of functions in the body's regulatory and metabolic processes. Sodium is essential for maintaining fluid balance (see Chapter 9). Sodium, potassium, and calcium have critical functions in nerve and muscle activity. Potassium and phosphorus play significant roles in acid-base balance. A disruption of the body's balance of any one of these minerals can be life-threatening.

Classification of Minerals

In nutrition, minerals are classified into two groups: major and trace. Major minerals, also called macrominerals, are present in the body in quantities greater than 5 grams (approximately 1 teaspoonful). The body needs a daily intake of 100 milligrams (approximately 1/50 teaspoonful) or more of each of the major minerals.

Trace minerals, often called microminerals or trace elements, are present in the body in amounts less than 5 grams. Humans need a daily intake of less than 100 milligrams of each of the trace minerals. The term "trace" does not mean unimportant. Trace minerals make vital and often unique contributions to the body's functioning.

MAJOR MINERALS

The seven major minerals include calcium and phosphorus, familiar to many people. The other five major minerals are sodium, potassium, magnesium, sulfur, and chloride.

Calcium

The body of a 150-pound adult contains approximately 3 pounds of calcium. Ninety-nine percent of this amount is in the bones and teeth. The remaining 1 percent of the calcium circulates in the body fluids. Of this 1 percent, 40 percent is bound to plasma proteins and thus is unavailable, while the other 60 percent is in free particles that carry an electrical charge (ions); see Chapter 9. The ionized calcium moves freely from one fluid compartment to another and serves several important functions in the body.

Functions of Calcium

Calcium, with phosphorus, forms the hard substance that characterizes bones and teeth. Bones continue to add minerals until age 30. Ample calcium and phosphorus alone will not guarantee strong bones and teeth, however. Vitamin D is necessary for calcium absorption. Exercise, particularly weight-bearing exercise, is also essential for strong bones. Very little calcium is deposited in fully formed teeth. Consequently, if calcium is lost from the teeth, it cannot be replaced. This is the reason dental cavities or caries cannot heal themselves.

Calcium also performs several vital metabolic functions in the nervous, muscular, and cardiovascular systems. (1) Calcium assists in the manufacturing of acetylcholine, a neurotransmitter, or chemical that enhances transmission of nerve impulses. (2) Calcium acts as a catalyst in initiating and controlling muscle contraction and relaxation; at the beginning of a muscle contraction, calcium is released from its storage area inside the muscle cell; at the end of a contraction, the calcium is again gathered into its storage area. (This function is vital to the heart muscle.) (3) Calcium is a catalyst in two steps of the clotting process: it aids in the conversion of platelets to thromboplastin and in the conversion of fibrinogen to fibrin. (4) Calcium controls the passage of substances across cell membranes by affecting membrane permeability. (5) Calcium activates certain enzymes such as pancreatic lipase and is necessary for absorption of vitamin B_{12}.

Control Mechanisms

Bone is the body's bank account or storage depot for calcium. As much as 700 milligrams of calcium is moved in and out of the bones each day. One reason for this is to maintain the serum calcium concentration within the normal limits of 8.5 to 10.5 milligrams per 100 milliliters of serum. Another reason for the movement of calcium in and out of the bones is to renew the bone tissue. In this process bone cells called **osteoclasts** produce enzymes to destroy the protein matrix that holds the calcium phosphate in place. Other bone cells, called **osteoblasts,** produce new matrix protein, which chemically attracts calcium and other nutrients to rebuild the bone.

Several hormones work together to accomplish all these activities. Vitamin D is one of these hormones. Parathyroid hormone and calcitonin are the

Osteoclasts— Bone cells that break down bone.
Osteoblasts— Bone cells that build bone.

other two. Vitamin D is actually a hormone because it regulates tissue functions. It increases calcium absorption by the intestine and increases calcium deposition in the bones and teeth.

Parathyroid hormone is secreted by tiny glands behind the thyroid gland in the neck. When the serum calcium level falls, the parathyroid glands secrete the hormone, which increases the withdrawal of calcium from the bone, thereby raising the serum calcium level. Additionally, parathyroid hormone increases the serum calcium level by stimulating the kidneys to return more calcium to the bloodstream instead of excreting it in the urine.

To balance the action of parathyroid hormone, **calcitonin,** another hormone is secreted by the thyroid gland. Calcitonin is released when the serum calcium level is high. It inhibits the release of calcium from bone.

Other hormones affect calcium utilization by the body. One prominent one is estrogen. Its exact mechanism of action in bone metabolism is unknown.

Parathyroid hormone—Hormone secreted by the parathyroid glands; regulates calcium and phosphorus metabolism in the body.

Calcitonin—Hormone produced by the C cells of the thyroid gland; it slows bone resorption when serum calcium levels are high.

Recommended Dietary Allowances

The RDAs for calcium are: infants—400 to 600 milligrams; children through age 10, women age 25 and older and men—800 milligrams; individuals aged 11 to 24 and pregnant and lactating women—1200 milligrams.

In one recent survey, only half the 1- to 5-year-old children consumed at least 769 milligrams per day (US Department of Health and Human Services, 1989).

Sources of Calcium

Even with the bones as a reservoir, daily intake of calcium is important. Calcium can be obtained from animal or vegetable sources, but animal sources are more readily absorbed.

ANIMAL SOURCES Milk and milk products are the best animal sources of calcium, followed by sardines, oysters, and salmon. In milk, calcium is combined with lactose, which increases absorption. Even so, we absorb only 28 percent of the available calcium in milk. Another advantageous component in milk is the protein the osteoblasts need to rebuild the bone matrix. In sum, milk is such an important source of calcium that it is virtually impossible to obtain adequate calcium without milk or dairy products. Figure 7–1 shows a child drinking milk with his meal.

Table 7–1 lists the quantity of foods containing approximately 300 milligrams of calcium, the amount in 1 cup of milk. "Bargain" foods listed that are high in calcium but low in fat include skimmed milk and plain yogurt. The "most expensive" sources of calcium, considering both fat and kilocalories, are hard and soft ice cream and large-curd, creamed cottage cheese. This table reveals that not all dairy products are equally beneficial as sources of calcium. It should not be interpreted as a call to abandon all fat intake. Consuming some fat with calcium increases the absorption of the mineral by slowing peristalsis.

Obtaining calcium from supplements is less desirable than obtaining it from foods. Milk products supply other nutrients, some of which, such as vitamin D and lactose, assist in calcium absorption. Milk is also a major source

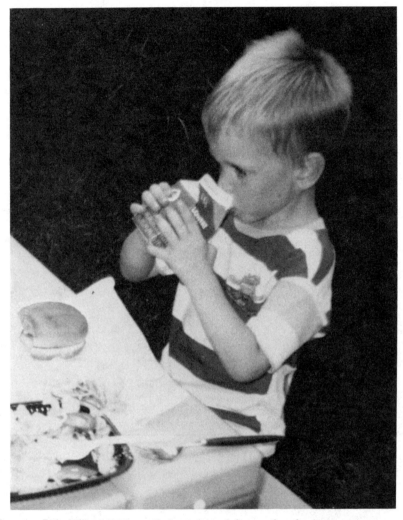

FIGURE 7–1. This child has a balanced meal from a fast food restaurant: a small hamburger, a salad, and milk. Growing bones and teeth need calcium from milk products.

of riboflavin and protein. Figure 7–2 shows the percentages of the RDAs for vitamins A and D, protein, thiamine, and riboflavin an adult woman could obtain from 3 cups of skimmed milk. Clinical Application 7–1 describes some of the contaminants in "natural" calcium supplements.

PLANT SOURCES   Good plant sources of calcium include beans, cauliflower, rhubarb, and green leafy vegetables such as chard, kale, and collards. Other vegetable sources include beets, broccoli, cabbage, carrots, celery, lettuce, rutabagas, spinach, and turnips. Some fruits which contain calcium in fair amounts are blackberries, dates, figs, and oranges. Almonds and brazil nuts are also fair sources.

TABLE 7–1 *Quantities of Food Containing Calcium Equal to One Cup of Milk**

Food	Amount	Kilocalories	Fat (Grams)
Cheese			
Blue	2 ounces	200	16
Cheddar	1.5 ounces	171	14
Cottage			
Creamed, large curd	2.25 cups	529	22
2 percent low-fat	2 cups	410	9
Grated Parmesan	4.3 tablespoons	99	6
Processed American	1.7 ounces	180	15
Swiss	1.1 ounces	118	8
Frozen Desserts			
Hard ice cream, vanilla	1.7 cups	459	24
Soft ice cream	1.3 cups	479	29
Sherbet	2.9 cups	786	11
Milkshake, vanilla	0.9 cups	273	9
Milk			
Skim	1 cup	86	0.4
2 percent	1 cup	121	5
Whole	1 cup	150	8
Yogurt, Low-Fat			
Plain	0.7 cups	101	2
With fruit	0.9 cups	199	2

*One cup of milk contains approximately 300 milligrams of calcium.

Factors Interfering with Absorption

The presence of calcium in a food does not mean that it is available for absorption. In general, the percentage of available calcium absorbed from vegetables is considerably less than that absorbed from milk. For example, only 5 percent of the total calcium found in spinach is absorbed. Several factors can interfere with the absorption of calcium: oxalates, phytic acid, and excessive intakes of protein, dietary fiber, or fat (see Table 7–2).

Some vegetables contain salts of oxalic acid called oxalates. Oxalates bind with the calcium present in the vegetable to produce calcium oxalate, an insoluble form of calcium which is excreted in the feces. The calcium content not bound to oxalates is available for absorption, however, and oxalates do not interfere with the absorption of calcium from other foods. Chard, spinach, beet leaves, rhubarb, cranberries, and gooseberries all contain oxalic acid. Unusually high intake of these foods may cause oxalic acid poisoning (see Clinical Application 7–2).

Cereals contain a substance that forms an insoluble complex with calcium. This interfering substance is <u>phytic acid.</u> The overall effect of oxalic

Oxalates—Salts of oxalic acid found in some plant foods; binds with the calcium in the plant, making it unavailable to the body.

% RDA

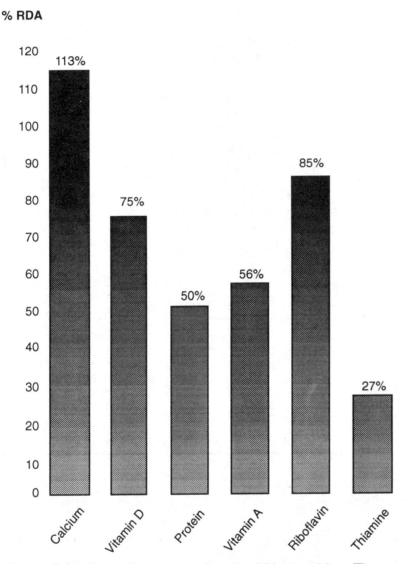

FIGURE 7–2. Milk supplies many nutrients in addition to calcium. Three cups of skimmed milk would give a woman more than 25 years of age 50 percent of her RDAs for vitamin D, protein, vitamin A, and riboflavin, as well as 27 percent of her RDA for thiamine. The caloric cost for all these nutrients is a minuscule 258 kilocalories. (Courtesy of Carroll A. Lutz.)

and phytic acids on calcium availability in most diets usually is not significant. Persons who avoid dairy products, however, may need careful attention to meal planning.

High-protein intake increases calcium absorption. Eating 100 grams or more of protein a day, however, not unusual for many Americans, increases

CLINICAL APPLICATION 7–1
Contents of Natural Calcium Supplements

Shells, bones, and dolomite are natural sources of calcium that are used as dietary supplements. Much of the calcium found in shells and bones is in the form of calcium phosphate, one of the most difficult calcium compounds to absorb. In addition, shells and bones often contain excessive amounts of mercury and lead.

Dolomite is a limestone that is rich in both calcium and magnesium. It also may contain lead, mercury, arsenic, and aluminum. Because of the possibility of contamination, it is best to obtain calcium from food sources whenever possible.

TABLE 7–2 *Factors Affecting Calcium Absorption*

Increase	Decrease
Acidity	Excess dietary fat
Estrogen	Poor absorption of fat
Lactose or sucrose	Alkalinity
Moderate fat	Dietary fiber
Protein	Oxalic acid
Vitamin D	Phytic acid
	Vitamin D deficiency

CLINICAL APPLICATION 7–2
Oxalic Acid Poisoning

It is possible to be poisoned by ingesting too much of one or more foods that contain oxalic acid. Cranberries, gooseberries, chard, spinach, beet leaves, and rhubarb are high in oxalic acid. For example, one normal serving of rhubarb contains one fifth the toxic dose. Rhubarb leaves contain three or four times as much as the stalks. A fairly small amount of leaves, then, can poison a child.

One way to minimize the chance of oxalic acid poisoning is to consume calcium-containing foods with any foods high in oxalic acid. The calcium combines with the oxalate, which then passes through the intestine harmlessly. However, calcium absorption will be decreased.

urinary excretion of calcium. When the protein is accompanied by a high phosphorus intake, the calcium loss is lessened considerably. Fortunately, in the American diet, foods high in protein usually are high in phosphorus as well.

Calcium absorption is hindered by excessive intake of dietary fiber or fat. Because dietary fiber is insoluble, it passes through the alimentary canal undigested. Any calcium that binds with dietary fiber suffers the same fate. Excess fat in the gut, whether from diet or malabsorption, combines with calcium to form insoluble soaps, which are excreted.

An alkaline environment decreases calcium solubility. Because the intestine is alkaline, any exaggeration of this quality will impair calcium absorption.

Calcium Deficiencies

Calcium deficiency in children can contribute to poor bone and tooth development. Rickets is more directly related to vitamin D deficiency than calcium deficiency except in premature infants, whose skeletons still need much added mineral. Two other conditions related to calcium balance are osteoporosis and tetany.

OSTEOPOROSIS   Osteopenia refers to a decreased bone mass per unit of volume. In osteoporosis the osteopenia is sufficient to allow fracture to occur after minimal trauma. Osteoporosis is most common in post-menopausal, fair-complected white women. A woman loses 2 to 5 percent of bone tissue per year immediately before and for about 10 years after menopause. The most rapid loss of bone occurs in the first five years after menopause. Black women and men lose bone mass also, but because their skeletons are generally heavier, the loss is less conspicuous.

Osteoporosis—A loss of bone mass.

The exact cause of osteoporosis is unknown, but it is more closely associated with a deficiency of calcium than with a deficiency of vitamin D. Furthermore, population studies have not demonstrated a relationship between calcium intake and osteoporosis in all countries.

Prevention of osteoporosis requires a two-pronged attack. First, an adequate intake of calcium throughout life is necessary. Second, a regular exercise program increases bone mass because weight bearing stimulates the deposit of bone.

TETANY   Despite the hormonal control of serum calcium and the large reservoir in the bones, serum calcium sometimes falls below normal. It may be caused by an actual lack of calcium or a lack of ionized calcium. A serum calcium level that is too low is called hypocalcemia. If the signs and symptoms described below appear, the condition is called tetany. Causes include parathyroid deficiency, vitamin D deficiency, and alkalosis.

Parathyroid deficiency can be caused by disease of the gland or accidental removal of the parathyroid glands during thyroidectomy. Tetany related to vitamin D deficiency can result from inadequate sunlight, malnutrition, or impaired kidney function. In alkalosis, the excessive alkalinity of body fluids, a greater number of calcium ions are bound to serum proteins, effectively inactivating the calcium. Therefore, nerve and muscle function is impaired. Alkalosis may be caused by the loss of acid (due to vomiting or gastric suction) or by the ingestion of alkalies (for example, sodium bicarbonate). Alkalosis can even be caused by breathing too rapidly, either in response to fear or through mechanical ventilation. The result is excessive loss of carbon dioxide. In the blood, carbon dioxide is transported as carbonic acid. Thus, when too much carbon dioxide is exhaled, the blood becomes more alkaline and produces tetany.

Early symptoms of tetany are nervousness, irritability, numbness and tingling of the extremities, and muscle cramps. Diagnostic signs are Trousseau's sign and Chvostek's sign. In Trousseau's sign, inflation of the blood pressure cuff causes ischemia of the peripheral nerves, increasing their excitability. What the examiner sees is muscle spasms of the forearm and hand. In Chvostek's sign, a tap over the facial nerve in front of temple causes a twitch of the facial muscles on that side. Figure 7–3 depicts these diagnostic signs.

Because of the many functions of calcium, tetany is a medical emergency. Untreated, it can progress to respiratory paralysis, seizures or coma, heart dilatation, and blood clotting problems.

Toxicity of Calcium

Hyperparathy-roidism—Excessive secretion of parathyroid hormone, causing changes in the bones, kidneys, and gastrointestinal tract.

A serum calcium level that is too high, above 10.5 milligrams per 100 milliliters of serum, is called hypercalcemia. Individuals taking 2 or more grams of calcium along with 25 micrograms of vitamin D per day for a period of time have developed hypercalcemia. These amounts are two and one-half times the adult RDA for calcium and five times their RDA for vitamin D.

Hypercalcemia can be caused by **hyperparathyroidism** and other diseases, by vitamin D poisoning, and by prolonged excessive intake of milk. Hypercalcemia is seen most frequently in infants of 5 to 8 months of age.

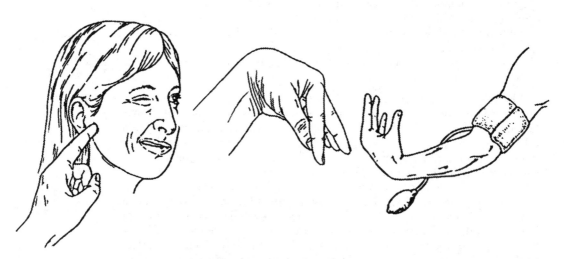

FIGURE 7–3. *A*, Chvostek's sign is a contraction of facial muscles in response to a light tap over the facial nerve in front of the ear. *B*, Trousseau's sign is (1) a carpal spasm (2) induced by inflating a blood pressure cuff above the systolic pressure. (From Lewis, SM, Collier, IC: Medical-Surgical Nursing, ed 2. Mosby Year Book, Inc. p 246, with permission.)

Phosphorus

An adult has about 2 pounds of phosphorus in the body. Eighty-five percent of this is in the bones, and the remaining 15 percent is in cells and body fluids. Phosphorus is closely associated with calcium both in interrelated metabolic functions in the body and in occurrence in foods. See Clinical Application 7–3 for information on phosphorus intake and calcium balance.

Functions of Phosphorus

Phosphorus occurs in bones and teeth as calcium phosphate. Phosphorus is also a component of DNA and RNA. The storage forms of energy, <u>ADP</u> and <u>ATP</u>, contain phosphorus. Phosphorus is an essential mineral in <u>phospholipids,</u> which are structural components of cells. Phospholipids contain glycerol, fatty acids, and phosphorus. Examples include lecithin, a part of cell membranes, and myelin, the insulating covering of many nerves. Phosphorus assists with the absorption of glucose and glycerol. Phosphorus compounds are used as a buffer system to maintain the pH of the blood between 7.35 and 7.45.

Control Mechanism for Phosphorus

A much higher proportion of dietary phosphorus is absorbed than is true of calcium. Seventy percent of dietary phosphorus is absorbed while the remaining 30 percent is excreted in the feces. Absorption occurs in the jejunum, the middle portion of the small intestine. The same factors affecting absorption of calcium are also at work for phosphorus.

Low levels of serum phosphorus stimulate the kidney to produce more active vitamin D. The vitamin D then increases the absorption of phosphorus from the intestinal tract. Excess phosphorus is excreted by the kidney in response to parathyroid hormone.

Recommended Dietary Allowances

The RDAs for phosphorus are: infants—300 to 500 milligrams; children, and men and women aged 25 and older—800 milligrams; individuals aged 11 to 24 and pregnant and lactating women—1200 milligrams.

 CLINICAL APPLICATION 7–3
Phosphorus Intake and Calcium Balance

In the past, the ratio of calcium to phosphorus was considered to be crucial to proper calcium balance. Now authorities believe that the calcium-to-phosphorus ratio is less important than the adequacy of calcium intake (US Department of Health and Human Services, 1989). Results of research indicate that a high phosphorus intake has little or no effect on calcium balance in humans: intake of 2 grams of phosphorus (two and one-half times the RDA) per day did not affect calcium balance in adult men regardless of calcium intake (Committee on Diet and Health, 1989).

Sources of Phosphorus

Phosphorus is widespread in foods simply because it is essential in plant and animal cells. Animal protein is the best source of phosphorus. Since ATP is an energy source in muscle, lean meat is a good source of phosphorus. Good plant sources include nuts and legumes.

Deficiency of Phosphorus

Hypophosphatemia—Too little phosphate per volume of blood; in adults, less than 2.4 mg per 100 ml.

Dietary deficiency of phosphorus is unlikely. Certain diseases or medications, however, will produce **hypophosphatemia.**

Hyperparathyroidism causes excess excretion of phosphorus. In this disease, parathyroid hormone causes withdrawal of calcium from the bones. Since, in the bones, the two are combined, phosphorus is lost along with calcium. Chronic kidney disease often produces the same result and is discussed in Chapter 18.

Toxicity from Phosphorus

Hyperphosphatemia—Abnormal amount of phosphate in the blood; in adults, greater than 4.7 mg per 100 ml.

Hyperphosphatemia caused by dietary overload is unusual. Cases have occurred in infants given only cow's milk during the first few weeks of life. Cow's milk has twice the phosphorus content of human milk and infant formula. That, coupled with an infant's immature kidneys, overtaxes the infant's ability to maintain homeostasis.

Sodium

The adult body contains about 90 grams of sodium, approximately 3 ounces. Two thirds of the sodium in the body is in the blood and other extracellular fluids. The other one third is in the bones.

Functions of Sodium

Sodium has a major role in maintaining fluid balance in the body. This balancing process is discussed in Chapter 9. Sodium also is necessary for the transmission of electrochemical impulses along nerve and muscle membranes and is a component of two phosphate buffers.

Control Mechanism for Sodium

The intestine readily absorbs sodium. Only about 5 percent of dietary sodium travels within the intestine to remain in the feces. To maintain a normal level of sodium in the blood, the kidney either reabsorbs sodium back into the bloodstream or allows it to be spilled in the urine. A hormone from the adrenal cortex, aldosterone, stimulates the kidney to return sodium to the bloodstream. Other control mechanisms for sodium are discussed in Chapter 8.

Recommended Sodium Intake

With sodium the chief concern is not a deficiency of the mineral but an excess of sodium in the diet. A safe minimum intake for infants and young children is considered to be 23 milligrams per kilogram of body weight. For adults, a safe minimum is regarded as 500 milligrams per day. Additional needs for pregnancy and lactation are estimated to be 69 milligrams and 139 milligrams, respectively, over the adult minimum (Subcommittee on the 10th Edition of the RDAs, 1989).

The average American intake is 4 to 6 grams of sodium per day. The maximum daily intake recommended is 2400 milligrams (Committee on Diet and Health, 1989).

Sources of Sodium

Table salt, which is sodium chloride, is the major dietary source of sodium. Table salt is 40 percent sodium and 60 percent chloride. One teaspoonful (5 grams) of salt contains over 2 grams of sodium.

Many foods, such as milk, milk products, and several vegetables, are naturally high in sodium. More often than not, though, the sodium we consume is from the salt in processed foods. Table 7–3 compares the sodium content of relatively unprocessed foods with processed versions.

Deficiency of Sodium

Deficiency of sodium is associated primarily with increased sodium loss. Conditions such as diarrhea, vomiting, heavy sweating, or kidney disease may cause low serum sodium. The technical name for low serum sodium is **hyponatremia.** A serum sodium which is low, not because of an absolute lack of sodium, but because of an excess of water is called dilutional hyponatremia (see Chapter 9).

Hyponatremia— Too little sodium per volume of blood; less than 135 mEq/L in adults.

Toxicity from Sodium

The reported 4 to 6 grams of sodium in the average American diet probably is underestimated. Frequently such surveys do not account for all sources of

TABLE 7–3 *Comparison of Sodium Content in Fresh and Processed Foods*

Fresh Food	Sodium (Milligrams)	Processed Food	Sodium (Milligrams)
Natural Swiss cheese, 1 ounce	74	Pasteurized, processed Swiss cheese, 1 ounce	388
Lean roast pork, 3 ounces	65	Lean ham, 3 ounces	930
Whole raw carrot, 1	25	Canned carrots, ½ cup	176
Tomato juice, canned without salt, 1 cup	24	Tomato juice, canned with salt, 1 cup	881

sodium. Healthy persons excrete excess sodium without adverse effects. For persons with hypertension, heart disease, or kidney disease, the control of sodium balance becomes an important issue. The dietary modifications necessary in these conditions are discussed in Chapters 17 and 18. An excess of sodium in the blood is called <u>hypernatremia.</u>

Potassium

The adult body contains about 270 grams of potassium, approximately 9 ounces. Ninety-eight percent of this amount of potassium is inside the cells, where it helps to control fluid balance.

Functions of Potassium

In addition to fluid balance, potassium is essential for the conduction of nerve impulses and the contraction of muscles, including one vital muscle, the heart. Potassium helps to maintain acid-base balance and is required for the conversion of glucose to glycogen.

Control Mechanism for Potassium

The kidney responds to systemic alkalosis by excreting potassium in order to conserve hydrogen. Retaining the hydrogen will make the blood more acidic and help to correct the alkalosis. Conversely, in acidosis, the body responds by excreting hydrogen and retaining potassium.

Estimated Minimum Intake for Potassium

There are no RDAs established for potassium. The estimated minimum amount for healthy adults is 2000 milligrams per day. The average American diet contains from 2000 to 4000 milligrams of potassium.

Sources of Potassium

Potassium is present in all plant and animal cells. Of all foods, only fats, oils, and white sugar have negligible potassium. The best single source is buttermilk. One cup contains 1910 milligrams. Other foods that supply almost half the minimum amount include: 1 cup of mashed winter squash, 1 cup of plain spaghetti sauce, 1 cup of chili with beans, or 1 potato with skin, baked in the microwave oven.

Deficiency of Potassium

A deficiency of potassium usually does not occur because of diet. Too little potassium in the blood, <u>hypokalemia,</u> can be fatal if prolonged or severe. Hypokalemia may be caused by diarrhea, vomiting, laxative abuse, alkalosis, and protein-calorie malnutrition. Deficiency symptoms include fatigue, muscle weakness, irregular pulse, nausea, vomiting, and decreased reflexes.

Toxicity from Potassium

High potassium levels in the blood, <u>hyperkalemia,</u> also can be fatal. Potassium toxicity is usually the result of diabetic acidosis, kidney failure, adrenal insufficiency, or severe dehydration. Hyperkalemia may also be caused by excessive destruction of cells in burns, crushing injuries, or severe infections. Symptoms include irritability, confusion, irregular slow pulse, diarrhea, and lower extremity weakness. For some conditions, dietary modification of potassium intake becomes an important part of the treatment plan.

Magnesium

The body contains about 1 ounce of magnesium. Up to 70 percent of this amount is combined with calcium and phosphorus in the bones. The remaining 30 percent is found in tissues and body fluids.

Functions of Magnesium

Magnesium is necessary for the transmission of nerve impulses and the relaxation of skeletal muscles after contraction. It activates enzymes for the metabolism of carbohydrates, fats, and proteins, including protein synthesis. Magnesium activates the enzymes that add the third phosphate group to ADP to form ATP. It also aids in the release of energy from muscle glycogen. As a cofactor in calcium utilization, magnesium not only aids bone formation but also helps to hold calcium in tooth enamel, thus preventing tooth decay.

Control Mechanism for Magnesium

Magnesium competes with calcium for absorption in the upper small intestine. As magnesium intake increases, the percentage absorbed decreases. The kidney selectively excretes excess magnesium.

Recommended Dietary Allowances

The RDAs for magnesium are: infants—40 to 60 milligrams; children—80 to 170 milligrams; adolescent boys—270 to 400 milligrams; adolescent girls— 280 to 300 milligrams; men aged 18 years and older—350 milligrams; women aged 18 years and older—280 milligrams; pregnant and lactating women— 320 to 355 milligrams.

Sources and Interfering Factors

Magnesium is widely distributed in foods, especially plant foods, because it is part of the chlorophyll molecule. Green vegetables are good sources of magnesium. For example, one cup of cooked spinach or cooked Swiss chard contains 150 milligrams. Other good sources are legumes, shrimp, and some bran cereals.

High intakes of some nutrients may interfere with the absorption of magnesium. Phosphorus, calcium, fat, and protein are four such nutrients.

Deficiency of Magnesium

Magnesium deficiency may occur with protein-calorie malnutrition, but deficiency usually is the result of increased magnesium excretion or decreased magnesium absorption. Excessive excretion of magnesium can result from vomiting, diarrhea, or diuretic therapy. Magnesium absorption is decreased in malabsorption syndromes and chronic alcoholism. Magnesium deficiency may be responsible for the hallucinations accompanying acute alcohol withdrawal.

Magnesium deficiency probably occurs more often than it is diagnosed. In one study, 20 percent of the patients admitted to a medical intensive care unit had a deficiency of magnesium (Reinhart and Desbiens, 1985). Insufficient magnesium impairs central nervous system activity and increases muscular excitability. Because magnesium metabolism is intricately linked to calcium metabolism, magnesium-deficient patients display the signs of tetany. Other signs include disorientation, convulsions, and psychosis.

Toxicity from Magnesium

Ordinarily, magnesium levels do not build up in the blood except as a result of kidney disease. A person with magnesium toxicity shows the following signs: lethargy, sedation, hypotension, slow pulse, and depressed respirations. Respiratory or cardiac arrest may ensue. Because of its close link to calcium, the effects of magnesium toxicity can be blocked by administering calcium.

Sulfur

Sulfur is a component of the cytoplasm of every cell. It is especially notable in hair, skin, and nails, where the disulfide linkages help to hold the amino acids in their distinct shapes. Sulfur is a component of thiamine, biotin, insulin, and heparin. A protective function of sulfur is that of combining with toxins to neutralize them.

Important sources of sulfur are cheese, eggs, poultry, and fish. Cases of deficiency of sulfur are unknown. Only persons with a severe protein deficiency will lack this mineral.

Chloride

Whenever an industrial accident involving chlorine occurs, such as the derailment of a chlorine tanker car, the surrounding area is quickly evacuated because of the chemical's toxic effects. A harmless form of chlorine, chloride, far from being poisonous, is a required nutrient. The body contains about 90 grams of chloride. Chloride is found in hydrochloric acid in the stomach, and in fluid outside of the cells. Chloride is involved in the maintenance of normal fluid and proper acid-base balance. The estimated minimum recommended intake for chloride ranges from 180 to 300 milligrams for infants and is 750 milligrams for adults. Table salt, 60 percent chloride, contains 3 grams of chloride in 1 teaspoon (5 grams).

Loss of gastrointestinal fluids through severe vomiting, nasogastric suctioning, or diarrhea is a common cause of chloride deficiency. In 1979, an outbreak of chloride deficiency occurred in infants because chloride was omitted from the formula they received.

See Table 7–4 for a summary of the main food sources of each of the major minerals. The foods are divided into five categories: mixed dishes/miscellaneous, meats, milk, fruits/vegetables, and grains.

TABLE 7–4 *Main Sources of Major Minerals by Food Groups*

Mineral	Mixed Dishes/ Miscellaneous	Meats	Milk	Fruits/ Vegetables	Grains
Calcium			All forms	Dark green leafy	
Phosphorus		Lean meat	All forms		
Sodium	Table salt	Processed meat		Canned vegetables	
Potassium	Chili with beans, Morton Salt Substitute or Light salt, plain spaghetti sauce	Meat		Winter squash, orange juice, bananas, dry beans	Whole grains
Magnesium		Shrimp		Green vegetables, legumes, nuts	
Sulfur		Poultry, fish, eggs	Cheese		
Chloride	Table salt	Processed meat		Canned vegetables	

TRACE MINERALS

Trace minerals are present in the body in amounts less than 5 grams and have a recommended intake of less than 100 milligrams per day. Many trace minerals occur in such small amounts that they are difficult to measure and analyze; thus their physiological functions and possible roles in nutrition are not completely understood. For example, lead, gold, and mercury are found in body tissue but only, as far as is known, as the result of environmental contamination. See Clinical Application 7–4 for a discussion on lead poisoning.

Eight trace minerals have probable, but as yet undetermined, functions in human nutrition. This group includes aluminum, arsenic, boron, cadmium, nickel, tin, silicon, and vanadium. Aluminum and its association with brain disorders is discussed in Chapter 18.

Of the other trace minerals, only ten have known bodily functions and have been assigned RDAs, estimated safe and adequate daily dietary intakes (ESADDIs), or estimated minimum requirements. Four of them are commonly recognized as being health related: iron, iodine, fluoride, and zinc. The other six include chromium, copper, cobalt, manganese, selenium, and molybdenum. These ten minerals are discussed individually in the sections below, starting with iron.

Iron

For a nutrient with functions as vital as those of iron, the amount in the body is very slight—about 4 grams. This is approximately the weight of a penny.

Function of Iron

Iron is essential to **hemoglobin** formation. Hemoglobin is composed of heme, the nonprotein portion that contains iron, and globin, a simple pro-

Hemoglobin— The iron-carrying pigment of the red blood cells; carries oxygen from the lungs to the tissues.

CLINICAL APPLICATION 7–4
Lead Poisoning

Lead is a contaminant in the human body. The effects of lead toxicity, such as neurological damage and retardation, can be devastating and permanent.

A 1981 survey of 535,000 children in the United States, aged 6 months to 5 years, revealed that 4.1 percent of them had symptoms of lead poisoning. Rural children were affected at a 2 percent rate, whereas inner-city children were affected at a 10 percent rate. Elevated blood lead levels were found in 12.2 percent of black children.

The chief sources of lead are not foods. Lead-based paint in older homes is the primary source for inner-city children. The chips of paint are sweet tasting. A piece the size of a penny may contain from 50 to 100 micrograms of lead. This amount ingested every day for 3 months amounts to 100 times the tolerable level for adults and could produce symptoms of lead poisoning.

Other sources of lead are automobile emissions from leaded gasoline, lead or lead glazes on serving utensils, and solder in metal cans. In addition, homemade stills fabricated from car radiators can produce moonshine whiskey that contains lead. Another possible source of lead contamination is the ink used on bread wrappers. Habitually turning the bags inside out and then using them for food storage could create a problem.

Hyperactivity has been linked to both lead poisoning and iron deficiency. There is evidence that suggests that these two conditions, not additives, allergens, or sugar, are the causes of hyperactivity.

Early diagnosis and treatment of lead poisoning are essential. Several chelating agents are available that will bind with lead. Even children successfully treated and kept away from further intake showed lasting brain damage in 25 percent of the cases.

Recently, concern about the lead content in aging municipal water pipes contaminating the water supply has resulted in action by the Environmental Protection Agency (EPA). The permissible lead level has been lowered from 50 parts per billion to 15 parts per billion. Many older homes also have plumbing that may contaminate the water. To decrease the chance of lead leaching into drinking or cooking water, (1) flush the system before drawing water and (2) use cold water. Local health departments should be able to direct people to appropriate laboratories if they wish to have their water tested.

Myoglobin—A protein located in muscle tissue that contains iron and stores oxygen.

tein. Iron is also a component of **myoglobin,** a protein located in muscle tissue. Myoglobin stores oxygen within the muscle cells. When the body needs an immediate supply of oxygen, as during strenuous exercise, myoglobin releases its stored oxygen. Iron is also present in enzymes that permit the oxidation of glucose to produce energy.

About 80 percent of the iron in a healthy body is available for carrying oxygen: 70 percent is contained in the hemoglobin, 5 percent in the myoglobin, and 5 percent in iron-containing enzymes. The remaining 20 percent is stored.

The main storage form of iron in the body is a protein-iron compound called **ferritin**. It is kept in the liver, spleen, and bone marrow for future use. When surplus iron accumulates in the blood due to the rapid destruction of red blood cells, the excess is stored in the liver in another compound, **hemosiderin**.

Absorption of Iron

The body tightly conserves its supply of iron. When red blood cells are destroyed after their life span of 120 days, the iron is stored for reuse. Once iron is absorbed, there is no mechanism for excreting excess. Fortunately, the body is selective about absorbing iron.

FACTORS AFFECTING AMOUNTS OF ABSORPTION As the body's need for iron increases, so does the proportion absorbed. In a healthy person, 5 to 15 percent of the iron in foods is absorbed. The anemic person, however, absorbs as much as 50 percent. In other words, the smaller the body stores, the more iron absorbed; the greater the body stores, the less iron absorbed.

The amount of iron that is absorbed is determined by the amount of ferritin already present in the intestinal mucosa (where ferritin is formed). The iron obtained from ingested food is bound to a protein called **apoferritin** to form ferritin. When the total supply of apoferritin has been bound to iron, any additional iron in the gut is rejected and eliminated in the feces.

Absorbed iron combines with a protein in the blood, **transferrin**, which transports iron to the bone marrow for hemoglobin synthesis, to the liver for storage, or to the body cells. Hemoglobin synthesis requires adequate protein and traces of copper, in addition to iron.

FACTORS AFFECTING RATES OF ABSORPTION Two types of iron are found naturally in food: heme iron and nonheme iron. **Heme iron** is bound to the hemoglobin and myoglobin in meat, fish, and poultry. Forty percent of the total iron in these animal sources is heme iron. Because heme iron is composed of ferrous iron, (Fe^{2+}), it is rapidly transported and absorbed intact. The other 60 percent of the total iron in meat, fish, and poultry, and all the iron in plant sources, is **nonheme iron.**

The absorption of nonheme iron is slow because it is closely bound to organic molecules in foods as ferric iron (Fe^{3+}). In the acidic medium of the stomach, the oxygen is removed from ferric iron during a chemical reaction called reduction. The end product is ferrous iron, which is more soluble. See Figure 7–4 for an overview of the steps involved in the process of iron absorption.

FACTORS ENHANCING THE ABSORPTION OF IRON Several factors increase the absorption of iron through very different mechanisms. Consumption of large amounts of alcohol damages the intestine, which then permits absorption of increased amounts of iron. A high calcium intake increases iron absorption because the calcium combines with phosphates and phytates so that they are not available to inhibit iron absorption. Vitamin C forms a soluble compound with iron. Drinking orange juice increased iron absorption two and one-half times in nine different breakfasts (Rossander, Hallberg, and Bjorn-Rasmussen, 1979). Lastly, an MFP (meat, fish, poultry) factor increases the absorption of iron. Nonheme iron absorption is increased when meat, fish, or poultry is consumed at the same time.

Ferritin—Form in which iron is stored in the tissues, mainly in liver, spleen, and bone marrow cells.

Hemosiderin—An iron oxide–protein compound derived from hemoglobin; a secondary storage form of iron.

Apoferritin—A protein found in intestinal mucosal cells that combines with iron to form ferritin; it is always found in the body attached to iron.

Transferrin—A protein in the blood that binds and transports iron.

Heme iron—Iron bound to hemoglobin and myoglobin in meat, fish, and poultry; 10 to 30 percent of the iron in these foods is absorbed.

Nonheme iron—Iron that is not bound to hemoglobin or myoglobin; all the iron in plant sources.

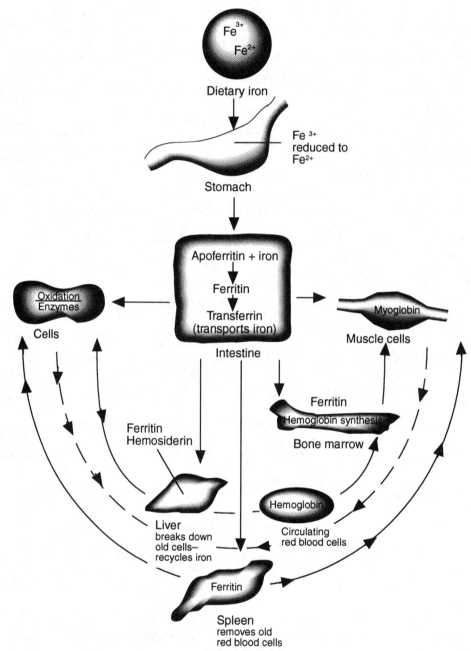

FIGURE 7–4. In the process of iron absorption, iron is absorbed primarily in the small intestine and may be transported or stored to meet the body's needs.

FACTORS INTERFERING WITH ABSORPTION OF IRON Some of these factors are the opposite of the enhancing factors. For instance, when less gastric acid is present, whether because of antacids or gastric resection, the absorption of iron is decreased. Both phytic acid from cereals and oxalic acid from certain vegetables combine with iron, reducing its availability. Other minerals compete with iron for binding sites. Excesses of copper, zinc, or manganese decrease absorption of each other and of iron.

Nonheme iron can be locked out of the absorption process by substances called tannates, which are found in tea and coffee. Tea contains more tannates than coffee, and is thus the more potent interfering agent. Tea with breakfast reduced iron absorption by one half (Rossander, Hallberg, and Bjorn-Rasmussen, 1979). Coffee decreases absorption of iron when taken during or within 1 hour after a meal. The stronger the coffee, the less iron absorbed (Morck, Lynch, and Cook, 1983). Table 7–5 summarizes the factors that affect iron absorption.

Excretion of Iron

No known mechanism exists to regulate the excretion of iron. Small amounts of iron are lost daily in sweat, hair, shed skin cells, and urine. Men lose 1 milligram per day, whereas women of reproductive age lose an average 1.5 to 2.4 milligrams per day, depending upon menstrual flow.

Recommended Dietary Allowance

The values set for the RDA are based on the assumption that only 10 to 15 percent of the iron in ingested foods is absorbed. The RDAs for iron are: infants up six months of age—6 milligrams; adolescent boys—12 milligrams; women of reproductive age and lactating women—15 milligrams; and pregnant women—30 milligrams. For everyone else the RDA is 10 milligrams.

Sources of Iron

In the United States, one third of dietary iron is supplied by grains, one third by meats, and one third by other sources. Absorption varies among the sources of iron also. Ten to thirty percent of iron is absorbed from liver and other meats; less than 10 percent is absorbed from eggs; and less than 5 percent is absorbed from grains and most vegetables. Spinach, iron supplements, and contamination iron are absorbed at a 2 percent rate. Clinical Application 7–5 describes one way iron is absorbed from nonfood sources.

TABLE 7–5 *Factors Affecting Iron Absorption*

Increase	Decrease
Large alcohol intake	Less gastric acid
High calcium intake	Coffee or tea (tannates)
Vitamin C	Phytic or oxalic acids
Meat, fish, or poultry	Excessive copper, manganese, or zinc

CLINICAL APPLICATION 7–5
Contamination Iron

It is possible to increase the iron content of foods by using iron cookware. Iron absorbed into food in this way is referred to as <u>contamination iron.</u> Little transfer of iron occurs during frying, but significant transfer does occur during the boiling or simmering of acidic foods, especially tomatoes. For instance, 3½ ounces of spaghetti sauce cooked for 3 hours in a cast iron pot contains almost 90 milligrams of iron. Compare this with the less than 5 milligrams of iron the sauce would contain if it were cooked in a glass container. Another acidic food, applesauce, acquires about fifty times the iron after cooking for 2 hours in iron cookware compared with glass cookware. Iron content of nonacidic foods can be increased in this way also, but to a much lesser extent. The absorption rate of contamination iron is the same as that of iron supplements, 2 percent at best.

Of the commercial cereals directed toward children, only Cap'n Crunch comes close to the 10-milligram RDA for children aged 1 through 10. It has 9.83 milligrams of iron per cup. Selected cereal products containing significant amounts of iron are listed in Table 7–6. As always, it is imperative to read labels when purchasing food. Although cereals and grains are nonheme sources, iron from grains is absorbed at a better rate than iron from supplements. Figure 7–5 illustrates some good sources of iron for the person who chooses not to eat liver.

Deficiency of Iron

Insufficient intake of iron, excessive blood loss, malabsorption, or lack of gastric hydrochloric acid can lead to iron deficiency anemia. This is the most common nutrient deficiency in the United States. The average United States diet contains 6 to 7 milligrams of iron per 1000 kilocalories. If men consume enough kilocalories and the diet is balanced, their iron needs are usually met. However, many women are deficient in both kilocaloric and iron intake.

TABLE 7–6 *Comparison of Iron Content of Cereal Products*

Cereal	Iron per Cup (Milligrams)
Kellogg's Raisin Bran	24
Product 19	21
Total	21
Kellogg's 40% Bran Flakes	11
Regular Cream of Wheat	11
Cap'n Crunch	9.83
Post Raisin Bran	9

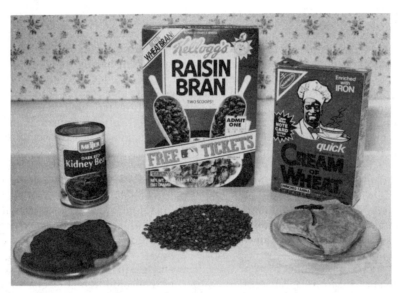

FIGURE 7–5. If a person does not like liver, there are other good sources of iron including (clockwise from top left): kidney beans, bran cereal with raisins, cream of wheat, and lentils.

OCCURRENCE   Iron deficiency anemia affects 10 to 20 percent of the world population. Iron deficiency is seen in 9.3 percent of 1- to 2-year-old children. Women 15 to 19 years old have a prevalence of 7.2 percent and those 20 to 44 years old, 6.3 percent. In sharp contrast, iron deficiency occurred in less than 1 percent of men aged 15 to 64.

RISK OF IRON DEFICIENCY   Individuals at greatest risk of iron deficiency are women of childbearing age and young children. Children 4 months to 3 years old, adolescents, and pregnant women should be monitored carefully for signs of iron deficiency because of increased needs. People with low incomes also are likely to be iron deficient. All women in their menstrual years are at risk, a risk that is increased if an intrauterine contraceptive device is being used. This device increases blood loss.

ASSESSMENT DATA   A common test to determine the hemoglobin level of the blood delivers valuable assessment data. The normal level for men is 14 to 18 grams per 100 milliliters of blood; for women it is 12 to 16 grams.

A second common laboratory test is the hematocrit. This test measures the percentage of red blood cells in a volume of blood. Normal hematocrit levels are 40 to 54 percent for men and 36 to 46 percent for women.

In early iron deficiency, before hemoglobin and hematocrit readings drop, serum transferrin levels rise. The person with early iron deficiency will, providing the body is attempting to compensate, manufacture more transferrin to increase iron-carrying capacity. For this reason, serum transferrin is the most reliable indicator of iron status.

After a person has been treated for iron deficiency, iron therapy should be continued for several months after hemoglobin and hematocrit levels return to normal. This prolonged therapy will enable the body to rebuild iron stores.

Toxicity from Iron

Iron toxicity can result from an oversupply of hemosiderin, iron metabolism disorders, chronic alcoholism, or iron poisoning. Surplus iron is stored in the liver as hemosiderin. When large amounts of hemosiderin are deposited in the liver and spleen, a condition called **hemosiderosis** results. If prolonged, it can lead to <u>hemochromatosis,</u> a disease of iron metabolism in which iron accumulates in the tissues. The person with this disease suffers from impaired liver function, blood sugar disturbances, joint pain, and skin discoloration. Cardiac failure and death may follow.

Hemosiderosis— Condition resulting from excess deposits of hemosiderin, especially in the liver and spleen; caused by the rapid destruction of red blood cells, which occurs in diseases such as hemolytic anemia, pernicious anemia, and chronic infection.

Chronic alcoholics have increased absorption of iron because of intestinal damage. Toxicity can occur if 75 milligrams of iron per day is ingested along with a regular intake of alcohol. Some alcoholic beverages themselves contain a significant amount of iron. For example, inexpensive red wines contain 10 to 350 milligrams of iron per liter. Thus, although the use of wine as a tonic may have certain merit, this is not the case when the user is an alcoholic.

Iron supplements present a significant hazard to children. Iron is second only to aspirin as a cause of poisoning in small children. Ferrous sulfate accounts for 6.2 percent of all acute poisonings in children. As few as six to twelve tablets of ferrous sulfate have been known to cause the death of a child. All nurses should teach safe storage of nutritional supplements.

Iodine

Iodine can be found in the muscles, thyroid gland, skin, and skeleton. The greatest concentration is in the thyroid gland, which is located in the neck. The body of the average adult contains 20 to 50 milligrams of iodine.

Function of Iodine

The thyroid gland secretes <u>thyroxine</u> (T_4) and triiodothyronine (T_3). Both of these hormones increase the rate of oxidation in cells, thereby increasing the rate at which the body's metabolism proceeds. The only known function of iodine is its participation in the synthesis of T_4 and T_3.

Control Mechanism for Iodine

Iodine is easily absorbed from all portions of the intestinal tract. Of the absorbed iodine, 33 percent is used by the thyroid cells for the synthesis of T_4 and T_3, and the remaining 67 percent is excreted in the urine. After performing their functions, T_4 and T_3 are degraded by the liver, and the iodine content is excreted in bile.

Recommended Dietary Allowance

The RDAs for iodine are: infants—40 to 50 micrograms; children—70 to 120 micrograms; adult men and women—150 micrograms; pregnant women— 175 micrograms; and lactating women—200 micrograms.

Sources of Iodine

Iodine can come from foods, either naturally present or fortified, or from incidental sources.

IODINE IN FOODS   Foods that are naturally high in iodine include saltwater fish, shellfish, and seaweed. The iodine content in plants varies with the mineral content of the soil in which they are grown. The amount of iodine present in eggs and dairy products depends on the animals' diets.

Table salt fortified with iodine (1 milligram of iodine in 10 grams of salt) has been available in the United States since 1924. You may have heard that sea salt is superior to regular table salt. However, because sea salt loses iodine during the evaporating (drying) process, it actually contains less iodine than fortified table salt.

INCIDENTAL IODINE   Sometimes we consume iodine that is present in the food as a side effect of processing. For example, iodine solutions are used to sterilize milk pasteurization vats; some iodine may remain on the vat and be mixed into the next batch of milk to be processed. Iodine is also used to improve the texture of bread dough. A third source of incidental iodine is FDA Red Dye #3.

Deficiency of Iodine

Because the normal function of the thyroid gland depends on an adequate supply of iodine, a deficiency may result in goiter, cretinism, or myxedema. Fortunately, thyroid function can be readily evaluated by measuring protein-bound iodine and the serum levels of T_4 and T_3.

GOITER   When the thyroid gland does not receive sufficient iodine, it increases in size, attempting to increase production. The gland may reach 1 to 1.5 pounds (500 to 700 grams). This enlargement of the thyroid is called **goiter.** Unfortunately, replacement of iodine does not reduce the goiter after the thyroid has enlarged.

Goiter has been known as a disease entity since 3000 BC. In Asia alone, 400 million people have goiter. Because of iodine-poor soil, the Great Lakes states and the Rocky Mountain states once were considered the "goiter belt." Now that food supplies are nationwide and iodized salt is readily available, goiter is less common in this country.

CRETINISM   Severe **hypothyroidism** during pregnancy results in cretinism in the newborn. As a consequence of the mother's thyroid deficiency, the infant exhibits mental and physical retardation. Cretinism is a congenital condition (present at birth). The acquired form of this disease, which occurs in older children and adults, is called myxedema.

Goiter—Enlargement of the thyroid gland caused by lack of sufficient iodine, thyroiditis due to infection or tumors, or hypofunction or hyperfunction of the thyroid gland.

Hypothyroidism—Undersecretion of thyroid hormones; reduces the metabolic rate.

Factors Interfering with Iodine

Substances called goitrogens may block the body's absorption or utilization of iodine. Goitrogens are found in vegetables belonging to the cabbage family, including cabbage, rutabaga, and turnips.

Toxicity from Iodine

Toxicity from iodine has occurred in Japan from the ingestion of seaweed. Some nutritionists have expressed concern that iodine is oversupplied in the American diet, which contains 4 to 13 times the adult RDA. Strangely, too much iodine causes an "iodine goiter" and may also cause skin lesions similar to acne.

Fluoride

Fluoride, an ionized form of the element fluorine, accumulates mostly in the bones and teeth. It seems to make bone mineral less soluble and hence less likely to be reabsorbed. As such, fluoride inhibits dental caries and has been investigated as possibly helping to prevent osteoporosis.

Function of Fluoride

Teeth are strengthened by the incorporation of fluoride into their structure and are thus better able to resist the bacterial acids that cause dental caries. For this reason, fluoride is often added to water supplies, mouthwashes, and toothpastes, or taken as a prescription supplement. In the past 20 years, the use of fluoridated water and fluoride supplements has resulted in a 30 to 50 percent decrease in children's caries. In addition, fluoridated mouth rinses and toothpastes have reduced the incidence of caries in children by about 40 percent.

Estimated Safe and Adequate Daily Dietary Intake

The ESADDIs that have been set for fluoride are: infants 0.0 to 0.5 years—0.1 to 0.5 milligrams; infants 0.5 to 1 year—0.2 to 1.0 milligrams; children 1 to 3 years old—0.5 to 1.5 milligrams; 4 to 6 years old—1.0 to 2.5 milligrams; 7 to 10 years old—1.5 to 2.5 milligrams; 11 years old to adult—1.5 to 2.5 milligrams; and adults—1.5 to 4 milligrams.

Sources of Fluoride

One of the main sources of fluoride is fluoridated water. About 50 percent of the community water supply in the United States is fluoridated, to a concentration of one part per million. This amount equals 1 teaspoonful of fluoride to 1,000,000 teaspoonfuls of water. Fluoridation costs only 30 cents per person per year. In Great Britain milk is fluoridated rather than water. Food sources of fluoride include fish, fish products, and tea. Also, foods prepared in fluoridated water will have increased levels of fluoride.

Toxicity from Fluoride

The excessive, prolonged ingestion of fluoride results in <u>fluorosis,</u> a condition that can cause mottled discoloration of the teeth in children (from birth to 8 or 10 years old). Fluorosis has been observed when the concentration of fluoride has reached 2 parts per million. The fluorosis produced by this dose may be cosmetically unacceptable, but the teeth are sound. Just as an excess of iodine causes the same symptoms as deficiency (i.e., goiter), a fluoride concentration of 4 parts per million is associated with increased dental caries.

Fluoride intake bears watching: some persons receive too little fluoride; others too much. For example, members of communities that do not have a fluoridated water supply may develop fluoride insufficiency, while the increased availability and excess use of fluoridated products (including water) may lead to toxicity.

Zinc

Zinc is a component of all body tissues, including pancreas, liver, kidney, lung, muscle, bone, eye, skin, and sperm. Greater concentrations are found in the eye, bone, and male reproductive organs.

Functions of Zinc

Zinc is essential for the growth and repair of tissues because it is involved in the synthesis of DNA and RNA. Zinc is incorporated into the structure of more than 200 enzymes for protein and DNA synthesis, and it is associated with the hormone insulin. It is also necessary for the metabolism of all the energy nutrients. The production of active vitamin A for the visual pigment rhodopsin requires zinc. It is necessary for the formation of collagen, a requisite material for wound healing. Zinc also protects against disease through its role in providing immunity.

Control Mechanism for Zinc

Zinc is absorbed from the small intestine through the same absorption sites as iron. No storage is available in the body for zinc.

Unabsorbed zinc and the zinc in pancreatic secretions are excreted through intestinal wastes. The liver removes excessive zinc effectively. An abnormal zinc metabolism has been observed in persons with diabetes, but zinc's role in the etiology of diabetes is as yet unknown. The healthy person excretes no zinc in the urine, but in catabolic conditions, zinc (as well as potassium, creatinine, and nitrogen) appears in the urine from the breakdown of muscle tissue.

Recommended Dietary Allowances

The RDAs for zinc are: infants—5 milligrams; children—10 milligrams; boys 11 years and older, men, and pregnant women—15 milligrams; girls and women—12 milligrams; lactating women—19 milligrams during first 6 months and 16 milligrams the second 6 months.

Sources of Zinc

The best dietary sources of zinc are shellfish, red meat, and liver. Three and one-half ounces of cooked Western oysters contain 48 milligrams of zinc. More popular foods provide smaller amounts: 3 ounces of lean roast beef or sirloin steak provide 5 milligrams; 1 cheeseburger contains 5.27 milligrams, and 1 cup of chili con carne with beans offers 4.15 milligrams of zinc. Other good sources include milk, eggs, and legumes.

Interfering Factors

Iron and zinc compete for the same absorption sites. Thus, if a person's intake of iron is two to three times that of zinc, the absorption of zinc is reduced. Decreased absorption of zinc has been noted when a 30-milligram supplement of iron is taken. As with iron, excessive copper or manganese decreases the absorption of zinc. Vitamin-mineral supplements with a

Chelating agent—Chemical compound that binds metallic ions into a ring structure, inactivating them; used to remove poisonous metals from the body.

greater than a 3-to-1 iron-to-zinc ratio inhibit zinc absorption. Calcium, excess folate, fiber, phytates, and **chelating agents** all reduce the absorption of zinc. Zinc itself is a chelating agent protecting the body from poisoning from lead and cadmium. If a person has marginal zinc status, high intakes of coffee, cocoa, tea, or whole grain products (especially if unleavened) may lower zinc levels because of their phytate content.

Deficiency of Zinc

In general, clinical zinc deficiency is not widespread in the United States. However, the American food supply provides only 12.3 milligrams per person per day. This amount is less than recommended for men and for pregnant and lactating women. Other groups at risk because of limited meat intake include the elderly, the poor, and vegetarians. Dietary changes begun for one reason may produce an unexpected result. For example, decreasing red meat intake to avoid heart disease and increasing fiber intake to avoid cancer are apt to reduce zinc levels.

Zinc deficiency in adults can also occur as a result of diseases that either hinder zinc absorption or cause excessive amounts of zinc to be excreted in the urine. Some of the clinical conditions that may precipitate zinc deficiency include acute myocardial infarction, alcoholic cirrhosis, celiac disease, Crohn's disease, and lymphoma.

Symptoms of zinc deficiency include abnormal fatigue, decreased alertness, impaired night vision, anorexia, and diminished sense of taste and smell. Signs include diarrhea and vomiting, retarded growth (dwarfism), delayed sexual maturation (if deficiency occurs during critical growth periods), low sperm counts, and delayed healing of wounds and burns.

Toxicity from Zinc

Because zinc can be toxic if consumed in excessive amounts, it should be obtained from foods in the diet and not from supplements. Supplemental doses only two to three times the RDA can interfere with copper absorption and lead to copper deficiency. Supplementation at the RDA level blocks the exercise effect of increasing serum levels of high-density lipoproteins (HDL), the "good cholesterol." Ten times the RDA, 150 milligrams per day, has been shown to impair white blood cells and decrease high-density lipoproteins (Subcommittee on 10th edition of RDAs, 1989).

Copper

The healthy adult body contains 80 milligrams of copper. Copper is absorbed in the stomach and upper intestine and is excreted in feces as a component of bile salts.

Functions of Copper

Copper is a cofactor for enzymes involved in hemoglobin and collagen formation. It helps to incorporate iron into hemoglobin and to transport iron to the bone marrow. As a component of Factor V, copper is necessary for blood clotting. It helps to oxidize glucose and release energy. Copper is necessary for melanin pigment formation and for maintaining myelin sheaths in the nervous system.

Estimated Safe and Adequate Daily Dietary Intake

The ESADDI for copper ranges from 0.4 to 0.6 milligrams for infants to 1.5 to 3 milligrams for adults. Intake in the United States, however, averages 1 to 2 milligrams for adults.

Sources of Copper

Unfortunately, data is lacking on the copper content of 30 percent of foods listed or programmed in databases. The best sources are organ meats, shellfish, nuts, and legumes. Three ounces of liver or ⅓ cup of oysters contain 3 milligrams.

High intakes of zinc, iron, and manganese interfere with copper absorption. Phytates hinder absorption by forming even more stable complexes with copper than with calcium or iron. An additional mineral with no known physiological function, cadmium, also decreases copper absorption.

Deficiency of Copper

Copper deficiency is not known in adults under normal conditions, but it has occurred as a result of the administration of **total parenteral nutrition** (TPN), for prolonged periods. Total parenteral nutrition is an intravenous feeding designed to meet all a person's nutritional needs. Copper deficiency also has occurred in premature infants fed exclusively on cow's milk.

Total parenteral nutrition(TPN)— An intravenous feeding that provides total nutrition.

Because of its link with iron utilization, copper deficiency produces signs of anemia. Other manifestations of copper deficiency are reduced growth, hypercholesterolemia, and impaired heart function.

Toxicity from Copper

Regular consumption of 10 milligrams or more per day produces toxicity. A genetic defect in excretion of copper causes Wilson's disease; copper then accumulates in various organs. Part of the treatment regimen is avoiding foods high in copper.

Selenium

The mineral selenium is part of an enzyme, glutathione peroxidase, which works with vitamin E to protect cellular compounds from oxidation. In this role, selenium functions as an antioxidant. Selenium and vitamin E have a reciprocal sparing relationship (i.e., each spares the other). Selenium forms part of the protein matrix of the teeth and also helps to protect the liver from cirrhosis. The highest concentrations of this mineral occur in the liver, kidneys, heart, and spleen.

The RDA for selenium ranges from 10 to 75 micrograms: 70 micrograms for adult men; 55 micrograms for adult women. Adolescence, pregnancy, and lactation increase the need for selenium and a high vitamin E intake reduces it.

The amount of selenium present in plant foods depends on the selenium content of the soil and water where the foods are grown. In Finland it is necessary to add selenium to the soil. Seafood, low-fat meats, whole grains, dairy products, and legumes are the best dietary sources of selenium.

Deficiencies of selenium have been produced in animals but are unlikely in humans if meat is consumed on a regular basis. Nevertheless, there are some exceptions. Several patients being maintained on total parenteral nutrition have developed heart disease that responded to selenium treatment. A deterioration of the heart due to selenium deficiency has occurred in residents of the province of Keshan, China. The fatality rate in what is called Keshan disease is as high as 80 percent.

Toxicity from selenium occurs in animals grazing on selenium-rich land. In humans, selenium toxicity occurred when the amount in a supplement was 125 times the correct dose. Signs and symptoms of selenium toxicity include fatigue, nausea and vomiting, garlic or sour-milk breath odor, and nail and hair loss. Animals who consume excessive selenium exhibit nervous system impairment and die of respiratory failure.

Chromium

This essential nutrient is the same chromium used in shiny automobile and appliance parts. Less than 6 milligrams of chromium is found in the body, with the highest concentrations occurring in the adrenal glands, brain, skin, muscles, and fat.

Chromium is associated with RNA and DNA and is a cofactor in the activation of enzymes involved in fat and cholesterol metabolism. Chromium increases the cellular uptake of glucose by helping to bind insulin to its receptor sites on the cell membranes. Chromium is a component of glucose tolerance factor (GTF), which stimulates the action of insulin.

Glucose tolerance factor
(GTF)—Organic compound containing chromium, which enhances the action of insulin, facilitating the uptake of glucose by the body's cells.

The ESADDI for chromium ranges from 10 to 200 micrograms. The estimated safe amount for adults ranges from 50 to 200 micrograms. Less than 5 percent of the dietary chromium is absorbed. The chief organ of excretion is the kidney.

Brewer's yeast and whole grains are good sources of chromium. Unprocessed foods are better sources than refined foods. Other sources are meats, especially oysters and liver; dairy products; and seasonings such as thyme and black pepper.

Chromium deficiency impairs the effectiveness of insulin and usually results in an elevated blood glucose or glucose intolerance. In some patients receiving total parenteral nutrition, chromium, not insulin, successfully lowered their blood sugar levels. Lack of sufficient chromium intake is also associated with coronary artery disease.

Toxicity from chromium usually occurs from eating contaminated foods. The characteristic symptom is a disagreeable metallic taste in the mouth.

Manganese

The body contains only 20 milligrams of manganese, found mostly in the bones and glands. Manganese is a cofactor of enzymes involved in energy metabolism and is required for hemoglobin synthesis, thiamin utilization, and tendon and bone formation. Unlike nutrients that fulfill unique functions, other minerals sometimes can substitute for manganese. One such mineral is magnesium.

The ESADDI for manganese ranges from 0.3 milligrams to 5 milligrams. The estimated safe and adequate level for adults is 2 to 5 milligrams. About 40 percent of the manganese ingested is absorbed. It is excreted in bile and pancreatic secretions.

The best sources of manganese are wheat bran, dried legumes, seeds, nuts, and leafy green vegetables. Other good sources are cereal grains, coffee, and tea. Excessive intakes of iron, zinc, or copper cause decreased manganese absorption.

Low serum manganese levels have been reported in diabetes, pancreatic insufficiency, protein-calorie malnutrition, and some types of epilepsy. The patient displays weight loss, hypocholesterolemia, nausea, vomiting, dermatitis, and color changes of the hair.

Toxicity due to dietary intake has not been reported. However, miners exposed to manganese dust over prolonged periods have suffered liver and central nervous system damage, muscle spasms, and monotone voice. The clinical picture of manganese toxicity resembles Parkinson's disease.

Cobalt

As an essential component of the vitamin B_{12} molecule, cobalt is necessary for red blood cell formation. An RDA for cobalt has not been established. Foods that provide vitamin B_{12} are also good sources of cobalt; these foods are meats, milk, cheese, and eggs.

Cobalt deficiency has not been reported in humans or animals. Very large pharmaceutical doses have produced an excess of red blood cells (polycythemia) in humans, and chronic high doses over time can produce goiter (Lindeman, 1987).

Molybdenum

Molybdenum, a cofactor for enzymes involved in protein synthesis, is found primarily in the liver, kidneys, bone, skin, and adrenal glands. It is equally excreted in the urine and the feces.

The ESADDI ranges from 15 to 250 micrograms. The estimated safe and adequate level for adults is 75 to 250 micrograms. Daily intake from the average diet provides from 200 to 500 micrograms. Sources of molybdenum are milk, organ meats, legumes, vegetables, and grains. Because molybdenum is a copper antagonist, high levels of copper decrease the absorption of molybdenum.

One patient on total parenteral nutrition was treated as molybdenum deficient. His signs and symptoms were caused by an inability to process sulfur-containing amino acids. His clinical picture was of increased pulse rate and respiratory rate, visual defects, night blindness, irritability, and coma. After discontinuation of sulfur-containing amino acid intake and supplementation with molybdenum, the symptoms disappeared (Committee on Diet and Health, 1989).

In Russia, intakes of 10 to 15 milligrams of molybdenum per day (40 times the US ESADDI) are associated with hyperuricemia and gout. No definite toxicity has been documented in humans.

A summary of the main food sources of each of the trace minerals discussed in this chapter appears in Table 7–7.

TABLE 7-7 *Main Sources of Trace Minerals by Food Groups*

Mineral	Mixed Dishes/ Miscellaneous	Meats	Milk	Fruits/ Vegetables	Grains
Iron	Fortified infant formulas, iron cookware	Meat, esp. liver, eggs	Seafood	Dark green leafy, nuts, legumes	Selected cereals, whole grains
Iodine	Fortified table salt	Saltwater fish	Milk*		Bakery products*
Fluoride	Fluoridated water, supplements, tea	Fish			
Zinc		Shellfish, red meat			
Copper		Organ meats, shellfish		Nuts, legumes	
Selenium		Lean meat, seafood	Milk products	Legumes	Whole grains
Chromium	Thyme, black pepper	Meat, esp. liver, oysters	Milk products		Brewer's yeast, whole grains
Manganese				Legumes, seeds, nuts, green leafy	Wheat bran
Cobalt		Meat, eggs	Milk, cheese		
Molybdenum		Organ meats		Legumes	Grains

*Contaminant Iodine

SUPPLEMENTATION

Excessive intake of nutrients can be as harmful as insufficient intake. For healthy people, obtaining minerals from food is preferred over medicinal supplementation. If supplements are elected by healthy people, the dose should not exceed the RDAs or ESADDIs for each mineral. For some minerals, toxicity is possible at levels slightly above the recommended or estimated intake amounts. In addition, an excess of one mineral may cause a deficiency of another.

Summary

Minerals are inorganic substances that are necessary for good health. Like vitamins, they help to regulate body functions without providing energy. Unlike vitamins, minerals become part of the body's structure and also part of its enzymes.

In human nutrition, minerals are classified as major or trace. Major minerals are present in the body in amounts of 5 grams (1 teaspoonful) or more and have a daily recommended intake of 100 milligrams or more. Of the seven major minerals, inadequate calcium intake and excessive sodium intake are considered actual public health problems, and inadequate potassium intake is considered a potential public health problem.

Trace minerals are those present in amounts smaller than 5 grams and have a daily recommended intake of less than 100 milligrams. Of the 10 trace minerals discussed in this chapter, only lack of iron intake is considered a public health issue in the United States. Intakes of fluoride and zinc are being monitored as potential problems by the federal government.

As is the case with vitamins, people can be adversely affected by either insufficient or excessive intakes of minerals. Strangely, some minerals produce the same symptoms in both cases. When a patient is nourished only by intravenous feedings for a long time, deficiencies of trace minerals may become apparent.

We are well advised to rely on food for our nutrients. To prevent possible toxicity, people who take supplements should limit intake to RDA or ESADDI levels. Pharmaceutical preparations are preferred to "natural" ones, which may have uncertain strengths and possible contaminants.

A case study and a sample plan of care appear below. They are both designed to show you how the information you have studied in this chapter can be used in nursing practice.

CASE STUDY 7–1

Mrs. B. is a 34-year-old woman who has related her fear of osteoporosis to the nurse. A recent visit to a 75-year-old aunt crystallized this fear. The aunt has become stooped and recently broke her hip. Mrs. B. is especially concerned because she has often been told she resembles this aunt. Mrs. B. asks, "Is there anything I can do to prevent this from happening to me?"

A 24-hour recall of dietary intake revealed a total of 1 cup of milk and no other dairy products. She did consume two 3-ounce servings of meat. Mrs. B. has three small children and stated that they are exercise enough for her. She sits outside and watches them play on every nice day.

Mrs. B. is 5 feet 3 inches tall and weighs 110 pounds. She is Caucasian with fair skin.

NURSING CARE PLAN FOR MRS. B.

Assessment:

Subjective

Fear of osteoporosis
Family history positive for osteoporosis
Less than RDA for calcium previous 24 hours
Meeting Food Pyramid guideline for meat group
No planned exercise program

Objective

Height: 5 feet 3 inches
Weight: 110 pounds
Caucasian, fair, slight build

Nursing Diagnosis

Knowledge deficit regarding preventive measures for osteoporosis related to fear of repeating aunt's experience as evidenced by request for information.

Desired Outcome/Evaluation Criteria

Patient will list appropriate actions to build a strong skeleton after teaching session.

Nursing Actions

1. Teach patient how to consume 800 milligrams of calcium daily: 3 cups of milk or equivalent.
2. Teach patient factors favoring calcium absorption: moderate protein and fat intake.
3. Teach patient role of exercise in making bones strong.

Rationale

1. One cup of milk contains approximately 300 milligrams of calcium.
2. High protein intake causes increased calcium excretion by the kidneys. High fat intake forms insoluble soaps with the calcium.
3. Weight-bearing exercise stimulates the osteoblasts to build bone.

STUDY AIDS

Chapter Review Questions

1. Like vitamins, minerals give no energy to the body. Unlike vitamins, minerals.
   a. Are completely absorbed from the intestinal tract
   b. Become part of the structure of the body
   c. Cause few clinical problems because of their great abundance in foods
   d. Cannot accumulate to such an extent to cause problems

2. Major minerals are those present in the body in amounts greater than 5 grams (1 teaspoonful) and have recommended intake levels of _____ milligrams or more per day.
   a. 10
   b. 50
   c. 100
   d. 250

3. Calcium is necessary for strong bones and teeth. It is also necessary for:
   a. Keeping the stomach acid
   b. Muscle contraction
   c. Preventing blood clots
   d. The production of insulin

4. To maximize absorption of calcium, the meal should also contain:
   a. Alcohol and nonacid fruits and vegetables
   b. Fiber and fat
   c. Protein and sugar
   d. Vitamins A and K

5. Present knowledge leads us to believe that the key to prevention of osteoporosis is:
   a. Lifelong adequate intake of calcium and regular exercise
   b. Postmenopausal estrogen therapy
   c. Supplemental vitamin and mineral therapy
   d. Weight control

6. Magnesium is necessary for the transmission of nerve impulses. Signs of magnesium toxicity would include:
   a. Delirium and hallucinations
   b. Petechiae and hemorrhage
   c. Nausea and vomiting
   d. Sedation and lethargy

7. From which of the following sources of iron is the greatest percentage of iron absorbed by the average person?
   a. Eggs
   b. Ferrous sulfate tablets
   c. Meat
   d. Vegetables

8. Which of the following beverages is known to increase the amount of iron absorbed from a meal?
   a. coffee
   b. milk
   c. orange juice
   d. tea

9. Deficiency or toxicity of iodine produces:
   a. Goiter
   b. Hypoparathyroidism
   c. Hyperthyroidism
   d. Mottling of the teeth

10. The most common nutrient deficiency in the United States is that of:
    a. Calcium
    b. Iodine
    c. Iron
    d. Zinc

NCLEX-Style Quiz

Situation One

Mrs. H. is a 30-year-old mother of three children all under 5 years of age. On her 6-week postpartum visit, her hemoglobin level was 10 grams per 100 milliliters of blood. She is given a prescription for ferrous sulfate and referred to the office nurse for nutrition counseling regarding her iron intake.

Mrs. H. tells the nurse that she eats what the children eat; cold cereal and milk for breakfast, peanut butter and jelly sandwiches and maybe a banana for lunch, and casseroles of tuna or hamburger for dinner. Mrs. H. is a heavy coffee drinker, consuming 10 cups per day, two with each meal and a total of four others during "coffee breaks."

The H. family is lower middle-class. Mr. H. is a long-distance truck driver and is away from home for long intervals. Mrs. H. has some knowledge of iron needs and sources because of her three pregnancies. She is reluctant to continue the ferrous sulfate she has been taking throughout her pregnancy. "It binds me up," she tells the nurse. Also, Mrs. H. maintains she cannot eat liver: "It gags me."

1. To maximize Mrs. H.'s iron intake with as little change in her habits as possible, the nurse would want to know:
   a. Whether Mrs. H. drinks regular or decaffeinated coffee
   b. What kinds of cereal Mrs. H. consumes
   c. At what time of day the H. family eats
   d. Whether or not Mrs. H. has tried veal liver

2. What other sources of iron are possibly acceptable to Mrs. H. but have not been assessed in the case thus far?
   a. Chicken and fortified margarine
   b. Cottage cheese, eggs, and milk
   c. Dried fruit and enriched or whole-grain products
   d. Fresh fruit and yellow vegetables

3. Which of the following beverage combinations have been shown to interfere with iron absorption by forming iron-tannate complexes?
   a. Apple juice and cranberry juice
   b. Beer and wine
   c. Cocoa and milk
   d. Coffee and tea

4. Which of the following statements by Mrs. H. would indicate she understood the nurse's instructions correctly?
   a. "I should eat a little meat, fish, or poultry with every meal containing grain and fruit and vegetable sources of iron."
   b. "I should increase the fiber in my diet because it will increase the absorption of iron."
   c. "If I want an alcoholic beverage, beer contains the most iron in a readily absorbable form."
   d. "Since I am taking an iron supplement, it is not important how I eat."

5. To meet the safety needs of the H. children, the nurse instructs Mrs. H. to keep her ferrous sulfate in a locked cupboard. The reason for this is:
   a. Oral pharmaceutical iron preparations are absorbed better than the iron in foods.
   b. The human body has no effective means of excreting an overload of iron.

c. Iron poisoning, although rare, can occur if a child ingests more than 30 tablets of ferrous sulfate.

d. Because iron binds with calcium, an overdose of iron would cause rickets.

BIBLIOGRAPHY

Brown, JE: The Science of Human Nutrition. Harcourt Brace Jovanovich, San Diego, 1990.

Cella, JH and Watson, J: Nurse's Manual of Laboratory Tests. FA Davis, Philadelphia, 1989.

Chandra, RK: Excessive intake of zinc impairs immune responses. JAMA 252:1443, 1984.

Chutkow, JG: Nutritional disturbances in neurology and psychiatry. In Halpern, SL (ed): Quick Reference to Clinical Nutrition, ed 2. JB Lippincott, Philadelphia, 1987.

Committee on Diet and Health. Food and Nutrition Board. Commission on Life Sciences. National Research Council: Diet and Health: Implications for Reducing Chronic Disease Risk. National Academy Press, Washington, DC, 1989.

Deglin, JH and Vallerand, AH: Davis's Drug Guide For Nurses, ed 3. FA Davis, Philadelphia, 1993.

Feldman, EB: Essentials of Clinical Nutrition. FA Davis, Philadelphia, 1988.

Goodwin, JS and Hunt, WC: Relationship between zinc intake, physical activity, and blood levels of high-density lipoprotein cholesterol in a healthy elderly population. Metabolism 34:519, 1985.

Green, ML and Harry, J: Nutrition in Contemporary Nursing Practice. John Wiley & Sons, New York, 1987.

Hay, EK. That old hip. Nurs Clin North Am 26(1):43–51, 1991.

Hui, YH: Human Nutrition and Diet Therapy. Wadsworth, Monterey, CA, 1983.

Kernstine, KH, Cerra, FB, and Buchwald, H: Enteral and parenteral nutrition. In Halpern, SL (ed): Quick Reference to Clinical Nutrition, ed 2. JB Lippincott, Philadelphia, 1987.

Lindeman, RD: Minerals in medical practice. In Halpern, SL (ed): Quick Reference to Clinical Nutrition, ed 2. JB Lippincott, Philadelphia, 1987.

McCarron, DA: Calcium and magnesium nutrition in human hypertension. Ann Intern Med 98:800, 1983.

Morck, TA, Lynch, SR, and Cook, JD: Inhibition of food iron absorption by coffee. American Journal of Clinical Nutrition 37:416, 1983.

National Institutes of Arthritis, Diabetes, and Digestive and Kidney Diseases (NIADDKD): Consensus conference: osteoporosis. JAMA 252:799, 1984.

Rossander, L, Hallberg L, and Bjorn-Rasmussen, E: Absorption of iron from breakfast meals. Am J Clin Nutr 32:2484, 1979.

Reinhart, RA and Desbiens, NA: Hypomagnesemia in patients entering the ICU. Crit Care Med 13:506, 1985.

Subcommittee on the 10th Edition of the RDAs. Food and Nutrition Board. Commission on Life Sciences. National Research Council: Recommended Dietary Allowances, ed 10. National Academy Press, Washington, DC, 1989.

Tamburro, CH: Nutritional management of alcoholism, drug addiction, and acute toxicity syndromes. In Halpern, SL (ed): Quick Reference to Clinical Nutrition, ed 2. JB Lippincott, Philadelphia, 1987.

US Department of Health and Human Services: Nutrition Monitoring in the United States. US Government Printing Office, Washington, DC, 1989.

Whitney, EB, Cataldo, CB, and Rolfes, SR: Understanding Normal and Clinical Nutrition, ed 3. West Publishing, St Paul, 1991.

Williams, SR: Nutrition and Diet Therapy, ed 6. Times Mirror/Mosby College Publishing, St Louis, 1989.

Chapter Outline

Key Terms

As a study aid, each key term is followed by the page number where the term is defined in the chapter. Terms that appear in **boldface** or <u>underscored</u> in the chapter text are located in the glossary.

Energy Balance

Learning Objectives

After completing this chapter, the student should be able to:

1. Describe energy homeostasis.
2. List two reasons why the body needs energy.
3. Describe how energy is measured both in foods and in the human body.
4. Discuss the effect of body composition on energy output.
5. Name the energy nutrient that has the highest kilocalorie density and identify two substances usually found in foods with a low kilocalorie density.

＿or about one half to three quarters of the population, the human body automatically regulates energy intake and/or expenditure to maintain energy balance. This is remarkable when you consider that individuals use varying amounts of energy daily and often have erratic food intake schedules. The body can also compensate for having less food fuel by conserving energy during food restriction or starvation.

This chapter describes the impact that energy intake and energy expenditure have on energy balance. Topics of discussion include energy measurements, factors that can influence the body's need for energy, energy consumption patterns, the kilocaloric and nutrient density of foods, energy allowances, and current recommendations concerning energy consumption.

HOMEOSTASIS

Homeostasis—Tendency toward balance in the internal environment of the body achieved by automatic monitoring and regulating mechanisms.

The human body seeks balance. **Homeostasis** means equilibrium or balance. Homeostasis, in terms of **energy balance,** results when the number of kilocalories eaten equals the number used to produce energy. An individual is usually in energy balance when a stable body weight is maintained.

Energy Intake

Energy balance—A situation in which kilocaloric intake equals kilocaloric output.

The typical adult eats between 500,000 to 850,000 kilocalories per year. Eating an excess of only 1 percent or 15 extra kilocalories per day would result in a weight gain of 1.5 pounds per year. This equals the kilocalories in 1/3 teaspoonful of butter or one fourth of a small apple. The individual at a stable healthy weight gives little thought to the amount of food eaten each day, yet the weight remains constant.

Energy Expenditure

Energy expenditure—The amount of fuel the body uses for a specified period.

Individuals also expend or use varying amounts of energy daily. **Energy expenditure** is measured by the number of kilocalories that an individual uses to meet the body's demand for fuel. A person uses many more kilocalories to run a marathon than to sleep all day. Physical activity costs energy. As mentioned above, about one half to three quarters of all adults are able to maintain a constant body weight despite daily fluctuations in energy output or expenditure.

Adaptive Thermogenesis

Adaptive thermogenesis—The adjustment in energy expenditure the body makes to either a large increase or a large decrease in kilocalorie intake of several days' duration.

Energy expenditure frequently adapts to either a large increase or a large decrease in food intake of several days' duration. This adaptive component of energy expenditure is called **adaptive thermogenesis.** Energy expenditure decreases during food restriction or starvation. The human body is trying to compensate for having less food fuel by conserving energy. Kilocalories are burned more efficiently. An individual trying to lose weight may either lose at a slower rate or stop losing weight. On the other hand, overeating for several days will cause an increase in energy expenditure. Energy expenditure has been found to be higher than predicted during the refeeding of previously starved patients (Krahn and Rock, 1993). Adaptive thermo-genesis is one example of how the human body evolved to cope with feast-or-famine conditions. When food was scarce, the human body adapted by conserving energy.

Energy Balance

Energy balance exists when energy expenditure equals energy intake. Most individuals are able to maintain a state of energy balance at a healthy body weight. Some people are able to achieve a stable body weight only after the deposition of an excessive amount of body fat. For example, a 120-lb individual (at a healthy body weight) can gain 100 lbs over a period of time and his or her weight will remain at 220 lbs indefinitely. The excessively lean person can also be in a state of energy homeostasis. Researchers do not understand why some people are unable to maintain energy homeostasis at their healthy body weights.

MEASUREMENT OF ENERGY

Both the energy (fuel) contained in foods and the amount of energy used by the body can be measured. The methods used to measure energy are fairly universal.

Units of Measurement

The energy content of food is measured in kilocalories, often abbreviated as kcalories or Kcal. A **kilocalorie** is the amount of heat required to raise 1 kilogram of water 1°C. Kilocalories are what lay people and the media call calories. Chemically, a <u>calorie</u> is the amount of heat required to raise 1 gram of water 1°C. One kilocalorie contains 1000 times as much energy as one calorie. Kilocalories are the terms used throughout this text.

The joule is another unit increasingly used to measure energy; you may encounter this term as you read scientific journals. One <u>kilojoule</u> is the energy required to move a mass of 1 kilogram with an acceleration of 1 meter per second. The kilojoule is equal to 0.239 kilocalories; a kilocalorie equals 4.184 kilojoules.

Kilocalorie (kcalorie or Kcal)—a measurement unit of energy; the amount of heat required to raise 1 kilogram of water 1°C.

Energy Nutrient Values

The energy nutrients are carbohydrate, fat, and protein. Alcohol (ethanol) also yields energy. A food's kilocalorie value is determined by its content of protein, fat, carbohydrate, and alcohol. To review:

- 1 gram of carbohydrate = 4 kilocalories (or 17 kilojoules)
- 1 gram of protein = 4 kilocalories (or 17 kilojoules)
- 1 gram of fat = 9 kilocalories (or 37.6 kilojoules)
- 1 gram of alcohol = 7 kilocalories (or 29.3 kilojoules)

Water, fiber, vitamins, and minerals do not provide kilocalories. Clinical Calculation 8–1 demonstrates how to determine the energy content of a food item.

Determination of Energy Values

Foods

The energy content of individual foods is measured by a device called a bomb calorimeter, illustrated in Figure 8–1. A bomb calorimeter is an insulated container that has a chamber in which food is burned. The amount of heat (kilocalories) produced by the burning of the food is determined by the change in the temperature of a measured amount of water that surrounds the chamber. All energy in food is in the form of chemical energy. In a bomb calorimeter, the chemical energy stored in the food sample is transformed into heat energy. The following equation may assist you in your understanding of this concept:

protein + oxygen = heat energy + water + carbon dioxide

(Carbohydrate or fat may be substituted for protein in the above equation.)

Human Body

A process similar to the combustion of food in the bomb calorimeter occurs in the body. The amount of energy the human body uses can be measured directly or indirectly. Direct measurement of energy used by the human body is expensive and used only in scientific research. Energy is measured directly by placing a person in an insulated heat-sensitive chamber and measuring the heat emitted by the body. Indirect measurement of energy is discussed in Clinical Application 8–1.

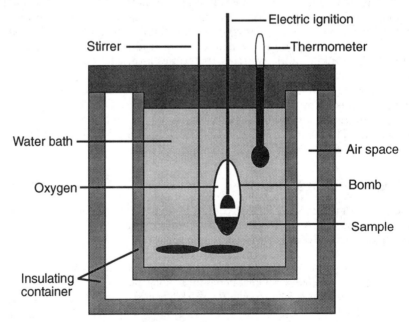

FIGURE 8–1. Cross-section of a bomb calorimeter showing essential features. Food sample is completely burned in the inner section; heat produced is absorbed by the known volume of water in the surrounding section. Change in temperature provides measure of heat produced. (Reproduced by permission from Guthrie, HA: Introductory Nutrition, ed. 7. Times Mirror/Mosby College Publishing, St. Louis, 1989.)

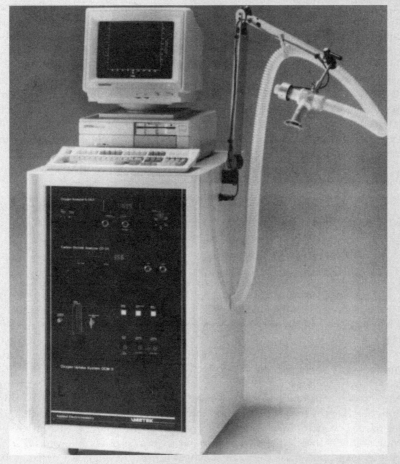

CLINICAL APPLICATION 8–1
Respiratory Gas Analyzer

The indirect method of measuring energy expenditure is done with a respiratory device called a respiratory gas analyzer or respirometer (Fig. 8–2). The amount of carbon dioxide exhaled and the amount of oxygen consumed for a given period are recorded. From this data, the number of kilocalories expended by the patient can be calculated. Kilocalorie expenditure, at rest, can be calculated from oxygen consumption and carbon dioxide production using the following equation (Cerra, 1984):

$$\text{kilocalories per day} = (3.8 \times \text{liter } O_2 \text{ used} + 1.2 \times \text{liter } CO_2 \text{ produced}) \times 1.4$$

In clinical practice, the indirect measurement of energy expenditure is only done for patients who are at a high nutritional risk. A respirometer is an expensive piece of equipment. The healthcare worker is most likely to observe this procedure being performed in the intensive care unit of an acute care hospital.

FIGURE 8–2. This device may be called a Respirometer, the Metabolic Measurement System, or a Respiratory Gas Analyzer. (Courtesy of Ametek, Inc., Pittsburgh, PA.)

COMPONENTS OF ENERGY EXPENDITURE

The human body requires energy (1) to meet resting energy expenditure needs and (2) to meet physical activity requirements. Resting energy expenditure includes not only the energy (kilocalories) needed to digest, absorb, transport, and utilize nutrients but also the energy required for other involuntary activities. Involuntary activities are those that cannot be consciously controlled. Physical activity includes the energy needed for voluntary activities, those that can be consciously controlled, such as running, walking, and swimming.

Resting Energy Expenditure

Resting energy expenditure (REE)—The amount of fuel the human body uses at rest for a specified period; often used interchangeably with basal metabolic rate (BMR).

Thermic effect of foods (diet-induced thermogenesis, specific-dynamic action)—The energy cost to extract and utilize the kilocalories and nutrients in foods; the heat produced after eating a meal.

Resting energy expenditure (REE) requires more total kilocalories than physical activity in *most people*. **Resting energy expenditure** represents the energy expended or used by a person at rest. Another term still in use in some scientific literature is basal metabolic rate (BMR). The major difference between resting energy and basal metabolic rate is that basal metabolic rate is always measured beginning at least 12 hours after the last meal and under certain conditions, such as controlled temperature and humidity. Clinical Application 8–1 discusses the measurement of REE in hospitalized patients. The energy cost to chew, swallow, digest, absorb, and transport nutrients is a component of REE. This component of REE is frequently referred to as the **thermic effect of foods.** In practice, BMR and REE differ by less than 12 percent and the terms are used interchangeably (Subcommittee on the 10th Edition of the RDAs, 1989).

The kilocalories necessary to support the following contribute to resting energy expenditure:

1. Thermic effect of foods
2. Contraction of the heart
3. Maintenance of body temperature
4. Repair of the internal organs
5. Maintenance of cellular processes
6. Muscular and nervous coordination.
7. Respiration (breathing)

REE makes up about 66 percent of total energy requirements in most people.

Body composition influences resting energy expenditure. Individuals of similar age, sex, height, and weight with a higher percentage of lean body mass have a higher REE than those with less lean body mass. It takes more energy, or kilocalories, to support lean body mass (protein) than to support body fat. This is because muscle tissue requires more kilocalories than does fat tissue, even when muscle tissue is resting. In other words, fat tissue is comparatively inactive and thus does not require as many kilocalories to support as lean body mass does. In practical terms, the higher a person's body protein content, the more kilocalories he or she can eat and still maintain a stable body weight.

Estimating a person's resting energy expenditure is commonly done by using the equations found in Table 8–1. These equations take into account age, sex, and weight but ignore differences in body composition, climate,

---

TABLE 8–1 *Equations for Calculating Resting Energy Expenditure*

Sex/Age Range (Years)	Equation to Obtain REE in Kilocalories per Day
Men	
0–3	(60.9 × weight in kilograms) − 54
3–10	(22.7 × weight in kilograms) + 495
10–18	(17.5 × weight in kilograms) + 651
18–30	(15.3 × weight in kilograms) + 679
30–60	(11.6 × weight in kilograms) + 879
greater than 60	(13.5 × weight in kilograms) + 487
Women	
0–3	(61.0 × weight in kilograms) − 51
3–10	(22.5 × weight in kilograms) + 499
10–18	(12.2 × weight in kilograms) + 746
18–30	(14.7 × weight in kilograms) + 496
30–60	(8.7 × weight in kilograms) + 829
greater than 60	(10.5 × weight in kilograms) + 596

SOURCE: Adapted from Subcommittee on the 10th Edition of the RDAs, 1989, p. 26.

---

and genetic variability (discussed below). Although these equations are not completely accurate for individuals, they can serve as a guide for menu planning. The ultimate test of how kilocalories eaten work in the body is to monitor body weight and kilocaloric intake over time.

Age

Resting energy expenditure varies with lean body mass, which varies with age. The highest rates of energy expenditure per pound of body weight occur during infancy and childhood. In adults, REE declines about 2 percent per decade because of a decline in lean body mass. This results in a reduced need for kilocalories. Individuals can retard the decline in lean body mass somewhat by increasing their exercise. An individual who fails either to adjust his or her kilocalorie intake to this reduced need for kilocalories or to increase his or her physical exercise will usually experience a slow weight gain.

Sex

Differences in body composition between men and women occur as early as the first few months of life. The differences are relatively small until the child reaches 10 years of age. During adolescence, body composition changes radically. Men develop proportionately greater muscle mass than do women, who deposit fat as they mature. Consequently, REE differs by as much as 10 percent between men and women.

Growth

Human growth is most pronounced during the growth spurts that take place during infancy, puberty, and pregnancy. Kilocalories required per kilogram of body weight are highest during these growth spurts. This is because the kilocaloric cost of anabolism is greater than the kilocaloric cost of catabolism.

Body Size

Persons with large bodies require proportionately more energy. A tall individual uses more energy to move his or her body mass over a given distance than a shorter one does. This is because a shorter person has less muscular tissue or lean body mass than a taller person.

Genetics

Recent evidence has shown that REE is strongly influenced by the genetic patterns of the individual. Each person is apparently programmed with a need to burn a certain number of kilocalories to meet energy balance. This fact will become apparent to healthcare workers when counseling two very similar patients. Both patients may be of the same sex, of equal weight, perform similar types of physical activity, and have about the same body fat content. Yet each patient may need to eat a different number of kilocalories to maintain a stable body weight. Many individuals have little control over the number of kilocalories required to meet the needs of REE.

Climate

Environmental climate affects REE because kilocalories are needed to maintain body temperature. This pertains to extreme differences in external temperatures, whether cold or hot.

In the United States, most individuals do not need to eat more kilocalories during colder months because the majority of living environments are in the 68°F to 77°F range. Outside, people usually protect themselves from extreme cold by wearing warm clothes. However, a relatively small increase in REE (2 to 5 percent) is associated with carrying the extra weight of winter clothing and boots. Shivering also causes an increase in REE.

Extra energy is needed to maintain thermal (heat) balance. Individuals performing heavy work at 99°F or higher have an increased REE. In practical terms, though, only individuals performing manual labor at 99°F or higher have been shown to need more kilocalories planned into their diets. The effect of high temperatures is minimized when the individual lives and works in an air-conditioned environment.

Extra kilocalories are also needed by feverish patients. Clinical Application 8–2 discusses the kilocaloric requirements for patients with fevers.

Thermic Effect of Food

The heat produced after eating a meal is called the **thermic effect of foods** (TEF). An older term for this energy cost is specific dynamic action (SDA). Energy is needed to chew, swallow, digest, absorb, and transport nutrients. Metabolism speeds up or increases after eating. As metabolism speeds up, more kilocalories are used. Clinical Calculation 8–2 demonstrates the calculation of a typical 18- to 30-year-old, 154-pound man's REE.

CLINICAL APPLICATION 8–2

Fever

Heat acts as a catalyst in most chemical reactions. A catalyst is a substance that speeds up a chemical reaction. Fever increases resting energy expenditure by about 7 percent for every 1°F increase in body temperature. Frequently, an individual with a fever is too ill to eat. Fruit juices with added glucose polymers or a nutritional supplement will give the patient needed energy.

According to the Food and Nutrition Board of the National Research Council, the consumption of protein and carbohydrate results in a much larger thermic effect than the consumption of fat. Fat in food is processed to body fat more efficiently than carbohydrate or protein. If an individual eats an equal number of kilocalories from carbohydrate as from fat, he or she will store fewer of the carbohydrate kilocalories as body fat. Thus, dietary fat, compared with dietary carbohydrate and protein, has the potential for harming a person's health if eaten in excess.

Physical Activity

For most of the US population, the second largest part of total energy expenditure is physical activity. Some very active individuals may need more kilocalories as a result of physical activity than as a result of resting energy expenditure. Figure 8–3 illustrates an athlete who may burn a large amount of kilocalories as a result of both training and engaging in competition. Activity factors associated with a range of activity patterns are provided in Table 8–2. The activity factor is multiplied by the REE to calculate kilocaloric

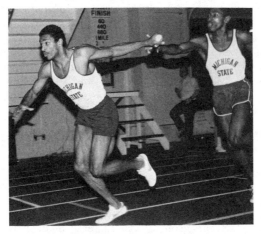

FIGURE 8–3. A trained athlete who may burn more kilocalories as a result of physical activity than as a result of his resting energy expenditure. (Courtesy of Sports Information, Michigan State University. East Lansing, Michigan.)

TABLE 8–2 *Factors for Estimating Daily Energy Allowances at Various Levels of Physical Activity for Men and Women (Ages 19–50)*

Level of Activity	Activity Factor	Description of Activity
Very Light		Sedentary: Inactive, institutionalized
Men	1.3	patient at bedrest
Women	1.3	
Light		Lightly active: Most professionals—
Men	1.6	teachers, doctors, housewives, office
Women	1.5	workers, unemployed persons
Moderate		Moderately active: Building workers
Men	1.7	(excluding laborers), many farm
Women	1.6	workers, active students, sales clerks
Heavy		Very active: Full-time athletes, unskilled
Men	2.1	laborers, army recruits, steel workers
Women	1.9	
Exceptional		Exceptional activity: Lumberjacks,
Men	2.4	blacksmiths, women construction
Women	2.2	workers, rickshaw pullers

Thermic effect of exercise—The number of kilocalories expended above REE as a result of physical activity.

requirements. The total kilocaloric need for a 70-kilogram, 19- to 50-year-old man who is moderately active is demonstrated in Clinical Calculation 8–3. The energy cost of physical activity is frequently referred to as the *thermic effect of exercise (TEE)*.

Healthcare workers can approximate a patient's kilocalorie allowance by first using the equations on Table 8–1 to calculate a patient's REE and then multiplying this result by the appropriate activity factor found on Table 8–2. However, calculations of such allowances are at best only approximations: kilocalorie allowances are not kilocalorie requirements. The most accurate method to determine a patient's kilocalorie requirement is to monitor both food intake and body weight over time (see Chapter 15).

Physical activity can greatly influence energy requirements. For example, a 154-pound man (70 kilograms) will require only 2406 kilocalories on a very sedentary day and up to 3938 kilocalories on a very active day. A 128-pound woman (58 kilograms) will require only 1856 kilocalories on a very sedentary day and up to 3038 kilocalories on a very active day. (Subcommittee of the 10th Edition of the RDAs, 1989).

Thermic Effect of Exercise

Energy expended *during* exercise is only a portion of the total energy cost of physical activity. Muscular work during exercise costs kilocalories. Exercise may also affect both REE and the thermic effect of foods. Some patients' REE increases for up to 48 hours after exercise.

Although the exact reason for this increase in REE is not known; the most plausible explanation is that the glycogen stores need to be refilled. Glycogen is the carbohydrate the body stores in the liver and muscle tissue. Because exercise depletes glycogen stores, there is an energy cost to refill these stores during the postexercise period.

Adaptive Response to Exercise

An individual with well-developed muscles uses fewer kilocalories to perform a given amount of physical work than an individual with less well developed muscles. As exercise is repeated, the body learns how to get the job done with the least effort. (This is the body's adaptive response to exercise.) A well-developed muscle performs more efficiently than a less well-developed muscle; thus it uses fewer kilocalories to perform a given physical activity. Also, if an individual loses weight due to increased exercise, he or she will eventually use fewer kilocalories to do a specific activity.

Lighter people require fewer kilocalories for a given amount of exercise than heavier people do. This is simply because it takes fewer kilocalories to move a smaller mass than to move a larger mass.

Exercise and Appetite

Many exercise researchers think that exercise decreases appetite. Appetite is defined as a strong desire for food or for a pleasant sensation, based on previous experience, that causes one to seek food for the purpose of tasting and enjoying. After exercise, (the individual) may be satisfied with less food. Some types of exercise release a chemical in the brain called beta-endorphin. Beta-endorphin has an effect similar to that of natural morphine. It produces a state of relaxation. In effect, exercise can substitute for overeating in those individuals who eat to decrease stress and tension.

Aerobic Exercise

Aerobic exercise is any activity during which the energy needed is supplied by the oxygen inspired. Aerobic exercises increase physical fitness and involve large muscle groups. Vigorous workouts that last at least 30 minutes, such as fast walking, cycling, swimming, skating, rope jumping, aerobic dancing, hiking, jogging, and rowing require inspired oxygen. Any exercise that raises your pulse to target heart rate is an aerobic activity. To determine your **target heart rate**, see Clinical Application 8–3.

There are many health benefits to aerobic exercise, including:

Target heart rate—Seventy percent of maximum heart rate (number of heartbeats per minute); the rate at which the pulse should be maintained for at least 20 minutes during aerobic exercise.

- Decreased risk of cardiovascular disease
- Better blood sugar control for the diabetic
- Decreased risk of obesity
- Reversal or prevention of varicose veins
- Decreased risk of osteoporosis
- Improvement in the quality of sleep
- Better control of hypertension

Anaerobic Exercise

Exercise during which energy needed is provided without the utilization of inspired oxygen is anaerobic exercise. Short bursts of vigorous activity, such as resistance or muscle strength training, are forms of anaerobic exercise. The typical example is weight lifting. Anaerobic exercise allows for muscle toning, the building of muscular strength and endurance, and the building of bone mass. This kind of training provides added strength and toughness, which helps to reduce injury during aerobic exercise, prevents lower back problems, and improves overall appearance.

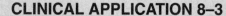

CLINICAL APPLICATION 8–3
Determining A Theoretical Target Heart Rate

The theoretical target heart rate is the rate you need to reach to achieve maximal aerobic effect. Determine your theoretical* target heart rate as follows:

1. Subtract your age from the number 220.
2. Multiply this number first by 65 percent and then by 80 percent. The two numbers should represent the range of heart beats per minute that you should try to maintain during aerobic exercise.

Example of an 18-year-old woman:

1. $220 - 18 = 202$
2. $202 \times 0.65 = 131$
3. $202 \times 0.80 = 161$

This individual should exercise sufficiently to reach a heart rate of between 131 and 161 beats per minute.

---

*To monitor your heart rate during exercise, count the number of times your heart beats for 6 seconds and multiply by 10.

ENERGY INTAKE

Historical Trends

Several recent surveys studied the kilocalorie intakes of men and women. Two different surveys found that the average daily energy intakes for men were between 2359 and 2639 kilocalories per day. The average daily reported intakes for women were between 1639 and 1793 kilocalories per day. The average reported intakes for women are of special concern because of the difficulty in incorporating all nutrients at recommended levels in a diet so low in kilocalories. (National Research Council, 1989). The need for the average woman to increase energy output or physical activity is well documented.

Information from the Nationwide Food Consumption Survey has been used to compare energy intakes in 1965 with those in 1977. This data suggests that energy intake declined for both sexes by approximately 10 percent during those 10 to 20 years (National Research Council, 1989). The percentage of overweight men and women has been increasing in spite of the decrease in energy intake. Many experts attribute increased obesity to decreased energy expenditure. We are becoming an increasingly sedentary society. The current recommendation is that the typical person should not decrease his or her kilocalorie intake below his or her recommended energy allowance. Instead the person should increase physical activity to achieve energy balance.

Kilocaloric Density of Foods

Some foods are more kilocalorically dense than other foods. Density is the quantity per unit volume of a substance. **Kilocaloric density** refers to the kilocalories contained in a given volume of a food. Figure 8–4 illustrates this concept. Foods with a high water and fiber content have a lower kilocaloric density. Fruits and vegetables such as lettuce, watermelon, and celery are high in water content and low in kilocalories. Grapes have fewer kilocalories than raisins in a given volume because grapes contain more water than raisins.

Fats or foods high in fat have the highest kilocaloric density. Whole-milk products, high-fat meat exchanges, and fat exchanges all contain appreciable fat. Table 8–3 lists several tips for decreasing the kilocalorie density of a diet.

Nutrient Density of Foods

Kilocaloric content alone should not be used to decide whether to include a food in one's diet. The nutrient density of a food is also an important consideration. The **nutrient density** of a food refers to the concentration of nutrients in a food compared with the food's kilocalorie content. If a food is high in kilocalories and low in nutrients, the nutrient density of the food is low. **Empty kilocalories** means that the food contains kilocalories and almost no nutrients. Table sugar is an example of such a food. If a food is low in kilocalories and high in nutrients, the nutrient density of the food is high. Cantaloupe is an example of a food with a high nutrient density—it is low in kilocalories, high in vitamin C, and contains a moderate amount

Kilocaloric density—The kilocalories contained in a given volume of a food.

Nutrient density—The concentration of nutrients in a given volume of food compared with the food's kilocalorie content.

Empty kilocalories—Food that contains kilocalories and almost no other nutrients.

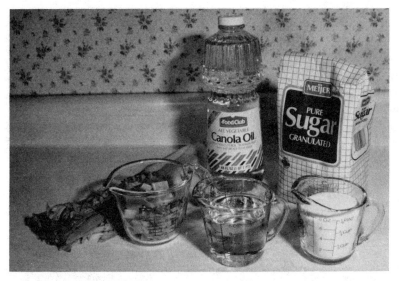

FIGURE 8–4. One cup of celery contains 17 kilocalories, 1 cup of sugar contains 770 kilocalories, and 1 cup of oil contains 1925 kilocalories. Celery is the least kilocalorically dense (of the foods pictured) and oil is the most dense. Sugar is between celery and oil in kilocaloric density.

TABLE 8–3 *Tips for Decreasing the Kilocaloric Density of a Diet*

- Use low-fat or nonfat dairy products including skimmed milk, cheese, and yogurt.
- Brown meats by broiling or cooking in nonstick pans with little or no fat. Avoid fried foods.
- Chill soups, stews, sauces and broths. Lift off and discard hardened fat.
- Trim all visible fat from meat before cooking.
- Use water-packed, canned foods such as fruits and tuna.
- Use fresh fruits and vegetables often. Try to eat at least 2½ cups of these foods each day.
- Use low-kilocalorie salad dressings.
- When you eat out, do not look at the menu. Instead, have an idea of what you would like to eat before you arrive at the restaurant. Explain to the waitress what you would like to eat.

---

of vitamin A. Please refer to Figure 8–5. Skimmed milk and whole milk are similar in nutrient content. Both types of milk contain about the same amounts of protein, calcium, and riboflavin. Eight ounces of skimmed milk provides about 90 kilocalories compared with 150 kilocalories in 8 ounces of whole milk. Skimmed milk thus has a higher nutrient density than whole milk.

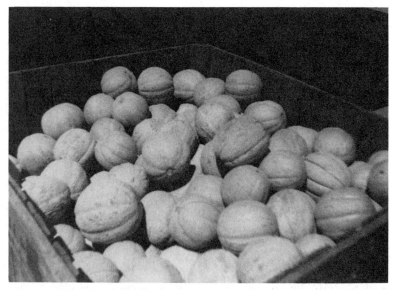

FIGURE 8–5. Cantaloupe is a food of high-nutrient density. One-quarter of an average melon contains only 47 kilocalories and is high in vitamin C and moderate in vitamin A.

ENERGY ALLOWANCES

The recommended dietary allowances for energy are shown in Table 8–4. Differences for age, sex, and body size are factored into the allowances. The kilocalories listed in the table are based on the reference man and woman. For example, the reference 15- to 18-year-old woman weighs 120 pounds and is 64 inches tall. Actual energy requirements may vary widely within any given age group. Genetics may play a role in determining a person's actual energy requirement.

Note in the table that the kilocalorie allowances for both the pregnant and lactating woman are increased. A pregnant woman's energy allowance is 300 kilocalories over and above her nonpregnant allowance; a lactating woman's energy allowance is 500 kilocalories over and above her nonlactating allowance.

TABLE 8–4 *Recommended Dietary Allowances for Energy*

Category	Age or Condition	Weight (Kilograms)	Height (Inches)	REE† (Kilocalories per Day)	Average Energy Allowance (Kilocalories)* Per Kilogram‡	Per Day
Infants	0–0.5	6	24	320	108	650
	0.5–1	9	28	500	98	850
Children	1–3	13	35	740	102	1300
	4–6	20	44	950	90	1800
	7–10	28	52	1130	70	2000
Males	11–14	45	62	1440	55	2500
	15–18	66	69	1760	45	3000
	19–24	72	70	1780	40	2900
	25–50	79	70	1800	37	2900
	51+	77	68	1530	30	2300
Females	11–14	46	62	1310	47	2200
	15–18	55	64	1370	40	2200
	19–24	58	65	1350	38	2200
	25–50	63	64	1380	36	2200
	51+	65	63	1280	30	1900
Pregnant	1st trimester					+0
	2nd trimester					+300
	3rd trimester					+300
Lactating	1st 6 months					+500
	2nd 6 months					+500

SOURCE: Adapted from Subcommittee on the 10th Edition of the RDAs, 1989, p. 33.

*Includes kilocalories needed for physical activity.

†Does *not* include kilocalories needed for physical activity.

‡Based on a median age, weight, height, and light-to-moderate activity level.

The 1989 edition of the National Research Council's RDA for energy (10th edition) is different from previous editions in one important detail. The heights and weights in each age/sex category for the reference individual have been changed. For example, according to the 1989 edition, the reference 25- to 50-year-old man weighs 174 pounds and is 70 inches tall. His energy allowance is 2900 kilocalories. In the 1980 edition, the reference 25- to 50-year-old male weighs 154 pounds and is 70 inches tall. His energy allowance is 2700 kilocalories. The actual energy allowance of a 25- to 50-year-old male has not increased from 2700 to 2900. Rather, the reference individual used to compute the new RDAs has changed: he is heavier by 20 pounds. The healthcare worker and patients may become confused if different tables are used in a facility or in individual practice. Consistency in the use of reference materials adds credibility to the healthcare worker's information.

DIETARY RECOMMENDATIONS

All the major national health organizations recommend that individuals maintain a healthy body weight. The American Heart Association recommends maintaining a healthy body weight to decrease the risk of heart and circulatory diseases. The American Cancer Society cites numerous studies suggesting that lower kilocalorie intake may lower the risk of cancer. Most individuals would benefit by monitoring their weight and increasing their energy expenditure and/or decreasing their energy intake as necessary to maintain a healthy body weight.

Summary

Energy balance exists when energy intake equals energy output. A person at his or her stable body weight is usually in energy balance. About one half to three quarters of the population have the capability of regulating energy intake and expenditure to accommodate daily variations. When an individual is not in energy balance, he or she is gaining or losing body weight.

The human body needs energy for resting energy expenditure and voluntary physical activity. Energy allowances are calculated by multiplying an individual's resting energy expenditure by a factor for physical activity.

Foods high in water and fiber are low in kilocaloric density. Foods high in fat are high in kilocaloric density. Individuals should try to consume nutritionally dense foods. These foods are low in kilocalories and contain substantial amounts of one or more nutrients.

Americans have been decreasing both their food intake and activity for the past 10 years. The current recommendation is that individuals who gain weight while consuming their energy RDA should increase their activity to maintain energy balance, rather than decrease intake.

A case study and a sample plan of care appear below. Both are designed to show you how the information you have studied in this chapter can be used in nursing practice.

CASE STUDY 8–1

The Fairview Nursing Home holds a weekly patient care conference. All the facility's residents have their nursing care plans reviewed on a rotating basis, with each patient's nursing care plan being reviewed once every 3 months. All members of the healthcare team are often present at the conference. Team members may include the administrator, the physician, the director of nursing, the staff nurse, the nursing assistant, the activities director, the social worker, the dietitian, and the patient or a family member representing the patient.

Mr. G., the patient, has been experiencing a slow weight gain. His weight history follows:

1/89	175 pounds
3/89	177 "
7/89	178 "
9/89	180 "
12/89	181 "

Mr. G. is 5 feet 8 inches tall and is 79 years old. He is alert, feeds himself, and has normal bowel and bladder function. He has good dentition and is on a regular diet. According to the appetite records kept by the nurse's aide, Mr. G.'s intake is good to excellent. He accepts all the major food groups. Mr. G. is concerned with his slow weight gain but claims he does not know what to do. To address the slow weight gain problem, the healthcare team and Mr. G. developed the following nursing care plan.

NURSING CARE PLAN FOR MR. G.

Assessment
Subjective: Patient expressed concern about his slow weight gain.
Objective: Height: 5 feet 8 inches
Weights and % HBW:
1/89   175 pounds   103% healthy body weight
12/89   181 pounds   106% healthy body weight

Nursing Diagnosis
Nutrition, altered: more than body requirements of energy related to knowledge deficit as evidenced by admitted lack of understanding and a gain in healthy body weight of 3 percent over the past year

Desired Outcome/Evaluation Criteria
1. Patient will maintain his present body weight over the next 3 months.
2. Patient will select fresh fruits for desserts at 50 percent of all social activities.
3. Patient will self-monitor his food intake by keeping a food diary 1 day per week for the next 3 months.
4. Patient will participate in the exercise program provided by the activities director at least three times per week for the next 3 months.

Nursing Actions
1. Weigh patient once per week
2. Provide encouragement to the patient to select fresh fruit at all social activities. Congratulate the patient when he is able to refrain from eating rich desserts. Remind the Dietary Department to serve fresh fruit at social functions.
3. Review the patient's food record with him each week. Note all empty kilocalories consumed. Discuss the patient's food selections with him. Document results.

4. Encourage the patient to attend the exercise program three times per week. Document attendance.
See Charting Tips 8–1 for patient-monitoring ideas.

Rationale

1. Monitoring body weight is necessary to determine the success or failure of the care plan.
2. Replacing kilocalorically dense cakes, pies, and cookies with fresh fruit will promote weight maintenance.
3. Self-monitoring of food intake will help the patient focus on his food behaviors. Nurse's review of food records with the patient while pointing out kilocalorically dense foods will educate the patient about his negative behaviors.
4. Exercise burns kilocalories and increases body protein content. A high body protein content is associated with increased energy expenditure.

CHARTING TIPS 8–1

✓ A simple work sheet for documenting exercise class attendance and eating behaviors at social functions would facilitate both documentation and evaluation.

✓ Do not be shy about asking other team members to assist in following a patient similar to the patient described in the case study. The dietitian, if asked, would most likely be willing to set up the monitoring forms. The activities director would probably be willing to monitor the patient's eating behavior at social activities and monitor exercise-class attendance. Quality patient care is not an accident. Close cooperation between team members is essential.

STUDY AIDS

Chapter Review Questions

1. One teaspoonful of butter contains 5 grams of fat. How many kilocalories does it contain?
   a. 20
   b. 45
   c. 70
   d. 73

2. The body uses all the following for energy *except:*
   a. Minerals
   b. Carbohydrates
   c. Lipids
   d. Alcohol

3. An individual's kilocaloric allowance is calculated by which of the following formulas?
   a. REE × activity factor
   b. 2(REE) + activity factor
   c. REE + activity factor
   d. REE + activity factor + a factor for genetic variability

4. One-half cup of orange juice contains 15 grams of carbohydrate. How many kilocalories does it contain?
   a. 15
   b. 25
   c. 60
   d. 90

5. Energy homeostasis exists when:
   a. Kilocalories from food intake = kilocalories used for energy expenditure.
   b. Kilocalories used for physical activity = kilocalories used for energy expenditure.
   c. An individual is gaining weight.
   d. Kilocalories from food intake = kilocalories used for resting energy expenditure.

6. A kilocalorie is a measure of:
   a. Weight
   b. Height
   c. Energy
   d. Fatness

7. When there is a greater energy intake than energy output the result is:
   a. Diabetes
   b. Hyperactivity
   c. Anorexia
   d. Weight gain

8. The kilocaloric value of alcohol is:
   a. 4 kilocalories per gram
   b. 7 kilocalories per gram
   c. 9 kilocalories per gram
   d. 25 kilocalories per gram

9. An individual having well-developed muscle tissue compared with a similar individual who has poorly developed muscles:
   a. Needs to eat less food
   b. Needs to exercise more

    c. May have a higher resting energy expenditure

    d. Will tend to remain in positive energy balance

10. Which of the following foods is the *least* kilocalorically dense?
    a. 1 cup of sugar
    b. 1 cup of margarine
    c. 1 cup of skimmed milk
    d. 1 cup of celery

NCLEX-Style Quiz

Situation One

Mr. I., resident of Sunnybrook Nursing Home, has been experiencing a undesirable slow weight loss. His weight history is as follows:

Feb	180 pounds
June	175 pounds
Oct	170 pounds

1. As Mr. I.'s nurse, you should first:
    a. Encourage Mr. I. to eat more fruits and vegetables.
    b. Call the doctor.
    c. Wait for the next patient care conference to act on this problem.
    d. Monitor Mr. I.'s food intake to determine what he is eating.

Situation Two

A teacher has noticed that many students in her fifth grade class are overweight. As a school project, the class kept food records for 3 days. The records were analyzed by a computer software program. Many students were eating less than their recommended dietary allowance for kilocalories. The teacher shared this information with the school nurse and asked her to speak to the class.

2. The school nurse correctly decided that:
    a. The teacher is overly concerned since the proportion of overweight students approximates the proportion of overweight adults in the community.
    b. The computer program must be in error.
    c. All the students need to increase their total intake, including foods from the major food groups.
    d. Many students would benefit from an increase in physical activity.

3. Which of the following suggestions would support your answer to question 2.
    a. Have the children keep activity records.
    b. Observe the children eating lunch.
    c. Enter the food intake into the computer a second time.
    d. Review attendance records for a sample of students.

Situation Three

A patient appears to be totally concerned with the kilocaloric density of foods and not at all concerned with the nutrient density of foods. You need to encourage the consumption of both types of foods.

4. Which of the following behaviors do you need to discourage?
    a. The substitution of skimmed milk for 2 percent milk
    b. The avoidance of all red meat
    c. Including dark green and yellow fruits and vegetables in the diet
    d. Including whole grains in the diet

CLINICAL CALCULATION 8–1

Calculating the Energy Content of a Food Item

If you know the carbohydrate, fat, and protein content of a food item, you can readily calculate the food item's kilocaloric content. Two examples are shown below. One starch exchange contains 3 grams of protein and 15 grams of carbohydrate. Adding the protein and carbohydrate content in the starch exchange together equals 18.

	Carbohydrate (grams)		Protein (grams)		Fat (grams)		Total (grams)
One starch exchange	15	+	3	+	0	=	18

There are 4 kilocalories in 1 gram each of carbohydrate and protein, so all you need to do to obtain the kilocaloric content of the starch exchange is to multiply 4 by 18. Thus there are 72 kilocalories in one starch exchange.

One fat exchange contains 5 grams of fat.

	Carbohydrate (grams)		Protein (grams)		Fat (grams)		Total (grams)
One fat exchange	0	+	0	+	5	=	5

There are 9 kilocalories in a gram of fat. To obtain the kilocaloric content of one fat exchange, multiply 5 by 9. Thus one fat exchange contains 45 kilocalories.

CLINICAL CALCULATION 8–2

Calculating Resting Energy Expenditure

Sample calculations for a 154-pound, 18- to 30-year-old man's resting energy expenditure:

1. Convert weight in pounds to kilograms.

$$\frac{\text{weight in pounds}}{\text{weight in pounds per kilogram}} = \text{weight in kilograms}$$

$$\frac{154}{2.2} = 70 \text{ kilograms}$$

2. Locate equation from Table 8–1 and perform the calculation

$$\text{REE} = (15.3 \times \text{weight in kilograms}) + 679$$

$$\text{REE} = (15.3 \times 70 \text{ kilograms}) + 679$$

$$\text{REE} = 1071 + 679$$

$$\text{REE} = 1750 \text{ kilocalories per day}$$

CLINICAL CALCULATION 8–3

Calculating Daily Energy Allowance

Sample calculation for a moderately active man weighing 70 kilograms who is 18 to 30 years old and has a resting energy expenditure of 1750 kilocalories per day.

1. The formula is:

$$\text{REE} \times \text{activity factor} = \text{daily energy allowance}$$

2. Locate the activity factor from Table 8–2.

The activity factor is 1.7

3. Perform calculations:

$$1750 \times 1.7 = 2975$$

Thus the daily energy allowance for this man is 2975 kilocalories.

BIBLIOGRAPHY

Cerra, F: Pocket Manual of Surgical Nutrition. CV Mosby, St Louis, 1984, p. 61.

Hands, ES: Food Finder Food Sources of Vitamins and Minerals. ESHA Research, Salem, 1990.

Hui, YH: Principles and Issues in Nutrition. Wadsworth Health Science Division, Arcata, CA, 1985.

Krahn DD, Rock C, Deckert MS, Nairn KK, and Hasse SA: Changes in resting energy expenditure and body composition in anorexia nervosa during refeeding. J Am Diet Assoc 93:4, 1993.

Poehlman, ET and Horton, ES: The impact of food intake and exercise on energy expenditure. Nutr Rev 47:129, 1989.

National Research Council: Diet and Health: Implications for Reducing Chronic Disease Risk. Report of the Committee on Diet and Health, Food and Nutrition Board, Commission on Life Sciences. National Academy Press, Washington, DC, 1989, p. 110.

Subcommittee on the 10th Edition of the RDAs. Food and Nutrition Board. Commission of Life Sciences. National Research Council: Recommended Dietary Allowances. National Academy Press, Washington, DC, 1989, pp. 24–38.

Thomas, PR (ed): Improving America's Diet and Health: From Recommendations to Actions. Food and Nutrition Board Institute of Medicine. National Academy Press, Washington, DC, 1991.

Chapter Outline

Key Terms

As a study aid, each key term is followed by the page number where the term is defined in the chapter. Terms that appear in **boldface** or <u>underscored</u> in the chapter text are located in the glossary.

Water and Body Fluids

Key Terms *(Continued)*

Homestasis (235)
Hydrostatic pressure (240)
Hypertonic (238)
Hypothalamus (241)
Hypotonic (238)
Insensible water losses (245)
Interstitial fluid (232)
Intracellular fluid (244)
Intravascular fluid (232)
Ion (230)
Ionic bond (231)
Isotonic (238)
Milliequivalent (237)
Milliosmole (238)

Obligatory excretion (242)
Osmolality (238)
Osmolarity (238)
Osmosis (237)
Osmotic pressure (237)
pH (242)
Renal (241)
Renin (241)
Sensible water losses (245)
Solute (234)
Solvent (234)
Systolic pressure (240)
Turgor (252)

Learning Objectives

After completing this chapter, the student should be able to:

1. Describe the locations and functions of water in the body.
2. Discuss the body's control mechanisms for maintaining fluid and electrolyte balance.
3. Recognize how acid-base balance is maintained by buffer systems.
4. List amounts of water usually gained and lost by adults in a day.
5. Differentiate insensible from sensible water loss.
6. Distinguish between heat exhaustion and heat stroke with respect to cause and first-aid treatment.

*A*lthough we have deferred the discussion of water until the ninth chapter in this book, the need for water is more urgent than the need for any other nutrient. Human beings can live a month without food but only 6 days without water. In this chapter we explain why water is so important in the body and discuss the ways in which water balance is achieved. We also describe the assessment and treatment of fluid volume deficit and fluid volume excess.

The distribution and movement of water in the body is intricately bound to certain elements. Understanding this relationship requires knowledge of the essentials of atomic structure. This chapter begins, then, with a discussion on how atoms interact with one another.

INTERACTIONS BETWEEN ATOMS

An element is a substance that ordinary chemical methods cannot divide into smaller units. There are more than 105 known elements. Oxygen is an element, as are sodium, chlorine, and the other minerals discussed in Chapter 7.

Atoms

Elements are composed of smaller parts, however. Together, these smaller parts make up an atom. In the center of an atom is the nucleus, which contains protons and neutrons. The nucleus gives an atom its weight and mass. Circling around the nucleus like satellites are electrons. These electrons are arranged in a consistent manner: a maximum of two in the orbit or shell closest to the nucleus, and a maximum of eight in each of the outer shells. The ability of an atom to react chemically depends on the number of "empty slots" in the outermost electron shell.

Chemical Bonding

A compound is a substance created by the chemical bonding, or joining, of two or more different kinds of atoms (elements). A chemical bond is actually the force that binds atoms together. A compound is formed when atoms either share electrons or when one atom donates one or more electrons to another atom. For example, water (a liquid) is formed when one atom of hydrogen (a colorless, odorless gas) is joined with two atoms of oxygen (another colorless, odorless gas).

Similarly, sodium chloride (table salt) is formed when an atom of sodium (an unstable, silvery white, waxy, soft metal) chemically bonds with an atom of chlorine (a greenish-yellow poisonous gas). How do these dissimilar elements combine to create a substance with totally different characteristics? To answer this question we will consider sodium and chlorine and explain how they combine to form sodium chloride.

Ion—An atom or group of atoms carrying an electrical charge; an ion with a positive charge is called a cation; an ion with a negative charge is called an anion.

A sodium atom has only one electron in its outer shell; a chlorine atom has seven. When placed together, the sodium atom donates the electron in its outer shell to the outer shell of the chlorine atom. With the loss of its electron, the sodium now has a positive electrical charge of +1 and is called a sodium **ion** (Na^+). Ions with positive charges are referred to as cations. The chlorine atom, which gained an electron, now has a negative charge of −1 and is called a chloride ion (Cl^-). Ions with negative charges are referred to as anions.

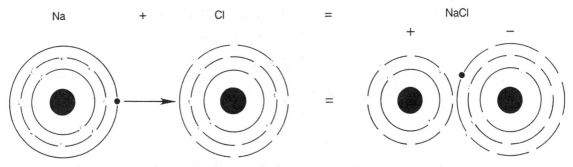

Na + Cl = NaCl

FIGURE 9–1. An ionic bond. The atom of sodium loses an electron to the atom of chlorine. After losing the electron, the sodium atom is a cation, carrying a positive charge and the chlorine is an anion, carrying a negative charge. These two opposites are attracted to each other, forming NaCl, sodium chloride, common table salt. (From Scanlon and Sanders, p. 27, with permission.)

Because both of these ions have opposite charges (+ and −) they are attracted to one another and unite, forming sodium chloride (NaCl). The chemical bond that holds the sodium and chloride ions together is called an ionic bond. There are other types of chemical bonds (not discussed here). Sodium can donate its single electron to other elements beside chlorine, and other elements can form ionic bonds as well. See Figure 9–1 for a diagram of the formation of sodium chloride from sodium and chlorine.

An **electrolyte** is an element or compound that when dissolved in water separates (dissociates) into ions that are capable of conducting an electrical current. These electrically charged particles are then available to take part in other chemical reactions in the body. Clinical Application 9–1 discusses examples of uses and hazards related to electrolytes in the body.

Electrolyte—An element or compound that when dissolved in water separates (dissociates) into ions that are capable of conducting an electrical current; acids, bases, and salts are common electrolytes.

CLINICAL APPLICATION 9–1
Diagnostic Uses and Potential Hazards of Electrolytes

Skin sensors attached to a device called an electrocardiograph can trace the electrical activity of the heart. The resulting graphic record is called an electrocardiogram (ECG). The machine's sensors on the skin can detect the electric current because the blood is an electrolyte solution and thus capable of conducting electricity. The same principle applies to the use of an electroencephalograph, a device that can trace brain-wave activity. The record obtained from this machine is called an electroencephalogram (EEG).

The same characteristic of electrolyte solutions that allows these machines to trace electrical activity can also be hazardous. A fluid-filled tube, such as a nasogastric tube or catheter, can conduct stray electricity from faulty electrical devices to the patient's heart, which could result in dysrhythmias. The amount of electricity in the shock may be minuscule, but enough to be fatal if it happens at the wrong time in the cardiac cycle. Always report equipment from which you receive shocks, or devices you suspect of being faulty.

DISTRIBUTION OF WATER IN THE BODY

All water within the body is continually in motion: it runs through the arteries, capillaries, and veins, and fills the cells and the spaces between the cells. It also forms the basic substance of lymph and body secretions. All tissues contain water.

Body Composition

Some tissues have significantly more water than others: muscle tissue is 70 percent water, fat tissue is 30 percent water, and bone tissue is 10 percent water. A man's body is 60 to 65 percent water and a woman's body is 50 to 54 percent water. Men have a higher water content as a result of their greater muscle mass.

Age affects the proportion of a body that is water, also. Compared with the 50 to 65 percent for women and men, an infant's body is 75 percent water. Premature infants may be 80 percent water by weight. Infants, especially those who are premature, are at high risk of fluid imbalances. The adult proportion of water to body weight is reached at about 9 to 12 months of age.

Fluid Compartments

Body fluids are held in compartments called intracellular and extracellular (*see* Figure 9–2). These compartments are separated by semipermeable membranes that allow some substances to pass through, while preventing passage of other substances. Water passes freely through the membranes.

Intracellular Compartment

The fluid inside the cells comprises that of the intracellular compartment. In adults, 60 percent of body water is found here. In infants, 46 percent of the body water is intracellular.

Extracellular Compartment

All fluid outside the cells is extracellular. In adults, 40 percent of the body's water is extracellular; in infants, 54 percent. Figure 9–3 illustrates the proportions of intracellular to extracellular fluid in men, women, and infants. The difference is important because extracellular fluid is more easily and rapidly lost to the outside of the body than is intracellular fluid. Extracellular fluid includes interstitial, intravascular, lymph, and transcellular fluid.

INTERSTITIAL FLUID   This is the fluid between the cells, or surrounding the cells. It assists in transporting substances between the cells and the blood and lymph vessels.

INTRAVASCULAR FLUID   This is the fluid within the blood vessels, arteries, arterioles, capillaries, venules, and veins.

LYMPH FLUID   The venous system cannot collect and return all the fluid from the tissues to the heart. Lymph vessels assist in returning the fluid part of the blood to the heart.

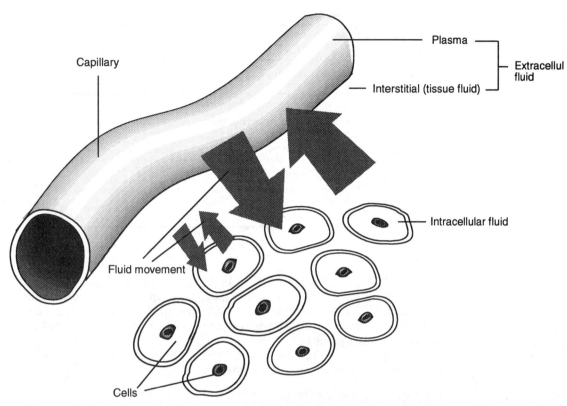

FIGURE 9–2. The three fluid compartments of the body. In distributing nutrients and disposing of waste, fluid moves from capillaries to interstitial fluid, to the cell, and vice versa. (From Scanlon, VC and Sanders, T: Essentials of Anatomy and Physiology. FA Davis, Philadelphia, p 443, with permission.)

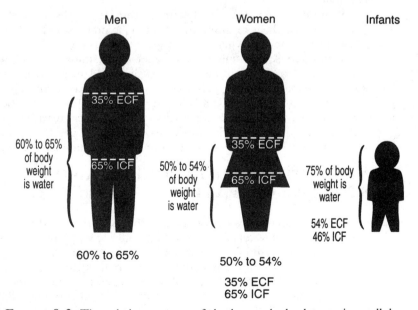

FIGURE 9–3. The relative amounts of the human body that are intracellular and extracellular water in men, women, and infants.

TABLE 9–1 *Functions of Water*

- Gives shape and form to cells
- Helps form the structure of large molecules
- Serves as a lubricant
- Helps to regulate body temperature
- Serves as a solvent
- Transports nutrients to cells
- Carries waste products away from cells
- Is a medium for chemical reactions
- Participates in chemical reactions

TRANSCELLULAR FLUIDS   These are fluids in many body cavities. This category includes cerebrospinal fluid, pericardial fluid, pleural fluid, synovial fluid, intraocular fluids, and gastrointestinal secretions. The transcellular fluids are constantly being secreted into their spaces and reabsorbed into the vascular system.

The solute in all these body fluids is water. Both intracellular and extracellular water serves a variety of essential functions.

FUNCTIONS OF WATER

Water has several important and vital functions in the body. As a component of cells, water gives the body shape and form. It helps to form the structure of many of the body's large molecules such as protein and glycogen. Some body water also serves as a lubricant, as in mucus secretions and joint fluid.

Water helps to regulate body temperature. It absorbs the heat produced by fever and the heat resulting from metabolic processes. The blood carries excess heat to the skin where it is dissipated by flushing or sweating.

Solvent—A liquid holding another substance in solution.
Solute—The substance that is dissolved in a solvent.

Water serves as a **solvent** for minerals, vitamins, glucose, and other small molecules. The substance that is dissolved in a solvent is called a **solute.** As a solvent, water is able to transport nutrients to the cells and carry waste products away from the cells. In addition, it becomes a medium for chemical reactions. Water also participates in chemical reactions, as may be seen in many of the digestive processes, such as the breakdown of proteins to amino acids. See Table 9–1 for a summary of the functions of water.

ABSORPTION, METABOLISM, AND STORAGE OF WATER

A small amount of water can be absorbed into the bloodstream from the stomach. A liter of water can be absorbed from the small intestine in an hour.

The metabolism of the energy nutrients produces water. Each energy nutrient produces a different amount of metabolic water: 1 gram of carbohydrate produces 0.60 gram, 1 gram of fat produces 1.07 grams, and 1 gram of protein produces 0.41 gram. One ounce of pure alcohol requires 8 ounces of water for its metabolism. Alcohol, rather than quenching thirst, causes dehydration and increased thirst.

No storage tanks for water exist in the body. Water continually moves from one body compartment to another, and is often reused by the body to perform different tasks.

Under conditions that have disrupted the individual's automatic adaptive mechanisms, water may be retained. The accumulation of excessive amounts of fluid between the cells (in the interstitial fluid compartment) is called **edema.** Hypothyroidism, congestive heart failure, severe protein deficiency, and some kidney conditions may cause such water retention. Excessive water can be dispersed throughout the body, also. This condition is called water intoxication. Many of the symptoms are caused by diluting the concentration of the electrolytes in the body's fluid compartments.

Edema—Accumulation of excessive amounts of fluid in interstitial spaces (between the cells).

WATER BALANCE

The last chapter discussed <u>homeostasis</u> in terms of energy balance. In this chapter, we consider homeostasis in terms of fluid and electrolyte balance. For optimum health, the water lost through the kidneys, skin, lungs, and large intestine must be continually replaced. This means that daily intake of water must equal daily output. The electrolyte content of fluids must also be maintained at the proper concentrations.

The movement, distribution, and composition of body fluids are influenced and controlled by electrolyte and plasma protein concentrations. Hormones control the amount of water retained or excreted and trigger the thirst response.

The Effect of Electrolytes on Water Balance

All body fluids contain electrolytes. Each fluid compartment has an electrolyte composition that best serves the needs of the cells in that particular compartment. Each of the fluid compartments has automatic mechanisms that are designed to keep it electrically neutral or balanced. The positive ions within a compartment must equal the negative ones. When shifts and losses occur, compensating shifts and gains take place to reestablish electroneutrality.

Regulation of Fluid Balance

Fluid balance is regulated by electrolytes because cells have no mechanism for holding onto water molecules, which pass freely through all membranes. However, cells can control the movement of electrolytes, and water tends to remain wherever the concentration of electrolytes is highest. In practical terms, this means that water will move to follow high concentrations of electrolytes such as sodium, the ion most closely associated with water balance. The body is quite tenacious in holding onto enough sodium. An abnormal serum sodium level is usually the result of gains or losses of water rather than gains or losses of sodium.

Important Body Electrolytes

The major mineral ions strongly influence not only water balance but also osmotic pressure, blood pressure, and acid-base balance. Osmotic pressure, blood pressure, and acid-base balance will be discussed later in the chapter.

Cations of importance in body fluids are sodium, potassium, calcium, and magnesium. Anions of importance include chloride, bicarbonate, phosphate, and sulfate. Sodium (Na^+) is the main electrolyte in extracellular fluid. Potassium (K^+) is the main electrolyte in intracellular fluid. Ionized sodium, potassium, and chloride are the solutes that maintain the balance between the intracellular and extracellular compartments. See Table 9–2 for a summary of the major body electrolytes.

Measurement of Electrolytes

Electrolytes are measured according to the total number of particles in solution rather than their total weight. This is because chemical activity is deter-

TABLE 9–2 *Major Body Electrolytes*

Electrolyte	Fluid Compartment*	Functions
Cations		
Sodium (Na^+)	Extracellular	Major cation in ECF. Na^+ concentration in fluids determines the distribution of H_2O by osmosis. With Cl^- and HCO_3^-, Na^+ regulates acid-base balance.
Potassium (K^+)	Intracellular	Major cation in ICF. K^+ with Na^+ maintains water balance. With Na^+ and H^+, K^+ regulates acid-base balance.
Calcium (Ca^{2+})	Extracellular†	Participates in permeability of cell membranes, transmission of nerve impulses, muscle action.
Magnesium (Mg^{2+})	Intracellular	Regulates nerve stimulation and normal muscle action.
Anions		
Chloride (Cl^-)	Extracellular	Major anion in ECF. Helps maintain water balance and acid-base balance.
Bicarbonate (HCO_3^-)	Extracellular	Most important ECF buffer.
Phosphate (HPO_4^{2-})	Intracellular	Within the ICF, phosphates and proteins buffer 95 percent of the body's carbonic acid and 50 percent of other acids.

*ECF and ICF both contain all of the cations and anions listed in this table, but are labeled as either ECF or ICF according to the concentration. For example, sodium ions make up 142 of the total 155 milliequivalents per liter (of the cations) in the ECF.

†Of the cations, 3 percent in ECF and 1 percent in ICF.

mined by the concentration of electrolytes in any given solution. The unit of measure used is the milliequivalent, expressed as milliequivalents per liter. The concentration of a pharmaceutical electrolyte in solution is also measured in milliequivalents per liter. Clinical Calculation 9–1 shows you how to convert milligrams of sodium chloride dissolved in water to milliequivalents.

Osmotic Pressure

Osmosis is the movement of water (or another solvent) across a semipermeable membrane from an area with fewer particles to one with more particles. The result, providing the difference is reasonable, is an equalization of concentration on either side of the membrane. Look at Clinical Application 9–2 for an experiment you can perform in your kitchen that demonstrates osmosis.

    Osmosis is a passive process. The movement of some substances, however, is active. Some substances require active transport mechanisms to push them through a membrane. Two such transport mechanisms are the "sodium pump" and the "potassium pump." Located in cell membranes, these pumps are actually proteins that can move ions. Sodium pumps move sodium ions out of the cells (and the water follows). Potassium pumps move potassium ions into the cells. In this manner, the electrolyte concentrations of the intracellular and extracellular fluid compartments are maintained. Unlike osmosis, which is a passive mechanism, active transport requires energy.

    DETERMINATION OF OSMOTIC PRESSURE   When two solutions with different concentrations are separated by a semipermeable membrane, pressure develops. This pressure, which is exerted on the semipermeable membrane, is called **osmotic pressure.** Osmotic pressure causes a solvent such as water to cross the membrane, while the solutes (particles) that are outside the membrane cannot go through.

    The size of the molecule and its ability to ionize determines the number of particles in a given concentration. Disaccharides and monosaccharides do not ionize. Without the appropriate enzymes to split the disaccharide into its component monosaccharides, the disaccharide molecule remains intact.

Osmosis—Movement of water across a semipermeable cell membrane from an area with fewer particles to one with more particles.

Osmotic pressure—Pressure that develops when a concentrated solution is separated from a less concentrated solution by a semipermeable membrane; only water crosses the membrane.

⚖ CLINICAL APPLICATION 9–2 ⚖
Osmosis in the Kitchen

    If you have ever made homemade sauerkraut, you have seen osmosis in action. The cabbage is sliced very fine and placed in the bottom of a crock. Salt is then added to the dry cabbage. This is repeated, layer after layer, until the crock is full. Upon completion, much liquid will already have gathered, pulled from the cabbage pieces by the concentrated salt. After the cabbage ferments for 5 or 6 weeks, the crock is really full of "extra" juice.

    You might try making a tiny batch of sauerkraut to see osmosis in action. If you do, use 2 teaspoonfuls of canning salt per pound of cabbage.

Just as there are more nails in a pound of tacks than in a pound of spikes, there are more particles in 100 kilocalories of glucose compared with 100 kilocalories of a disaccharide in a given volume. A large number of particles per unit volume exerts more osmotic pressure, which tends to draw water into an area of greater particle concentration.

OSMOLARITY OF BODY FLUIDS   The measure of the osmotic pressure exerted by the number of particles per volume of liquid is referred to as its **osmolarity** The unit of measure for osmotic activity is the milliosmole. Clinically, osmolarity is usually reported in milliosmoles per liter.

Osmolality, in contrast, is the measure of the osmotic pressure exerted by the number of particles per weight of solvent. Clinically, osmolality is usually reported in milliosmoles per kilogram.

The osmolality of human blood serum is about 300 milliosmoles per kilogram. (Laboratory texts list various ranges between 280 and 310 milliosmoles per kilogram.)

Most serum osmolarity is contributed by sodium, potassium, and chloride. In the extracellular fluid, sodium is the primary determinant of osmolality.

Within the cells, potassium helps to maintain the correct volume of intracellular fluid. Whenever cells are being built up, potassium moves into the cells. Tissue repairs after burns, trauma, or starvation increase the need for potassium.

OSMOLALITY AND NUTRITION   Fluids are designated as **isotonic** if they approximate the osmolality of the blood serum. Fluids exerting less osmotic pressure than serum are labeled **hypotonic.** Those exerting greater osmotic pressure than blood serum are called **hypertonic.**

Achieving the correct osmolality of fluids administered intravenously is very important. A solution that is too concentrated pulls water out of the red blood cells and the cells shrivel and die. Too weak a solution allows water to be pulled into the red blood cells until the cells burst.

Examples of isotonic fluids are 5 percent glucose in water and 0.9 percent sodium chloride. Only isotonic sodium chloride is given with red-blood-cell products to avoid shrinking or bursting the red blood cells.

Less concentrated solutions of glucose and sodium chloride and plain water are hypotonic. Stronger solutions are hypertonic. Total parenteral nutrition solutions are so strong that they must be infused into a large vein in the chest so that they are diluted quickly by the liberal volume of blood flowing past the infusion port or catheter.

Oral fluids also can be categorized as to their osmotic pressure. Plain water is hypotonic. Whole milk at 275 milliosmoles per liter is close to isotonic. Two fluids often taken to soothe a digestive upset are ginger ale and 7-Up. Since ginger ale has 510 milliosmoles per liter and 7-Up 640, both are hypertonic.

SERUM ELECTROLYTES   The electrolytes in blood plasma are also reported in milliequivalents per liter. Normal serum sodium is 135 to 148 milliequivalents per liter. In most cases, because sodium is the most influential extracellular ion, osmolarity of the extracellular fluid can be estimated clinically by doubling the serum sodium value. Normal serum sodium doubled would be 270 to 296 milliosmoles per liter. Normal osmolality of the serum is about 300 milliosmoles per kilogram. This simple method gives a close approximation.

The other ion that is monitored carefully is potassium. Most of the potassium in the body is inside the cells. Potassium concentration is 150 milliequivalents per liter in the intracellular fluid. By contrast, potassium concentration in the blood is only 3.5 to 5.0 milliequivalents per liter. Even slight variations above or below these values can produce severe consequences. The heart muscle is particularly sensitive to high or low levels of potassium. Either abnormally high or abnormally low levels can produce cardiac arrest.

Table 9–3 lists the normal values for serum sodium and serum potassium, along with the technical names and some of the signs and symptoms for deviations from the normal. Many other signs, including the direct measurement of serum electrolytes and the results of electrocardiograms, assist in the diagnosis of electrolyte imbalances. Note that all four of the conditions mentioned in the table produce dangerous illnesses. If the nurse recognizes and reports early signs and symptoms, the need for drastic treatment measures may be averted.

Electrolyte Imbalances

In the clinical chapters, more information will be presented on electrolyte imbalances commonly accompanying various disease conditions. Look for

TABLE 9–3 *Signs and Symptoms of Abnormal Serum Sodium and Potassium Levels*

	Low	Normal	High
Sodium			
Lab value	Less than 135 milliequivalents per liter	135–148 milliequivalents per liter	Greater than 148 milliequivalents per liter
Condition	Hyponatremia		Hypernatremia
Symptoms	Irritability Anxiety		Thirst Fatigue
Signs	Muscle twitching Seizures Coma		Flushed skin Agitation Coma
Potassium			
Lab value	Less than 3.6 milliequivalents per liter	3.6–5.0 milliequivalents per liter	Greater than 5.0 milliequivalents per liter
Condition	Hypokalemia		Hyperkalemia
Symptoms	Nausea/vomiting Paresthesias, esp. lower extremities		Irritability Abdominal cramps Weakness, esp. lower extremities
Signs	Decreased bowel sounds		Irregular pulse Cardiac arrest if greater than 8.5 milliequivalents per liter
	Weak, irregular pulse Coma		

more material on sodium and potassium balance in Chapter 17 (Diet and Cardiovascular Disease). More details on potassium levels appear in Chapter 16 (Diabetes Mellitus and Hypoglycemia) and Chapter 18 (Diet in Renal Disease).

The Effect of Plasma Proteins on Water Balance

Hydrostatic pressure—Pressure created by the pumping action of the heart on the fluid in the blood vessels.

Colloidal osmotic pressure (COP)—Pressure produced by plasma and cellular proteins.

The body has a highly developed mechanism that maintains the constant flow of water and nutrients to the cells and the flow of water and waste materials from the cells. Water and nutrients in the blood are pushed out through the very thin walls of the capillaries into the interstitial fluid by **hydrostatic pressure** (blood pressure). The heart provides the force that does the pushing. From the interstitial compartment, the water and nutrients cross cell membranes to bathe and nourish the cell. Plasma proteins, including albumin, remain in the capillaries because they are too large to squeeze through the capillary wall. Inside the blood vessels, the plasma proteins exert **colloidal osmotic pressure** (COP). The COP, now greater than the hydrostatic pressure, pulls water and waste materials from the cells back into the blood capillaries. Thus these two opposing forces control the movement of water and solutes across capillary membranes. However, osmotic pressure within the cell is still being maintained by the balance of fluid and electrolytes as described above.

Plasma proteins protect the volume of fluid in the blood. Clinical Application 9–3 describes a condition in which a low serum protein is the cause of water imbalance.

Blood Pressure

Blood pressure is the force exerted against the walls of the arteries. It is reported in two numbers, such as 120/80 (measured in millimeters of mercury). The top number is the pressure when the heart beats. It is called the systolic pressure. The bottom number is the pressure between beats. It is called the diastolic pressure. One of the factors necessary to maintain an adequate blood pressure is a sufficient volume of blood in the arteries and veins.

 CLINICAL APPLICATION 9–3
Protein-Energy Malnutrition and Water Balance

Perhaps you have seen photographs of starving children who look plump. The plumpness is caused by edema. These edematous starving children are victims of kwashiorkor, a disease of protein-energy malnutrition. It occurs most often in children just after weaning when there is not enough protein in their diets to replace their mothers' milk.

Protein plays a crucial role in maintaining the volume of fluid in the blood vessels. These children develop edema because they do not have enough plasma proteins remaining in the capillaries to pull water back into the circulatory system. Thus, it accumulates in the interstitial spaces.

Body Regulation of Water Intake and Excretion

The body has mechanisms that regulate both the intake and the excretion of water. Thirst governs water intake. The excretion of water is controlled mainly by two hormones: antidiuretic hormone causes the body to reabsorb (retain) water; aldosterone causes the body to retain sodium.

Thirst Mechanism

Thirst is the desire for fluids, especially water. Thirst occurs when 10 percent of the intravascular volume is lost or when cellular volume is reduced by 1 to 2 percent. When there is too little water in the blood (or, put another way, when the solutes are too concentrated), there is an increase in the osmotic pressure of the blood. Special sensors in a part of the brain called the **hypothalamus** monitor the osmotic pressure of the blood as it circulates in the brain. When the hypothalamus detects an increase in the osmotic pressure, it triggers the mechanism that sets into motion the desire to drink.

Hypothalamus— A portion of the brain that helps to regulate water balance, thirst, body temperature, carbohydrate and fat metabolism, and sleep.

Antidiuretic Hormone

If thirst is not alleviated, the sensors in the hypothalamus increase the secretion of **antidiuretic hormone** (ADH) from the posterior pituitary gland at the base of the brain. ADH causes the kidneys to return more water to the bloodstream rather than spilling it into the urine. Antidiuretic hormone, also named vasopressin, has an additional effect of arterial vasoconstriction. By constricting blood vessels, it increases blood pressure. When someone places a finger over the end of a garden hose, the amount of water flowing is the same as before, but the smaller outlet increases the pressure.

Not surprisingly, sometimes the ADH mechanism goes awry. In diabetes insipidus the hypothalamus does not secrete ADH or the kidneys do not respond appropriately. Diabetes insipidus can be caused by brain injury or tumor. If the hypothalamus is not secreting ADH, a pharmaceutical preparation can be given. Clinical Application 9–4 tells about a condition called Syndrome of Inappropriate Secretion of Antidiuretic Hormone (SIADH).

Antidiuretic hormone (ADH)— Hormone formed in hypothalamus and released from posterior pituitary in response to blood that is too concentrated; effect is return of water to the bloodstream by the kidneys.

Aldosterone

The release of **aldosterone,** a hormone secreted by the adrenal glands, is another water-balancing mechanism in the body. It causes sodium ions to be returned to the bloodstream by the kidneys rather than to be spilled into the urine. As the most influential extracellular ion, sodium will pull water along with it.

The trigger for the release of aldosterone is thought to be a decrease in the blood pressure in the **renal** arteries. Aldosterone then stimulates the kidneys to produce <u>renin.</u> Renin acts as an enzyme to split angiotensinogen, a serum globulin secreted by the liver, to form angiotensin I. Enzymes in the lungs convert angiotensin I to <u>angiotensin II.</u> Angiotensin II constricts blood vessels and stimulates the secretion of aldosterone. Aldosterone then increases sodium retention. Water follows sodium; thus the blood volume is maintained.

Another side of sodium retention is potassium loss. Within compartments, positively charged particles must equal negatively charged ones. When sodium is retained, to maintain electroneutrality the kidney excretes more potassium.

Aldosterone—An adrenocorticoid hormone that increases sodium and water retention by the kidneys.

Renal—Pertaining to the kidney.

CLINICAL APPLICATION 9–4

Syndrome of Inappropriate Secretion of Antidiuretic Hormone (SIADH)

Normally, increased osmolality of the blood stimulates the posterior pituitary gland to release ADH. When enough water is returned to the bloodstream by the kidney, the ADH secretion stops.

Several situations cause ADH to be released inappropriately. Certain lung tumors produce an ADH-like substance. Other lung conditions such as pneumonia, tuberculosis, and asthma have caused SIADH. Stress, surgery, some anesthetics, pain, and morphine have been implicated in increased release of ADH. Medications such as chlorpropamide and oxytocin have precipitated SIADH. Conditions directly affecting the brain (including the hypothalamus and the pituitary gland) such as meningitis, brain tumors, and subarachnoid hemorrhage have been linked to SIADH.

The signs and symptoms of SIADH are those of hyponatremia. In this case it is called a dilutional hyponatremia. The patient has enough sodium, but it is diluted in too much retained water. Initially, the patient becomes apprehensive. When the serum sodium drops to 120 to 125 milliequivalents per liter, neurological signs appear, owing to edema of the brain cells. The patient becomes irritable, apathetic, and displays personality changes. Other signs of hyponatremia include tremors, hyperactive reflexes, muscle spasms, and convulsions. Increased intracellular fluid produces edema, which can be detected when pressure over a bony surface leaves the mark of the examiner's fingertip visible. When the serum sodium drops to less than 115 milliequivalents per liter, seizures, coma, and permanent neurological damage can occur.

Effective treatment of SIADH is based upon discovering and removing the cause of the condition. Beyond that, or in the instance of a postoperative or stress reaction, treatment involves diuretic therapy and fluid restriction. The patient is given precisely prescribed amounts of fluids throughout the day. Over a period of several days, through <u>obligatory excretion,</u> the patient's body will excrete the extra water.

ACID-BASE BALANCE

Electrolytes also play an important role in maintaining the acid-base balance of body fluids. Acids are compounds that yield hydrogen ions when dissociated in solution. The more hydrogen ions a solution contains, the more concentrated the acid. Bases, or alkalies, are substances that accept hydrogen ions. The acidity or alkalinity of a substance is measured according to a scale called **pH**. The pH scale ranges from 0 to 14: acids are rated from 0 to 6.999; 7 is neutral; bases are above 7.

The balance between too much and too little acid in body fluids is maintained by the action of buffer systems in the blood and other body fluids, the lungs, and the kidneys. The purpose of buffer systems is to minimize significant changes in the pH of the body fluids by controlling the

pH—A scale representing the relative acidity or alkalinity of a solution; a value of 7 is neutral, less than 7 is acidic, and greater than 7 is alkaline.

hydrogen ion (H^+) concentration. **Buffers** are substances that can neutralize both acids and bases. **Bicarbonate** (HCO_3^-) is the most important buffer in the extracellular fluid. Phosphate (HPO_4^{2-}) and proteins are two important buffers in the intracellular fluid.

Extracellular Fluid

The normal pH of the extracellular fluid (including the blood and interstitial fluid) is 7.35 to 7.45. This is slightly alkaline, although most of the body's waste products are acid. The body is continually working to maintain the correct pH of its fluids. If the serum pH drops below 6.8 or rises above 7.8, death is usually the result.

Extracellular fluid contains both positive sodium ions (Na^+) and negative bicarbonate ions (HCO_3^-). When a strong acid is introduced to the fluid, a chemical reaction takes place. The end products of this reaction are sodium chloride (a salt), which is neutral, and carbonic acid (a weak acid). The carbonic acid breaks down to carbon dioxide and water. The carbon dioxide is excreted by the lungs (exhaled) and the water is excreted by the kidneys.

Another chemical reaction takes place when a strong base (alkali) is introduced into the fluid system. When a strong base enters the system, carbon dioxide and water (the two main waste products of cellular metabolism) react to form carbonic acid to counteract the alkaline effect of the base. The end products of this reaction are water and a weak base that will not drastically affect the pH.

Respiratory System

The lungs help maintain pH by varying the amount of carbon dioxide (CO_2) exhaled. Excess carbon dioxide makes the body fluids more acidic because it reacts to form carbonic acid, a source of hydrogen ions. Too much carbonic acid, or any acid, will result in **acidosis.** When this happens, the lungs automatically increase the rate and depth of breathing, eliminating more carbon dioxide and water.

This respiratory response to acidosis begins within minutes of an increase in acidity. Respiratory compensation for acidosis is 50 to 75 percent effective and is an extremely important component in the regulation of pH. Normally, the respiratory system has one or two times the buffering power of all chemical buffers in the body.

Renal System

The respiratory system acts quickly but it can only eliminate carbonic acid. Other acids, as well as excess carbonic acid, must be eliminated in the urine. The kidney spills or retains hydrogen, sodium, and bicarbonate ions as necessary to maintain an acceptable pH in the blood. For example, in response to acidosis, the kidneys excrete hydrogen ions and reabsorb sodium and bicarbonate ions. Ketoacidosis, a form of acidosis resulting from diabetes mellitus, is discussed in detail in Chapter 16. In response to alkalosis, the kidneys conserve hydrogen ions and excrete sodium and bicarbonate ions. The kidneys initiate these actions within 24 hours but require 3 to 4 days to compensate for changes in blood pH.

Buffer—A substance that can react to offset excess acid or excess alkali (base) in a solution; blood buffers include carbonic acid, bicarbonate, phosphates, and proteins, including hemoglobin.

Bicarbonate—Any salt containing the HCO_3 anion; blood bicarbonate is a measure of alkali (base) reserve of the body; bicarbonate of soda is sodium bicarbonate, $NaHCO_3$.

Acidosis—Condition that results when the pH of the blood falls below 7.35; may be caused by diarrhea, uremia, diabetes mellitus, and certain drug therapies.

Intracellular Fluid

The normal pH of the intracellular fluid is 6.8 to 7.0, slightly acid to neutral. Within the intracellular fluid, organic phosphates and proteins are the most important buffers. These substances buffer 95 percent of the body's carbonic acid and 50 percent of other acids. Protein is the most powerful and plentiful buffer system in the body. Of the body's proteins, hemoglobin has the largest buffering capacity. Thus the red blood cells have 70 percent of the buffering power of the blood. This buffering capacity allows large quantities of carbon dioxide to be transported from the tissues to the lungs with only a small change in venous pH compared with arterial pH.

When the blood contains excessive hydrogen ions, they move into the cells to be buffered. Then, to maintain electroneutrality, potassium moves from the intracellular compartment to the extracellular (intravascular), raising serum potassium levels.

RECOMMENDED DIETARY ALLOWANCE

There is no RDA for water. Unless they are taking a high-salt or high-protein diet, adults need one milliliter per kilocalorie per day. So a person on a 1500-kilocalorie diet should take in 1½ liters of liquid. Adults require 2 to 4 percent of their body weight as water daily. The 154-pound person would need 3 to 6 pounds of water. A pint is approximately a pound, so 2 to 4 percent of 154 pounds would be 1½ to 3 quarts of liquid. Of this amount, at least 60 percent should be consumed as water and the remainder obtained from foods and metabolic water (Fig. 9–4).

Infants have a greater need for water than adults do. Their basal heat production per kilogram is twice that of adults. To rid their bodies of the heat and waste products, 1.5 milliliters of water per kilocalorie are needed. This means that infants must drink 10 to 15 percent of their body weight as water to maintain health.

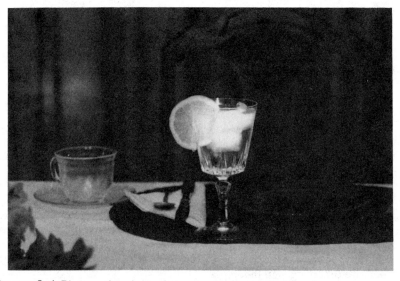

FIGURE 9–4. Place setting shows that water can be an appealing beverage.

SOURCES OF WATER

Much of our water is consumed disguised as other beverages. Adults consume 6 cups of water per day in beverages. Water may contain other nutrients as well. Hard water has calcium, magnesium, and often iron. Water conditioners used to soften water replace the calcium, magnesium, and iron with sodium. For some people, drinking softened water increases their sodium intake excessively. In fact most experts recommend that the cold water faucet at the kitchen sink be plumbed for unsoftened water.

We obtain about 4 cups of water per day in foods. It is probably not surprising that skimmed milk is 91 percent water, and whole milk is 88 percent water. Some foods that are solids also have a high water content: head lettuce is 96 percent water, celery is 95 percent water, and raw carrots are 88 percent water. Other foods that contain a large percentage of water include apples (84 percent), grapes (81 percent), bananas (74 percent), hard-cooked eggs (75 percent), drained tuna (61 percent), and chicken breast or thigh (52 percent). Whole wheat bread is 38 percent water, which drops to 29% when it is toasted.

Water is also a product of metabolism. The average person acquires 1 cup of water per day from this process.

LOSSES OF WATER

We lose water in obvious ways, such as in perspiration and urine. We also lose water in less obvious ways, such as through breathing. The obvious ways are called **sensible water losses**. The less obvious ways are called **insensible water losses**.

Sensible water loss—Visible water loss through sweat, urine, and feces.

Insensible water loss—Water that is lost invisibly through the lungs and skin.

Sensible Water Losses

Sensible water losses include losses of the major extracellular ions, sodium and chloride. Three important routes commonly account for sensible water losses: through the skin as perspiration, through the kidney as urine, and through the gastrointestinal tract in the feces.

Perspiration

To produce 1 liter of perspiration requires 600 kilocalories. In extreme cases, a person may perspire at the rate of 2 liters per hour. For example, during a race, marathon runners may lose 6 to 7 percent of their body weight, primarily as perspiration.

Sweat is not pure water. It is salty to the taste. Perspiration is hypotonic. One liter of perspiration contains 45 milliequivalents of sodium, 5 milliequivalents of potassium, and 58 milliequivalents of chlorine. In this instance, the milliosmole value is the same as the milliequivalent value (because all the ions are monovalent) so the milliequivalents can be added to obtain an osmolarity of 108 milliequivalents per liter of perspiration.

Urine

In the normal, healthy person, urine output is roughly equal to liquid intake. Often this amount equals 1200 to 1500 milliliters per day.

Obligatory excretion—Minimum amount of urine production necessary to keep waste products in solution, amounting to 400 to 600 milliliters per day.

A minimum amount of urine must be excreted each day to carry away the waste products resulting from metabolic processes. This is called **obligatory excretion.** Obligatory excretion of urine amounts to 400 to 600 milliliters per day.

For seriously ill patients, hourly urine output is monitored. These amounts must be interpreted in relation to the patient's whole situation. Even if a person is losing massive amounts of fluid through disease, such losses do not rid the body of metabolic wastes as efficiently as the kidney does. Adults should excrete between 40 and 80 milliliters of urine per hour. Clinical Calculation 9–4 shows a method of determining a desirable hourly urine output for children.

Gastrointestinal Secretions

Abnormal gastrointestinal function can cause extensive fluid loss. When the secretion lost is high in the gastrointestinal tract, the resulting symptoms differ from those that occur when the secretion is lost from lower in the tract. Gastric juice is acid, or high in hydrogen ions. Intestinal juices are alkaline, or low in hydrogen ions. Therefore, gastrointestinal losses are divided into those lost above the outlet of the stomach and those lost below the stomach. The opening between the stomach and the small intestine is called the pylorus.

ABOVE THE PYLORUS   The common causes of these losses are vomiting or stomach suctioning. Two organs secrete digestive juices above the pylorus. They are the salivary glands in the mouth and the gastric glands in the stomach. Both of these secretions are isotonic, so their loss threatens electrolyte balance to a greater extent than loss of an equal amount of perspiration would. The ions lost in secretions above the pylorus are sodium, potassium, chlorine, and hydrogen.

About 1 liter of saliva per day is mixed with food or just swallowed. The stomach secretes about 1.5 to 2.5 liters of gastric juice per day. If gastric juices are lost, hydrogen ions in the hydrochloric acid are also lost. The person is in danger of alkalosis.

BELOW THE PYLORUS   The usual causes of these losses are diarrhea or intestinal suctioning. Gastrointestinal secretions below the pylorus also are isotonic. They contain sodium, potassium, and bicarbonate. About 2 to 3 liters of intestinal secretions per day flow into the bowel to digest the food intake. Normally, bile is released from the gallbladder into the small intestine at the rate of 1 liter per day. The total gastrointestinal secretions amount to 6.5 to 8.5 liters per day. Yet, because water is absorbed back into the blood from the large intestine, normal feces from an adult contain only 100 to 200 milliliters of water.

See Clinical Application 9–5 for a discussion of two conditions resulting from exposure to extreme heat: heat exhaustion and heat stroke.

Insensible Water Losses

Although we do not see it go, water is lost through the lungs and the skin. These are insensible losses. We lose between 800 and 1000 milliliters of water each day through the insensible losses via the lungs and skin.

CLINICAL APPLICATION 9–5
Heat Exhaustion and Heat Stroke

Exposure to extreme heat may overtax the body's adaptive capabilities. Depending on the body's response, two very different clinical conditions appear: heat exhaustion or heat stroke. The patient should seek medical attention if either condition occurs.

HEAT EXHAUSTION

In this condition, which is more common, the patient suffers the loss of water and sodium chloride in sweat. The patient's temperature is normal or below. The pulse is weak, thready, and rapid. Respirations are shallow and quiet. The skin is cool, clammy, and sweaty. First aid treatment consists of moving the patient to a cooler environment. The patient should lie down with the feet elevated and clothing should be loosened. If the person can drink it, ½ teaspoonful of salt in ½ glass of water will begin to replace the water and sodium chloride lost. The salt-in-water treatment should be repeated every 15 minutes until the emergency team arrives.

HEAT STROKE

In this condition, the patient fails to perspire because the body can no longer regulate body temperature. The patient has an extremely elevated temperature, 105°F or above. The pulse is full and bounding. Breathing is difficult and respirations are loud. The skin is flushed, hot, and dry. The patient is not sweating. First aid treatment of heat stroke includes complete quiet with the head elevated, removal of clothing, and bathing with cool water. Of the two conditions, heat stroke is more likely to be life-threatening.

Lungs

We "see our breath" only in very cold weather. It appears as steam coming out of our mouths and noses. Even in warmer weather and indoors, breathing causes the loss of 400 milliliters of water per day. This is average; deep respirations or a dry climate increase the amount of water lost.

Skin

The insensible loss of water through the skin is evaporative. It is almost pure water and nearly electrolyte-free. This insensible water loss amounts to 6 milliliters per kilogram of body weight in 24 hours.

This is a baseline amount. Look at Clinical Calculation 9–2 to see how it is determined for a patient. Burns, phototherapy, radiant warmers, or fever will increase the amount of insensible water loss. Fever increases evaporative losses by about 12 percent per Celsius degree of temperature elevation. Clinical Calculation 9–3 shows how evaporative water losses are calculated.

CLINICAL APPLICATION 9–6
Replacing Insensible Water Losses

Although the patient in kidney failure puts out very little urine, he or she still loses water insensibly through the lungs and skin. These losses are roughly 800 milliliters per day. To replace insensible water losses the physician will sometimes prescribe 800 milliliters of fluid intake per day plus an amount equal to the previous day's urine output. Careful evaluation of the patient's electrolyte status is also made. Nutrition for patients with kidney disease is covered in detail in Chapter 18.

Clinical Application 9–6, discusses the replacement of evaporative water losses. It is especially pertinent in kidney disease, the subject of Chapter 18.

Figure 9–5 illustrates the sources and routes of loss of body fluids. Table 9–4 lists the average fluid gains and losses for adults in a 24-hour period.

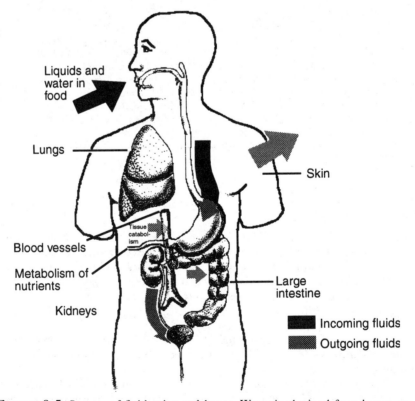

FIGURE 9–5. Sources of fluid gains and losses. Water is obtained from beverages, water in foods, and energy metabolisms. It is lost through the lungs, skin, kidney, and bowel. (Adapted from Scanlon, VC and Sanders, T: Essentials of Anatomy and Physiology. FA Davis, Philadelphia, p 445.)

TABLE 9–4 *Average Fluid Gains and Losses in Adults in 24 Hours*

Fluid Gains		Fluid Losses*	
Energy metabolism	300 milliliters	Kidneys	1200–1500 milliliters
		Skin	500–600 milliliters
Oral fluids	1100–1400 milliliters	Lungs	400 milliliters
Solid foods	800–1000 milliliters	Intestines	100–200 milliliters
Total	2200–2700 milliliters	Total	2200–2700 milliliters

*Includes sensible and insensible losses.

Assessment of Water Losses

Gathering data on water losses is quite straightforward. Because water is more than 50 percent of body weight, a loss of water will be exhibited in the patient's weight. Recording the liquid a patient takes in and puts out is a second means of tracking water balance.

Weight

Rapid weight changes usually are a reflection of fluid balance. Daily weight is the single most important indicator of fluid status. An easy way to relate volume to weight is to remember "A pint is a pound the world around." One liter is 1 kilogram or 2.2 pounds. Acute weight loss in adults is rated as follows: mild volume deficit—2 to 5 percent loss; moderate volume deficit—5 to 10 percent loss; and severe volume deficit—10 to 15 percent loss. A loss of greater than 15 percent can be fatal.

Fluid balance in the infant is much more precarious. Because a greater proportion of body water is in the extracellular space in infants, they can lose it more rapidly than an adult. Therefore, a loss of 5 percent of body weight in an infant merits medical attention.

Sudden weight changes are not always due to fluid shifts. If a patient receives no oral, enteral, or parenteral nutrition, the loss of body tissue may amount to 0.3 to 0.5 kilogram per day. Enteral and parenteral nutrition are discussed in Chapter 13.

Recording Intake and Output

In addition to monitoring weight, we often record liquid intake and output. In the healthy person, liquid intake and output should be approximately equal. If you refer again to Table 9–4, you will see that the intake from oral fluids and the output through the kidney are within 100 milliliters of being equal. Of course, variations in the other gains and losses affect the liquid totals. Measuring intake is easier than measuring output. See Charting Tips 9–1 for ideas on how to keep a more accurate record of output.

CHARTING TIPS 9–1

Intake and Output

✓   Record intake and output immediately so that the information is not forgotten.

✓   Most institutions post the amounts that food and beverage containers hold. Ice chips should be recorded as one half of their volume. When 1 cup of ice chips melts, you will see only ½ cup of water.

✓   Fluid that is lost into a dressing or a diaper presents a problem for the nurse who is recording output. Dressings and diapers can be weighed. The weight of the dry material is subtracted from the total. One gram of weight equals 1 milliliter of water. Specific gravity, is the weight of a substance compared with distilled water. Normal specific gravity of urine is 1.010 to 1.025. So, although the diaper weight from urine is not exactly the same as if it were wet with water, this method of recording incontinent urine is adequate in most situations.

In the sick person, the totals may not balance every day. The patient's intake and output should be analyzed over a period of several days; a one-day evaluation could prove misleading. Of utmost importance is the ability to see the big picture. See Charting Tips 9–2 for teaching and documentation tips.

CHARTING TIPS 9–2

Be Specific in Teaching and Document It

✓   Be specific when teaching patients.

✓   Record both the content and the patient's response to the material.

One patient was told to "drink a lot of fluid" when he was discharged from the hospital. He interpreted this to be 3 to 4 gallons per day! His kidneys did their best, but kidneys cannot produce plain water. In a few days, the patient was back in the hospital for correction of electrolyte imbalance. This outcome could have been prevented if the patient had been taught to drink a specific amount of fluid rather than "a lot."

WATER IMBALANCES

Because water is being discussed in this chapter, electrolytes are included only to the extent necessary to understand water balance. Two common imbalances are fluid volume deficit and fluid volume excess.

Fluid Volume Deficit

In fluid volume deficit, the individual experiences vascular, interstitial, or cellular dehydration. In the body's effort to compensate, fluid moves from one compartment to another. This means that the patient's situation is constantly changing.

Losses of Fluid

Fluid losses can be external or internal. Treatments may differ, but the signs and symptoms of fluid volume deficit are similar regardless of the cause.

EXTERNAL LOSSES   Fluids lost to the outside of the body are called external fluid losses. Gastrointestinal losses are the most common. Vomiting or diarrhea are just two of the ways in which gastrointestinal fluids are lost. But medical treatments such as gastrointestinal suctioning or surgical rerouting of intestinal contents also produce fluid deficit. Hemorrhage produces not only fluid loss but also the loss of blood cells.

INTERNAL LOSSES   It may be hard to imagine, but fluids can be "lost" inside the body. Excessive fluid accumulation in the interstitial fluid compartment is edema. Although the same amount of fluid is inside the body, any fluid outside the blood vessels is lost to the circulation.

As a result of injury or trauma, capillary permeability increases so that more fluid and cells can travel to the site of the injury to begin repairs or healing. It also causes the swelling, or edema, at the site of an injury. Think of what happens when you burn yourself badly enough to cause a blister. Fluid leaves the vessels and accumulates in the skin. Thus, correct fluid replacement is a high priority for severely burned patients.

There are also several places in the body where vast amounts of fluid can accumulate. These losses are called "third-space" losses. Several liters of fluid can accumulate in the bowel when a person has a bowel obstruction. Certain diseases can cause ascites, the accumulation of fluid (often amounting to several liters), not within the bowel but around it in the abdominal cavity. Other third-space losses involve internal bleeding or the collection of fluid in the chest cavity.

An alert nurse can spot an early clue to third-space losses. Decreasing urine output in spite of seemingly adequate fluid intake demands further assessment.

Assessment of Fluid Volume Deficit

Loss of fluid may be mild and corrected easily if the patient obeys the body's thirst command to drink. On the other hand, the patient's life may be threatened if the fluid loss is severe or sudden.

SYMPTOMS The thirst response is triggered when 10 percent of intravascular volume is lost or when cellular volume is reduced by 1 to 2 percent. Thus, thirst is a symptom of fluid volume deficit. The patient may also suffer a loss of appetite or be nauseated because of decreased blood flow to the intestines.

SIGNS Vital signs are correctly named. Variations in vital signs signal changes in the patient's condition. The individual with fluid volume deficit will be less able to maintain his or her blood pressure immediately after rising from a lying or sitting position. This is called orthostatic hypotension. The nurse measures the blood pressure with the patient lying or sitting, asks the patient to stand, and immediately retakes the blood pressure. A drop of 15 millimeters or mercury in either systolic or diastolic blood pressure upon standing suggests fluid volume deficit. A narrowing of pulse pressure (the difference between systolic and diastolic readings) also occurs with fluid volume deficit. In an effort to maintain perfusion of the tissues, the body compensates for a lowered blood pressure by an increase in pulse rate. Taking a pulse when lying or sitting and immediately after rising is another method of assessing fluid volume deficit. An increase of 20 beats per minute upon standing merits further assessment.

Turgor—Resistance of the skin to being pinched; in a healthy young person the effect of the pinch disappears rapidly; in a dehydrated or elderly person, the pinched skin remains elevated longer.

Decreased skin **turgor,** or elasticity, is a sign of fluid volume deficit. To assess skin turgor, pinch the skin on the forearm, over the sternum, or on the back of the hand. If the skin stays pinched, suspect fluid volume deficit. This is a less reliable sign in the elderly person, whose skin has lost much of its elasticity.

Another sign of fluid volume deficit can be found in the patient's mouth. Besides dry mouth, many longitudinal furrows of the tongue may be seen to replace the single one in the well hydrated adult.

Delayed filling of hand veins is a sign of fluid volume deficit. To assess vein filling, raise the hand above the heart. Normally, the veins will collapse in 3 to 5 seconds. Then lower the hand below the heart. The veins should refill in 3 to 5 seconds. A person with fluid volume deficit will require more than 5 seconds for the veins to refill.

The symptoms of loss of appetite and nausea may progress to the sign of vomiting. Here, too, the cause is decreased blood flow to the intestines.

Fluid volume deficit produces changes in certain laboratory readings. The patient will show increases in hemoglobin level and hematocrit unless he or she has lost red blood cells through hemorrhage.

Special attention must be given to the assessment of infants. Because 75 percent of the infant's body weight is water and 54 percent of the water is extracellular, dehydration from fluid loss can occur rapidly. Signs to assess in the infant, in addition to poor skin turgor and dry mucous membranes, are depressed fontanel ("soft spot" in skull), sunken eyes, and lack of tears when crying.

SHOCK If fluid volume deficit continues, the patient will go into shock. The loss of 20 to 25 percent of intravascular volume produces shock. Shock is an acute peripheral circulatory failure due to loss of circulatory fluid or derangement of circulatory control. Signs of shock are a decreased blood pressure and an increased pulse. The person's skin is pale, cool, and clammy from perspiration. Urine output is decreased to less than 15 milliliters per hour.

Treatment of Fluid Volume Deficit

When treating fluid volume deficit, it is essential to correct the cause of the fluid depletion. In addition, to replace fluid volume and correct electrolyte imbalances, hypotonic fluids are given. If possible, oral rehydration is used. See Clinical Application 9–7 for an example of a commonly used oral rehydration solution.

If hypertonic solutions were given to correct fluid loss, the concentrated solution would draw fluid from the bowel wall into the lumen; the result would be diarrhea. This is called osmotic diarrhea. Some commercial laxatives and enemas are hypertonic solutions that work in this way.

Maximal sodium and water absorption is thought to occur with a glucose concentration of 10 to 25 grams per liter. Higher concentrations allow less sodium and water to be absorbed, in addition to causing osmotic diarrhea. Cola beverages, ginger ale, and apple juice are poor choices for rehydration in prolonged diarrhea, owing to their high glucose and low electrolyte concentrations.

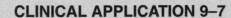

CLINICAL APPLICATION 9–7
Oral Electrolyte Solutions

Originally, oral electrolyte solutions were designed to combat diarrheal diseases in developing countries. They proved so useful that they have since been modified for use in Western nations.

One commonly used oral electrolyte solution is Pedialyte. It is available over the counter without a prescription. One liter of Pedialyte contains:

> 45 milliequivalents of sodium
> 20 milliequivalents of potassium
> 35 milliequivalents of chloride
> 30 milliequivalents of citrate, a base

The total osmolarity of Pedialyte is mildly hypotonic, about 243 milliosmoles per liter. Pedialyte also illustrates electroneutrality. The sodium and potassium are cations carrying positive charges. The chloride and citrate are anions carrying negative charges.

45 milliequivalents Na^+	35 milliequivalents Cl^-
+ 20 milliequivalents K^+	+ 30 milliequivalents $citrate^-$
65 cations	65 anions

Pedialyte is designed for maintenance of an infant or child experiencing vomiting or diarrhea. If the patient becomes dehydrated, medical attention is needed. Intravenous fluids or an oral rehydration solution of different composition from Pedialyte may be prescribed for the dehydrated patient. Loss of 5 percent of body weight indicates dehydration.

Pedialyte also has the ideal concentration of glucose to promote sodium and water absorption, 25 grams per liter.

CLINICAL APPLICATION 9–8

Hyperkalemia following Blood Transfusion

A person who has hemorrhaged may need blood replacement. Red blood cells do not live as long in the blood bank as they do in the human body. Potassium is the major cation in red blood cells (intracellular). When the red blood cells die and their cell walls rupture, potassium is spilled into the serum.

Blood that has been stored for a prolonged period may contain up to 30 milliequivalents per liter of potassium due to the destruction of the red blood cells. This may not sound like a lot, but potassium is usually administered intravenously at a concentration of 40 milliequivalents per liter to a person who is potassium depleted. The person receiving a blood transfusion may have a serum potassium level that is nearly normal, and the old blood containing a higher concentration of potassium may push him or her into hyperkalemia.

Hyperkalemia, as well as hypokalemia, can be life-threatening. The nurse should always be alert for patients at risk of electrolyte imbalances, whether due to disease, diet, or treatments.

Another electrolyte imbalance is a possibility if the patient in shock requires blood transfusions. Look at Clinical Application 9–8 to learn about this complication.

Fluid Volume Excess

This situation is the opposite of fluid volume deficit. The individual is retaining fluid intracellularly or extracellularly. A fluid compartment does not operate in isolation: if one is out of balance, the other compartment eventually will be affected as the body attempts to equalize osmotic pressure across the compartments.

Gains of Fluid

If the kidney and the hormones from the adrenal and pituitary glands are functioning normally, excess water is excreted from the body in the urine. The amount of urine excreted in 24 hours is roughly equal to the amount of liquids consumed. When a person becomes ill and these control mechanisms stop working, fluids shift from the intravascular and interstitial spaces to the intracellular space so as to equalize osmotic pressure throughout.

Inflammation increases the fluid in interstitial space, causing edema. In most cases, localized edema is not life-threatening. However, the accumulation of fluid in the brain (cerebral edema) or in lung tissue (pulmonary edema) are life-threatening conditions. Cerebral edema may result from tumors, toxic chemicals, or infection. Pulmonary edema can be a consequence of a failing heart or irritation of the lung, as when a patient inhales toxic gases.

Assessment of Fluid Volume Excess

Many of the presenting signs and symptoms of fluid volume excess are oppo-site those of fluid volume deficit. One common symptom is loss of appetite.

SYMPTOMS   The patient with fluid volume excess complains of loss of appetite and nausea. Here the symptoms are due to edema of the gastroin-testinal tract, rather than decreased blood flow as in fluid volume deficit.

SIGNS   Because the brain cells are so sensitive to changes in the internal environment, the person with fluid volume excess exhibits deteriorating consciousness. The same edema of the gastrointestinal tract causing the anorexia and nausea causes the sign of vomiting.

Because increased fluid in the blood decreases the proportion of red blood cells to total volume, the hematocrit reading is decreased. The increase in blood volume causes an increased pulse pressure. The same technique described under fluid volume deficit is used to assess hand veins. With fluid volume excess the veins will not empty 3 to 5 seconds after rais-ing the hand above the heart.

Increased blood flow to the kidneys causes increased urine output if the kidneys are functioning. The increased systolic blood pressure due to the excessive fluid pushes more fluid into the interstitial space, causing edema. Firm pressure over a bone, the ankle, or the top of the foot, forces some of the fluid aside. An indentation remains visible for a short time. This is called pitting edema. Table 9–5 lists signs and symptoms for fluid volume deficit and fluid volume excess.

Treatment of Fluid Volume Excess

As with fluid volume deficit, the remedy for fluid volume excess is to treat the cause. Osmotic diuretic drugs such as mannitol remain in the extracellu-lar spaces. By increasing the osmotic pressure there, these drugs pull excess fluid from the cells.

Nutritionally, the patient may be on a restricted fluid regimen. The physician may prescribe an intake of no more than 1000 milliliters in 24 hours. This amount will compensate for insensible losses through the skin and lungs. It is essential for the nurse to supply fluid as prescribed and to teach the patient the reason for the restriction. Over a period of several days, the obligatory urine output and any diuretic therapy will help the patient's body to excrete the excess fluid.

Summary

Water is our most essential nutrient. It comprises at least half of every-one's body weight. The amount of water varies with the type of tissue, with gender, and with age. Body fluids are held in two compartments: intracellu-lar fluid is the water within the cells; extracellular fluid is the water outside the cells. The latter includes intravascular fluid, lymph, interstitial, and transcellular fluid.

Water has many vital functions in the body. It gives shape and form to the cells, helps form the structure of large molecules, serves as a lubricant, and helps regulate body temperature. As a solvent, water transports solutes to and from the cells, is a medium for chemical reactions, and participates in chemical reactions.

TABLE 9–5 *Signs and Symptoms of Abnormal Fluid Volume*

	Fluid Volume Deficit	Fluid Volume Excess
Symptoms		
Gastrointestinal	Thirst	Loss of appetite (edema of the bowel)
	Loss of appetite (decreased blood to intestines)	Nausea
Signs		
General	Weight loss	Weight gain
	Depressed fontanel (infant)	Edema
	Sunken eyes (infant)	
	Lack of tears when crying (infant)	
Skin and mucous membranes	Dry mucous membranes	
	Decreased skin turgor	
Cardiovascular System	Orthostatic hypotension (pressure decrease of 15 millimeters of mercury in systolic or diastolic)	Increased hematocrit values
	Increased pulse rate upon standing	Increasing pulse pressure
	Increased hematocrit values (unless RBCs also lost)	Emptying of hand veins takes longer than 5 seconds
	Narrowing pulse pressure	
	Filling of hand veins takes longer than 5 seconds	
Urinary	Decreased urine output	Polyuria
	Concentrated urine	Dilute urine
Gastrointestinal	Vomiting (decreased blood to intestines)	Vomiting
	Longitudinal furrows on tongue	
Central nervous system	Confusion, disorientation	Deteriorating consciousness

The human body has no storage tanks for water. When necessary, the body can absorb water rapidly. Although some water can be absorbed from the stomach, 1 liter per hour can be absorbed from the small intestine.

The movement, distribution, and composition of body fluids are influenced and controlled by electrolyte and plasma protein concentrations. In the extracellular fluid, sodium is the major cation and chloride is the major anion. The major cation in the intracellular fluid is potassium. Ionized sodium, potassium, and chloride are the solutes that maintain the balance between the extracellular and intracellular compartments.

A complex system regulates the amount of water retained or excreted by the kidney. Aldosterone and ADH are hormones that cause retention of sodium and water, respectively. The hypothalamus stimulates the thirst mechanism when fluids inside the cells become too concentrated (with solutes).

Acid-base balance is maintained in the body by the action of buffer systems in the body fluids, the lungs, and the kidneys. Buffer systems act to minimize drastic changes in the pH of body fluids. Bicarbonate is the most important buffer in the extracellular fluid. Phosphate and protein are two important buffers in the intracellular fluid.

The body's sources of water include beverages, foods, and water from the metabolism of the energy nutrients (except alcohol). Water can be lost through the skin, lungs, kidneys, and intestinal tract. Although still present in the body, fluid can be lost to circulation in "third spaces." The single most important measure of fluid balance is daily weight.

Since most fluid losses are hypotonic, the fluids usually used to correct fluid volume deficits and electrolyte imbalances are hypotonic. The use of hypertonic fluids would have the opposite effect, pulling more water out of the tissues and into the bowel or bloodstream.

Fluid volume excess can be local or generalized. The most dangerous sites for local edema are the brain and the lungs. Generalized fluid volume excess can make exorbitant demands on the heart.

A case study and a sample plan of care appear below. Both are designed to show how the information in this chapter can be used in nursing practice.

CASE STUDY 9–1

Mr. N., a 75-year-old retired office worker, recently arrived from his summer home in the North to his winter home in Florida. He had anticipated enjoying the 85°F weather. He left temperatures in the forties. Although Mr. N. had hired someone to care for his small yard while he was away from Florida, he identified a number of chores to be done. These he tackled with a vengeance.

After an 1½ hours, Mr. N. began to get a headache. He felt a bit weak and dizzy, but continued his work. He was nearly finished with the outside tasks.

Half an hour later, Ms. N. found her husband lying on the ground. She called their neighbor, who is a retired nurse.

The nurse noted that Mr. N.'s skin was pale and cool but that he was perspiring profusely. He was conscious and coherent but said he felt weak. The nurse took Mr. N.'s pulse. It was 90 beats per minute, regular but weak. His respirations were 12 per minute and shallow.

The nurse provided the emergency care described in the following nursing care plan. (Of course, she did not write it all out before helping Mr. N.)

NURSING CARE PLAN FOR MR. N.

Assessment

Subjective

Has worked outside in 85°F heat 2 hours

Headache, weakness, dizziness

Recently arrived from colder climate

Objective

Conscious, coherent

Skin pale, cool, wet with perspiration
Pulse 90, regular and weak
Respirations 12 and shallow

Nursing Diagnosis

Fluid volume deficit related to excessive loss of hypotonic fluid (sweat) as evidenced by wet, pale skin and weak, rapid pulse

Desired Outcome/Evaluation Criteria

Patient will remain conscious and oriented, with a pulse no greater than 90, until the emergency team arrives.

Nursing Actions

1. Instruct Ms. N. to call emergency medical services and return to help.
2. Loosen Mr. N.'s clothing.
3. With Ms. N., move patient to shade.
4. Keep patient lying down with legs elevated slightly.
5. Send Ms. N. to kitchen for ½ glass of water with ½ teaspoonful of salt in it. Administer salty water to Mr. N.

Rationale

1. In an emergency situation, the nurse stays with the patient. Potential electrolyte imbalance requires medical care.
2. Mr. N. is already in a state of shock. Loosening the clothing will allow maximum air exchange and permit relaxation.
3. Mr. N. must get out of the sun. Depending on the situation, he might be moved indoors, but perhaps the two women could not manage to move him.
4. Lying down permits maximum blood circulation to the brain. Raising the legs increases the return of blood to the heart. The head should not be lowered because this causes venous congestion in the brain.
5. Although this is a hypertonic solution, sodium is readily absorbed by the intestine, so it is unlikely to cause osmotic diarrhea. Only 5 percent of consumed sodium remains in the feces (see Chapter 7). Sodium levels in the blood are controlled by the kidneys. This patient has lost water and sodium chloride in perspiration.

STUDY AIDS

Chapter Review Questions

1. Which of the following persons would have the greatest percentage of body weight as water?
   a. A 3-pound premature infant
   b. A 154-pound man
   c. A 120-pound woman
   d. All of them would have an equal percentage.

2. A 0.9 percent solution of sodium chloride is isotonic. This means it is:
   a. More acid than blood plasma
   b. A more concentrated solution than blood plasma
   c. A less concentrated solution than blood plasma
   d. Equal in concentration to blood plasma

3. The passive movement of water across a semipermeable membrane from the side with the less concentrated solution to the one with the more concentrated solution is called:
   a. Diffusion
   b. Active transport
   c. Osmosis
   d. Hydrostatic pressure

4. Antidiuretic hormone (ADH) causes the kidney to return more water to the bloodstream. The organ that secretes ADH is the:
   a. Adrenal gland
   b. Kidney
   c. Posterior pituitary
   d. Pancreas

5. The substance that has the most influence on extracellular fluid osmolality is:
   a. Chlorine
   b. Sodium
   c. Calcium
   d. Potassium

6. When aldosterone secretion is increased, _____ is retained by the kidney and _____ is excreted to maintain electroneutrality.
   a. Sodium, potassium
   b. Potassium, sodium
   c. Calcium, hydrogen
   d. Hydrogen, potassium

7. If a person's body is too acid, the automatic response of the body is to:
   a. Increase sweat production
   b. Retain water
   c. Decrease rate and depth of breathing
   d. Increase rate and depth of breathing

8. An adult who is not on a high-salt or high-protein diet should consume _____ of water per kilocalorie per day.
   a. 1 ml
   b. 5 ml
   c. 10 ml
   d. 15 ml

9. The amount of urine required to excrete metabolic wastes is:
   a. 200 to 300 ml per day
   b. 400 to 600 ml per day

   c. 800 to 1000 ml per day
   d. 1200 to 1500 ml per day

10. Water loss severe enough to cause shock will produce:
   a. Flushed skin, increased pulse, increased blood pressure, and increased urine output
   b. Decreased urine output, decreased pulse, decreased blood pressure, and cool and clammy skin
   c. Decreased urine output, increased pulse, decreased blood pressure, and cool and clammy skin
   d. Increased urine output, flushed skin, decreased pulse, and increased blood pressure

NCLEX-Style Quiz

Situation One

Baby I., a 4-month-old boy, has developed diarrheal stools within the past 2 days. At birth he weighed 7 pounds 8 ounces. Since then he has gained steadily to 12 pounds 8 ounces three days ago. Baby I.'s present weight is 12 pounds 2 ounces.

   Mrs. I. has been feeding the baby his usual formula. He drinks eagerly but then has an explosive bowel movement with loud crying. Baby I. has had six bowel movements per day instead of his usual two.

1. With this history, what physical assessment measures would the nurse include initially?
   a. Skin turgor, fontanel fullness, moisture of mucous membranes
   b. Condition of hair, strength of grasp, presence of sucking reflex
   c. Heart sounds, lung sounds, blood pressure
   d. Urine specific gravity, observation of diaper rash

2. Which of the following nursing diagnoses is best supported by the history provided?
   a. High risk for fluid volume deficit
   b. Fluid volume deficit
   c. Diarrhea
   d. Nutrition, altered: less than body requirements

3. Which of the following recommendations by the nurse would show understanding of supportive care of this patient?
   a. Give Baby I. whole milk to maintain nutrition.
   b. Continue, as Mrs. I. has been doing, to allow the bowel to empty itself.
   c. Substitute orange juice for the formula for 3 days.
   d. Start Baby I. on an oral rehydration solution.

4. The nurse instructs Mrs. I. to return for additional care for Baby I. if one of the following events takes place. Which one would indicate the need for reassessment of Baby I.?
   a. The baby sleeps soundly and has to be awakened for a night feeding.
   b. The baby has three loose bowel movements the day after beginning treatment.
   c. The baby continues to lose weight or passes blood in the stool.
   d. The baby gains more than 2 ounces per day.

5. To assess the health education needs of Mrs. I., the nurse would review the way in which Mrs. I.:
   a. Launders Baby I.'s diapers
   b. Prepares the formula
   c. Holds Baby I. for feeding
   d. Weighs Baby I

CLINICAL CALCULATION 9–1

Converting Milligrams to Milliequivalents

Milligram is a measure of weight. Milliequivalent is a measure of the concentration of electrolytes (number of particles) per volume of solution. The usual amount of solution on which electrolytes are reported is 1 liter.

In order to convert milligrams to milliequivalents, it is necessary to know the number of milligrams per liter, the molecular weight of the substance, and its valence. Valence, a number indicating the combining power of an atom, is the number of dictionaries.

A teaspoonful of table salt in 1 liter of water will produce a 0.5 percent solution. (Isotonic sodium chloride is 0.9 percent.) How would the electrolytes be reported in milliequivalents? A teaspoonful is roughly 5 grams. Since table salt is 40 percent sodium and 60 percent chloride, the liter of 0.5 percent salt water would contain 2 grams of sodium and 3 grams of chloride.

Two other values are needed: atomic or molecular weights, and valences. The atomic weight for sodium is 22.9898. Sodium has a valence of 1.

The formula for converting milligrams to milliequivalents is:

$$\text{milliequivalents per liter} = \frac{(\text{milligrams per liter}) \times \text{valence}}{\text{molecular weight}}$$

Filling in the sodium values we know for this case, we have:

$$\text{milliequivalents per liter} = \frac{2000 \text{ milligrams per liter} \times 1}{22.9898}$$

$$= 87 \text{ milliequivalents per liter of sodium}$$

Continuing, we can use the same formula with different values to calculate the milliequivalents of chloride. The automic weight for chlorine is 35.453. Chlorine has a valence of 1.

Filling in the values for chloride, we have:

$$\text{milliequivalents per liter} = \frac{3000 \text{ milligrams per liter} \times 1}{35.453}$$

$$= 85 \text{ milliequivalents of chloride}$$

Then, adding the sodium and chloride, we have:

$$87 + 85$$
$$= 172 \text{ milliequivalents per liter in the 0.5 percent solution}$$

CLINICAL CALCULATION 9–2

Insensible Water Loss through the Skin

The rule of thumb for insensible water loss through the skin is 6 milliliters per kilogram per 24 hours. Let us look at the 154-pound reference patient to see what his or her amount of water loss would be in a 24-hour period. First, convert pounds to kilograms:

Then, multiply the patient's weight (in kilograms) by the amount of water loss per kilogram:

70 kilograms × 6 milliliters per kilogram
= 420 milliliters

Thus, this patient's insensible water loss in a 24-hour period is expected to be 420 milliliters.

CLINICAL CALCULATION 9–3

Evaporative Water Loss in Fever

Fever increases the amount of evaporative loss by 12 percent for every degree Celsius of fever. How much of an elevation would this be on the Fahrenheit scale? How much water would be lost by a person with this degree of fever over a 24-hour period?

Let us take 98.6°F as normal. This is equal to 37°C. So an increase of 1°C of fever would give a reading of 38°C. To change Celsius to Fahrenheit add 40 and multiply the result by $9/5$:

38 + 40 = 78 × 9/5 = 100.4°F

Now, consider the 154-pound patient in Clinical Calculation 9–2 whose evaporative losses were 420 milliliters in 24 hours. If he were feverish, he would lose additional water. We find an increase of 12 percent for the 1°C fever this way:

420 milliliters × 0.12
= 50.4 milliliters additional evaporative loss

420 milliliters + 50.4 milliliters
= 470.4 total insensible loss through the skin

CLINICAL CALCULATION 9–4

Hourly Urine Output in Children

Children should excrete between 0.5 and 2 milliliters of urine per kilogram of body weight per hour. What would be a normal hourly urine output for a child who weighs 50 pounds?

First convert pounds to kilograms. There are 2.2 pounds per kilogram.

$$\frac{154 \text{ pounds}}{2.2 \text{ pounds per kilogram}} = 70 \text{ kilograms}$$

To find the desirable range of output, multiply the child's weight in kilograms by the desired factors of 0.5 and 2 milliliters per kilogram.

$$22.7 \times 0.5 = 11.4 \text{ milliliters per hour}$$

$$22.7 \times 2 = 45.4 \text{ milliliters per hour}$$

Thus the 50-pound child normally should excrete between 11 and 45 milliliters of urine per hour.

BIBLIOGRAPHY

Borowitz, D: Pediatric nutrition. In Feldman, EB: Essentials of Clinical Nutrition. FA Davis, Philadelphia, 1988.

Brown, JE: The Science of Human Nutrition. Harcourt Brace Jovanovich, San Diego, 1990.

Cella, JH and Watson, J. Nurse's Manual of Laboratory Tests. FA Davis, Philadelphia, 1989.

Deglin, JH and Vallerand, AH: Davis's Drug Guide For Nurses, ed 3. FA Davis, Philadelphia, 1993.

Fischbach, F: A Manual of Laboratory Diagnostic Tests, ed. 3. JB Lippincott, 1988.

Horne, MM, Heitz, UE, and Swearingen, PL: Fluid, Electrolyte, and Acid-Base Balance. Mosby Year Book, St Louis, 1991.

Lederer, JR, et al: Care Planning Pocket Guide, ed 5. Addison-Wesley Nursing, Redwood City, CA, 1993.

Members of the Research Committee, greater Milwaukee Area chapter of the AAC–CN. Fluid volume deficit: Validating the indicators. Heart Lung 19(2):152, 1990.

Pagana, KD and Pagana, TJ: Mosby's Diagnostic and Laboratory Test Reference, Mosby Year Book, St Louis, 1992.

Physicians' Desk Reference, Medical Economics, Montvale, NJ, 1992.

Scanlon, VT and Sanders, T: Essentials of Anatomy and Physiology. FA Davis, Philadelphia, 1991.

Shlafer, M and Marieb, E: The Nurse, Pharmacology, and Drug Therapy. Addison-Wesley, Redwood City, CA, 1989.

Thorp, FK, Pierce, P, and Deedwania, C: Nutrition in the infant and young child. In Halpern, SL (ed): Quick Reference to Clinical Nutrition, ed 2. JB Lippincott, Philadelphia, 1987.

Whitney, EB, Cataldo, CB, and Rolfes, SR: Understanding Normal and Clinical Nutrition, ed 3. West, St Paul, 1991.

Williams, SR: Nutrition and Diet Therapy, ed 6. Times Mirror/Mosby, St Louis, 1989.

Yucha, C and Suddaby, P. David could have died of thirst, yet he never felt thirsty. Nursing 91 21(7):42, 1991.

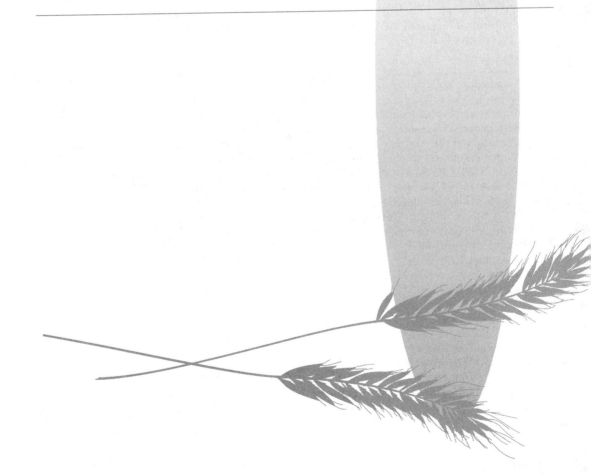

Unit Two

Family and Community Nutrition

Key Terms

As a study aid, each key term is followed by the page number where the term is defined in the chapter. Terms that appear in **boldface** or <u>underscored</u> in the chapter text are located in the glossary.

Life Cycle Nutrition:
Pregnancy, Infancy, Childhood, and Adolescence

Learning Objectives

After completing this chapter, the student should be able to:

1. Compare the nutritional needs of a pregnant woman with those of a nonpregnant woman the same age.
2. Describe the normal growth pattern for a full-term infant.
3. List several qualities of breast milk that make it uniquely suited to the human infant's capabilities.
4. Discuss the rationale for the sequence in which semisolid foods are introduced into an infant's diet.
5. List the common areas of concern for an adolescent's diet.
6. Identify the psychosocial developmental task to be achieved at each stage of growth.

*O*ur need for many nutrients changes as we enter different stages of our lives. Social, economic, and psychological circumstances have an impact on our nutritional status as we grow, develop, and age. Human beings are most vulnerable to the impact of poor nutrition during the stages of rapid growth. If the essential nutrients are not present to support growth, permanent damage to tissues and organs can occur. This chapter focuses on the periods of rapid growth: pregnancy (including lactation) infancy, childhood, and adolescence. In addition to nutritional needs for all periods of rapid growth, we will also discuss the physical and psychosocial development that should occur during infancy, childhood, and adolescence.

PSYCHOSOCIAL DEVELOPMENT

Psychologists have defined developmental tasks which should be mastered by each individual in the course of his of her lifetime. Developmental needs also impact nutritional practices. In this chapter, we discuss the developmental tasks to be achieved by the infant, toddler, preschooler, school-age child, and adolescent. The developmental tasks for the young, middle, and older adult are discussed in the next chapter.

Erikson's Theory

An American psychoanalyst, Erik Erikson, developed a theory of human development that linked psychological development with interactions with other people. Erikson understood life as divided into eight stages. Each stage has a psychosocial developmental task to be mastered, and an opposite negative trait that comes to the fore if the task is not mastered. Of course, even when the task is not successfully mastered, the individual continues in life. "Repeating the grade," as schoolchildren do, is not an option. We cannot see stunted psychosocial growth as readily as stunted physical growth. Even if a developmental task was successfully mastered, a new situation may arise challenging the person to reaffirm his or her mastery. A brief listing of Erikson's developmental tasks appears in Table 10–1. Throughout this chapter and the next we integrate psychosocial development for each age group, especially in relation to nutritional practices.

TABLE 10–1 *Erikson's Theory of Psychosocial Development*

Stage of Life	Developmental Task	Opposing Negative Trait
Infancy	Trust	Distrust
Toddler	Autonomy	Doubt
Preschooler	Initiative	Guilt
School-age child	Industry	Inferiority
Adolescent	Identity	Role confusion
Young adult	Intimacy	Isolation
Adult	Generativity	Stagnation
Older adult	Integrity	Despair

NUTRITION DURING PREGNANCY

A mother's nutritional status can affect the outcome of pregnancy. For example, during the first month of **gestation,** it is crucial that the mother be well nourished so that a healthy **placenta** will form. Also, within 2 to 3 months of conception all the major body organs are being formed in the **embryo.** From the beginning of the third month until birth, the embryo is called a **fetus.** Because the fetus obtains nutrients from the mother, from either her diet or her body stores, the health of the fetus depends on her nutritional intake.

Poor outcomes of pregnancy include spontaneous abortion (miscarriage), premature delivery, a low-birth-weight (LBW) infant, and mental and physical abnormalities in the newborn. The best insurance an expectant mother can provide for her unborn child is to enter the pregnancy with good nutrient stores, to consume a well-balanced diet while pregnant, and to avoid harmful substances, such as alcohol and illicit drugs.

From **implantation** to birth, the fertilized <u>ovum</u> (which weighs less than 100 micrograms) develops into an infant that weighs about 3.2 kilograms (7 lb). During this period of rapid growth and development the mother needs additional nutrients, including kilocalories, protein, and certain vitamins and minerals.

Increase in Energy Needs

Increased energy is needed for the development of the mother, the fetus, and the placenta. From the third through the sixth month, much of this energy supports the growth of the uterus (womb) and other maternal tissues. During the seventh through ninth months, the third trimester, much of the energy supports the fetus and the placenta. To meet this increased metabolic workload and to spare protein for tissue building, the pregnant woman needs an additional 300 kilocalories per day.

Increase in Protein Needs

Building fetal tissue requires protein. The mother also needs adequate protein for growth of her tissues. Her blood volume increases in anticipation of blood loss at delivery. Her breasts develop in preparation for lactation. The uterus enlarges and fills with **amniotic fluid.** For these reasons, an additional 10 grams of protein per day are needed. Translating this to the exchange system, 1 extra cup of milk (8 grams of protein) and 1 additional ounce of meat (7 grams of protein) would more than meet the increased protein requirement.

A complication arises if a woman with phenylketonuria (PKU) consumes a regular diet during pregnancy. (Review Clinical Application 4–3.) The high level of phenylalanine in a woman's bloodstream can cross the placenta and cause fetal malformations and defects. Careful monitoring of blood levels of phenylalanine and provision of a special medical food are begun before conception and continued throughout the pregnancy. Because women of childbearing age with PKU may have been taken off the special diet after age 4 to 6, they may have little memory of this part of their medical history. The healthcare worker should investigate further when a woman cites a history of troubled pregnancies: congenital abnormalities, a mentally

Gestation—The time from the fertilization of the ovum until birth; in humans, the length of gestation is usually 38 to 42 weeks.

Placenta—The organ in the uterus through which the unborn child exchanges carbon dioxide for oxygen and wastes for nourishment; lay term is afterbirth.

Embryo—Developing infant in the prenatal period between the second and eighth weeks inclusive.

Fetus—The human child in utero from the third month until birth.

Implantation—Embedding of the fertilized egg in the lining of the uterus.

Amniotic fluid—Albuminous liquid that surrounds and protects the fetus throughout pregnancy.

retarded infant, spontaneous abortion, or stillbirth. This is especially true if the woman is intellectually slow or is subject to seizures.

Increase in Vitamin Needs

Increased amounts of certain B-vitamins, including folic acid, and vitamin C are needed during pregnancy. For pregnant women 25 years of age or older, an adequate diet normally provides the additional requirements for vitamins D, E, and K. Supplementation with vitamins and minerals should be approached carefully in the pregnant woman. The fetus can be harmed by deficiencies or excesses.

To prevent megaloblastic anemia, folic acid supplements may be ordered by the physician if the diet lacks sufficient amounts. Special attention should be given to the assessment of the pregnant teenager. Teenagers of both sexes commonly have low folic acid intakes.

Due to increased metabolic demands, some of the other B-vitamins are also required in additional amounts. These include thiamine, riboflavin, niacin, and vitamin B_6. The B-vitamins are all coenzymes involved in the metabolism of carbohydrates, fats, and proteins.

There is a greater need for vitamin C during pregnancy because it (1) converts folic acid to an active form, (2) enhances the absorption of iron, and (3) helps form connective tissues. These functions of vitamin C are essential for the body's proper utilization of iron, a mineral required by the pregnant woman in great amounts.

Because of the risk of fetal deformities, vitamin A supplementation is contraindicated during the first trimester. In fact, there is no increase in the RDA for vitamin A for pregnant women. Because vitamin A sometimes is used to treat acne, the fetus of the teenager who did not plan to become pregnant may be at special risk. This risk involves only preformed vitamin A. There is no need to restrict carotene. See the RDA table in Appendix E for the specific amount recommended for each vitamin during pregnancy.

Increase in Mineral Needs

Minerals differ from vitamins in that minerals become part of the structure of the body whereas vitamins do not. Both the mother and the fetus are building new tissues.

Iron

The mother's need for iron is enormous. The mother's volume of red blood cells increases by 21 to 26 percent. Iron is also needed for the hemoglobin in the red blood cells in the fetus, placenta, and umbilical cord. Iron is transported to the fetus regardless of the mother's iron status.

Fortunately, absorption of iron is enhanced in the second and third trimesters. From 6.5 percent at the beginning of pregnancy, the rate of absorption increases to 14.3 percent at term if the woman is not taking an iron supplement. This rate drops to 8.6 percent with an iron supplement. The body knows when its sources are limited and when they are abundant.

Women who receive prenatal care usually are given an iron supplement because meeting the increased demand for iron by dietary means is difficult. One common preparation is ferrous sulfate. A 150-milligram dose of ferrous sulfate contains 30 milligrams of iron, the RDA for pregnancy. If iron needs are not met, the pregnant woman may develop iron-deficiency anemia. Even when supplements are taken, the woman's hemoglobin and hematocrit should be monitored every 2 to 3 months.

Calcium

Calcium is the chief mineral in the adult body, with the bones serving as a storage depot. When serum calcium is low, the bones demineralize to restore the serum level. The requirement for calcium during pregnancy is 1.5 times the amount required for the nonpregnant woman. Almost all of the additional amount is used by the fetus, mostly in the third trimester, for the development of skeletal tissue. More calcium is accumulated during pregnancy than any other mineral. As with iron, intestinal absorption of calcium increases during pregnancy. Early in the pregnancy, intestinal absorption doubles and remains high. Normally only 10 to 30 percent of calcium is absorbed. One reason for this increased absorption is the ability of the placenta to convert inactive vitamin D to the active form.

The RDA for calcium for pregnant and lactating women is 1200 milligrams. This can be obtained from four servings of milk or milk products equivalent in calcium.

Iodine

With the increase in energy requirements, resting energy expenditure also increases. During the second half of pregnancy it increases by as much as 23 percent. Iodine is necessary for the formation of the thyroid hormones. A pregnant woman's usual need for iodine is met, as with other adults, by the use of iodized salt.

Fluoride

The fetus begins to develop teeth at the 10th to 12th week of pregnancy. Fewer dental caries have been found in infants of mothers whose diets were supplemented with 1 milligram of fluoride daily (Glenn, Glenn, and Duncan, 1982).

Zinc

Zinc is not mobilized from the mother's tissues. To provide for the fetus, the mother needs constant intake. Zinc deficiency has been associated with abnormally long labors and delivery of small and malformed infants. Three servings of meat or meat substitute per day will provide for the pregnant woman's zinc needs.

Other Minerals

In addition to calcium, two other minerals involved in skeletal formation are also in great demand during pregnancy. These are phosphorus and magnesium. For pregnant women 25 years of age and older, the allowance recommended for phosphorus is 1.5 times the amount allowed for nonpregnant women. See the RDA table in Appendix E for the specific amount recommended for each mineral during pregnancy.

Water and Weight Gain

The pregnant woman should drink about 6 glasses of water per day. Fear of excessive weight gain should not interfere with the consumption of adequate fluid.

The amount of weight a woman was expected to gain during pregnancy has varied over the years. The current recommendation is made based on a Body Mass Index (BMI), which incorporates the woman's height and weight before pregnancy. Clinical Calculation 10–1 shows how Body Mass Index is determined and applied to the pregnant woman.

Meal Pattern

Relatively few modifications in the Food Pyramid recommendations for adults are needed for the mature woman who becomes pregnant. She can meet the needs of the fetus and herself by consuming one additional serving of milk, an additional ounce of meat, and one additional source of vitamin C each day. Instead of a fruit or vegetable high in carotene every other day, she should eat one every day. Vitamin A also contributes to normal bone growth.

The pregnant teenager needs even more nutrients to provide for her own growth as well as that of the fetus. She should have an additional serving from each of the milk and starch/bread groups over and above the number of servings recommended for the mature pregnant woman. Table 10–2 can be used as a food guide for pregnant adult women and adolescents and during lactation.

Substances to Avoid

Women are urged to eliminate certain substances from their diets while they are pregnant. Alcohol and caffeine are two such substances that merit special mention.

TABLE 10–2 *Daily Food Guide in Pregnancy and Lactation*

	Pregnant Adult	Pregnant Adolescent*	Lactation
Milk, cups	3–4	4–5	3–4
Meat, ounces	6	6	6
Fruit, servings			
High vitamin C	2	2	2
Other	2	2	3
Vegetable, servings			
High vitamin A	1	1	1–2
Other	2–4	2–4	2–4
Starch/Bread, servings	10	11	10
Other foods	To meet kilocaloric needs	To meet kilocaloric needs	To meet kilocaloric needs

*Meets adolescent RDA except for iron and folic acid.

Alcohol

More is known now than ever before about the effects of alcohol on the fetus. Fetal alcohol syndrome (FAS), first recognized in 1973, occurs in 30 to 50 percent of alcoholic mothers' offspring. In FAS, alcoholism is defined as the ingestion of more than 3 ounces of alcohol per day. The fetus is most vulnerable to FAS during the first trimester when basic structural development occurs. Often, the woman does not even know that she is pregnant until late in the first trimester.

Children with FAS are malformed and suffer from mental retardation (Fig. 10–1). This condition is completely preventable. Because research has not been able to determine how much alcohol is safe to ingest during pregnancy, women who are planning a pregnancy should abstain from alcohol for the good of the fetus.

Caffeine

In contrast to the evidence linking alcohol consumption with fetal defects, the connection between caffeine and defects is inconsistent and fragmentary (Subcommittee on Nutritional Status and Weight Gain during Pregnancy and the Subcommittee on Dietary Intake and Nutrient Supplements during Pregnancy, 1990). When alcohol, smoking, maternal age, and pregnancy history are controlled, heavy coffee drinking has minimal, if any, adverse effect on the outcome of pregnancy (Feldman, 1988). However, caffeine intake should be moderated to maximize the mother's rest. Sleepiness is a message

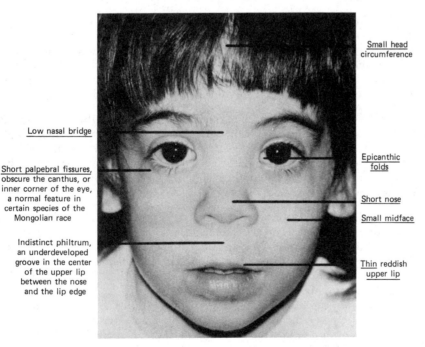

FIGURE 10–1. Characteristic facial features of a child with fetal alcohol syndrome (FAS). Children with FAS also suffer from hampered growth and mental retardation. (From Feldman, p 164, with permission.)

from the body. Responding to it by jolting the body with caffeine is not a healthy practice.

Common Problems and Complications of Pregnancy

The physiological changes that take place in a woman's body during pregnancy may cause a variety of possible medical conditions. Some of the more common problems such as morning sickness and leg cramps are usually annoying but only occasionally require medical intervention. Other conditions, such as pregnancy-induced hypertension and gestational diabetes, are more complicated and must have medical treatment.

Common Problems of Pregnancy

Four of the most common problems of pregnancy are morning sickness, leg cramps, constipation, and heartburn. Pica (see below) is a regional complaint that is mostly influenced by culture.

MORNING SICKNESS   Hormonal changes cause the nausea and vomiting of pregnancy. The occurrence and duration of morning sickness vary widely, but it is not confined to mornings. Control of the signs and symptoms without medication is the goal. Eating dry crackers before getting out of bed is the classic treatment. Other suggestions include (1) avoiding fatty foods in favor of fruits and complex carbohydrates taken in small, frequent meals; (2) consuming cold foods rather than hot foods; (3) drinking liquids between rather than with meals; and (4) eating a high-protein snack at bedtime. In most cases, morning sickness subsides after the first trimester.

LEG CRAMPS   Pregnant women often complain of leg cramps. One theory postulates the cause to be neuromuscular irritability due to low serum calcium. Increasing calcium intake is the prescribed treatment. Another theory postulates the cause to be a high serum phosphorus level in relation to calcium. Here the treatment prescribed is to substitute a calcium supplement for some of the milk intake, thus decreasing serum phosphorus.

CONSTIPATION   The increasing size and weight of the uterus presses on the intestines, causing constipation. Adequate fluid intake and a high-fiber diet should relieve this condition. The suggested amount of fiber intake, 30 grams per day, should be accomplished by consuming food rather than pharmaceutical preparations. Table 10–3 lists foods high in fiber but relatively low in kilocalocies.

HEARTBURN   Hormonal changes cause relaxation of the cardiac sphincter, located between the esophagus and the stomach. This, coupled with the upward pressure of diaphragm from the enlarging uterus, causes reflux of gastric contents into the esophagus. The name heartburn comes from the effect of the reflux, which is described as a burning sensation beneath the breastbone.

Heartburn can be controlled by avoiding spicy or acidic foods and taking small, frequent meals. Sitting up for an hour after a meal may help. Treatments often used by the nonpregnant individual are ill-advised during pregnancy. The pregnant woman should not self-medicate with sodium bicarbonate or antacids. The bicarbonate can be absorbed, producing alkalo-

TABLE 10–3 *Nutrient-Dense Foods High in Fiber*

Food	Quantity	Grams of Dietary Fiber	Kilocalories
Grains			
All Bran	⅓ cup	10	70
Bran Buds	½ cup	11.5	109
100% Bran	½ cup	10	89
Fruits			
Applesauce, unsweetened	1 cup	4	106
Orange sections, raw	1 cup	4	85
Pear, D'Anjou, raw with skin	one each	6	120
Prunes, cooked, unsweetened	½ cup	4.5	114
Strawberries, fresh	1 cup	4	45
Vegetables			
Baked beans, in tomato sauce with pork	½ cup	7	129
Lima beans, cooked from frozen	½ cup	8	94
Broccoli, raw	one spear	6	42
Brussels sprouts, cooked from raw	1 cup	6	60
Kidney beans, canned	½ cup	8.5	108
Navy beans, cooked from dry	½ cup	8	130
Black-eyed peas, cooked from dry	½ cup	10.5	99

sis. The antacids decrease iron absorption by decreasing gastric acids, thus increasing the risk of anemia.

PICA   Pica is the craving to ingest nonfood substances. The practice occurs in certain geographic areas and cultural groups. Non-nutritive items commonly ingested are laundry starch and clay. The women say these substances "taste good." Nurses should be aware that women transplanted to other areas take their cultural practices with them. The hazard to nutritive status is the substitution of these nonfood items for nutritious foods.

Complications of Pregnancy

The student is referred to an obstetrical nursing text for a comprehensive discussion of the complications of pregnancy. In this chapter we will introduce two such ailments with nutritional ramifications: pregnancy-induced hypertension and gestational diabetes.

PREGNANCY-INDUCED HYPERTENSION   This pathology, involving edema, proteinuria, and hypertension, occurs in 5 to 7 percent of preg-

Pregnancy-induced hypertension (PIH)—A potentially life-threatening disorder that may develop after the 20th week of pregnancy; includes pre-eclampsia and eclampsia.

nancies. The signs and symptoms appear after the 20th week of pregnancy, usually in the 2 months before term. **Pregnancy-induced hypertension** (PIH), also called <u>preeclampsia-eclampsia syndrome,</u> is potentially life-threatening for both the mother and the fetus. The cause is unknown. Excesses or deficiencies of magnesium, calcium, polyunsaturated fatty acids, zinc, cadmium, and sodium have been investigated as contributing factors. The syndrome occurs most frequently in women under 20 or over 35 years old, pregnant for the first time, and in women who have had five or more pregnancies. Also increasing the risk of this syndrome are personal or family histories of diabetes, hypertension, or vascular or renal disease.

Preeclampsia—Hypertension, edema, and pro-teinuria, appearing after the 20th week of preg-nancy.

Pregnancy-induced hypertension may progress from mild preeclampsia to severe preeclampsia to eclampsia. The signs of **preeclampsia** are hypertension, edema, and proteinuria (protein in the urine). When the patient's condition declines to eclampsia, her brain is sufficiently edematous to cause convulsions and coma.

Mild preeclampsia is characterized by a systolic blood pressure increase of 30 millimeters of mercury or a diastolic increase of 15 millimeters of mercury over prepregnancy levels. It is treated with bed rest and possibly a high-protein diet to replace urinary losses. Diuretics are not used; they would aggravate the condition by increasing the permeability of the kidney's filtering system, causing greater losses.

Severe preeclampsia is characterized by a systolic blood pressure greater than 160 millimeters of mercury or a diastolic pressure greater than 110 millimeters of mercury. This patient is hospitalized to provide rest and to monitor the mother and the fetus. Sedative drugs may be prescribed to lessen the irritability of the brain.

Eclampsia—An obstetrical emer-gency involving hypertension, edema, protein-uria, and convul-sions, appearing after the 20th week of preg-nancy.

Eclampsia is an obstetrical emergency, which occurs in 1 of 200 cases of preeclampsia. The mother is in immediate danger of convulsing, if not already doing so. She requires intensive nursing care because she is at high risk of cerebral hemorrhage, circulatory collapse, or kidney failure. The fetus, too, is in grave danger.

The preferable method of dealing with pregnancy-induced hypertension is to prevent it. Good prenatal care, including weight and blood pressure monitoring and urine testing, and early intervention are the keys to minimizing the hazard of pregnancy-induced hypertension.

Gestational dia-betes—An exag-geration of the natural resistance to insulin that develops in the pregnant woman's tissues late in pregnancy.

GESTATIONAL DIABETES   Pregnancy may precipitate the onset of diabetes in some women. This condition, known as **gestational diabetes,** is detected by glucose tolerance tests. Gestational diabetes is discussed in detail in Chapter 16.

THE BREAST-FEEDING MOTHER

Later in the chapter, the advantages breast milk confers on the infant will be discussed. Here, the nutritional implications of breast-feeding for the mother are presented.

Nutritional Needs

The birth of the baby does not end the concern for proper nutrition for the mother. All mothers must replenish their body stores after childbirth. The breast-feeding mother also has to produce the infant's milk.

Energy

Thirty ounces of breast milk a day at 20 kilocalories per ounce amounts to 600 kilocalories. Another 150 kilocalories are allowed for the energy needed to make the milk. The RDA allows for 500 of these 750 kilocalories from food. The other 250 kilocalories are expected to be taken from fat stores laid down for this purpose during pregnancy (see Table 10–2).

Effect of Maternal Deficiencies

Even if a mother lacks some nutrients in her current diet, her milk contains the correct level of nutrients. The lack of nutrients in the mother's diet ultimately will affect her nutrient stores, but while she nurses, she usually will produce good quality milk, but in less quantity. However, if the mother's diet is low in vitamin C, her milk also will be deficient. In an otherwise well-nourished mother, the use of a vitamin supplement does not increase the vitamin content of her milk.

Benefits to the Mother

Several advantages to the mother are associated with breast-feeding. It helps the uterus return to its nonpregnant state more quickly. Breast feeding is convenient and less costly than bottle feeding, and may be protective against later breast cancer.

Aids Uterine Involution

During breast-feeding, the sucking of the infant stimulates the release of <u>oxytocin</u> from the posterior pituitary gland in the brain. Oxytocin causes the uterine muscles to contract. This aids in returning the uterus to its normal nonpregnant size.

Convenience at Less Cost

Breast milk is always ready at the correct temperature. There is no formula to make or contamination problems to worry about. Clinical Calculation 10–2 compares the cost of the added nutrients needed for the breast-feeding mother's diet against the cost of infant formula. Notice in the Clinical Calculation that the extra meat exchange is postulated as two eggs. Substituting other meat exchanges will cause the cost to vary significantly. The example compares annual costs, since most women do not breast-feed for an entire year, the cost of formula for the later months would be substituted for the mother's additional food.

Lessens Risk of Breast Cancer

Over the long term, breast-feeding is associated with a decreased risk of breast cancer later in life. This is a statistical projection for the group, not an individual guarantee.

Techniques of Breast-Feeding

The medical and nursing staff at the place of delivery will assist in getting the infant and mother started breast-feeding. However, some general principles have been established.

If at all possible, the mother and infant should not be separated during the first 24 hours after birth. This practice permits bonding of infant and mother. Some areas encourage fathers to "room in," also, to bond with the baby.

The correct position for breast-feeding is shown in Figure 10–2. It's tummy to tummy. The infant should face the breast squarely. If the breast is

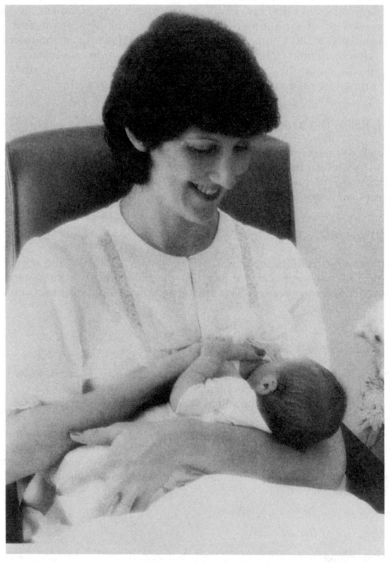

FIGURE 10–2. Correct breast-feeding position, tummy to tummy. The infant takes the entire areola in its mouth. (Used and reprinted with permission of Ross Laboratories, Columbus, Ohio.)

very large, care must be taken not to block the infant's nose, which may otherwise cause the infant to have trouble breathing. When nursing, the infant should grasp the entire areola (the colored portion around the nipple) to prevent the nipples from becoming sore.

Most infants will take 80 to 90 percent of the milk from each breast in the first 4 minutes of nursing. Because nursing stimulates further milk production, the mother should alternate which breast is first offered to the infant. This method allows the infant to empty the first breast offered and to finish feeding on the other breast if it is still hungry or is just enjoying the experience. At the next feeding, the mother should start with the breast the infant finished on the time before.

Maternal Contraindications to Breast-Feeding

Several situations make breast-feeding inadvisable. These include the mother's exposure to toxic chemicals, the mother's use of medications, and illness in the mother. The physician is the best source of guidance in a particular case. A contraindication due to a metbolic defect in the infant is discussed later in the chapter.

Exposure to Toxic Chemicals

Certain chemicals, such as DDT and PCB, have been shown to be **teratogenic.** If the mother has consumed food contaminated with the chemical, she may transmit it to the infant in breast milk. The contaminants are stored in her adipose tissue and, as mentioned earlier, the lactating mother's fat stores are mobilized to produce milk.

> **Teratogenic—** Capable of causing abnormal development of the embryo; results in a malformed fetus.

Some experts believe that the risk is minimal unless the mobilization of the mother's fat is due to inadequate intake. Others say that there is no hazard unless the woman has had occupational exposure or has consumed a large amount of fish from contaminated waters.

Medication Use

Many medications are secreted in breast milk. The physician should be consulted about both prescription and nonprescription drugs taken by the mother.

Substances that are often not thought of as drugs may also affect the breast-fed infant. These include alcohol and caffeine. Here again, experts offer opposite advice to the breast-feeding mother. While some recommend abstinence, others think that the moderate use of alcohol and caffeine is acceptable.

Maternal Illnesses

Absolute contraindications to breast-feeding include AIDS and active tuberculosis. Acute or chronic diseases in the mother may preclude breast-feeding. Some of these are heart disease, severe anemia, and nephritis. If the woman becomes pregnant again, she will have to stop breast-feeding. In some parts of the world, breast-feeding is used as a means of birth spacing, but this is not a reliable practice. If a couple wants to delay the birth of another child, they should use more effective methods of birth control.

NUTRITION IN INFANCY

Infancy refers to the first year of life. To be more specific, for the first 28 days of life, the baby is a newborn. From day 29 to the first birthday the baby is an infant.

Growth

Growth refers to an increase in size. During infancy, certain milestones are used to judge the adequacy of the baby's growth. The first year of life is critical for the growth of essential organs.

Expected Milestones

The only time human beings grow faster than in the first year after birth is the 9 months before birth. A baby's birth weight should double by age 4 to 6 months and triple by age 1. Thus an infant who weighs 7 pounds at birth should weigh 14 pounds at 6 months and 21 pounds at 1 year. From a birth length of about 20 inches, the baby grows to about 30 inches by age 1.

The rate of growth is more significant than absolute values. Is the infant progressing at a reasonable pace? A gain of 5 to 8 ounces per week is expected during the first 4 or 5 months. Thereafter, a gain of 4 or 5 ounces per week until the first birthday would be reasonable.

Immediately after birth, the baby loses weight as it adjusts to its new environment and food supply. The amount of weight lost should not exceed 10 percent of the birth weight. The newborn usually regains to its birth weight within 14 days.

Critical Tissue Growth

The period most critical to brain development extends from conception into the second year of life. Brain cells increase most rapidly before birth and during the first 5 or 6 months after birth. To reach the maximum brain growth, the baby needs optimal nutrition. Once this period of brain cell division and growth is completed, no further growth is possible. Improved nutrition after age 2 will not increase the number of brain cells. Conversely, severe protein-calorie malnutrition in the last trimester of pregnancy or the first 6 months of life may decrease brain cells by as much as 20 percent.

Development

Development refers to the process of changing to a mature individual. It involves psychosocial and physical development, usually including an increase in size.

Psychosocial Development

The infant's developmental task is to learn to trust. The parent who responds promptly and lovingly to the infant's cries is teaching the baby to trust. If the caregiver handles the infant gently one time and roughly the next, the baby learns to mistrust. In situations where physical care is provided, but no tender relationships, infants may actually suffer stunted physical growth. This occurs often enough so that <u>failure to thrive (FTT)</u> has become a medical diagnosis for severely underweight infants. The developmental task of trust, if achieved, lays the foundation for future human relationships. If not accomplished, it lays a foundation also, but for mistrust and suspiciousness.

An infant can explore the world through feeding and foods. New foods encourage experimentation. Babies like to poke their fingers in the food. They attempt to feed themselves but turn the spoon upside down on the way to their mouths. Consistent acceptance from the parent will teach the infant to trust his world. The same behavior should not receive a laugh one time and a scolding the next.

Physical Development

Development proceeds at a different pace in various tissues and organs. Proper feeding practices are based on the maturation rate of body organs.

GASTROINTESTINAL SYSTEM   Not until it is 3 or 4 months old does an infant develop a sense of taste. Its salivary and pancreatic amylases are inadequate for several months. Consequently, complex carbohydrates are indigestible at birth.

Anyone having the slightest contact with infants knows that they have to be fed often. A newborn's stomach holds about an ounce. By 1 year of age, the stomach will hold about 8 ounces. An adult's stomach, on the other hand, can hold about 2 quarts.

An infant's intestinal tract is also immature. In some ways it is more like a chain-link fence than like a sieve. It allows whole proteins to be absorbed into the bloodstream. The more mature intestine permits absorption of amino acids but not whole proteins. This has major ramifications for the feeding of infants.

NERVOUS SYSTEM   Nervous tissue, bile, and hormones all require fat and cholesterol for their growth and development. Because of the rapid growth of the brain and the nervous system, the infant requires adequate fat and even cholesterol in its diet.

The <u>term infant</u> does have some well-developed reflexes. One of these is the <u>rooting reflex.</u> When the infant's cheek is stroked, the head turns toward that side to nurse.

For the first 3 or 4 months, the infant suckles by using an up-and-down motion of the tongue. If semisolid food is offered at this time, the natural motion of the tongue tends to spit it out. This, too, affects wise choices of food for infants.

After 4 months, the infant can suck using orofacial muscles. The tongue moves back and forth instead of up and down. At this point, semisolid food is more likely to be swallowed than spit out.

By 6 months of age, the infant has enough hand-to-eye coordination to put food and other objects into its mouth. A 7-month-old infant can chew appropriate foods.

URINARY SYSTEM   An infant's kidneys are immature. This means they have limited capacity to filter solutes. Not until the end of the second month can the infant's kidneys handle the waste of semisolid foods. As is discussed later, however, feeding of semi-solids often is delayed another 2 months for different reasons. By the infant's first birthday, the kidneys have reached full functional capacity.

Nutritional Needs of the Term Infant

Because breast milk is naturally suitable for human infants, its characteristics are the standard for infant formulas, which are designed to copy many of the qualities of breast milk.

Protein

Because of the extensive tissue building that occurs, an infant needs 2.5 to 3.5 grams of protein per kilogram of body weight. The 1-year-old infant requires only 2 grams of protein per kilogram of body weight. Compare this with the recommended amount of protein for an adult, 0.8 grams per kilogram of body weight. Proportionately, the infant needs 250 percent of the adult requirement.

The protein in breast milk is easy for the infant to digest. Sixty percent of the protein in breast milk is lactalbumin, with an amino acid pattern much like that of the body tissues. The infant's body can absorb it easily and, without much processing, can use it for building tissue.

Energy

Infants have high metabolic rates. Normal pulse rate is 120 to 140 per minute; normal respiratory rate is 20 per minute. Because of the large proportion of skin surface to body size, temperature regulation takes significant energy. Crying may double the metabolic rate.

A newborn requires 100 to 120 kilocalories per kilogram of body weight per day. If our 154-pound (70-kilogram) man consumed at the rate of a newborn, he would take in 7000 to 8400 kilocalories per day. By the end of the first year of life, the infant requires only 80 to 100 kilocalories per kilogram of body weight.

CARBOHYDRATE As is the case with protein, the carbohydrate in breast milk is easily digested by the infant. The lactose in breast milk is a source of galactose, which is necessary for brain cell formation. One source of carbohydrate the infant should not have is honey (see Clinical Application 10–1).

FAT An infant needs 30 to 55 percent of kilocalories from fat. With the small stomach capacity, the infant requires a concentrated source of energy. Fat contains 9 kilocalories per gram, compared with 4 kilocalories per gram of carbohydrate or protein. The developing nervous system also requires fat. Since breast milk contains the necessary lipase to begin digestion for the infant, about 95 to 98 percent of the fat in human milk is absorbed. Because of their need for fat, children less than 2 years old should receive whole milk, not low-fat milk.

EVALUATION The best indicator of adequate kilocaloric intake is a normal growth rate according to standard growth charts. These measurements should be made every 3 months. They can be graphed on growth charts such as those that appear in Appendix C. See Charting Tips 10–1 for suggestions on obtaining these measurements.

CLINICAL APPLICATION 10-1
Honey Is a Danger to Infants

No honey should be given to an infant until after the first birthday. There are frequently organisms in honey that an infant cannot fight off.

Bees may contaminate honey with botulism spores acquired from plants or the soil. These spores are not destroyed by processing. If ingested by the infant, the spores become active in its intestinal tract and produce a toxin. This is a potentially serious, even fatal situation because the toxin affects the nervous system.

Botulism spores hide in many places. Honey is not the only source. Other foods and even dust contain botulism spores. In fact, in only 20 percent of the reported cases of infant botulism had the infant been fed honey. However, keeping honey out of the infant's diet lessens the risk considerably. The child's intestinal tract is better able to expel the botulism spores once the child reaches the age of 1 year.

Vitamins

In the RDA table, vitamins are specified for infants aged 0 to 6 months and 6 to 12 months (see Appendix E). Infants need all the vitamins that other humans need, but in different amounts.

VITAMIN C   Human beings cannot manufacture vitamin C, and deficiency produces scurvy. Human breast milk contains more vitamin C than cow's milk. This is because most animals can synthesize vitamin C; thus it is unnecessary in their milk.

VITAMIN D   Breast milk contains less vitamin D than cow's milk. However, vitamin D is present in the milk we buy because it has been fortified.

CHARTING TIPS 10-1

Throughout infancy and childhood the rate of growth is an essential objective sign of a child's nutritional status. Thus measurements of weight and height should be as accurate as possible. The following tips may be helpful in obtaining accurate measurements of growth:

✓ Balance the scale before weighing the child.
✓ Weigh the child in approximately the same clothing each time.
✓ Record measurements of growth accurately, promptly, and legibly.

One advantage to the presence of cholesterol in breast milk is its function as a precursor of vitamin D, which is produced in the skin. For infants who receive some exposure to sunlight, this is a benefit. Because of other hazards of exposure to sun, however, a vitamin D supplement may be a wiser choice.

Special situations demand vitamin supplements. These are discussed in a later section of this chapter.

Minerals

Infants also require the same minerals as other human beings. Breast milk contains only one third the sodium, potassium, and chloride and one eighth the phosphorus of cow's milk. This dilution accommodates the limited function of the infant's kidneys. Breast milk also contains less iron than cow's milk. The infant absorbs 49 percent of it, however, compared with 10 percent from cow's milk. Likewise, 50 to 60 percent of the calcium in breast milk is absorbed by the infant, compared with 25 to 30 percent of the calcium in cow's milk. The zinc in breast milk is absorbed better than that in cow's milk as well.

These differences in mineral content affect the osmolality of the milk. See Clinical Application 10–2 for additional information on the extra minerals' effect on the workload of the kidneys. The data will show why unmodified cow's milk is inappropriate for young infants.

CLINICAL APPLICATION 10–2
Renal Solute Loads

When considering selecting a formula, it is important to distinguish two measures of osmolality or osmolarity. One is the osmotic pressure the formula presents to the gut. The other measure examines what remains to be excreted by the kidney after digestion and absorption have taken place. These leftovers are excess electrolytes and by-products of protein metabolism. The osmolality or osmolarity of these leftovers presented to the kidney for disposal is called the renal solute load. It varies considerably from one method of feeding to another. When dealing with an infant's immature digestive and urinary systems, selecting an appropriate formula may be crucial to health. Below is a comparison of several infant feedings with the intestinal osmolality and the renal solute load listed. As always, the standard of comparison is human breast milk.

Milk/Formula	Intestinal Osmolality (milliosmoles per kilogram)	Renal Solute Load (milliosmoles per liter)
Human breast milk	300	101
Similac 60/40	260	96
Similac	290	105
Isomil	250	122
SMA	300	128
3.3% Cow's milk	275	275

Water

The infant's body is 75 percent water. By the age of 1, the body has converted to the adult proportion of 60 percent water. Water, therefore, is a critical need in the infant. The daily turnover of water in the infant is 15 percent of body weight. Breast milk contains more water than cow's milk. Even in hot desert climates, an infant can be adequately hydrated on breast milk alone. An infant will regulate its intake of formula to obtain sufficient energy. If the formula is dilute, the baby will take more of it; if concentrated, less. This self-regulating mechanism is not perfect, however, since the infant may consume excess formula to quench its thirst.

The Breast-Fed Infant

Infancy is the only time in life when a single food is the entire diet. You will see that all breast milk is not alike but rather adjusts to the infant's needs. Breast milk varies from mother to mother and even in one mother with the time of day.

Composition of Breast Milk

We have already mentioned some of the ways that breast milk compensates for the shortcomings of the infant's digestive system. Now you will see how breast milk varies within a feeding and during the weeks an infant is nursing.

COLOSTRUM   The first milk secreted after the birth of the baby is colostrum. It is a thin, yellow, milky fluid. Colostrum is high in proteins such as immunoglobulins, in fat-soluble vitamins, in minerals, and is low in fat.

TRANSITIONAL MILK   By the second week after delivery, breast milk changes. It contains lactose, fat, and water-soluble vitamins at the level of mature milk. It is also produced in larger quantities.

MATURE MILK   As breast-feeding becomes established, the mother produces mature milk. It varies in composition. At 3 months, for instance, immunoglobulins comprise a smaller portion of the proteins than was true when the baby was younger.

During a feeding, the constituents of the milk change. The milk contains more fat at the end of a feeding than in the beginning. Mature breast milk is 2 percent fat at the beginning of a feeding and 7 percent at the end. Fat provides satiety, or a feeling of fullness or satisfaction. If the infant received high-fat milk at the beginning of a feeding, it might become contented and stop nursing. The variation in content also provides the infant with a variety of taste experiences. Fear of heart disease in the infant should not deter women from breast-feeding. Despite the fact that some of their milk contains 7 percent fat, breast-fed infants at 1 year have serum cholesterol levels equal to formula-fed infants.

Unique Advantages to Breast-Feeding

There are two advantages to breast-feeding that cannot be duplicated by formulas. The first is the protection against disease provided by a mother's milk. The second is the lessening of the possibility of allergies in the infant.

PROTECTION AGAINST DISEASE   Breast-fed infants are sick less frequently than formula-fed babies. This is most important in developing countries. Gastrointestinal infections are the leading cause of infant mortality worldwide. In fact, fluid and electrolyte imbalances caused by infection kill more children than any other disease or disaster.

Breast-feeding promotes a particular kind of bacteria, *Lactobacillus bifidus,* in the baby's intestine rather than *Escherichia coli.* Although the normal adult intestine harbors *E. coli,* it can cause diarrhea in children. The *L. bifidus* also suppresses the growth of other organisms, such as staphylococci, shigella, and protozoa, which can cause disease.

Among the infection-fighting agents in breast milk are white blood cells (WBCs). Each cubic millimeter contains 4000 WBCs. This concentration is nearly as much as occurs in the blood. Most of these WBCs are macrophages that kill microorganisms.

Breast milk also contains immunoglobulin A (IgA), an antibody against viruses and bacteria. Many proteins, if taken orally, would be digested. IgA is resistant to acidity and enzymes that break down protein, so it is effectively transferred to the infant in the mother's milk. Moreover, IgA is supplied in the greatest amount during the first 3 months of lactation when an infant's immune system is weakest.

PREVENTION OF ALLERGIES   The infant's gastrointestinal tract can permit the passage of whole proteins into the bloodstream. These proteins can stimulate an allergic response in susceptible infants. Contrary to earlier opinion, infants can be allergic to their own mother's milk. The occurrence rate is less than that in infants who become allergic to cow's milk. Once an infant becomes allergic to cow's milk, the risk of other allergies developing increases. Fortunately, most infants outgrow food allergies by age 2.

Often a mother cannot make a long-term commitment to breast-feed an infant. Although it is possible to pump the breasts and then bottle the milk for someone else to feed the baby while the mother is at work, this is not desirable for some women. However, even a few weeks of breast-feeding would confer some of these important health benefits on an infant.

Galactosemia Precludes Breast-Feeding

The lack of an enzyme to metabolize galactose is an absolute contraindication to breast-feeding. This condition of galactosemia occurs once in every 40,000 to 50,000 live births. The infant is fed a substitute formula containing no lactose or galactose.

The Formula-Fed Infant

As good as it is, even breast-feeding has some disadvantages. Among them is the inability of others, including the father, to feed the infant. Infants can be well nourished with commercial formulas, which are modified cow's milk products made to nearly duplicate breast milk. Earlier, when we compared breast milk to cow's milk, we were comparing it with unmodified cow's milk, not to commercial baby formulas.

Characteristics of Formulas

The processing of infant formulas in the United States has been regulated by law since 1980. These products have been so well received that 95 percent of formula-fed infants receive commercial products rather than a home-made formula. Formulas for full-term infants must contain 20 kilocalories per ounce. The formula osmolality may be no more than 400 milliosmoles per kilogram. Commercial formulas are designed to imitate human breast milk but they differ from it in protein, fat, and mineral content.

Formulas contain more protein than breast milk. The cow's milk proteins do not contain the optimal amino acids for human infants, so enough protein is included in the formula to provide a sufficient distribution of amino acids.

The saturated fats of cow's milk are poorly digested by the infant. In infant formulas, the saturated fats are removed and replaced by vegetable oils.

Formulas are treated to lower the sodium content of the cow's milk, but most formulas still contain more sodium than breast milk. SMA is the lowest in sodium, with 6.5 milliequivalents per liter. This is a trifle lower than breast milk, with 7 milliequivalents per liter.

Formulas can be purchased with or without added iron. Formulas without iron contain less than 1 milligram per quart, and formulas with iron contain 12 milligrams per quart.

Formula Preparations

Commercial formulas come in three forms: powder (to mix with water), liquid concentrate, and ready-to-feed. In practice, there is less waste with the powdered formula. A smaller amount can be mixed for the young infant. Opened cans of liquid formula may be stored covered in the refrigerator but must be used within 48 hours. Prepared bottles of formula should be discarded once they have been out of the refrigerator 1 hour.

In Western countries with safe drinking-water supplies, the use of clean rather than sterile technique often is sufficient. The parents will receive specific instructions from their healthcare workers. Nevertheless, separate utensils should be kept for formula preparation. Parents should be cautioned that equipment cannot be adequately sanitized in a microwave oven.

Parents must be impressed with the need to feed the infant the correct strength formula. Either too concentrated or too dilute a formula can cause severe electrolyte imbalances, even death.

Feeding Techniques

Contrary to the rigid feeding practices of some years ago, the current practice is to feed the infant when it is hungry. Most of the time the infant evolves a schedule whereby it demands a feeding approximately every 4 hours. By the age of 2 to 3 months, the baby probably will have eliminated one feeding so the schedule is five times a day. By 6 months most infants are feeding four times a day.

The baby is positioned in the crook of the arm almost as if breast-feeding. The parent's or caregiver's touch is important to the infant's development. The nipple hole should be large enough for milk to drip out without shaking. The bottle should be tipped so that the nipple is kept full of milk at all times. This prevents the infant from swallowing air while feeding. "Propping" an infant with a bottle is never acceptable because (1) choking is a real hazard and (2) the infant needs to be held in order to develop a closeness with the parent or caregiver. Figure 10–3 shows the infant and caregiver concentrating on each other during the feeding.

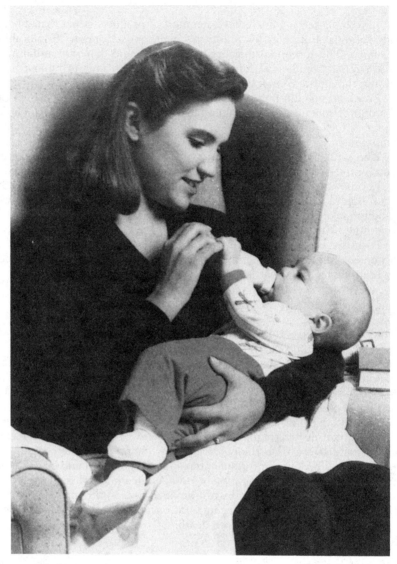

FIGURE 10–3. Babies are held close to the caregiver for bottle feeding so that its psychological as well as physical needs can be met. (Used and reprinted with permission of Ross Laboratories, Columbus, Ohio.)

The daily intake for an infant should be 1.5 to 2 ounces of formula per pound of body weight. At this rate, a 7-pound baby would take 10.5 to 14 ounces a day. This small an infant would be feeding six times a day, so it would take 1.75 to 2.3 ounces per feeding. A 14-pound baby would be taking 21 to 28 ounces in four feedings of 5.25 to 7 ounces. Each single feeding should never exceed 8 ounces.

Special Formulas

Manufacturers have devised formulas for special needs. We have mentioned a few possibilities as we discussed the infant's digestive capacity. Infants

CLINICAL APPLICATION 10–3
Soy Protein Formulas

Several formulas based on soy protein are available for infants with special needs. Most of them contain no lactose. Two commonly used soy products are ProSobee and Isomil SF. Many others are available. Soy formulas are prescribed when an infant is allergic to cow's milk or has a lactose or sucrose intolerance. Temporary lactose intolerance sometimes follows diarrhea because of damage to the intestinal mucosa.

In this situation, soy formulas may be useful temporarily until the infant's intestinal function returns to normal.

who are allergic to cow's milk, those with galactosemia or lactose intolerance, and those with fat absorption problems all need special formulas. See Clinical Application 10–3 for a brief description of soy formulas. Unfortunately, soy proteins may also cause allergies.

We consider the term infant's digestive, nervous, and urinary systems immature. How, then, do we meet the challenge of feeding the littlest humans, the premature infants? Clinical Application 10–4 summarizes some of the nutritional problems and interventions used with "preemies."

Hazards of Formula-Feeding

On a few occasions, improperly manufactured formulas have been responsible for vitamin and mineral deficiencies in infants. This is unacceptable, certainly, but rare. A more common hazard, and one an individual nurse can monitor, is the improper preparation and use of formulas by the parent. Formulas can be prepared with too much or too little water. Parents may not be aware of sources of contaminated water. A third hazard is holding a bottle of formula at feeding temperature too long. Body temperature is "just right" for bacteria to multiply, whether in the body or in a formula bottle.

Choice of Breast or Bottle

In this country, infants can be well nourished whether breast- or formula-fed. Of course, to raise a child successfully takes more than simply "fertilizing" with the correct ratio of nutrients. No mother should be forced into breast-feeding because it meets the physician's or nurse's needs. Her decision should be supported enthusiastically.

Semisolid Foods

Contrary to folklore, no proof exists that the early feeding of solid food to infants promotes their sleeping through the night. At 3 months, 75 percent of infants sleep all night long, regardless of diet.

When to Start

If solid foods are introduced too early, the infant may develop allergies because of the permeability of the intestine, which at this age permits whole

CLINICAL APPLICATION 10-4
Premature Infants

Premature infants are born before 37 weeks gestation. A low-birth-weight (LBW) infant weighs less than 2500 grams at birth. A very low birth-weight (VLBW) infant weighs 1000 grams (2.2 pounds) or less. An infant can be both premature and LBW or VLBW. Not all premature infants weigh less than 2500 grams. Nor are all LBW infants premature. Nevertheless birth weight is the most potent single predictor of an infant's future health status. LBW infants are 20 times more likely to die as normal-weight infants. Although LBW infants make up just 7 percent of the births in the United States, they comprise almost 66 percent of deaths in the first year of life. There is a substantial association between intellectual function and LBW, even greater with VLBW.

Compared with full-term infants, premature infants have an even larger proportion of their bodies as water. They have less protein and fat. Their bones are poorly calcified and their muscles are poorly developed. There is almost no glycogen. The sucking reflex is not developed prior to the 32nd or 34th week of gestation, so often premature infants require tube feeding through the gastrointestinal tract, or parenteral feeding. Tube feeding will conserve energy even in an infant who is able to suck. Esophageal peristalsis is absent and the esophageal sphincter is weak, leading to increased danger of aspiration. The liver is immature in enzyme systems and in iron stores. Fat digestion is limited by decreased activity of pancreatic lipase. Fat absorption is limited by a deficiency of bile salts.

However, protein digestion and absorption functions are relatively intact. Carbohydrate absorption also is intact, but digestion is limited by decreased pancreatic and salivary amylase activity and delayed development of lactase.

Special formulas for premature infants are designed to provide for the infant's growth needs despite the immature digestive system. Glucose polymers and medium-chain triglycerides are used to construct a formula that will take advantage of the infant's digestive capabilities. The premature infant has high energy needs. If given 120 kilocalories per kilogram of body weight enterally, the infant will grow at about the same rate as if still in the uterus. Special growth grids for premature infants are available. These are based on conceptual age or the expected due date.

Vitamin supplements are needed because the infant's intake is so small. Maximal transfer of vitamin E across the placenta occurs just before full-term delivery. Vitamin E stabilizes red blood cell membranes. If deficient, the infant suffers from hemolytic anemia. The other function of vitamin E is the possible contribution to preventing retrolental fibroplasia in infants receiving oxygen.

Premature infants may need to have their diet supplemented with the minerals calcium, phosphorus, and sodium. A rickets of prematurity can occur in the second postnatal month due not to the lack of vitamin D but to the lack of calcium and phosphorus. Sodium needs will increase as the infant grows. Monitoring serum and urine sodium levels will alert the physician to the infant's changing needs.

Continued on next page.

CLINICAL APPLICATION 10–4 *(Continued)*
Premature Infants

Not all mothers of premature infants can establish lactation. The milk of those who do differs significantly from the milk of mothers who deliver at term: the breast milk of the mother of a premature baby has more protein and sodium but insufficient calcium, phosphorus, and magnesium. As is true with full-term infants, the mother's antibodies cannot be duplicated by formula. Figure 10–4 compares a premature infant born 24 years ago with the adult of today.

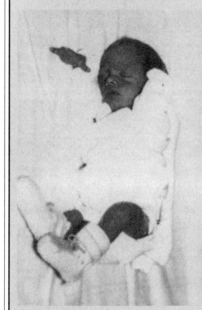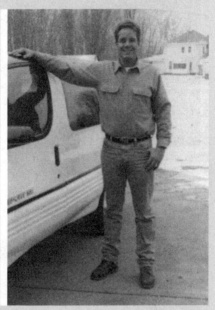

FIGURE 10–4. *(Left)* Premature infants can grow into large, normal adults. *(Right)* This man started life as a 3-pound 12-ounce premature infant, 17 inches long.

proteins to be absorbed. Most physicians recommend starting semisolid foods at about 4 to 6 months of age. Figure 10–5 shows an infant trying cereal for the first time.

The infant should achieve voluntary control of swallowing at about 3 to 4 months. Before being offered solid food, the infant should be able to control his or her head and trunk. With this ability the baby can turn away when satisfied. By this time the infant has doubled its birth weight, is drinking 8 ounces of formula, and yet becomes hungry in less than 4 hours.

In introducing solid food it is important to follow the infant's lead. To avoid later feeding problems, solid foods should be started when the baby is interested. Babies this age are hungry and not fussy about tastes. They learn from adults, though, so the parent should avoid showing distaste for particular foods.

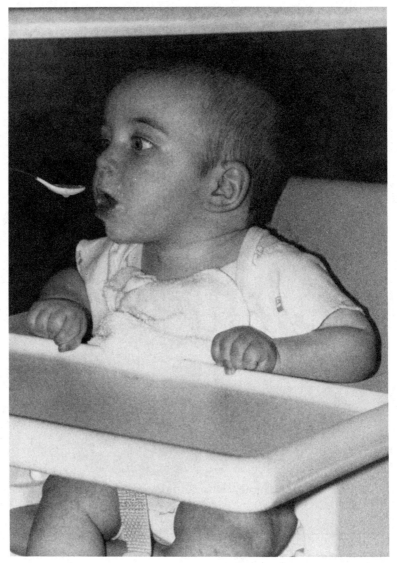

FIGURE 10–5. This 5-month-old baby is experiencing semisolid food for the first time. His readiness is clear. Notice how eager he is, how focused on the spoon.

How to Feed

New foods should be introduced one at a time, so if a problem develops, it can be readily identified. A food should be tried for 3 to 5 days before the infant is permitted to reject it. Only a taste or two is sufficient for the first try. Even if the baby takes the food eagerly, small amounts should be given to keep a sufficient appetite for milk.

The parent should heat a small amount to serve the infant. Food that has been heated and not consumed should be discarded. This will prevent possible contamination with salivary enzymes and bacteria. Food that has been opened but not heated can be stored in the covered jar in the refrigerator if it will be used in 2 to 3 days. A commonly used schedule for introducing new foods appears in Table 10–4. The baby's physician may modify this to meet individual needs.

This is a critical time in the infant's life. Eating adult foods is a skill that the baby must learn. However, the foods must be items the infant can chew and swallow safely. See Clinical Application 10–5 for tips on how to avoid choking accidents.

Weaning the Infant

Teaching the infant to use a cup is a gradual process. Often the baby will show an interest in the cup at 4 to 6 months. For these early experiments water can be offered.

Most mothers will begin serious weaning when the breast-fed infant is 7 to 8 months old. The best advice is to wean the child to formula and not to unmodified cow's milk.

The bottle-fed infant may not be ready to give up the bottle until 12 to 14 months of age. If bedtime bottles have not been used, weaning will proceed more rapidly.

It is best to change one feeding period at a time. Use the new schedule for 5 days or so, and then substitute the new method for a second feeding. Allowing the infant to set the pace will make the task easier.

TABLE 10–4 *Suggested Schedule for Infant Foods*

Age of Infant	Food	Rationale/Precautions
4 months	Infant cereal mixed with formula	Because of risk of allergies, rice offered first; wheat after age 12 months. Read labels: some mixed infant cereals contain wheat.
5 to 6 months	Strained vegetables	Less sweet than fruits; less likely to be rejected if offered first.
6 to 7 months	Strained fruits	Will be well accepted; humans have strong preference for sweets.
6 to 8 months	Finger foods (bananas, crackers)	Encourages self-feeding. Different textures may aid speech development.
7 to 8 months	Strained meats	Offer variety. See Clinical Application 10–5.
10 months	Strained or mashed egg yolk	Start with ½ teaspoonful. Due to possible allergy, delay egg white till 1 year old.
10 months	Bite-sized cooked foods	Select appropriate foods. See Clinical Application 10–5.
12 months	Foods from adult table	Select suitable foods, prepared according to baby's abilities.

CLINICAL APPLICATION 10–5
Avoiding Choking Accidents

Each year several hundred infants are asphyxiated by food. This is a hazard for older children as well. On average, one death every 5 days is reported in children from infancy to 9 years of age.

Hot dogs, or frankfurters, are involved most often. Hot dogs, apples, cookies, and biscuits cause choking most often in infants. Peanuts and grapes are the most dangerous for 2-year-old children, while 3-year-olds still face a risk from hot dogs.

Other foods that are often implicated in choking accidents are listed below. Because there are many other foods the child can eat safely, the prudent course is to avoid all of the foods listed. If a choking incident occurs, any caregiver needs to be able to administer cardiopulmonary resuscitation (CPR) should it become necessary. Training in CPR should be sought by all parents or parents-to-be. Small children should always be supervised while they are eating.

Hard Foods	Stringy Foods	Sticky Foods	Plug-shaped Foods
Apples	Beans	Bread	Grapes
Carrots	Celery	Chewing gum	Hot dogs
Cookies		Peanut butter	
Corn			
Hard candy			
Nuts			
Peanuts			
Popcorn			
Raisins			
Raw vegetables			
Seedy items (e.g., watermelon)			

Nutritional Problems in Infancy

Iron-deficiency anemia is the most prevalent nutritional deficiency in children in the United States. Other problems related to nutrition are allergies, cow's milk protein–induced intestinal injury, colic, and diarrhea. Additional problems of nutrition in infancy are summarized in Table 10–5. Some home remedies are included. If the infant does not improve rapidly, however, medical attention should be sought.

Iron-Deficiency Anemia

Sometimes a child drinks so much milk that he or she does not take in enough iron-rich foods. The result is iron-deficiency anemia.

OCCURRENCE It is estimated that 24 percent of children between the ages of 6 months and 2 years have iron-deficiency anemia. This deficiency is ten times more prevalent in poor families than those with a higher socioeconomic status.

TABLE 10–5 *Nutritional Problems in Infancy*

Problem	Intervention	Comments
Regurgitation	Handle baby gently. Burp well; sit up after feeding.	Very common for first 6 months; not serious unless vomiting is projectile or bile-tinged
Hiccoughs	Offer water to drink. Continue regular feedings.	May be caused by swallowed air
Constipation	½ ounce prune juice with ½ ounce water; or ½ teaspoonful dark corn syrup per feeding	Rare in breast-fed infants
Burns to mouth	Shake formula after heating; test well.	Formula warmed in microwave oven continues to increase in temperature after removal.
Nursing-bottle syndrome	Do not use milk or juice as bedtime bottle. Do not put sweetener on pacifier.	See Clinical Application 2–1

EARLY DIAGNOSIS To be sure that iron deficiency is diagnosed promptly in infants and toddlers, routine monitoring of the hemoglobin level is necessary through the infant's second birthday. Normal hemoglobin levels are 14 to 24 grams per 100 milliliters in the newborn, 10 to 15 grams per 100 milliliters in the infant.

TREATMENT OF IRON-DEFICIENCY ANEMIA Treatment may be medication, iron-fortified foods, and/or foods naturally high in iron. Red meats, especially liver, are high in iron. The parent should offer the iron-rich foods at the beginning of the meal when the infant is hungry. After the baby has eaten the strained or pureed foods, breast milk or formula may be given.

To help prevent iron-deficiency anemia, tea should only be offered to a child after the first birthday, if at all. As little as 1 cup of tea per day decreases the absorption of iron from both plant sources and milk in 6- to 12-month-old infants. (Merhav et al., 1985).

A number of special circumstances make vitamin and/or mineral supplementation desirable. Some of these situations appear in Table 10–6.

Allergies

Allergies have been referred to a number of times throughout the chapter. Introducing certain foods too early increases the likelihood of allergies developing.

COMMON FOOD ALLERGENS IN INFANCY An **allergen** is a substance that provokes an allergic response. One common allergen is cow's milk protein. Although it affects only 1 to 3 percent of children, an allergy to cow's milk can be a big problem for the affected families. Special formulas without cow's milk protein are available.

Allergen—A substance that provokes an allergic response.

TABLE 10-6 *Vitamin-Mineral Supplementation for Infants*

	Prescribed for	Situation
Vitamin		
D	Breast-fed infants	If sunlight exposure to head, arms, hands is less than 1 hour per week
E	Premature infants	See Clinical Application 10-4.
K	All infants	Given immediately before birth to mother or after birth to baby
C	2-week-old formula-fed infants, if vitamin is not in formula	Synthetic preferable to juices. Orange juice, especially, may be allergen.
Folic acid	Evaporated milk formula–fed infant	Sterilizing heat destroys folic acid.
B_{12}	Breast-fed if mother is strict vegetarian	
Minerals		
Calcium	Premature	See Clinical Application 10-4.
Phosphorus	Premature	See Clinical Application 10-4.
Iron	When birth weight has doubled	Iron-fortified formula available
Fluoride	All, shortly after birth, unless fluoride is in water used for formula or in supplemental fluid given breast-fed infant.	Fluoride is not secreted in breast milk.

The identification of allergies to orange juice has stimulated a major change in infant feeding. Formerly, infants were given orange juice (to provide vitamin C) as the first food to complement evaporated milk formulas. However, there is enough vitamin C in both breast milk and commercial formulas to prevent scurvy. Currently, if additional vitamin C is needed, a synthetic product is usually prescribed to avoid the allergens in orange juice.

Wheat protein and egg-white protein can also be allergens to infants. Other foods that have caused allergies in infants are peanut butter, other nuts, butters, and chocolate.

Hives (urticaria)—Sudden swelling and itching of skin or mucous membranes, often caused by allergies; if the respiratory tract is involved, may be life-threatening.

SIGNS AND SYMPTOMS   Allergies to foods may produce signs and symptoms beyond the gastrointestinal tract. Food allergies can cause skin and respiratory problems. The infant may have **hives,** eczema, or other rashes; asthma, bronchitis, wheezing; or a runny nose, called allergic rhinitis.

The signs and symptoms of food allergies may appear as long as 5 days after exposure to the allergen. Thus, if 5 days are allowed to elapse between the introduction of each new food, chances are that the allergen will be identified more readily.

TREATMENT OF ALLERGIES   It is easier to prevent allergies than to diagnose and treat them. If there is a family history of allergies, the best course may be for the mother to breast-feed for 6 months. Ironically, the soy formula used to treat children allergic to cow's milk protein also can cause allergies.

Many infants outgrow these food sensitivities by age 1 or 2. It is important not to permanently exclude foods from the diet based on the first year's experience. The physician should be reminded of the diet limitation so that an appropriate time can be chosen to reintroduce the offending foods.

Cow's Milk Protein–Induced Intestinal Injury

Approximately 1 percent of infants incur intestinal injury from cow's milk protein. The signs include failure to thrive, fever, vomiting, diarrhea that may test positive for blood, and anemia resulting from the blood loss. Treatment consists of removing cow's milk protein from the diet.

Colic

Infantile colic frustrates parents but generally resolves by the time the baby is 3 months old. The infant with colic is unhappy and fussy. It may cry for hours, starting late in the afternoon, just when its caregivers are also tired and cranky.

POSSIBLE CAUSES   Any time multiple, diverse treatments are proposed, it is likely that the basic cause of a condition is unknown. This is the case with colic. Spasms of the muscles of the colon are blamed, hence the name colic. The baby's abdomen is tense and its legs are drawn up to the abdomen. Distention may result from swallowing air. The pain seems to be relieved by the passage of gas or flatus.

For the bottle-fed baby the nipple holes may be too big or too small, increasing the amount of air swallowed. If the infant is overfed, bacteria will ferment the excess milk in the intestine, forming gas.

The breast-fed infant might be swallowing air because its nursing position is incorrect. Breast-fed infants seem to get gas from some of the same foods that give adults gas. Garlic, onion, broccoli, brussels sprouts, cabbage, and sauerkraut intake by the mother have all been suggested as contributing to infantile colic. Other foods that may cause problems, particularly if eaten in excess, are pickles, nuts, berries, citrus fruits, and chocolate. It is also possible that the baby may be allergic to antigens in the mother's milk. In one study, colic stopped when the breast-feeding mother stopped drinking cow's milk.

Other contributing factors may include fatigue or chilliness in the baby or tensions or emotional upsets in the mother. Allergies or lactose intolerance should be ruled out first.

TREATMENT OF COLIC   Because of the lack of knowledge as to specific causes, many treatments have been devised. Holding the baby upright, burping, or giving it some warm water sometimes helps. Diluting the formula or offering cold formula has been successful with some babies.

Even though their baby's condition is stressful for them, the parents should try not to be overly concerned. Most infants grow and gain weight despite the colic. And, as was stated earlier, colic usually disappears with or without treatment at about 3 months of age.

Diarrhea

Seventy-five percent of an infant's body weight is water, 54 percent of it extracellular. For this reason, an infant is at special risk of rapid dehydration when it suffers from diarrhea.

CAUSES OF DIARRHEA   Infants are subject to osmotic diarrhea. Both overfeeding and food intolerances are common causes of diarrhea. Apple juice may produce diarrhea in infants, owing to carbohydrate malabsorption.

PATHOPHYSIOLOGY   As a result of diarrhea, the wall of the intestine may become inflamed. This diminishes the amount of lactase produced, so the infant exhibits a temporary lactose intolerance. Distension, cramps, and osmotic diarrhea ensue.

TREATMENT OF DIARRHEA   Electroyte solutions are life-saving not only in developing countries but in this country as well. An infant should take 120 milliliters of fluid per kilogram of body weight per day plus an amount equal to the liquid lost in the stools. Liquids at room temperature are often better tolerated than warm or cold beverages. This intake should maintain fluid balance unless the insensible water losses due to fever or environmental heat or humidity are excessive. Loss of 5 percent of body weight indicates dehydration and demands medical attention.

After 12 hours, if the diarrhea seems to be lessening, half-strength formula can be offered. If the diarrhea returns, the infant may have developed a temporary lactase insufficiency. Lactose-free formula may be needed.

WHEN TO CALL THE PHYSICIAN   Although diarrhea is common in infants, it can be life-threatening. When should the physician be called? A parent should seek medical treatment immediately if the child has lost 5 percent of body weight, or if the diarrhea amounts to ten or more stools or is marked by a large volume of fluid loss. Other signs requiring immediate medical attention are a fever of 101°F or higher, vomiting, or a lack of improvement after 24 hours of home care.

NUTRITION IN CHILDHOOD

Childhood covers the growth periods of the toddler (1 to 3 years), the preschool child (3 to 6 years), and the school-age child (6 to 12 years). Nutritional needs and the rate of growth and development are different for each period. Psychosocial development varies with each age group as well.

Nutrition of the Toddler

Fortunately, the child's nutritional needs become more like those of adults after the first birthday. Fewer modifications of foods are necessary to accommodate the child's organs than during infancy.

The toddler is 1 to 3 years old. During these years growth is slower and, although activity increases, the need for kilocalories decreases compared with infancy. So the child's appetite slackens.

Nevertheless, the child has to eat. How and what the family eats will influence the child's tastes for many years. How family members treat one another and the toddler at mealtimes and at other times is more important than the precise amount of food the toddler swallows at each meal.

Psychosocial Development

The psychosocial development task of the toddler is to build <u>autonomy,</u> or independence. The child still lives a sheltered life. Parents must take the toddler to playmates or bring playmates home. Toddlers generally do not travel far unaccompanied. In many ways the toddler is still very dependent.

Between 1 and 3 years come the "terrible twos." In Erikson's terms the child is learning to be autonomous. Every 2-year-old knows the word "No." One way toddlers show their budding autonomy is in strong food preferences. They may eat only a few foods for weeks on end. Then later, they cannot stand and adamantly refuse foods they previously "loved." Parents must be flexible. If the parent insists on the consumption of certain items, the child may learn to use food rejection as a means of gaining attention. Later, more serious eating problems may result from such interactions.

Physical Growth and Development

Growth slows. The expected weight gain in the second year may be just 4 to 6 pounds. Height may increase by about 4 inches. By age 2, though, head circumference reaches two thirds of its final size and the brain cells stop reproducing.

The toddler is aptly named. One of the skills being acquired during this time is walking upright. As this skill is being perfected, the child's muscles of the back, buttocks, and thighs are enlarging. The bones are becoming more mineralized. The baby fat disappears.

Along with the gross motor skill of walking, the toddler's fine motor control improves. Eating utensils can be used with more finesse. The spoon is likely to reach the mouth with the correct side up.

The toddler's mouth is more sensitive than an adult's mouth. Foods are eaten better at lukewarm temperatures rather than hot. Thus, dawdling at the table may have a physiological basis.

Nutrition Fundamentals

The toddler needs all the essential nutrients. The need for many nutrients increases proportionately with body size throughout the growth years. These needs, plus the poorer appetite and behavior patterns of toddlers, stretch the parents' ingenuity and patience.

FOOD LIKES Toddlers like finger foods. From a variety of finger foods, the child learns about texture. Toddlers prefer plain foods to most mixtures. Familiar combinations, though, may be relished. Some popular dishes are macaroni and cheese, spaghetti, and pizza.

To help the toddler develop autonomy, parents need to understand and accept that the child is an individual. Whenever possible, the child's preferences should be honored. This does not mean that separate meals have to be prepared for the toddler. Appropriate choices can be given the child. Not "What do you want to eat?" but "Would you rather have spaghetti or pizza?" honors the child's opinion but does not have the parent on a leash.

MEALTIMES Toddlers are learning social skills as well as good nutritional habits. Eating is a social experience for adults most of the time; toddlers appreciate company also.

Keeping to a regular schedule will help maintain the child's intake. A 1-year-old's stomach holds just 1 cup. Eating regular meals and nutritious snacks helps to avoid fatigue and controls the appetite. However, if high-sugar snacks are used to assuage hunger before a meal, the more nutritious foods at the meal may be taken poorly.

NEW FOODS After the pureed foods of infancy, parents will be pleased to offer more attractive plates to the toddler. Brightly colored foods are appealing. Nevertheless, chewing may not be well developed. Tough meat is not for the toddler. Grinding the meat several times may make it safer and easier to eat.

All of the foods that were delayed until after the first birthday are allowed now. These include unmodified cow's milk, egg white, wheat, citrus fruits, seafood, and chocolate. Nut butters are allowed also, but review Clinical Application 10–5 before choosing to include them. The careful parent will continue to introduce foods one at a time and watch for reactions.

Because of the toddler's small stomach capacity, small servings are all that can be tolerated. A serving is one fourth to one fifth the size of an adult serving. A good rule of thumb is to serve 1 tablespoonful for each year of age.

Daily intake should include one serving of a vitamin C-rich fruit or vegetable and one serving of a green leafy or yellow vegetable. Difficult as it may be, the parent should limit sugar and encourage consumption of fiber in cereals as well as in other foods. Iron-enriched cereals are the best choices.

Offering three meals and three nutritious snacks daily will increase the likelihood of the toddler obtaining sufficient nourishment. Because there are so many choices, the wise parent will avoid hazardous foods (review Clinical Application 10–5). Sometimes all that is necessary is chopping the food into very tiny pieces. Still, the toddler who is eating should not be left alone.

Because the kidneys become mature about age 1, the toddler may have salt in moderation. The liking for salty foods is an acquired taste. Because of the association between salt and high blood pressure later in life, the prudent parent will discourage the consumption of heavily salted foods.

MILK INTAKE Because iron-deficiency anemia is common in toddlers, milk intake may have to be curtailed to no more than 1 quart per day to maintain the appetite for iron-enriched cereals, meats, and iron-rich fruits and vegetables. The term "milk anemia" refers to iron deficiency anemia caused by overconsumption of milk and underconsumption of iron-rich foods.

Nutrition of the Preschool Child

The preschool child requires all the nutrients necessary for other human beings. This is a delightful time of enthusiastic learning, much of which concerns food, since it is of course consumed every day.

Psychosocial Development

Erikson's theory postulates <u>initiative</u> as the psychosocial task to be mastered by the preschool child. Within their capabilities, children should be encouraged to set and achieve some goals of their own.

In the realm of nutrition, children can participate in planning and preparation of meals. They should be prompted to help in the kitchen, but not just with the cleanup. Preschool children love to make fancy cookies and showy relishes. Making even simple things like gelatin desserts gives the child a sense of accomplishment.

By making the meal a social time and eating slowly themselves, parents can encourage the same behavior in the child. Children learn by imitating adults. Exemplifying good manners will be more productive than criticizing the child's manners. Having company their own age is helpful. Children have been observed to stay at the table longer and to eat more in company of their peers. Exchanging visits with a friend's child will begin to broaden the child's horizons.

Physical Growth and Development

From the third to the sixth year, a child continues to gain 4 to 5 pounds per year. A gain in height of about 2 inches per year is average. Adequacy of growth should be assessed every 6 to 12 months. Growth charts remain the standard against which a given assessment is judged.

Nutrition Fundamentals

Preschool children are very active. A 3-year-old may need 1300 to 1500 kilocalories per day. But the child may have little appetite. Food jags similar to those displayed by toddlers are common through age 4.

An adaptation of the Food Pyramid for preschoolers appears in Table 10–7. A serving of meat, fruit, or vegetable is 1 tablespoonful per year of age. A serving of breads & cereals is a half to one slice of bread or ½ cup of cereal or pasta. A serving of milk is still 1 cup.

DEVELOPING GOOD HABITS   The preschool child responds best to regular mealtimes. When the adult meal will be served late, the parents have to decide if it would be better to allow the child to socialize with adults at a late meal or to feed the child early.

But these children, like the toddlers, cannot eat enough three times a day to meet their needs. By age 3, a child is able to verbalize hunger. A good supply of wholesome snacks will serve the conscientious parent well. Such items as cottage cheese, low-fat yogurt, fresh fruit, raw vegetables, milk, fruit juices, graham crackers or fig bars all are nutrient dense and low in fat.

TABLE 10–7 *Food Pyramid for the Preschool Child*

Food Group	Number of Servings	Serving Suggestions
Bread/Cereal	six or more	
Fruit	two or more	Include 4 ounces of orange juice or other food high in vitamin C.
Vegetable	three or more	Include one vegetable high in vitamin A. Crisp-cooked, warm rather than hot vegetables preferred
Meat	two servings	Child-size servings of red meat essential for RBC synthesis
Milk	three servings	Not to be overdone at expense of blood-forming nutrients. Low-fat milks now permissible

So long as the parent still has control over the child's world, concentrated sweets such as candy and soda pop should be strictly limited.

Tableware appropriate for the preschool child will ease tensions during mealtimes. Unbreakable dishes that are designed for stability, with deep sides to permit scooping the food onto a spoon or fork, are a practical choice. Small glasses and cups, also unbreakable, with a squat design and low center of gravity, will serve the child's and the parents' needs well.

It is not too early to emphasize the importance of cleanliness. Regularly washing hands before meals and brushing teeth after meals will cultivate good health habits.

NEW FOODS   As with younger children, new foods should be offered one at a time in small amounts. Trying something new is most acceptable at the beginning of the meal when the child is hungriest. A taste or two is sufficient if new foods are offered at regular intervals.

Parents have the advantage over their children in being able to select the food. Items the parents dislike will not grace the family table with regularity. Children, too, should be permitted their preferences. This advice is not permissive, just practical. If an argument over food develops into a power struggle, as sometimes happens, the child will never admit to liking it, even when it turns out to be quite tasty.

Nutritional Problems

Iron-deficiency anemia continues to be a significant problem for children of this age. The other concern is that of dental caries.

IRON-DEFICIENCY ANEMIA   Children in low-income families are particularly subject to iron-deficiency anemia. Black and Hispanic children in the United States have been found to be low in iron, vitamin C, and vitamin A. Fortunately, the situation is improving. In 1985, 3 percent of the 6-month to 6-year-old-children in low-income households were anemic compared with 8 percent in 1975. This change is attributed to the Women, Infants, and Children's Program (WIC). The WIC program provides specific goods and nutritional services to low-income pregnant women and young children.

DENTAL CARIES   The destruction of tooth enamel by dental caries is a problem for all economic groups. The "baby" teeth, as well as the permanent teeth, deserve care and professional attention. Brushing the teeth correctly may mean that the parent has to do it. Regular dental checkups should be a part of the preschool child's routine.

Nutrition of the School-Age Child

By this time, few modifications in foodstuffs are necessary to accommodate the child. A balanced diet suitable for adults, emphasizing protein, vitamins, and minerals will also be good for a school-age child.

Psychosocial Development

The developmental task of the school-age child is to develop <u>industry.</u> These are the years to build competence in many different skills. School work, sports, hobbies, and chores at home permit the child to recognize the worth of work. Making and keeping commitments is part of this learning process.

An older child can participate in planning menus, shopping for food, preparing the meals, and, yes, cleaning up afterwards. As with younger children, though, limiting the child to a scullery role will be more likely to foster a sense of inferiority than habits of industry.

Basic dietary habits are formed by the time a child enters school. Peer-group acceptance and approval is very important. Interactions with other children and school experiences expose a child to different foods and different cultures.

Growth and Health

By age 6, the child should weigh twice as much as at age 1. Suppose that our 7-pound infant who weighed 21 pounds at 1 year gained 5 pounds in the second year and 4 pounds per year through age 6. At age 6, the child would weigh 42 pounds, an amount that is twice the 1-year weight.

By school age, the effects of good or poor nutrition will begin to be apparent. The well-nourished child will display most of the qualities listed in Table 10–8. The poorly nourished child will be lacking in a significant number of these qualities.

Nutrition Fundamentals

School-age children, especially those 8 to 10 years old, generally have good appetites and they like almost all foods. However, vegetables are the least liked of the food groups. Parents sometimes invent novel strategies to persuade children to eat vegetables (Fig. 10–6).

Breakfast is very important. The child needs energy and other nutrients to last till lunch. Breakfast should contain one fourth to one third of the day's nutrients. Unfortunately, it is the meal most likely to be skipped. A common excuse is "lack of time." Girls are more likely than boys to skip breakfast (Burtis, Davis, and Martin, 1988).

The school-age child needs adequate protein intake for developing muscle and laying down bone matrix. Calcium is necessary to build dense bones. The body anticipates the adolescent growth spurt. The greatest retention of

TABLE 10–8 *Indications of Good Nutrition in the School-Age Child*

General appearance	Alert, energetic
	Normal height and weight
Skin and mucous membranes	Skin smooth, slightly moist; mucous membranes pink, no bleeding
Hair	Shiny, evenly distributed
Scalp	No sores
Eyes	Bright, clear, no fatigue circles
Teeth	Straight, clean, no discoloration or caries
Tongue	Pink, papillae present, no sores
Gastrointestinal system	Good appetite, regular elimination
Musculoskeletal system	Well-developed, firm muscles; erect posture, bones straight without deformities
Neurological system	Good attention span for age; not restless, irritable, or weepy

Calvin & Hobbes

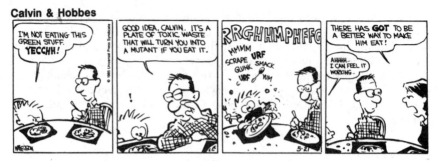

FIGURE 10–6. Calvin is tricked into eating green vegetables. (From Universal Press Syndicate.)

calcium and phosphorus precedes the rapid growth of adolescence by 2 years or more. Therefore, a liberal intake of milk and milk products before the age of 10 gives a child a great advantage. An adequate calcium intake is closely correlated with the consumption of milk and milk products.

Exercise

Exercise can help the school-age child achieve growth and development in several areas. Weight-bearing exercise stimulates the osteoblasts, the bone-building cells. Exercise balances intake and activity for weight control. Conversely, lack of exercise and excessive time spent watching television have been correlated with fatness. If long hours spent with television are accompanied by consumption of multiple snacks, the risk for obesity rises greatly. Exercise, especially team sports, fosters interactions with peers. Activities that are likely to become lifetime interests should be especially encouraged. Not many adults play football. A skill at tennis, though, may provide an outlet for many years.

Problem Areas

School-age children are generally so active that they may have trouble sitting still. Requiring 15 to 20 minutes at the table for meals will increase the likelihood of a complete meal being eaten. One study found 10 percent of school-age children skipped breakfast.

Vitamin A and C deficiencies are common in school-age children. Carefully selected fruits and vegetables should be served regularly. Finding creative ways to prepare, cook, and serve vegetables will be a challenge for the cook in this family.

Some children are bothered by caffeine. One cup of hot chocolate or 12 ounces of cola contains 50 milligrams of caffeine. Two such beverages in a 60-pound child are the equivalent of 8 cups of coffee in a 175-pound man. If the child has difficulty sleeping or has an irregular pulse, the first factor to investigate is caffeine intake.

Puberty—Period of life at which the physical ability to reproduce is attained.

NUTRITION IN ADOLESCENCE

Adolescence is the period that extends from the onset of **puberty** until full growth is reached. For most individuals, adolescence occurs between the ages of 12 and 20. Adolescence is second only to infancy in the nutritional requirements necessary for normal growth and development.

Psychosocial Development

The developmental task of adolescents is to achieve their own identity. With all the changes that take place in their bodies and in their feelings and with the pressures from peers to conform, shaping their identities is a monumental task. In this process, teenagers "try on" various identities. These years can be trying for parents, as well. Adolescents pick up fads instantly and drop them just as suddenly. Food fads are part of the same pattern.

Physical Growth and Development

For adolescents, growth charts are useless. The term growth spurt is accurate. A teenager who may seem not to grow as much as others the same age will suddenly sprout like a weed, seemingly overnight. Boys commonly will grow 4 inches and gain 20 pounds in a year.

Boys and girls differ in the timing and completion of the growth spurt. Look at Table 10–9 for a summary of adolescent growth spurts. Be aware that growth is not completed at ages 15 to 19, only the growth spurt.

Zinc is essential for male sexual maturation. Before eliminating red meat from the diet, consider the best sources of zinc—shellfish and red meat.

Nutrient Needs of the Adolescent

Because of their growing and developing bodies, adolescents need more energy, vitamins, and protein than the school-age child or the adult.

Energy

The adolescent may require 60 to 80 kilocalories per kilogram of body weight per day. This amounts to 2700 to 3600 kilocalories for a 100-pound teenager. Men need more kilocalories than women. A 15-year-old girl requires 2100 kilocalories compared to a 15-year-old boy's requirement of 3000 kcalories. The boy may be in a growth spurt, whereas the girl has probably completed hers.

Vitamins

Emotional or physical stress can increase the utilization of vitamin C by three or four times. Change is stressful. At no other time of life is an individual who is capable of introspection changing so fast and so dramatically.

TABLE 10–9 *Adolescent Growth Spurts*

Status	Age in Years	
	Boys	Girls
Begins	12 to 13	10 to 11
Peaks	14	12
Completed	19	15

The adolescent athlete may need up to 6000 kilocalories per day. Thiamin and niacin are related to energy expenditure and riboflavin is needed for protein utilization. Therefore, the need for these B-vitamins is increased in the athlete. A training table laden with extra whole-grain or enriched bread and milk, should meet these vitamin needs.

Food Pyramid Modification

Foods should consist of the adult distribution except that three servings of milk or milk products should be ingested. Since one fourth the adolescent's kilocalories come from snacks, these "between-meal meals" should be nutritionally dense and chosen to balance the diet.

Nutrient Deficiencies

Adolescent girls have the dubious distinction of being the worst nourished population group in the United States. Sixty percent of adolescent females eat only two thirds of their needed nutrients. As many as 80 percent are iron deficient, and as many as 50 percent are calcium deficient. Vitamin C also has been found to be lacking in the diets of adolescent girls. Unfortunately, pregnancy in a teenage girl escalates her nutritional needs (Clinical Applications 10-6).

Both girls and boys have low intakes of vitamin A and folic acid. This is due to the inadequate ingestion of green and deep yellow vegetables.

Common Nutritional Problems

Two common nutritional problems of teenagers are overenthusiastic weight control and poor choices of foods.

CLINICAL APPLICATION 10–6
Teenage Pregnancy

A nutritional crisis can result when a teenage girl becomes pregnant. This happens, by accident or intention, to 1 million teenagers in the United States every year. Forty percent of these girls are under 18 years of age. Three percent are girls under age 15. Sixty percent of teenagers continue the pregnancy to delivery and 25 percent become pregnant again within a year.

The pregnant or lactating teenager has the highest nutritional requirements of any healthy human being. The average girl does not reach her full height or attain gynecological maturity until age 17. She herself is still growing and now has a fetus to nourish besides.

Nutrients most often lacking in the pregnant teenager's diet are calcium, iron, vitamin A, and niacin. (In addition, kilocalorie intake is usually insufficient to meet daily needs.) The 11- to 14-year-old expectant mother requires 2700 kilocalories per day, the 15- to 18-year-old, 2400 kilocalories. Teenage mothers are at increased risk of complications of pregnancy, such as preeclampsia and premature delivery. The cause is not solely age, however. Complications of pregnancies are more strongly associated with poor nutrition than with maternal age.

Reduction Diets

Self-prescribed reduction diets are the bane of American women. Teenagers are no exception. Achieving and maintaining a healthy body weight is an admirable goal. Unfortunately, Americans also are lured by the "quick fix." We want instant results. Most often the diet consultants who promise quick results do so with an unbalanced diet. The principles laid out in Chapter 15 on proper weight control methods are as applicable for teenagers as for adults. Two disorders of young adolescents, especially girls, that are related to food consumption and/or weight control are bulimia and anorexia nervosa.

Poor Choices of Foods

Fast-food restaurant chains have made remarkable changes in their selections. They are now offering items such as salads, lower fat salad dressings, and low-fat milks. There are some healthy choices possible. However, the old standbys on the fast-food menus are generally higher in kilocalories, fat, sugar, and sodium than are similar items prepared at home.

As undesirable as a steady diet of fast food might be, it cannot be blamed for causing acne. About 80 percent of adolescents suffer from acne, starting about age 12 to 13 in girls and 14 to 15 in boys. Acne is caused by sex hormones stimulating the sebaceous glands. The skin becomes oilier and the ducts to the glands sometimes plug up, permitting the accumulation of harmful bacteria. There is as yet no convincing evidence that dietary indiscretions cause acne.

Summary

During periods of rapid growth such as pregnancy, infancy, childhood, and adolescence, the need for nutrients is critical. The lack of nutrients or the excessive intake of certain substances during such periods may cause serious, permanent damage in the individual. Each growth period has different nutritional requirements.

During pregnancy, to supply the mother, fetus, and placenta, there is an increased need for kilocalories, protein, and certain vitamins and minerals. Pregnant women are urged to avoid alcohol and to moderate caffeine intake. Some of the more common problems of pregnancy that may be resolved through dietary measures include morning sickness, leg cramps, constipation, and heartburn. Complications of pregnancy such as pregnancy-induced hypertension and gestational diabetes require medical treatment.

While infants require the same nutrients as adults, they need them in different amounts. Breast milk is especially suited to the human infant. Because the protein, fat, and carbohydrate in breast milk are tailored to the infant's digestive capabilities, they are readily usable. After the age of 4 months, semisolid and then solid foods are added to the diet gradually. Nutritional problems in infancy include iron-deficiency anemia, allergies, colic, and diarrhea.

Childhood includes the growth periods of the toddler, the preschool child, and the school-age child. Growth and development during childhood are not as rapid as during infancy. However, total amounts of nutrient recommended continue to increase with age so that the body's needs are met. Preschoolers often lack vitamin A in their diets and have a need for additional vitamin C. Along with adults, school-age children are the best nourished in the United States. However, iron deficiency is common in children and also in adolescent girls.

During adolescence, the final growth spurt of childhood occurs. Physical growth and development are rapid and sexual maturity is attained. Energy, protein, vitamins, and minerals are needed in increasing amounts. Because adolescents often have erratic eating habits and make poor food choices, their intake of vitamins A, C, and folic acid may be low. In addition to a deficiency of iron, adolescent girls may also be deficient in calcium.

A case study and a sample plan of care appear below. Both are designed to show you how the information you have studied in this chapter can be used in nursing practice.

CASE STUDY 10–1

Baby L., a 9-month-old girl, is being evaluated in a well-baby clinic. Her birth weight was 8 pounds 4 ounces. Her present weight is 20 pounds 8 ounces.

Mrs. L. states that the baby is taking 10 ounces of formula four times a day. The baby sleeps a lot between feedings. Mrs. L. gives the baby cereal or fruit after the formula three times a day. She has not offered the baby vegetables or meats. The formula she is using contains 1 milligram of iron per quart.

The nurse notes that Baby L. is pale. Her mucous membranes, including the conjunctiva on the lower eyelid, are very light pink. Laboratory test results show that Baby L.'s hemoglobin is 8 g per 100 ml.

The physician may prescribe medical interventions. In addition, the nurse begins to implement the following nursing care plan.

NURSING CARE PLAN FOR BABY L.

Assessment
Subjective
Inactive for age
Taking 40 ounces of formula per day
Few solids taken after formula
Objective
Pale skin, mucous membranes
Hemoglobin 8 grams per 100 milliliters

Nursing Diagnosis
Nutrition, altered: less than body requirements
Related to limited access to iron-rich foods as evidenced by pale skin and mucous membranes, hemoglobin 8 grams per 100 milliliters

Desired Outcome/Evaluation Criteria
1. Will take one serving of meat per day and one serving of vegetable per day in 3 weeks
2. Will increase hemoglobin to 9 grams per 100 milliliters in 3 weeks

Nursing Actions/Interventions with Rationales in Italics

1. Teach Mrs. L. to offer semisolid food to Baby L. before offering formula. *Offering the semisolid food when the baby is hungry increases the amount consumed.*
2. Teach Mrs. L. to limit Baby L. to 32 ounces of formula per day. *Limiting the amount of milk the infant takes will increase its appetite for iron-rich foods.*
3. Instruct Mrs. L. to change to the iron-fortified preparation of the baby's formula. *Changing preparations will increase the available iron from 1 milligram per quart to 12 milligrams per quart. The RDA for a 6- to 12-month-old infant is 10 milligrams.*
4. Instruct Mrs. L. to introduce one iron-rich vegetable or meat to Baby L. every 5 days. *Adding iron-rich foods will increase the iron available for absorption. The baby should be taking vegetables and meats, but the 5-day trial period should be maintained to monitor for allergies.*

STUDY AIDS

Chapter Review Questions

1. A nurse in a clinic would identify which of the following infants as needing additional assessment of growth?
   a. Baby girl A., 4 months old, birth weight 7 pounds 6 ounces, present weight 14 pounds 14 ounces
   b. Baby boy B., 2 weeks old, birth weight 6 pounds 10 ounces, present weight 6 pounds 11 ounces
   c. Baby boy C., 6 months old, birth weight 8 pounds 8 ounces, present weight 15 pounds 0 ounces
   d. Baby girl D., 2 months old, birth weight 7 pounds 2 ounces, present weight 9 pounds 10 ounces

2. Which of the following are advantages of breast milk that formula does not provide?
   a. Less fat and cholesterol
   b. More antibodies and less risk of allergy
   c. More fluoride and iron
   d. More vitamin C and vitamin D

3. Mothers should be instructed not to give infants plain cow's milk. The reason underlying this advice is that:
   a. The vitamin C content of cow's milk may reach toxic levels.
   b. The infant's kidneys cannot adequately filter the excess minerals in cow's milk.
   c. The infant lacks lipase to digest fat.
   d. The pasteurization process destroys essential amino acids in the cow's milk.

4. Mrs. T. is having her 2-month-old son checked in the well-baby clinic. She tells the nurse that the baby is not sleeping through the night yet. Mrs. T.'s mother advised her to start the infant on cereal to "fill him up" at bedtime. Despite the nurse's instructions, Mrs. T. says she is going to try her mother's idea. Which of the following would be most important if Mrs. T chooses to start the cereal?
   a. Following the cereal with a bedtime bottle to wash it down
   b. Making cream of wheat very thin and feeding the baby with an eyedropper
   c. Putting infant cereal into a bottle and enlarging the nipple hole
   d. Using infant rice cereal mixed with formula

5. Which of the following combinations of foods are appropriate for a 6-month-old infant?
   a. Cocoa-flavored wheat cereal, orange juice, and strained chicken
   b. Graham crackers, strained prunes, and stewed tomatoes
   c. Infant cereal, mashed banana, and strained squash
   d. Mashed potatoes, strained beets, and chopped hard-cooked egg

6. To avoid choking accidents, which of the following groups of foods would be considered safest for a toddler?
   a. Apple quarters, green beans, and chicken noodle casserole
   b. Grapes, carrot strips, and macaroni and cheese
   c. Diced peaches, mashed potatoes, and spaghetti
   d. Watermelon chunks, cheese-stuffed celery, and sliced frankfurters

7. If a family is following the dietary guidelines of the National Research Council, which of the following is it important not to eliminate from the school-age child's diet?
   a. Caffeine

    b. Fat

    c. Salt

    d. Sugar

8. Which of the following individuals is at greatest nutritional risk?

    a. 3-month-old infant being fed commercial formula

    b. 3-year-old child who drinks 3 cups of milk a day

    c. 8-year-old child who eats four chocolate chip cookies and drinks 2 glasses of milk after school

    d. 16-year-old girl who is pregnant

9. Which of the following nutrient supplements is most commonly prescribed for pregnant women?

    a. Calcium

    b. Iron

    c. Vitamin A

    d. Vitamin C

10. Which of the following substances is contraindicated during pregnancy?

    a. Alcohol

    b. Cocoa

    c. Coffee

    d. Tea

NCLEX-Style Quiz

Situation One

Ms. T. is a 15-year-old girl who thinks that she is 2 months pregnant. She confides to the school nurse that she is not sure if she should have an abortion. She has not told anyone else of the pregnancy. Her purpose in disclosing the information to the school nurse is to obtain assistance with weight control so she has more time to make up her mind.

1. Based on the above information, which one of the following interventions would be of highest priority at this time?

    a. Designing a weight control program that is high in calcium

    b. Giving information on the desirability of breast-feeding the infant

    c. Instructing the girl regarding substances that are likely to harm the fetus

    d. Scheduling a visit with a social worker to help the girl decide on a course of action

2. Knowing that adolescents are often lacking in certain nutrients, the nurse would want to assess the girl's intake of:

    a. Cola, coffee, and tea

    b. Fruits, vegetables, milk, and red meat

    c. Fried foods and pastries

    d. Poultry, seafood, and white bread

3. If this girl is average, she is _____ years away from attaining gynecological maturity.

    a. 1

    b. 2

    c. 3

    d. 4

4. Ms. T. complains of morning sickness. The nurse instructs her to:

    a. Eat breakfast later in the morning.

    b. Drink at least two glasses of liquid with every meal.

c. Increase her intake of whole-grain breads and cereals to two servings per meal.

d. Take a large glass of skimmed milk at bedtime.

5. Prenatal care is important for every expectant mother, but especially for teenagers because of the increased risk of:
   a. Hemorrhage during delivery
   b. Excess weight gain
   c. Preeclampsia
   d. Rickets in the newborn

CLINICAL CALCULATION 10–1

Determining Recommended Weight Gain during Pregnancy

$$\text{Body mass index (BMI)} = \frac{\text{Weight in kilograms}}{\text{Height in meters}^2}$$

Suppose a woman is 5 feet 4 inches tall and weighs 125 pounds.

$$5 \text{ feet } 4 \text{ inches} = 64 \text{ inches}$$

$$1 \text{ meter} = 39.371 \text{ inches}$$

$$\frac{64}{39.371} = 1.6 \text{ meters}$$

$$\frac{125 \text{ pounds}}{2.2 \text{ pounds per kilogram}} = 56.8 \text{ kilograms}$$

$$\text{BMI} = \frac{56.8}{(1.6)^2}$$

$$\text{BMI} = \frac{56.8}{2.56} = 22.2$$

Looking at the table below, we see that 22.2 is in the normal category. Recommended weight gain for this woman is 25 to 35 pounds.

BMI Category	Recommended Weight Gain for Pregnancy	
	Kilograms	Pounds
<19.8 = Low	12.5–18	28–40
19.8–26 = Normal	11.5–16	25–35
26–29 = High	7–11.5	15–25
>29 = Obese	6	15

Young adolescents and black women should strive for gains at the upper end of the recommended range. Women whose height is less than 157 centimeters (62 inches) should strive for gains at the lower end of the range.

Reprinted with permission from Nutrition During Pregnancy, © 1990 by the National Academy of Sciences. Published by National Academy Press, Washington, DC.

CLINICAL CALCULATION 10–2

Cost of Breast-Feeding versus Infant-Formula Feeding

Method of Feeding	Unit Purchased	Price per Unit	Cost
Breast			
2 cups milk	1 gallon	$2.25	$.28
2 eggs	1 dozen	.79	.13
4 ounces orange juice	12 ounces concentrate	1.69	.14
			Per Day $.55
			× 365
			Per Year $200.75
Infant Formula			
Concentrated Similac	13-ounce can	$1.83	
	1 can per day for 3 months		$164.70
	1.5 cans per day for 6 months		494.10
	2 cans per day for 3 months		329.40
			Per Year $988.20
Powdered Similac	16-ounce can (makes 116 fluid ounces)	$7.36	
	32 fluid ounces per day for 3 months		$182.73
	48 fluid ounces per day for 6 months		548.19
	64 fluid ounces per day for 3 months		365.46
			Per Year $1,096.38

Box continued on next page.

CLINICAL CALCULATION 10–2 *(Continued)*

Cost of Breast-Feeding versus Infant-Formula Feeding

Ready-to-feed
Similac
 1-quart can $2.83
 1 can per day
  for 3 months $257.70
 1.5 cans per day
  for 6 months   764.10
 2 cans per day
  for 3 months   <u>254.70</u>
      Per
      Year $1,276.50

BIBLIOGRAPHY

Acosta, RB and Wright, L: Nurses' role in preventing birth defects in offspring of women with phenylketonuria. JOGNN 21(4):270, 1992.

Beckholt, AP. Breast milk for infants who cannot breastfeed. JOGNN 19(3):216, 1990.

Benenson, AS (ed): Control of Communicable Disease in Man. American Public Health Association, Washington, DC, 1985.

Brown, JE: The Science of Human Nutrition. Harcourt Brace Jovanovich, San Diego, 1990.

Borowitz, D: Pediatric nutrition. In Feldman, EB: Essentials of Clinical Nutrition. FA Davis, Philadelphia, 1988.

Burtis, G, Davis, J, and Martin, S: Applied Nutrition and Diet Therapy. WB Saunders, Philadelphia, 1988.

Deglin, JH and Vallerand, AH: Davis's Drug Guide for Nurses, ed 3. FA Davis, Philadelphia, 1993.

Glenn, FB, Glenn, WD, and Duncan, RC: Fluoride table supplementation during pregnancy for caries immunity: A study of the offspring produced. Obstet Gynecol 143:560, 1982.

Gortmaker, SL, Dietz, WH, Jr, and Cheung, LWY. Inactivity, diet, and the fattening of America. J Am Diet Assoc 90(9):1247, 1990.

Graham, MV and Uphold, CR. Health perceptions and behaviors of school-age boys and girls. Journal of Community Health Nursing 9(2):77, 1992.

Hamilton, EMN, Whitney, EN, and Sizer, FS: Nutrition Concepts and Controversies, ed 2. West, St Paul, 1991.

Jacobsson, I and Lindberg, T: Cow's milk proteins cause infantile colic in breast-fed infants: A double-blind crossover study. Pediatrics 71:268, 1983.

Jaffin, H and Hayworth, SD: Nutrition in pregnancy. In Feldman, EB: Essentials of Clinical Nutrition. FA Davis, Philadelphia, 1988.

Klish, WJ and Montandon, CM: Nutrition and upper gastrointestinal disorders. In Feldman, EB: Essentials of Clinical Nutrition. FA Davis, Philadelphia, 1988.

Lankford, TR and Jacobs-Steward, PM: Foundations of Normal and Therapeutic Nutrition. John Wiley & Sons, New York, 1986.

Merhav, H, et al: Tea drinking and microcytic anemia in infants. Am J Clin Nutr 41:1210, 1985.

Morse, JM, et al: The effect of maternal fluid intake on breast milk supply: A pilot study. Can J Public Health 83(3):213, 1992.

Muecke, L, et al: Is childhood obesity associated with high-fat foods and low physical activity? J Sch Health 62(1):19, 1992.

Newman, V and Fullerton, JT. Role of nutrition in the prevention of preeclampsia. Journal of Nurse Midwifery 35(5):282, 1990.

Pemberton, CM, et al: Mayo Clinic Diet Manual, ed 6. BC Decker, Philadelphia, 1987.

Reeder, SJ and Martin, LL: Maternity Nursing, ed 16. JB Lippincott, Philadelphia, 1987.

Robinson, CH, et al: Normal and Therapeutic Nutrition, ed 17. Macmillan, New York, 1986.

Steinmetz, G. Fetal alcohol syndrome. National Geographic 181(2):36, 1992.

Subcommittee on Nutritional Status and Weight Gain During Pregnancy and the Subcommittee on Dietary Intake and Nutrient Supplements During Pregnancy of the National Academy of Sciences: Nutrition During Pregnancy. National Academy Press, Washington, DC, 1990.

Thorp, FK, Pierce, P, and Deedwania, C: Nutrition in the infant and young child. In Halpern, SL (ed): Quick Reference to Clinical Nutrition, ed 2. JB Lippincott, Philadelphia, 1987.

Whitney, EB and Cataldo, CB: Understanding Normal and Clinical Nutrition, ed 3. West, St Paul, 1991.

Williams, SR: Nutrition and Diet Therapy, ed 6. Times Mirror-Mosby, St Louis, 1989.

Key Terms

As a study aid, each key term is followed by the page number where the term is defined in the chapter. Terms that appear in **bold face** or <u>underscored</u> in the chapter text are located in the glossary.

Life Cycle Nutrition:
The Young, Middle, and Older Adult

Learning Objectives

After completing this chapter, the student should be able to:

1. Compare average dietary intakes of adults with dietary guidelines
2. Discuss several obstacles to good nutrition in adults.
3. Identify the food groups most likely to be lacking in the diets of adults and foods which are often eaten in excess.
4. Describe the changes in the older adult's body that impact nutritional status.
5. List several suggestions to improve food intake for older persons in a variety of living situations.

*T*he life cycle of human growth and development continues throughout the adult years. Both psychosocial and physical development proceeds as a person matures. This chapter discusses the impact upon nutrition of the physiological and psychosocial changes that occur during young, middle, and older adult years. Because much of the material in this book is based on the nutritional needs of the average adult, the main focus of the present chapter is the older adult.

YOUNG ADULTHOOD

We define young adulthood as ages 18 through 39. Not all 18-year-olds are adults, developmentally. Nor are all 40-year-olds middle-aged in thought or behavior. Chronological age is a convenient means of sorting people but has limited applicability to an individual's interests and abilities.

Developmental Task of Young Adulthood

When identifying the patient's stage of psychosocial development, chronological age is not as important as a person's life situation. During the early years of young adulthood, the individual may be completing the adolescent task of identity. In many cases, our educational system demands dependency past the age of 18. According to Erikson, the developmental task of young adulthood is <u>intimacy.</u> For example, couples who delay commitment to a life partner until their thirties and forties will probably be working at achieving intimacy, whereas other 40-year-old persons may be tackling the task of generativity.

To achieve intimacy, the individual strives to build reciprocal, caring relationships. Intimacy suggests sexuality, but these relationships are not necessarily sexual. Solid friendships are based on intimacy, the revealing of oneself to another. The negative side of intimacy is isolation. Here, perhaps more than with the other developmental tasks, you can see that a person chooses what he or she is to become.

Nutrition in the Young Adult

Throughout this book, the RDAs for individual nutrients, as well as dietary guidelines, have been specified. How well do the dietary intakes of young adults conform to these standards? The age categories cited in the literature differ from our division into young, middle, and older adulthood. Across all the age groupings, however, most adults do not consume recommended intakes.

Fat and Fiber

Women aged 19 to 50 have decreased their average (mean) fat intake from 40.8 percent of kilocalories in 1977–78 to 36.8 percent in 1985 (Thompson, et al, 1992). This still is above the recommended 30 percent.

Because fiber is valuable in assisting the excretion of cholesterol, a high-fiber intake would be desirable if cholesterol intake is high. White women and Hispanic women surveyed consumed less than the maximum recommended 300 milligrams of cholesterol daily; black women consumed 313 milligrams. None of the groups averaged even half the recommended 25 grams of fiber daily.

Fruits and Vegetables

Fruits and vegetables are good sources of fiber as well as vitamins and minerals. Recent survey data indicates only 6 percent of adults aged 19 to 29 consumed at least two servings of fruit and three servings of vegetable on the day recorded (Patterson, et al, 1990).

Consumption of recommended levels of either fruit or vegetable was slightly better: 25 percent of adults aged 19 to 29 consumed three servings of vegetables, and 22 percent had two servings of fruit. This compares with 27 percent of those aged 30 to 54 for vegetables and 26 percent of the same group for fruits (Patterson, et al, 1990).

Although 24-hour recall data is insufficient to evaluate an individual's nutritional status, data from large groups can serve to identify problem areas. The conclusion here is that the average young adult does not eat well. If these adults feed their children the same limited fare, the next generation will learn no better.

MIDDLE ADULTHOOD

We define the middle adult years as those between ages 40 and 65. Mandatory retirement rules in the past designated age 65 as the beginning of old age. Now the entry and exit points for middle age are more flexible.

Developmental Task of Middle Adulthood

To achieve generativity, the person guides the next generation to adopt similar values and follow a path parallel to the mentor's. In this way, a middle-aged adult can attain a measure of immortality. This can be accomplished through influencing not only one's own children, but also one's students or one's protégé at work.

Nutrition in Middle Adulthood

As is true of the young adult, only a small minority of middle-aged adults report meeting or exceeding their RDAs or dietary guidelines on a given day. Middle-aged adults consumed a slightly better diet in regard to fruits and vegetables than did young adults.

Compared with 6 percent of adults 19 to 29, 8 percent of those aged 30 to 54 consumed at least two servings of fruit and three servings of vegetable on the day recorded. This compares with 13 percent of adults aged 55 to 74 (Patterson, et al, 1990).

Consumption of recommended levels of either fruit or vegetable: 27 percent of adults aged 30 to 54 consumed three servings of vegetables and 26 percent had two servings of fruit. This compares with 28 percent of those aged 55 to 74 for vegetables and 40 percent of the same age group for fruits (Patterson, et al, 1990).

The data indicates the average adult does not meet the RDAs or abide by the Food Pyramid Guidelines. Only 9 percent of all adults consumed three servings of vegetables and two servings of fruits on the survey day. The proportion of adults who did so increased with age. Of the subgroups studied, none of the 19- to 54-year-olds were better than the average at consuming three servings of vegetables and two servings of fruit. White men and women aged 55 to 74 were the only subgroups of whom more than 9 percent met or exceeded the guidelines: 12 percent of the men, and 13 percent of the women.

OLDER ADULTHOOD

Older adults traditionally have been defined as those over the age of 65. For years, that was the typical retirement age. It is still recognized by various governmental units as the gateway to Social Security benefits, Medicare coverage, extra income tax deductions, and property tax reductions.

Changes in the Elderly Population

Our older population is changing demographically. These changes and underlying causes are discussed next.

Population Characteristics

Life expectancy—The probable number of years that persons of a given age may be expected to live.

Saying that the older population has changed since the benchmark of age 65 was established grossly understates the case. In 1900, the **life expectancy** was 45 years. Currently, the life expectancy for women is 78 years and for men it is 71 years. In 1900, 4 percent of the population was over age 65; now the percentage is at 12 percent and growing. Barring major calamities, by early in the next century 20 percent of the population will be over 65 years of age; 11 percent will be over 75 years of age.

Reasons for the Changes

This transformation is attributed to improved sanitation, increased concern about safety, and control of communicable diseases. In 1900, 1 in 10 infants died; now the figure is 1 in 100, despite the fact that smaller infants are surviving. In the days of the "Wild West," a woman usually died before her youngest child left home, and a man could have a horse that lived as long as he did. The average life span of horses is 25 years. The work world was harsh. Children worked in heavy industry. The death of one miner a week in a relatively small mining operation was commonplace.

Today the major causes of death in adults are heart disease, cancer, and stroke. All of them are linked to lifestyle, including a nutritional component.

DISTINCTIONS AMONG OLDER ADULTS

As a group, older adults display a wide range of interests and abilities. Some will be content to stay at home and work in the garden. Others will travel extensively. Only 10 percent are confined in any serious way. A roomful of 3-year-old children will be more like one another than a roomful of 70-year-old adults. Figure 11-1 shows a man whose image we hope you will retain as a symbol of the uniqueness of each individual's life experience.

Lifelong Habits

In old age, people become more like themselves, accentuating traits they have had all along. Many older persons have difficulty changing their behavior patterns, including those related to food.

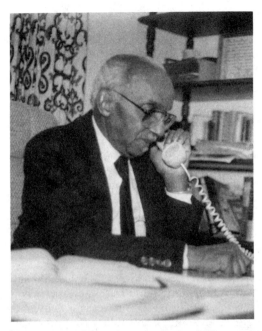

FIGURE 11–1. This man represents the uniqueness of life experiences of all elderly people. Although the elderly may share a few characteristics in common, it is grossly unfair to say that they are all alike.

Economic Differences

Financially, too, a broad range is evident. The average income of older men is $10,000 per year, of older women $5,000 per year. Half of older black women have incomes of less than $1,000 per year. Despite these low averages, 50 percent of older Americans need no financial assistance from the government.

Inaccuracy of Stereotypes

The stereotype of the old folks in a nursing home is just that, a stereotype. Only 5 percent of older adults live in nursing homes. However, that 5 percent represents more than 1 million patients. This subgroup of the older population has special nutrient needs. Up to 50 percent cannot feed themselves. Often they have very low calcium intakes and low intakes of vitamin A, vitamin C, thiamin, riboflavin, and iron. If they do not get sufficient sun exposure or do not consume fortified dairy products, they are at increased risk for vitamin D deficiency.

PSYCHOSOCIAL DEVELOPMENT

The developmental task for older adults to achieve is <u>integrity.</u> Those who accomplish this task will look back on their lives as worthwhile. Although they may have suffered some failures and have some regrets, they are able to see their lives in perspective. They can forgive themselves for their faults because they know they did the best they could with what they had.

Socially, the older adult faces tremendous adjustments when a spouse of many years dies. The accompanying depression and new responsibility for tasks the spouse performed may significantly affect food intake.

THE AGING BODY

Just as adolescents face a changing body image, so do older adults. Even without frank disease, the physical abilities of the older adult diminish. Middle-age spread gives way to dwindling bulk and waning strength. Living with the bodies they have challenges the old to adjust. Among the body systems significantly changed in the aging process are the integumentary, sensory, gastrointestinal, urinary, musculoskeletal, nervous, endocrine, and cardiovascular systems.

Integumentary System

Many changes take place in the skin as a person ages. As subcutaneous fat is lost, the skin becomes dry and wrinkled. Less elasticity is present to spring back after a pinch, so using this method to test for dehydration is unreliable. The older adult also loses some of the ability to synthesize vitamin D from sunshine. Compared with a younger person, someone over 65 produces only one half the vitamin D from a given dose of sunshine as a younger person does (MacLaughlin and Hollic, 1985).

Sensory System

Four senses become markedly less acute as a person ages: vision, hearing, taste, and smell. Because the sense receptors do not deteriorate equally, some of the sense loss is attributed to changes in the central nervous system. Again, extensive variations exist among individuals.

Eyes

Cataract—Clouding of the lens of the eye.

Vision is reduced. The person sees reds, oranges, and yellows better than blues and violets. Clouding of the lens of the eye, a **cataract,** decreases overall vision. The fine print labeling food items may be illegible to the elderly. Older eyes do not adjust well to glare. These changes in vision may make grocery shopping burdensome. Food preparation may become not only difficult but also hazardous if the person cannot see adequately.

Ears

The sound receptors in the inner ear deteriorate. First to be lost is the ability to perceive high tones. The older person with poor hearing usually will pick up men's voices better than women's. Hearing aids do not fully compensate for the hearing loss. In fact, they often magnify sideline noise to the point of distraction. The result may be social isolation when it becomes too laborious to interact with others. Socializing at meals may become embarrassing or frustrating, and thus avoided.

Nose and Tongue

For the sense of taste to function well, the sense of smell must also be intact. Food tastes bland when your nose is plugged up with a head cold. Older adults have dulled senses of smell and taste. The peak acuity of the sense of smell is between 20 and 40 years of age. In the tongue, receptors for sweet and salty taste deteriorate before those for bitter and sour. For this reason, older persons may start to lavish sugar and salt on their food.

Gastrointestinal System

Particularly crucial to nutriture is the gastrointestinal system. Hundreds of processes are required for the proper digestion, absorption, and metabolism of foods. Many functions of the gastrointestinal system decline significantly in older people.

Half of Americans lose their teeth by the age of 65. The term for being without teeth is **edentulous.** The major cause of tooth loss in the older adult is not dental caries but **periodontal disease,** which affects the gums. Dentures, like hearing aids, only partially substitute for the real thing. Furthermore, a denture cannot be effective if the underlying tissue is in poor condition.

The production of saliva decreases sharply in the older adult. This results in **xerostomia.** Chewing and swallowing become more difficult and food intake may be affected. Also with age, less mucus and smaller quantities of enzymes are secreted. Decreased amounts of gastric acid are secreted after the age of 50. An extreme case, **achlorhydria,** the absence of hydrochloric acid in the stomach, may interfere with protein digestion and with vitamin and mineral absorption. Vitamin B_{12} and iron are of special concern.

Intestinal **motility** decreases because of lessened muscle tone. Medications may interfere with electrolyte balance, also diminishing muscle tone. By the age of 70, the liver loses 18 percent of its weight and has reduced capabilities.

Edentulous—The state of having no teeth.

Periodontal disease—Any disorder of the supporting structures of the teeth.

Xerostomia—Dry mouth caused by decreased salivary secretions.

Achlorhydria—Absence of free hydrochloric acid in stomach.

Motility—Ability to move spontaneously.

Urinary System

The kidneys lose about 10 percent of their weight by the time an adult reaches the age of 70. At age 80, the blood flow to the kidneys is one half of what it was at age 35. This compromised kidney function makes reliance on urine samples for nutrient analyses less reliable in the elderly. Renal function can be measured by a **blood urea nitrogen (BUN)** test. An increase in the BUN level usually indicates a decrease in function. Patients with even slightly elevated BUNs may not be able to excrete the waste products from protein metabolism. Thus care must be taken when giving high-protein nutritional supplements to older persons with elevated BUNs.

Blood urea nitrogen (BUN)—The amount of nitrogen present in the blood as urea.

Musculoskeletal System

The major loss of body mass in the older adult is loss of muscle mass. By age 70, skeletal muscle diminishes by 40 percent. Because muscle is a more active tissue than fat, energy needs decline with the diminished muscle mass.

Perhaps more noticeable than the overall loss of muscle is the loss of height in older people. The average lifetime loss of height amounts to 2.9 centimeters (1.16 inches) in men and 4.9 centimeters (1.96 inches) in women. A major cause of this loss of height is osteoporosis, the loss of bone mass.

An estimated one third of postmenopausal women have osteoporosis. This condition is more conspicuous in women than in men because women have smaller skeletons than men. For the same reason, white women are affected more often than black women. Women who develop osteoporosis begin to lose bone at the approximate age of 35. The loss amounts to about 8 percent per decade, so that by the age of 70, 25 percent of the bone structure is gone.

One hazard of the weakened skeleton is the possibility of fractures. **Kyphosis,** or humpback, is characteristic of osteoporosis. In these patients kyphosis is caused by fractures of the spine but other pathologies are possible. Two other fractures often due to osteoporosis are those of the femur (commonly called a broken hip) and of the wrist. About 200,000 cases of fractured hip are recorded each year in the United States. Almost 30 percent of those patients die within a year.

Kyphosis—Exaggerated thoracic curvature of spine; humpback.

Up to the age of 80, women are afflicted with osteoporosis four times as often as men. After age of 80, occurrence by sex is equal. In men, bone loss begins later, at about age of 50. Men lose about 3 percent per decade.

Joint surfaces are roughened by **arthritis.** By the age of 50, one half of all adults have this degenerative joint disease. Arthritis impairs the use of the hands for opening jars, chopping raw foods, and cutting cooked foods at the table. Arthritis also impairs the operation of the mandibular joint of the jaw for chewing.

Arthritis—Inflammatory condition of the joints, usually accompanied by pain and swelling.

Nervous System

By the time a person reaches old age, the brain has endured a lifetime of stressors. Brain cells are not replaced as they are destroyed. Consequently, the number of brain cells is decreased. Blood flow to brain decreases due to narrowing of the arteries. Thirst sensation becomes less operative, increasing the risk of uncompensated dehydration. Adaptation to stress is less effective as people age. For instance, **mortality** from heat stroke rises sharply after age 60.

Mortality—The death rate; number of deaths per unit of population.

Endocrine System

The older person is slowing down. Resting energy expenditure (REE) decreases, especially in the brain, skeletal muscle, and the heart. The older adult's REE may be 10 to 12 percent less than a younger person's. Lost muscle mass is replaced, if at all, by adipose tissue which is less active metabolically than muscle.

Cardiovascular System

As the older adult continues to age, there is (1) a decrease in cardiac output and (2) a slower heart rate. In response to exercise, the heart rate does not increase as effectively as in youth, nor does it return to normal as rapidly. Because of these diminishments, the elderly are at risk for diseases of the heart. Dietary modifications for heart disease are discussed in Chapter 17.

NUTRITIONAL NEEDS OF THE OLDER ADULT

Available evidence suggests that older persons need almost the same intake from all nutrients as do other adults, with the exception of kilocalories. Energy needs decrease with age. Thus, there is less leeway for indiscretions and empty kilocalories in the diet.

Energy Nutrients

Energy needs take priority in the utilization of nutrients. When necessary, glucose can be manufactured from proteins or fats.

Energy Needs Decrease with Age

Estimates of the decrease in energy needed by older adults average about 5 percent per decade after the age of 40. As with younger people, the simplest criterion for the suitability of intake is the maintenance of normal weight.

Desirability of Exercise

Older persons do benefit from exercise. Old age is not necessarily a detriment to good health. The current recommendation is that older adults should have 20 minutes of aerobic exercise three or four times per week. Besides contributing to weight control by increasing muscular metabolism, exercise increases circulation to the brain. Measurable training effects can be seen almost immediately. In one study, after 8 weeks of weight training a small group of 90-year-old men and women showed an increase in muscle bulk and strength (Fiatrone, et al, 1990). Functional abilities improved. Two subjects no longer used canes to walk at the conclusion of the study. Another person, unable to rise from a sitting position without using the arms, did so before the end of the training period.

Distribution of Energy Nutrients

The proportion of energy to be obtained from each of the energy nutrients is changed slightly for older adults. They should derive 50 to 60 percent of their kilocalories from carbohydrates. Fats should contribute 20 to 30 percent of the kilocalories. Limiting fats should also increase comfort, mainly because fat absorption is delayed in older persons, causing early satiety.

An intake of protein at the level of 0.8 gram per kilogram of healthy body weight still should amount to 12 percent of total kilocalories. Some authorities suggest increasing the protein allotment for the elderly. No consistent relationship between protein intake and serum albumin level has been found in elderly people, however (Freedman and Ahronheim, 1985). One reason for this may be related to liver function. A normally functioning liver is necessary to construct albumin molecules from the ingested protein and resulting amino acids. If liver function is impaired, no amount of intake will produce normal blood albumin levels. An additional reason for moderate protein intake concerns calcium use. A high protein intake also increases calcium loss in the urine.

Vitamins

Vitamin intake and usage are potential problems for the elderly. Deficiencies of vitamins A, D, C, and niacin, and B_{12} are most frequently of concern. Excesses are possible, also, especially in persons who self-medicate on megadoses of vitamins.

Fat-Soluble Vitamins

Because fat-soluble vitamins are stored in the body, it may take a long time for a deficiency to present clinical signs. Although common findings for groups of the elderly will be discussed here, survey data are not applicable to individual cases. Assessment of the individual is the only means to pinpoint a person's practices and risks.

VITAMIN A   Vitamin A plays a role in bone metabolism. Children with vitamin A deficiency have erratic bone growth, stunting of some bones and overgrowth of others. In the elderly, excessive levels of vitamin A are associated with increased bone loss.

VITAMIN D   Most of a person's vitamin D is synthesized in the skin. This process is substantially reduced in the older adult. Milk is an excellent source of vitamin D because of fortification. The elderly person who is likely to be deficient in vitamin D, then, is the one who stays indoors and does not consume enough milk or milk products.

Water-Soluble Vitamins

Water-soluble vitamins are not stored in the body to any great extent. Consequently, it is imperative that everyone, including the elderly, have vitamin C and the B-complex vitamins supplied regularly.

VITAMIN C   The RDA for older adults is the same amount of vitamin C, 60 milligrams, as for younger adults. Older adults living at home generally have a better vitamin C status than those living in institutions. The independent elderly may spend more on fruits and vegetables than institutions do, or the vitamin C in foods may be destroyed by poor cooking and serving practices in institutions.

B VITAMINS   Older adults who eat little meat and consume little milk or milk products containing tryptophan are at risk for niacin deficiency. Older adults have decreased gastric juice, which contains intrinsic factor. Because of this, senior adults may develop a vitamin B_{12} deficiency. In one study, 12 percent of the subjects displayed vitamin B_{12} deficiency (Cooley, et al, 1991).

Minerals

Minerals become embedded in the structure of the body. The chief mineral in the body is calcium. It should come as no surprise that calcium levels are an area of concern in caring for the elderly.

Calcium

It is estimated that more than 80 percent of adult women and 50 percent of adult men do not consume the RDA for calcium. For both sexes, the RDA is

800 milligrams, or 2.7 milk exchanges. Experts are still debating whether or not the postmenopausal woman needs more than this amount. Until the issue is resolved, older women should be encouraged to consume foods containing the RDA for calcium. Remember that the calcium in supplements is very poorly absorbed.

Skeletal demineralization may be lessened by taking 1500 milligrams of calcium per day and exercising for 1 hour four times a week. This program has not been shown to remineralize bone, but fracture frequency decreased as much as with estrogen therapy (Feldman, 1988). Estrogen replacement therapy is advocated by some physicians because it may retard bone loss after menopause. Such a program for an individual woman should be adopted only after careful consultation with her physician. Nurses should also refer questions about calcium supplementation to the physician.

Iron

Decreased gastric acidity, whether due to aging or to antacid use, impairs iron absorption. Despite this fact, average iron intake is generally adequate until age 75. After that, less meat and more cereal is eaten. Heme iron in meat is absorbed much more readily than nonheme iron in grains and vegetables. As some cereals are fortified with iron, deficiency need not be the inevitable result of eating more cereal if selections are appropriate.

Groups at higher than average risk for iron deficiency are members of lower socioeconomic groups and black women. Anemia is not always the result of aging or nutritional deficits. Hidden blood losses should be suspected and their sources sought in the anemic elderly person, just as in younger patients.

Water

Many older persons have problems maintaining fluid balance. Sometimes the difficulty is self-inflicted. Loss of sphincter muscle tone in women and difficulty urinating in men may prompt older people to limit fluids. Older adults need 6 to 8 glasses of water per day, enough to produce about 1.5 liters of urine (see Clinical Application 11–1).

Dehydration in the elderly can result in abnormal functioning. One of the signs of dehydration in the elderly is confusion. If no one is alert to these mental changes, the person may compound his or her difficulties by forget-

---

✿ CLINICAL APPLICATION 11–1 ✿
Tallying Fluid Intake at Home

The person who is truly motivated will think of a way to obtain needed nutrients, even water. One person takes six glasses out of the cupboard every morning and places them by the sink. During the day, each drink of water is taken from a clean glass. Afterwards, the glass is put in a different location. When all the clean glasses are used, the person has achieved the desired water intake for the day without having to count the number of glasses.

TABLE 11–1 *Signs of Dehydration in the Elderly*

Body System	Sign
Skin and mucous membranes	Warm and dry
	Decreased turgor (pinch test); may be inaccurate due to loss of elasticity in aging skin
	Furrowed tongue
	Elevated temperature
Cardiovascular	Elevated pulse
Urinary	Increased specific gravity
	Increased urinary sodium
Musculoskeletal	Weakness
Neurological	Confusion

ting to take medications or eat meals. Table 11–1 lists the signs of dehydration in the elderly.

Patients who are immobilized may need as many as 12 to 14 glasses of water per day. Immobility increases the calcium loss from bones. The high serum calcium level is controlled by the kidney. A large fluid intake keeps the urine dilute so that the calcium does not form stones.

COMMON PROBLEMS RELATED TO NUTRITION

Although constipation, obesity, and low protein intake are common problems that are not unique to the elderly, they do represent special geriatric concerns. *Geriatric* means of or related to the aged, and **geriatrics** is the branch of medicine involved in the study and treatment of diseases in the elderly.

Geriatrics—The branch of medicine involved in the study and treatment of diseases in the elderly.

Constipation

A person may complain of acute <u>constipation,</u> which is the lack of stools, or chronic constipation, which is general difficulty passing bowel movements. Customary methods used to achieve bowel regularity include increasing fluid intake, consuming high-fiber foods, taking time for elimination, and exercising.

Doubling the person's water intake, medical conditions permitting, is the first place to start. Loading the diet with fresh fruits and vegetables is the second. Time should be set aside every day to have a bowel movement, preferably in the morning after drinking a warm beverage. Lastly, exercise is noteworthy in promoting regular bowel movements.

Older adults sometimes adopt the routine use of laxatives to correct bowel habits. For such persons, the program mentioned above will not provide instant resolution. However, if the regimen is adhered to, it is possible to overcome even long-standing constipation. Occasionally, a person who is passing liquid stool is actually constipated (Clinical Application 11–2).

CLINICAL APPLICATION 11–2
Distinguishing Diarrhea from Fecal Impaction

If a patient usually is constipated and then has diarrhea, the nurse should check the rectum for impacted stool. The stool will be dry and hard and the patient will not be able to pass it unassisted. The diarrheal stool is passed around the impaction. This type of constipation is not treated with diet. As in many cases, prevention is preferable to diagnosis and treatment. Institutionalized patients should be monitored for elimination problems. Frequency and consistency of bowel movements should be charted.

Obesity

Since weight control is the subject of Chapter 15, only brief mention of obesity in the elderly appears here. For a person to have lived more than 65 years, some correct lifestyle choices must have been made. Weight reduction should be pursued if it is needed to treat current problems, such as diabetes mellitus, but not to prevent new ones (Feldman, 1988). Only modest changes should be suggested and these should be introduced gradually. Concentrating on changing one behavior at a time may help avert further weight gain. For example, you could encourage a patient who is gaining weight to substitute skimmed milk for whole or 2 percent milk.

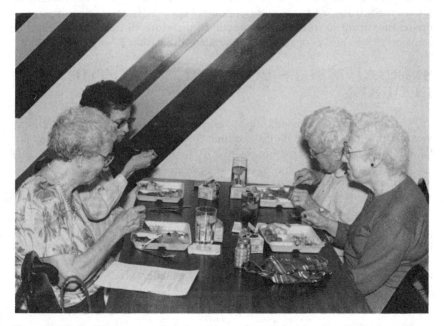

FIGURE 11–2. This group of senior citizens is participating in a federal meal program. The program provides not only food, but also a social activity and a regular schedule.

CLINICAL APPLICATION 11–3

Learning to Eat with Dentures

Persons need to learn to use dentures one step at a time. The steps are in exactly the same order as those used by infants learning to eat. The person should first practice swallowing liquids with the dentures in place. After this is mastered, soft foods can be chewed. Lastly, the person should learn to bite regular foods with the dentures. Splitting up the learning process into manageable units helps to make this process less frustrating for the new denture wearer.

Low Protein Intake

The main reason older adults do not eat enough protein is the lack of money. To rectify the situation, the federal government, with an amendment to the Older Americans Act, established meal programs for senior citizens. Low-cost meals are offered at central gathering places and/or delivered to the homebound. Figure 11–2 illustrates a group of senior citizens participating in one such meal program.

Again, individual assessment is the key to planning nutritional care. For example, milk-based supplements that are both nutrient-dense and easy to consume might be a dietary recommendation for the person who cannot chew. To accommodate dentures, the person may reduce his or her intake of meats, fresh fruits, and vegetables, and may need assistance selecting appropriate substitute items. A recommended procedure for learning to eat and drink with dentures is discussed in Clinical Application 11–3.

SPECIAL ISSUES FOR SCREENING THE ELDERLY

Although elderly persons are not all alike, they do share some problems in common that occur frequently enough to bear special mention. These are listed as topics to be assessed in the elderly in Table 11–2.

INTERVENTIONS

Suggestions to increase the nourishment of elderly patients appear in Table 11–3. Keep in mind that there is no single answer suitable for every problem. The nurse's role in nourishing the hospitalized elderly patient is discussed in Clinical Application 11–4. Obtaining adequate food for a patient undergoing many diagnostic procedures may tax the nurse's ingenuity.

NUTRITION EDUCATION FOR ADULTS

Because none of the age groups of adults are remarkable in complying with the recommended food intake, some general suggestions for improve-

TABLE 11-2 *Topics to be Assessed in the Elderly**

Oral Cavity Function
- Difficulty tasting, changes in taste perception
- Bleeding gums, dry mouth
- Difficulty chewing, toothaches, poorly fitting dentures
- Foods patient is unable to eat

Meal Management
- Who shops? Where? Ease of making food decisions?
- Transportation problems?
- Budgeting a concern? Knowledge to make informed choices?
- Who cooks? Knowledge and skill level?
- Refrigeration, storage, and cooking facilities?
- Ability to manage containers: jars, cans, bottles

Psychosocial Factors
- Where are most meals eaten?
- Mealtime companions?
- Recent change in living conditions?
- Satisfaction with situation?

*In addition to the normal assessment, that is, appetite or weight changes, bowel habits.

TABLE 11-3 *Increasing Food Intake in the Elderly*

Get the Person Ready for Meals
- Provide oral hygiene before meals to freshen and moisten mouth.
- Suggest smokers refrain for 1 hour before meal to increase appetite.
- Allow 4 to 5 hours between meals and supplements to permit hunger to develop.

Promote Social Interaction
- Encourage potluck meals with friends for those who live alone.
- Combine meal at senior center with an activity of interest.
- Encourage alert nursing home residents to choose compatible mealtime companions.
- Control the noise in the dining room to avoid overstimulating those with hearing aids.

Serve Food Attractively
- Vary textures, colors, flavors.
- To increase vegetable intake, offer raw, crisp-cooked, or marinated as appetizers.
- Use "good" dishes and flatware, centerpieces, tablecloths, or place mats.
- Provide enough nonglaring light to see food clearly.

Obtain Outside Help
- Home health aide to shop, do basic fix-ahead preparations
- Meals on Wheels for homebound
- Food stamps, surplus commodity programs for those eligible
- Instructional materials on food purchasing, storage, cooking from county extension service

CLINICAL APPLICATION 11–4
Hospitalization of the Elderly

Regardless of where you choose to practice nursing, with the exception of obstetrics and pediatrics, you will have elderly patients under your care. Eighty percent of the elderly, compared with 40 percent of people less than 65 years old, have one or more chronic diseases.

Change is stressful. Hospitalization is a change for anyone but is especially stressful for the elderly. Older persons are unable to stand starvation for more than 5 days because they lack nutritional reserves (Feldman, 1988). Serving no food to a patient because of diagnostic tests is starvation. The conscientious nurse obtains meals or feedings for the patient who was NPO (i.e., who was allowed "nothing by mouth") for breakfast and lunch. There is nothing magical about the times of 8 AM–12 NOON–6 PM for meals. The committed nurse will arrange for adequate nourishment for patients, despite scheduling difficulties. Dietary staff have no idea when an individual patient is finished with tests for the day until notified as such by the nurse.

ment are pertinent to the majority of adults. As always, for individual counseling an individual assessment is needed.

Fat consumption is excessive, especially in the poor. Modifications in food preparation techniques could decrease these fat kilocalories. For example, an estimated 71 percent of the time, poultry is eaten without efforts to minimize its fat content. For pork the estimate is 68 percent of the time (Thompson, et al, 1992).

Fruits and vegetable consumption is very low. Neither fruit nor vegetable was consumed by 11 percent of adults surveyed. Almost half of the adults, 45 percent, reported having no servings of fruit or juice, and 22 percent had no servings of vegetables. Even when two servings of vegetables were reported, 21 percent of the adults consumed two servings of the same vegetable (Patterson, et al, 1990).

Most adults could benefit from instruction in the key concepts of nutrition: balance, variety, and moderation. The alert nurse has an important contribution to make in identifying knowledge deficits and impaired health practices related to nutrition. This responsibility applies to all patients receiving nursing care, not only those with obvious nutrition-related medical diagnoses.

Summary

Surveys have indicated that a majority of adults do not follow the Food Pyramid guidelines or the RDAs for some nutrients. Of special concern is excessive fat intake, despite recent declines in consumption. Low fiber intake is another problem. Adequacy of vitamin and mineral intake is in question when 91 percent of persons did not consume the recommended two servings of fruits and three servings of vegetables in the period surveyed. Consequently, the need for nutrition education among adults is apparent. Healthcare workers who are motivated to seek optimal health for their patients will use every opportunity to teach better food selection and practices.

Changing social, economic, and physical circumstances affect the nutritional status of the elderly patient. When a spouse dies, grief, depression, and poor appetite often overcome the widow or widower. Learning to live on Social Security benefits, pensions, and savings may place a strain on some elderly persons.

With age, secretions decrease along the entire gastrointestinal tract. Nutrients that require an acid medium for maximum utilization, including vitamins C and B_{12}, will be affected. Lack of outdoor activity, dislike for milk, and decreasing effectiveness of the skin's synthesis of vitamin D all place the older person at risk for vitamin D deficiency. The senses of taste and smell become less keen. Having to wear dentures may compound the problem of inadequate intake. Decreased mobility and declining vision can cause food procurement and preparation to become even more difficult.

However, all elderly persons are not affected equally by the aging process. This makes an individual assessment crucial to providing adequate nutritional care.

A case study and a sample plan of care appear below. Both are designed to show you how the information you have studied in this chapter can be used in nursing practice.

CASE STUDY 11–1

Mr. E. is a 75-year-old widower. He recently had surgery for cataracts and subsequently gave up driving his car. His home is two blocks off the bus route and eight blocks from the nearest supermarket. Mr. E. has moderately painful knees from arthritis. He has been taking the bus to the supermarket every other day so that he could manage one package on the way home. He has confided to the nurse in his doctor's office that he is ready to "just give up. It's too much trouble to eat any more." Mr. E.'s weight today is 160 pounds, 5 pounds less than last month.

Assessment
Subjective
Restricted vision led to inability to drive a car safely
Dependent on public transportation
Painful knees
Verbalized discouragement with procuring food
Objective
Weight loss of 5 pounds in past month

Nursing Diagnosis
Health maintenance, altered: related to impaired mobility outside of home, as evidenced by verbalization to nurse and weight loss of 5 pounds in past month

Desired Outcome/Evaluation Criteria
1. Mr. E. will acknowledge need for assistance with meals to stop losing weight by end of visit today.
2. Given several options of community support, Mr. E. will select one and begin to implement the change within 3 days.

Nursing Actions/Interventions with Rationales in Italics

1. Discuss Mr. E.'s weight change with him. Determine what kind of assistance he would accept. *Patients are likely to change behaviors only if the new behavior is acceptable to them.*

2. Describe Senior Citizen Nutrition Program, Meals on Wheels, home health aide shopping service, and door-to-door Care-a-Van service. Explore social support available from family and less restricted friends. *Patients may know about these programs but prefer to remain independent. Allowing the patient some time to choose makes the choice more his own.*

3. Nurse to follow-up with telephone call in 3 days. *Following up with a telephone call shows the nurse is committed to working through this problem with Mr. E.*

STUDY AIDS

Chapter Review Questions

1. The sense of taste diminishes with age. Which of the following sensations usually are missed first?
   a. Bitter and sour
   b. Salty and sour
   c. Salty and sweet
   d. Sour and sweet

2. The major cause of tooth loss in the elderly is:
   a. Dental caries
   b. Periodontal disease
   c. Scurvy
   d. Vitamin D deficiency

3. Which of the following changes contribute to the danger of dehydration in the elderly?
   a. Constipation and atherosclerosis of the brain
   b. Decreased REE and decreased skeletal muscle mass
   c. Diminished gastrointestinal mucus and slowed peristalsis
   d. Less active thirst mechanism and impaired kidney function

4. A nurse making a home visit routinely screens for dehydration in elderly patients. Which of the following would the nurse assess?
   a. Body temperature and urine specific gravity
   b. Tongue condition, pulse rate, and muscle strength
   c. Skin turgor and heart and lung sounds
   d. Patient's Intake and Output records

5. Which of the following conditions is likely to contribute to vitamin D deficiency in older adults?
   a. Atrophied skin, dislike for milk, and indoor life
   b. Lack of exercise, failing hearing and vision
   c. Slowed peristalsis, diminished secretion of intrinsic factor
   d. Achlorhydria and inability to chew meats

6. Osteoporosis is related to:
   a. Consumption of toxic chemicals
   b. Fat and cholesterol intake
   c. Lack of exercise and low vitamin D intake
   d. Race, sex, and lifetime health practices

7. The person who is recently widowed may have anorexia. Which of the following suggestions would address the psychosocial cause of this lack of appetite?
   a. Attending group activities and meals at a senior citizens' center
   b. Ordering Meals on Wheels
   c. Encouraging the person to make a "company" meal for herself or himself
   d. Vigorous exercise before meals

8. Which of the following proportions of kilocalories from the energy nutrients are recommended for elderly people?
   a. 45 percent carbohydrate, 40 percent fat, 15 percent protein
   b. 50 percent carbohydrate, 35 percent fat, 15 percent protein
   c. 55 percent carbohydrate, 33 percent fat, 12 percent protein
   d. 60 percent carbohydrate, 28 percent fat, 12 percent protein

9. Which of the following statements is true?
   a. Young adults have built up enough reserve nutrients so that poor intake in the years 18 to 29 is unimportant.
   b. Sources of dietary protein should be increased in the diets of most older adults.
   c. Older adults have the largest proportion of their group meeting or exceeding the Food Pyramid guidelines for fruits and vegetables.
   d. Black people adequately compensate for a high cholesterol intake by consuming a higher-than-recommended fiber intake.

10. Nutritional treatment of constipation in the elderly includes all of the following except one. Identify the *exception*.
   a. Eliminating seedy foods
   b. Increasing fluid intake
   c. Increasing the amount of raw vegetables consumed
   d. Taking a warm beverage in the morning

NCLEX-Style Quiz

Situation One

Ms. O. is a 66-year-old retired schoolteacher who suffered a stroke 8 months ago. For the past 7 months she has resided in a nursing home. Ms. O is paralyzed on her right side. She has not mastered the use of tableware with her left hand. Her nurse is concerned because Ms. O weighs 125 pounds, compared with 135 pounds upon admission to the nursing home. The nursing assistants report that Ms. O. takes a little of most foods but refuses to eat more than half of any of the foods.

1. Which of the following areas should the nurse assess first to try to resolve Ms. O.'s weight loss problem?
   a. Possible allergies to the preservatives used in dried foods
   b. The medical chart for history of fad dieting
   c. The meaning of food in Ms. O.'s life just now
   d. Ms. O.'s abdomen for evidence of distention

2. The nurse discovers that a contributing factor in Ms. O.'s refusal to eat is embarrassment over her inability to control her lips. Which of the following outcomes would be appropriate in this case?
   a. Patient will gain 5 pounds in the next 2 weeks.
   b. Patient will consume ¾ of the food served within 1 week.
   c. Patient will feed herself with her left hand within the next 3 weeks.
   d. Physician will prescribe a tube feeding for Ms. O.

3. Which of the following nursing actions is appropriate initially to minimize Ms. O.'s embarrassment?
   a. Allowing her to eat her meals alone in her room
   b. Ordering finger foods that she can eat with her left hand
   c. Assigning her to a table with other stroke patients who feed themselves
   d. Instructing the nursing assistants to feed Ms. O. privately

4. Which of the following activities could reasonably be expected to increase Ms. O.'s appetite?
   a. Participating in a craft session before lunch
   b. Taking a nap before dinner
   c. Practicing walking before lunch or dinner
   d. Watching television with her roommate after breakfast

5. The next routine care conference for Ms. O. is 2 months from now. The nurse correctly decides to:
   a. Put Ms. O. on the agenda for this week's interdisciplinary care conference.
   b. Refer the problem to Administration.
   c. Ask Ms. O.'s family to come in at mealtimes to feed her for 2 months.
   d. Discuss Ms. O.'s problem with the physician tomorrow.

BIBLIOGRAPHY

Ali, NS: Teaching osteoporosis prevention. Advancing Clinical Care 6(2):32, 1991.

Bortz, WM: Disuse and aging. JAMA 248:1203, 1982.

Brown, JE: The Science of Human Nutrition. Harcourt Brace Jovanovich, San Diego, 1990.

Coodley, G, et al: Malnutrition in the elderly. Geriatric Medicine Today 10(2):45, 1991.

Eliopoulos, C: Caring for the Elderly in Diverse Care Settings. JB Lippincott, Philadelphia, 1990.

Feldman, EB: Essentials of Clinical Nutrition. FA Davis, Philadelphia, 1988.

Fiatrone, MA, et al: High intensity strength training in nonagenarians. JAMA 263:3029, 1990.

Freedman, ML and Ahronheim, JC: Nutritional needs of the elderly: Debate and recommendations. Geriatrics 40:45, 1986.

Hamilton, EMN, Whitney, EN, and Sizer, FS: Nutrition Concepts and Controversies, ed 2. West, St Paul, 1991.

Hay, EK: That old hip. Nurs Clin North Am 26:43, 1991.

Koehler, KM, Hunt, WC, and Garry, PT: Meat, poultry, and fish consumption and nutrient intake in the healthy elderly. J Am Diet Assoc 92(3):325, 1992.

MacLaughlin, J and Hollic, MF: Aging decreases the capacity of human skin to produce vitamin D_3. Journal of Clinical Investigation 76:1536, 1985.

MacLean, TB: Influence of psychosocial development and life events on the health practices of adults. Issues in Mental Health Nursing 13(4):403, 1992.

Miller, CA: Nursing Care of Older Adults. Scott, Foresman/Little, Brown Higher Education, Glenview, IL, 1990.

Patterson, BH, et al: Fruit and vegetables in the American diet: Data from the NHANES II survey. AJPH 80(12):1443, 1990.

Pritikin, N and Cisney, N: Dietary recommendations for older Americans. In Dychtwald, K (ed): Wellness and Health Promotion for the Elderly. Aspen Systems, Rockville, MD, 1986.

Russell, RM, Sahyoun, NR, and Whinston-Perry, R: Nutritional assessment. In Calkins, E, Davis, PJ, and Ford, AB (eds): The Practice of Geriatrics. WB Saunders, Philadelphia, 1986.

Stutte, RC. Health promotion in the young adult: Instrument development. Texas Women's University, Denton, TX, 1990. Thesis.

Thompson, FE, et al: Sources of fiber and fat in diets of US women aged 19 to 50: Implications for nutrition education and policy. APHJ 82(5):695, 1992.

Verdery, RB: 'Wasting Away' of the old old: Can it be—and should it be treated? Geriatrics 45(6):26, 1990.

Whitney, EB and Cataldo, CB: Understanding Normal and Clinical Nutrition, ed 3. West, St Paul, 1991.

Williams, SR: Nutrition and Diet Therapy, ed 6. Times Mirror-Mosby, St Louis, 1989.

Chapter Outline

Key Terms

As a study aid, each key term is followed by the page number where the term is defined in the chapter. Terms that appear in **boldface** or <u>underscored</u> in the chapter text are located in the glossary.

Food Preparation, Storage, and Safety

Learning Objectives

After completing this chapter, the student should be able to:

1. Describe the conditions under which microbiological food illnesses can occur.
2. Identify foods that are likely to harbor disease-producing microorganisms.
3. Describe how to prevent foodborne illness through the proper storage, handling, and preparation of foods.
4. Discuss one important way nurses can minimize the threat of microbiological hazards.
5. List, in descending order from the most dangerous to the least dangerous, threats to food safety as determined by the Food and Drug Administration.

*E*ach American eats over 1000 pounds of food each year. Considering the number of people involved in the growth, distribution, preparation, and service of food, our food safety record is excellent. The US food supply is as safe, wholesome, and nutritious as any in the world.

Our food delivery system is the envy of many countries. Many of our farmers use highly sophisticated scientific methods and controls. Food moves from the farmer to the consumer under conditions of controlled temperature and sanitation. One reason starvation exists in many third world countries is the lack of a comparable food delivery system. Efforts to transport food grown in the United States to starving nations have often failed. In part, this is due to the lack of roads, trucks, stores, and refrigeration facilities to transport the food from the airports or shipping docks to the starving people.

Our food distribution system and technology enable high standards of quality control. One example is our ability to produce a consistent product. For example, the American consumer expects each new package of cornflakes to be the same as the last one purchased. On the other hand, food processing in foreign countries may lack this consistency. For instance, the McDonald's Company had difficulty planning and building their first McDonald's restaurant in the former Soviet Union. One problem was that each batch of beef purchased in that country was slightly different. Different grains were used to feed the cattle, and thus the flavor and fat content of the meat varied. This affected the taste of each hamburger sold.

Food turns over relatively quickly in American stores. If a particular item does not sell, it usually is not restocked. Highly perishable items are labeled with expiration dates. Products are removed from the stores' shelves when outdated. Such procedures increase the food's safety.

Although the overall food safety record in the United States is excellent, careless handling of our food supply does sometimes occur. Death from botulism (a food poisoning) provides headlines in newspapers, featured stories on radio and television. Milder forms of illness from food poisoning afflict millions each year. As you will learn, the symptoms of food poisoning or food intoxication are very similar to those of the common flu. For this reason, most cases of mild food poisoning go unreported and unnoticed. Food poisoning that is mild in healthy adults can be fatal in infants, in unhealthy adults, and in many elderly people. Since healthcare workers frequently work with these groups, it is important for them to know about food safety.

RECENT CONCERNS

Food meets not only a biological need but also psychological and social needs. Many experts feel food safety issues will be the focus of many consumers' attention in the next decade. Thus healthcare workers should expect many questions about food safety.

Why do experts feel that food safety will increasingly be on the American consumer's mind? First, food is a very personal commodity. Our ancestors used to grow, store, and prepare most of what they ate. This provided them a degree of control and thus of comfort. Many modern people are dependent on others to grow, store, and prepare their food. This lack of control promotes a feeling of insecurity. Second, more individuals live farther away from their food sources than ever before in history. Our ancestors decided that a food was safe to eat if they first observed an animal eating the food. Many people now lack that opportunity. Third, our methods of analyzing chemicals in foods has improved. Laboratory analysis can detect very small amounts of compounds in our food. Our ancestors did not know rhubarb contained oxalic acid (a naturally occurring food intoxicant). Today, we know that oxalic acid is present in rhubarb because we can detect and measure it by laboratory analysis. All of these reasons are increasing consumers' desires to know about the food they purchase.

Changing lifestyles have created an increased demand for partially prepared food items. Consumers are purchasing more convenience or partially prepared food to save time. However, partially prepared foods may increase the likelihood of food poisoning.

One of the basic principles of food safety is that the longer a food is held at room temperature, the greater the likelihood of contamination. Frozen foods such as convenience foods frequently require more handling at room temperature than foods prepared homemade. Convenience foods are initially prepared at room temperature in the factory and again when reheated in the consumer's kitchen. Another principle of food safety is that the more people involved in preparing a menu item, the greater the likelihood of contamination. Convenience foods are usually prepared by more than just one person. This increases the potential for foodborne illness.

Safety Ranking

The Food and Drug Administration (FDA) has set up a list of food safety problems. Problems were ranked in descending order of importance, considering the number of people affected by a problem and the severity of the problem. The FDA's list of food safety priorities is:

1. Microbiological hazards
2. Nutritional hazards
3. Environmental pollutants
4. Natural food intoxicants
5. Food additives

MICROBIOLOGICAL HAZARDS

Microbiological hazards include single-cell and multiple-cell organisms such as bacteria, viruses, molds, and parasites that can invade the food supply through direct, indirect, or intermediary means. These microorganisms may be carried from one host to another through animal sources, air, contact infections, food or water, insects, inanimate objects, soil, and humans. Many microorganisms cause disease. Under certain conditions, food can turn into a vehicle for disease transmission.

Most foodborne diseases infect the tissues of the digestive tract, resulting in gastric distress. Symptoms of gastric distress include abdominal pain, nausea, vomiting, diarrhea, and cramps. If prolonged, the resultant diarrhea can lead to dehydration or other complications, some of which can be fatal. More severe symptoms include fever and neurological disorders. Foodborne disease can last for a few hours or for several days.

Bacterial Foodborne Disease

Bacteria are everywhere. Doorknobs, countertops, hands, eyelashes, mouths, some water supplies, and food are a few of the many places where bacteria can be found. The type of food, the presence or absence of oxygen, the moisture content of the food, and the acidity or alkalinity of the food's environment determine bacterial growth rates. The length of time food is held at a given temperature also affects bacterial growth rates. Given sufficient time, bacteria can frequently adapt to all types of foods and to all conditions of moisture, acidity, oxygen, and temperature. Most bacteria can get used to a new environment in about 4 hours. For this reason, vulnerable foods should not be eaten if held at room temperature for more than 4 hours.

Bacterial growth refers to an increase in the numbers of organisms. Under ideal conditions, cell numbers can double every half hour: one becomes two, two become four, four become eight. A single bacterial cell can multiply to 33 million after 12 hours.

The following conditions are necessary for microbiological food illness to occur:

Source of bacteria—The bacteria must come in contact with the food.

Food—The food must permit the bacteria to grow and either increase in number or produce a poisonous toxin.

Temperature—The temperature must be favorable for the growth of bacteria. 45°F to 140°F is the temperature range in which most bacteria multiply rapidly. (Note: room and body temperature are in this range.)

Time—Enough time must elapse for bacteria to grow and/or produce a toxin.

Ingestion—An unsuspecting person must eat the food that contains the toxin or bacteria.

Bacteria are frequently odorless, tasteless, and colorless. Without laboratory analysis there is no way to tell whether a food will cause illness. For this reason, proper food handling to prevent the growth of bacteria is the best insurance against food poisoning. Bacterial foodborne diseases are usually subdivided into two groups, food infections and food intoxications.

Food Infections

Food infection— An illness acquired through contact with food or water contaminated with disease-producing microorganisms.

A **food infection** is an illness caused by eating food containing a large number of disease-producing bacteria. Symptoms of food infections occur 12 to 36 hours after consumption of the offending food.

SALMONELLA   Probably the best known genus of bacteria responsible for foodborne illness is *Salmonella.* The infection, called **salmonellosis,** is transmitted by the consumption of contaminated foods or contact with an infected person. Some foods support the growth of *Salmonella* better than others (Table 12–1).

Salmonellosis— A bacterial infection manifested by the sudden onset of headache, abdominal pain, diarrhea, nausea, and vomiting. Fever is almost always present.

Elderly persons, infants, pregnant women, and people with illnesses that impair their ability to fight infections are at highest risk. In these persons, a relatively small number of bacteria could cause severe illness. Please refer to Clinical Application 12–2 for a discussion of patients with suppressed immune systems. A healthy person would require a much larger number of bacteria to cause illness. Most of the recent deaths caused by *Salmonella* have occurred among the elderly in nursing homes (Department of Health and Human Services, 1990).

Typhoid fever is caused by one type of *Salmonella* bacteria. This illness

TABLE 12–1 *Food-Handling Tips Related to Specific Infective Agents and Susceptible Foods*

Infective Agent and Susceptible Foods	Food-Handling Tips
Salmonella species Meat, eggs, poultry, milk, and products made with these foods	Never serve raw eggs. (see Clinical Application 12–1) Cook eggs until thoroughly done. Do not allow infected people to handle food.
Typhoid Fever Any food or water	Wash hands after urination and/or defecation. Avoid contaminated water.
Staphylococcus aureus Bruised poultry, processed meats, cheese, ice cream, mixed dishes such as potato salad and spaghetti	Personal hygiene: hand-washing; avoid handling food when you have infected cuts, boils, and burns. Temperature control: Store food between 40°F and 140°F (see Fig. 12–1); do not eat food held at room temperature for longer than 4 hours.
Clostridium perfringens Meats, stews, sauces, gravies, large masses of food	Cool food rapidly in shallow containers that are no more than 4 inches deep. Heat all leftovers to at least 165°F Hold all hot food above 140°F
Clostridium botulinum Canned foods Large masses of food with an air-free center	Never taste food from a bulging container. Do not serve home-canned food to institutionalized patients. Follow manufacturer's directions when home canning food and use only equipment that has been carefully cleaned. Avoid improperly home-smoked fish. Do not store home-smoked fish in plastic bags.
Trichinella spiralis Pork and pork products	Feed swine only cooked garbage. Use pest control measures. Cook all pork to an internal temperature of 170°F.
Tapeworms Raw seafood and undercooked beef and pork	Do not eat raw seafood (sashimi) and meat.
Hepatitis A virus Water and any food	Infected people should not handle food. Avoid contaminated water and shellfish harvested from fecally contaminated water. Use pest control measures.

CLINICAL APPLICATION 12–1
Guidelines for the Safe Handling of Eggs

FACTORS THAT INCREASE THE RISK OF SALMONELLOSIS

- Cracking a large number of eggs at one time and combining them (frequently referred to as pooling).
- Exposing eggs to time and temperature abuse (leaving pooled eggs unrefrigerated for more than 1 hour).
- Eating raw or undercooked eggs.
- Partial cooking, chilling, holding, and reheating of egg dishes (allows too much opportunity for bacteria to multiply).
- Using eggs with cracks or leaks. Shell contamination and penetration has not been ruled out as a possible source of the bacteria.
- Practices that mix the shell and its contents. Examples include using centrifuge egg-breaking machines and using a mixer to break eggs and then straining the contents from the shell.
- Blending eggs in blenders that have not been properly washed and sanitized, and the use of unpasteurized raw eggs in blenderized foods.
- Adding undercooked scrambled eggs to "old" eggs on a buffet or cafeteria line service.
- Using raw eggs in sauces or dressings (e.g., hollandaise, Caesar) that are undercooked and held at warm (less than 140°F) temperatures.

FACTORS THAT DECREASE THE RISK OF SALMONELLOSIS

- Prepare eggs individually. For example, individually prepared and immediately served poached, soft-cooked, and over-easy eggs with a soft yolk are a low-risk way to eat eggs.
- Serve eggs soon after preparation. Do not hold longer than necessary. Do not cook, chill, hold, and reheat unless temperature is tightly maintained (below 50°F or greater than 140°F).
- Refrigerate eggs. Keep eggs at less than 45°F, both shell eggs and mixtures. Egg should not remain out of refrigeration for more than 1 hour.
- Do not use eggs with cracks or leaks. Inspect each egg individually.
- Use a pasteurized egg product if procedures require pooling or undercooked/raw eggs. Pasteurized is safer, but be aware that pasteurized eggs must also be handled with care. Time/temperature abuse is still a factor: They must be thawed under refrigeration or kept refrigerated—the egg is still a perfect medium for bacteria.
- Cook eggs adequately. Cooking for any amount of time reduces the number of bacteria present. In general, cook eggs until the white is set and the yolk begins to thicken. The white coagulates between 144°F and 149°F and the yolk between 149°F and 158°F. Eggs are pasteurized at 140°F for 3½ minutes.

Source: Adapted from Morris, 1990.

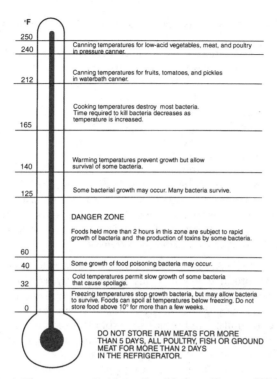

°F

250
240 — Canning temperatures for low-acid vegetables, meat, and poultry in pressure canner.

212 — Canning temperatures for fruits, tomatoes, and pickles in waterbath canner.

165 — Cooking temperatures destroy most bacteria. Time required to kill bacteria decreases as temperature is increased.

140 — Warming temperatures prevent growth but allow survival of some bacteria.

125 — Some bacterial growth may occur. Many bacteria survive.

DANGER ZONE

Foods held more than 2 hours in this zone are subject to rapid growth of bacteria and the production of toxins by some bacteria.

60

40 — Some growth of food poisoning bacteria may occur.

32 — Cold temperatures permit slow growth of some bacteria that cause spoilage.

0 — Freezing temperatures stop growth bacteria, but may allow bacteria to survive. Foods can spoil at temperatures below freezing. Do not store food above 10° for more than a few weeks.

DO NOT STORE RAW MEATS FOR MORE THAN 5 DAYS, ALL POULTRY, FISH OR GROUND MEAT FOR MORE THAN 2 DAYS IN THE REFRIGERATOR.

FIGURE 12–1. A Temperature Guide to Food Safety. (Source: US Department of Agriculture.)

☙ CLINICAL APPLICATION 12–2 ❧
Food Safety and Immunosuppressed Patients

All patients receiving <u>immunosuppressive agents</u> need counseling on food safety and sanitation. These patients have an inability to fight infections, so a relatively small number of bacteria could cause illness. Immunosuppressive agents are drugs that interfere with the body's ability to fight infections. These drugs are used in tissue and organ transplantation procedures, such as a kidney transplant. They are also used in controlling certain diseases.

AIDS (acquired immune deficiency syndrome) is caused by a virus. This virus permits infections, malignancies, and nervous system disorders to develop out of control. According to the FDA, AIDS patients are 300 times more likely than healthy persons to contract a *Salmonella* infection if the organism is present. Preventing food illness from occurring in the first place will save these patients much expense and suffering. All AIDS patients need instruction on the importance of good handwashing and personal hygiene. Proper instruction on food selection, storage, and preparation is also indicated.

is spread by food and water contaminated by feces and urine of patients and carriers.

Other types of bacteria cause food infections. *Shigella* and *Campylobacter* are other examples of disease-producing bacteria.

Food Intoxication

Food intoxication—An illness caused by the consumption of a food in which bacteria have produced a poisonous toxin.

Food intoxication is an illness caused by the consumption of a food in which bacteria have produced a poisonous toxin. The onset of symptoms is very rapid (1 to 8 hours) since the bacteria have already produced the offending toxin before food consumption. Also, because a toxin causes the illness rather than an infection, there is often no fever. Symptoms of this disorder last for a day or two but are usually so severe that exhaustion and dehydration can produce serious aftereffects. Three organisms are responsible for the majority of reported cases of food intoxication: *Staphylococcus aureus*, *Clostridium perfringens*, and *Clostridium botulinum*.

STAPHYLOCOCCAL POISONING   One of the most common species of bacteria that produce a poisonous toxin is *Staphylococcus aureus*, often referred to as staph. Staph have been reported to be in the noses of 30 to 50 percent of healthy people and on the hands of 20 percent of all healthy people. Infected cuts, boils, and burns also harbor this organism.

Good personal hygiene prevents contamination of the food. Heat destroys the bacteria but not the toxin the bacteria already have produced. Because heat does not destroy the toxin produced by the staph organism, control of temperature alone will not provide protection. Prevention of staph poisoning must include *both* good personal hygiene and temperature control (see Table 12–1).

Signs and symptoms of staphylococcal poisoning appear suddenly after 2 to 6 hours and generally subside within 24 hours. These include abdominal cramps, nausea, vomiting, diarrhea, fever, headache, and sweating. The extent to which a person may suffer the effects of the staph toxin depends on (1) how much is ingested and (2) the person's susceptibility.

CLOSTRIDIUM PERFRINGENS   *Clostridium perfringens* are bacteria that produce a toxin that causes lower gastrointestinal colon distress. Careful control of a food's temperature can protect a person against this food infection (see Table 12–1).

Botulism—An often fatal form of food intoxication caused by the ingestion of food containing poisonous toxins produced by *Clostridium botulinum*.it

BOTULISM   *Clostridium botulinum* is another organism that produces a toxin. The toxin produces a disease called **botulism**. The organism is found in soils throughout the world and may be found in the intestinal tract of domestic animals. Vegetables grown in soil may harbor this organism. The spores of *C. botulinum* grow under anaerobic (without air) conditions. A spore is a one-celled organism produced by plants and a few other organisms. The spores of bacteria are difficult to destroy because they are very resistant to heat and require prolonged exposure to high temperatures to destroy them.

Botulin, the toxin produced by *C. botulinum*, is so highly poisonous that a single ounce is enough to kill the world's human population. The onset of symptoms usually occurs after 12 to 36 hours but may be as early as 3 hours. The toxin affects the nervous system, leading to dizziness, headache, double vision, and paralysis of muscles. The paralysis leads in turn to respiratory and heart failure. Food tips to avoid exposure to the botulism organism can be found in Table 12–1.

In summary, bacteria need food, moisture, warmth, and time to grow. Usually we cannot control the food source (the food is the source) or moisture content of food to decrease bacterial growth. We can control both how long and at what temperature food is held and handled. The longer food is held at room temperature and the more food is handled, especially between 45°F and 140°F, the more likely the food houses harmful bacteria.

Parasitic Infections

A **parasite** is an organism that lives within, upon, or at the expense of a living host without providing any benefit to the host. There are several parasites that can live in animals used for food by human beings. When a person eats an animal infected with a parasite, he or she also consumes the parasite. This can result in illness. The parasites discussed in this text are *Trichinella spiralis* and tapeworms.

Parasite—An organism that lives within, upon, or at the expense of a living host.

Trichinella spiralis

Trichinella spiralis is a worm that becomes embedded in the muscle tissue of pork (Fig. 12–2). A pig may eat meat from an animal that harbors the worm in its muscle. The worm produces a larva that is protected from animal (including human) digestion. The larvae mature in the animal's stomach in 5 to 7 days. The adult worms then invade the lining of the small intestine, where they reproduce. The original worm's larvae enter the bloodstream of the animal and are carried to all parts of the body. They then penetrate the muscles, form cysts, and remain alive and infective for months. The cycle is completed when another animal eats the muscle containing the live *Trichinella spiralis* larvae.

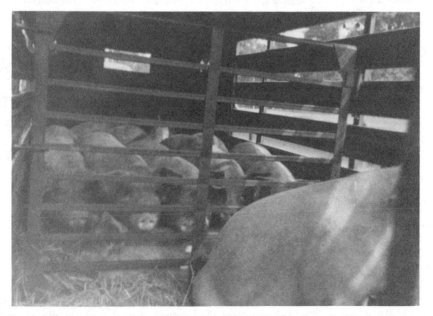

FIGURE 12–2. Swine may harbor *Trichinella spiralis,* which can easily be destroyed by cooking pork to an internal temperature of 160°F.

Trichinosis—The infestation of *Trichinella spiralis*, a parasitic round-worm, transmitted by eating raw or insufficiently cooked pork.

Incubation period—The time it takes to show disease symptoms after exposure to the offending organism.

When a human being eats the larvae, usually in undercooked pork, he or she develops **trichinosis**. The symptoms of trichinosis usually appear 9 days after eating the infected meat, but this time can vary from 2 to 28 days. This period of time is called the **incubation period**. The incubation period is the length of time it takes to show disease symptoms after exposure to the offending organism. The first symptoms, which mimic food poisoning, are nausea, vomiting, and diarrhea. When the larvae migrate into the muscles, systemic symptoms develop. These include fever, swelling of the eyelids, sweating, weakness, and muscular pain. Death due to heart failure may result.

Tapeworms

Tapeworms are acquired by humans through the ingestion of raw seafood or undercooked beef and pork. Hogs and steers become intermediate hosts when they graze on sewage-polluted pastures. Tapeworm infestation can occur when human wastes contaminate freshwater streams and lakes, animal pastures, or feed.

Viral Infections

Virus—Very small noncellular para-site that is entirely dependent on the nutrients inside host cells for its metabolic and reproductive needs.

A **virus** is a microscopic parasite that is entirely dependent on the nutrients inside host cells for its metabolic and reproductive needs. Viruses may invade the cells of people, animals, plants, and bacteria to survive and thereby cause disease. Food frequently serves as a vehicle for some viruses, including those that cause influenza and infectious hepatitis. Food can become contaminated in its growing environment or during processing, storage, distribution, or preparation. Some viruses are found in the intestinal tract of infected humans. If an infected person neglects to wash his or her hands after defecation and then handles food, the virus can contaminate the food (see Table 12–1).

Hepatitis A virus

The hepatitis A virus causes infectious hepatitis, a liver disease. This virus can be found in water that has been contaminated with raw sewage and in shellfish harvested from fecally contaminated water. During food processing, hepatitis A can be transmitted when polluted water is used or by fecal contamination by insects or rodents. Infected workers can transmit the virus through sandwiches, baked goods, or any other food that is handled. Thus there are three ways the virus can be spread: polluted water, insects and rodents, and infected food handlers (see Table 12–1).

Substances Made Poisonous by Other Organisms

The consumption of toxic fish and plants can cause illness. Molds can also produce disease. Some molds, however, are beneficial.

Toxic Seafood

The tissue of fish and shellfish can be naturally toxic to humans even when the fish is fresh. The fish may not show any outward signs of illness and there is usually no way to tell whether the fish is toxic or not. Because most fish toxins are stable to heat, they are not destroyed by cooking. <u>Paralytic</u>

shellfish poisoning outbreaks have been reported after the consumption of poisonous clams, oysters, mussels, and scallops. Ciguatera is the name of a toxin produced by an organism which frequently infects larger fish such as, snapper, grouper, and barracuda. From time to time the concentration of this toxin occurs in large amounts and causes the ocean to appear red. Coastal waters are routinely monitored for the presence of the organism which produces ciguatera. If excessive numbers of the organism are found, a "red tide" alert is made. The best prevention is to avoid eating fish caught during a red tide.

Another illness, called scromboid fish poisoning, is caused by the presence of undesirable bacteria. This poisoning occurs in fish such as tuna, mackerel, bonito, and skipjack. The bacteria produce a toxin on fish flesh after they have been caught. Scromboid fish poisoning can be prevented by the adequate refrigeration of freshly caught fish.

Molds

Molds are the most widely encountered microorganism. Molds are spread by air currents, insects, and rodents. Like bacteria, molds are often involved in food spoilage and are a nuisance in the food industry. A number of molds grow well in cold storage but are easily destroyed by a mild heating process where temperatures of 140°F or higher are reached.

Molds grow on bread, cheese, fruits, vegetables, starchy foods, preserves, grains, and a wide variety of other products. Some molds can cause severe problems when they grow on foods. Certain molds produce poisons called **mycotoxins,** which can cause liver and kidney disease. *Claviceps purpurea,* a parasitic fungus from which the drug ergot is obtained, produces mycotoxins that can cause death if infected foods made from rye or wheat are ingested. Taking an overdose of the drug or eating foods contaminated will result in ergot poisoning. *Aspergillus* molds produce a series of mycotoxins called aflatoxins that may be present in peanuts or peanut products. Many experts believe aflatoxins to be the most potent liver toxin and cancer-producing agent known (Christian and Greger, 1985).

Mycotoxin—A substance produced by mold growing in food; can cause illness or death when ingested by humans or animals.

The best advice is to discard moldy bread as the mold may have penetrated the rest of the item and not be visible to the naked eye. Mold on natural cheese can be safely removed and the remainder of the cheese eaten. The mold is not as likely to have penetrated the rest of the cheese.

Some molds are beneficial. For example, molds are used to manufacture several types of cheese and soy sauce.

NUTRITIONAL HAZARDS

Although problems associated with an unbalanced diet occur frequently, clinical symptoms of illness are not as acute and severe as those arising from microbiological hazards. Illness from a food infection or food intoxication poses an immediate danger.

ENVIRONMENTAL POLLUTANTS

A great many people are concerned about environmental pollution. Although the problem is widespread, situations that pose a severe and immediate danger to health are uncommon.

Chemical Poisoning

Chemical poisoning is caused when people eat toxic substances that may be intentionally or accidently added to foods during growing, harvesting, processing, transporting, storing, or preparing foods. Two general types of chemical poisoning may occur. They are heavy-metal and chemical-product contamination pesticides.

Heavy Metals

Several metals can be toxic. Sources of metals in the soil include parts of rocks and minerals that have weathered to produce soil; water erosion of soil particles; metals as added ingredients or impurities in fertilizers; pesticides containing metals; metals in manure and sludge; and metals in airborne dust. The origin of airborne dust is industrial and mining waste, fossil fuel combustion products, radioactive fallout, pollen, sea spray, and meteoric and volcanic material. Airborne dust eventually settles to the ground and becomes part of the soil. Plants may grow normally but contain levels of selenium, cadmium, molybdenum, or lead that are toxic to humans.

The toxic action of metals is believed to be important in enzyme poisoning. For example, mercury, lead, copper, beryllium, cadmium, and silver have been found to inhibit the enzyme alkaline phosphatase. One function of alkaline phosphatase is in the mineralization process of bone. Some disease states associated with the consumption of toxic minerals include rickets and bone tumors.

Mercury is extremely toxic and is widely distributed over the surface of the earth. In the 1950s, a well-publicized incident occurred in Japan. A large chemical plant poured industrial waste containing mercury into a bay. Area residents who ate fish from the bay complained of numbness of the extremities, slurred speech, unsteady gait, deafness, and visual disturbances. Mental confusion and muscular incoordination were apparent in all the patients. The death rate among those afflicted was 33 percent.

Chemical Products

Chemical foodborne illness is also associated with chemical products such as detergents, sanitizers, pesticides, and other chemicals that may enter the food supply. After consumption, the symptoms of chemical poisoning appear in a few minutes to a few hours, but the reaction time is usually less than 1 hour. Patients may complain of nausea, vomiting, abdominal pain, and diarrhea. The individual may also complain of a metallic taste in his or her mouth.

We all keep many chemicals around our homes. When compounds such as detergents and cleaners are used for the wrong purpose or in excessive amounts, they can cause illness and death. Chemical poisoning can be prevented by:

1. Using each product for its intended use and in the amounts recommended
2. Reading the label before use
3. Keeping chemicals in their original containers
4. Never storing or transporting chemicals in containers used to store food. They may be mistaken for food.

Pesticides are chemicals used to kill insects or rodents. Improperly used pesticides have caused poisonings when they were accidentally mixed with food. The use of pesticide-containing aerosols around foods and packaging materials and in food preparation areas can be dangerous.

According to a 1989 survey by the Food Marketing Institute, pesticide residues in food appear to be the number one concern to the public. Residues are trace amounts of any substance remaining in a product at the time of sale. Three governmental agencies are involved in the regulation of products that enter the US food supply:

- The Environmental Protection Agency (EPA)
- The Food and Drug Administration (FDA)
- The United States Department of Agriculture (USDA) Food Safety and Inspection Service (FSIS)

The EPA regulates the use of potentially harmful pesticides that are used in food production. Included among its duties is that of establishing tolerance levels for pesticides.

The FDA, in addition to its other functions, regulates animal drugs, including food additives, and environmental contaminants. This includes setting tolerance levels for these residues in edible foods. In setting a tolerance level, the FDA determines the highest dose at which a residue causes no ill effects in laboratory animals. This is called the **tolerance level.** The tolerance level is then divided by a factor ranging from 100 to 1000 to account for possible differences between animals and humans. This assumes that humans are 10 times more sensitive than the most sensitive animal species tested. In addition, a further assumption is made that children and the elderly are 10 times as sensitive as others. This is the 100-fold safety factor, which is derived by multiplying 10 times 10. A large margin of safety is built into residue limits established for compounds involved in the production of human food.

Tolerance level— The highest dose at which a residue causes no ill effects in laboratory animals.

The Food Safety and Inspection Service (FSIS) enforces the residue limits in meat and poultry. The FDA is responsible for foods other than meat and poultry. When an illegal residue is found, the FDA can conduct an investigation and the FSIS can detain future shipments from the violating producer.

NATURAL FOOD INTOXICANTS

Many foods (unprocessed or uncooked) contain natural components that can harm health. All foods are made up of chemicals, some of which can alter the way the body uses nutrients. For example, some foods contain chemicals that inactivate vitamins. Table 12–2 lists several natural intoxicants, common food sources, and the toxic effects. Healthy people who eat well-balanced diets should not worry about natural food intoxicants. Illness from naturally occurring toxic compounds in foods is not common in this country. However, if an individual eats large amounts of a single food at one time, he or she may experience the effects of natural food intoxicants. The best protection against the effects of natural food intoxicants is to eat a wide variety of foods. This will limit exposure to any one toxic compound.

TABLE 12–2 *Natural Food Intoxicants*

Natural Food Intoxicant	Food Source	Toxic Effect
Ascorbic acid oxidase	Vegetables, fruits	Destroys vitamin C
Avidin	Raw egg whites	Biotin antagonist
Goitrogen	Cabbage, broccoli, brussels sprouts, horseradish, kale, turnips, rutabagas, cauliflower, carrots	Causes goiter by interfering with the body's use of iodine
Oxalic acid or oxalate	Spinach, rhubarb, cocoa, beet greens, Swiss chard, collard greens, almonds, cashews, chocolate	Prevents calcium and zinc absorption
Nitrates and nitrites	Green beans, asparagus, beets, celery, greens, smoked meats	Potential association between cancer and consumption
Phytic acid or phytate	Oatmeal, whole-grain cereals	Prevents calcium and iron absorption
Solanine	Green immature spots on potatoes	Vomiting and diarrhea
Tannins	Tea and red wine	Interferes with the body's use of iron, thiamine, and vitamin B_{12}
Thiaminases	Raw brussels sprouts, red cabbage, and some berries	Destroys thiamine

Toxic Plants

There are many types of poisonous plants. Illness and death can result from eating toxic mushrooms. This form of poisoning can be prevented by purchasing foods from inspected and approved sources. Households with young children should place all indoor plants out of the reach of toddlers. Toddlers should not be allowed to play outside in wooded areas without adult supervision. They might eat poisonous berries or plants. Patients should be cautioned against making tea leaves from outside foliage; the foliage may be toxic.

FOOD ADDITIVES

Additive—A substance added to food to increase its flavor, shelf life, characteristics such as texture, color, aroma, and/or other qualities.

Additives may be introduced into food deliberately or accidentally.

Intentional Use of Additives

Additives are intentionally added directly to food during processing, for several reasons. Steroids and antibiotics are intentionally used in animal production for various reasons.

Reasons for the Use of Additives

There are four reasons additives are intentionally used:

1. To maintain or enhance a food's nutritional value: frequently vitamins, minerals, and different forms of fiber are added to food.
2. To maintain a food's quality: many additives are used to prevent the growth of microorganisms and extend a product's shelf life. Some additives, called antioxidants, are used to prevent fats in food from deteriorating. Antioxidants are substances that prevent chemical breakdown by preventing or inhibiting the uptake of oxygen. Many researchers believe antioxidants protect an individual from cancer.
3. To assist in processing, transporting, or holding a food: one additive that helps facilitate the processing of food is an <u>emulsifier.</u> An emulsifier helps to evenly distribute the molecules of two liquids that normally do not mix. Mayonnaise is an example of an emulsified product. Baking soda and baking powder are other commonly used additives. These substances cause such products as cakes to rise and improve their texture and volume as well.
4. To improve the way a food tastes, looks, or smells: artificial colors, flavors, and sweeteners all fall into this category.

Table 12–3 lists the types of common food additives.

TABLE 12–3 *Common Food Additives*

Type of Additive	Reasons Used	Examples
Acidity control agents	Influence flavor, texture, and shelf life	Sodium bicarbonate Citric acid Hydrogen chloride Sodium hydroxide Acetic acid Phosphoric acid Calcium oxide
Antioxidants	Prevent discoloration Prevent fats from rancidity	Vitamin C Vitamin E BHT and BHA
Flavors	Food enhancers	Hydrolyzed vegetable protein Black pepper Mustard Monosodium glutamate
Leavening agents	Used to make dough rise	Sodium acid phosphate Sodium aluminum phosphate Monocalcium phosphate Yeast
Preservatives	To extend shelf life	Sulfur oxide Benzoic acid Propionic acid EDTA
Stabilizers and thickeners	To enhance texture	Sodium caseinate Gum arabic Modified starch Pectin

Use of Steroids in Animal Production

Hormones or steroids have been approved by the FDA for use in beef cattle and sheep. Currently, the only FDA-approved hormones for animal use are the anabolic (growth-promoting) steroid implants. Steroids are given to the animal in the form of implants, which are deposited underneath the skin on the back side of the animal's ear. Implants improve feed efficiency (the animal's ability to grow on a given amount of food), reduce the cost of meat production, and result in the production of carcasses with more lean meat and less fat. The implants are composed of natural or synthetic steroid sex hormones: estrogens, androgens, progestins, and combinations thereof (Ritchie, 1990).

Many consumers are concerned about the health hazards of eating beef and sheep with steroid residues. Implantation results in some increase in the hormone content of beef tissue. Beef muscle from an implanted steer contains 0.022 nanograms per gram of steroids compared to 0.015 nanograms per gram in the muscle of nonimplanted steer. (A nanogram equals one billionth of a gram.) These numbers really do not mean much unless you compare them with the amount of the same steroid produced daily in the human body. Before puberty, a boy produces 41,000 nanograms of estrogen and progesterone daily. A pregnant woman produces 20 million nanograms. These steroids are also present naturally in our food supply. A 3-ounce serving of potatoes contains 225 nanograms and a 3-ounce serving of cabbage contains about 2000 nanograms of these steroids. The fact is that the hormone content of beef, whether implanted or not, contains very low levels of steroids as compared with levels naturally produced by the human body or naturally present in foods.

Use of Antibiotics in Animals

Many consumers are also concerned that using antibiotics in animal production poses a human health risk. These compounds are used in animal production in two basic ways: (1) to treat specific diseases, and (2) to maintain health and well-being, thus promoting growth and feed efficiency. The antibiotics penicillin and tetracycline have received the most attention. The three issues raising the most controversy are (Ritchie, 1990):

1. Do antibiotic residues in meat consumed by humans cause development of resistant bacteria in the human body?
   Most experts think not, because the residues of antibiotics in meat are very low.
2. Does the feeding of antibiotics to animals increase levels of disease-resistant bacteria, which may be transferred to humans via bacteria-contaminated meat?
   The use of antibiotics does appear to increase the proportion of resistant bacteria in the animal's body. However, the transfer of resistant bacteria from animals to humans, resulting in illness, has not been adequately studied.

In summary, the controversy on the use of antibiotics in meat remains unresolved.

Accidental Use of Additives

Some additives have entered the food supply accidentally. For example, chemicals may be added to food through contact with surfaces that have been cleaned with solutions that contained the chemical.

FOOD SELECTION, STORAGE, AND HANDLING GUIDELINES

Even experts have difficulty monitoring all the toxic substances in the food supply. Thus, it is impossible for the average consumer to be aware of all the poisonous substances found in foods. This section of the chapter offers some guidelines that, if followed, will help decrease the risks of food-borne disease.

Food Selection

The greater the variety of foods consumed, the less likelihood of exposure to contaminants of any single food item. Remember that contaminants of natural origin are present in foods.

Food Storage

Proper storage of food helps ensure that there will be minimal contamination of the food from any source. The following guidelines should be followed when storing food:

- Containers used to store food should be covered to provide physical protection for the food.
- Food should be stored in locations that provide minimal risk of contamination from other foods.
- Stored food should be properly labeled to prevent confusion due to similar appearances.
- Proper temperature control of stored food is important to control the growth of disease-producing organisms. The use of thermometers in refrigerators and freezers is recommended.
- Food storage immediately following food preparation is important. Hot food items should be stored in such as manner that they can cool quickly. Allowing hot food to cool to room temperature prior to placing it in the refrigerator is an unsafe practice.

Sanitation and Personal Hygiene

The cleanliness of people involved in food handling and a clean working environment are essential to the prevention of foodborne disease. An unclean person cannot handle food in a sanitary fashion. Smoking and eating while preparing food may result in food contamination. Personal practices such as scratching the head, placing fingers in or about the mouth or nose, and sneezing may contaminate food. Work surfaces in the food preparation area should be clean. Food handlers should always wash their hands after touching themselves. The wearing of soiled clothing while preparing food increases the risk of foodborne disease. Frequent hand-washing with soap is the best insurance against food contamination (see Figure 12–3). In fact, the most common way sources of disease are transmitted from a food handler to food is by the hands. Needless to say, it is essential to always wash your hands after using the toilet.

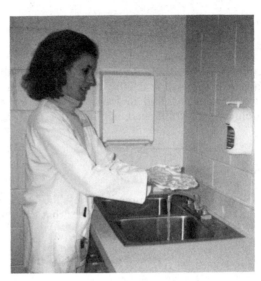

FIGURE 12–3. A Nurse Washing Her Hands. Proper hand washing is the best way to prevent the spread of infection. Proper hand washing requires the right equipment and the right technique: the basic needs are soap, water, and paper toweling; the basic technique involves sudsing, friction, and flushing.

Preventing Cross-Contamination

Cross-contamination—The spreading of a disease-producing organism from one food, person, or object to another food, person, or object.

Cross-contamination refers to the spreading of a disease-producing organism from one food to another. This may happen when a food preparer handles raw meat, eggs, or milk and then handles fruit, lettuce, or bread products that will be served uncooked. The cook transfers the offending substance or organism to the uncooked food item. Organisms can also be transferred to nonfood items such as a cooking utensil and then passed on to the food or a person.

Cooked meat should not be allowed to come in contact with raw meat. This includes the drippings of raw meat. For example, storing raw meat above cooked meat in the refrigerator is inviting trouble. As raw meat drips, the drippings could fall on the cooked meat, thus contaminating it. Nor should consumers use the same utensils for raw meat and foods intended to be served uncooked. Never use the same platter to carry raw meat to the grill and then to carry cooked meat to the table. Instead the platter should be washed in hot, soapy water between uses.

Safe Food Preparation

Food is the least protected during actual food preparation because of necessary handling, possible contamination from the environment, and the room's temperature. Food should always be prepared with the least amount of hand contact. Cooking utensils should be used whenever possible. Raw fruits and vegetables should be thoroughly washed. Potentially hazardous foods requiring cooking should be cooked to heat all parts to at least 140°F. In addition, poultry, poultry stuffings, stuffed meats, and stuffings containing meat should be cooked to at least 165°F. Fresh pork needs to be cooked until at least 170°F.

Safe Cooling and Reheating

Food should be thawed properly. This can be done in refrigerated units at a temperature that should not exceed 45°F. This can also be accomplished under running water at a temperature of 70°F or below. Using the microwave oven to thaw food is a safe method as long as the thawing is part of a continuous cooking process. After thawing the food should be cooked immediately. All foods that have been cooked and then refrigerated should be reheated to a safe temperature of 165°F.

Frozen food items will soon bear a new kind of label that is designed to turn a special color if the food item undergoes an undesirable increase in temperature during transit. The label will thereby warn both food retailers and consumers that the food may be unsafe to eat.

Summary

Thousands of substances besides nutrients are present in foods. Most of these substances are harmless in the amounts typically eaten if the food item

---

CLINICAL APPLICATION 12–3
The Power of the Consumer

Consumers exercise substantial power when they make a food-purchasing decision. This power can be seen by examining the public response after the "Alar incident." Alar is a pesticide that had been used on apples to keep them on the trees longer and make them look better. During the early part of 1989, the television program "60 Minutes" ran a segment on Alar. Alar breaks down into a substance called UDMH, which can cause cancer. Because children eat apples, the implication was that children are especially vulnerable to the effects of UDMH. The public response was enormous. The New York City Board of Education canceled its program of handling 13 million apples annually. Schools in Los Angeles, Chicago, and elsewhere did the same. Customers returned apple juice, apple sauce, and fresh apples to grocery stores demanding a refund. Grocery stores posted signs that their apples were "Alar-Free." The financial cost to the apple industry was staggering.

The government had various responses to the charges made by environmental groups. The California state health director charged the originators of the Alar claim to be "toxic bogeymen." On March 16, 1989, in an unusual joint statement, the EPA, FDA, and Agriculture Department said, "The federal government believes it is safe for Americans to eat apples." Government officials pointed to the 100-fold safety factor in discussing pesticide residues. The government's data showed very little Alar residue on apples. The environmental groups' data showed that after analyzing 32 samples of apple juice on the market only 9 had no detectable Alar. These examples point up a common problem in discussing food safety issues—opposing sides use different data to argue a position. This makes any intelligent discussion of the subject difficult. The net result of the Alar incident was a statement by the International Apple Institute. They recommended that "all growers stop using Alar, a pesticide in diminishing use on the domestic apple supply, until the EPA makes a final determination on the continued use of this product."

is selected, stored, and prepared under recommended conditions. Many foods contain toxic substances naturally. Only in recent years have we been able to detect and measure these toxic substances. It stands to reason that a particular food is safe if our ancestors have eaten it for countless generations with no resulting disease. The human body appears able to safely handle small amounts of toxic substances without injury.

The FDA ranks pathogenic (disease-causing) microorganisms as the most dangerous food-related public health threat. An individual is more likely to suffer from a foodborne illness due to microbiological contamination than from any other source. Most microbiological hazards can be controlled by following good principles of food handling. Selecting a wide variety of foods, storing the foods appropriately, and preparing foods correctly all help prevent illness. Consumers perceive chemical residues to be the most dangerous food-related threat and rank pesticides as the most dangerous chemical residue. Healthcare workers should address microbiological and residual chemical hazards of foods with their patients.

A case study and a sample plan of care appear below. Both are designed to show you how the information you have studied in this chapter can be used in nursing practice.

CASE STUDY 12–1

Ms. N. is a 95-year-old woman who is 5 feet tall and weighs 122 pounds (dressed without shoes). She has just been admitted to the nursing home. During the routine nursing admission process, Ms. N. requested an eggnog every night at 8:00 PM. She stated she dislikes package mixes and would prefer her eggnog made with whole milk, ice cream, and a raw egg. Ms. N.'s physician has ordered an eggnog at HS (Latin for hour of sleep, or just before bedtime) q.d. (every day). Ms. N. stated she has always drunk a homemade eggnog every night for a the past 50 years. The patient's daughter has stated she makes her mother an eggnog each day from raw eggs.

NURSING CARE PLAN FOR MS. N.

Assessment

Subjective: Patient stated she drinks an eggnog made with a raw egg each day. Patient's daughter stated she makes her mother such a beverage.

Objective: Height: 5 feet 0 inches Weight: adm 122 pounds 100 percent RBW Age 95

Nursing Diagnosis

Infection, potential for: unsafe food behavior related to knowledge deficit as evidenced by patient's statement, "I eat one raw egg each day," and the patient's age.

Desired Outcome/Evaluation Criteria

1. The patient will state that raw eggs can make one ill.
2. The patient will accept an eggnog made from pasteurized egg.

Nursing Actions/Interventions with Rationales in Italics

1. Provide verbal and written information to the patient and the patient's daughter on the relationship between food illness and *Salmonella* infection. *Elderly patients are particularly at risk from salmonellosis.*

   Have the patient and the patient's daughter state that raw eggs are hazardous. *Verbal recognition of a hazard is the first step in behavorial change.*

2. Request the dietitian send an eggnog made with pasteurized eggs to patient at bedtime each day. *The risk of salmonellosis from pasteurized eggs is lower than from raw eggs.*

   Chart acceptance or rejection of the beverage. *Acceptance of the modified eggnog will increase long-term compliance.*

STUDY AIDS

Chapter Review Questions

1. Trichinosis is most frequently transmitted by:
   a. Raw milk
   b. Infested pork
   c. Raw vegetables
   d. Wild mushrooms

2. Foods commonly contaminated with *Salmonella* are:
   a. Eggs
   b. Raw vegetables
   c. Canned foods
   d. Breads and cereals

3. The most common way agents of disease are transmitted from food handlers to foods are:
   a. Outer garments
   b. Hair
   c. Hands
   d. Coughing and sneezing on foods

4. Safe ways of thawing food include:
   a. Under refrigeration
   b. Under cold running water
   c. Cooking from the frozen state
   d. All of the above

5. The primary reason that chemicals should be stored away from food is:
   a. They may be mistaken for food.
   b. Poisonous vapors from the chemicals will invade and contaminate food.
   c. Chemicals decrease air circulation around food.
   d. Chemicals may leach out of the containers and contaminate food.

6. The FDA ranks which of the following as the most dangerous threat to food safety?
   a. Food additives
   b. Chemical residues including pesticides
   c. Environmental pollutants
   d. Microbiological hazards

7. Consumers rank which of the following as the most dangerous threat to food safety?
   a. Food additives
   b. Microbiological hazards
   c. Chemical residues including pesticides
   d. Nutritional hazards

8. A major factor in chilling a hot liquid food is the:
   a. Depth of food in the container
   b. pH of the food
   c. Food's moisture content
   d. Amount of time the food has been held above 140°F

9. Rodents, insects, and other pests contaminate food because they:
   a. Track in dirt
   b. Carry disease-producing organisms
   c. Bite
   d. Distract food handlers

10. The best method to control the spread of foodborne illness is by:
    a. Wearing gloves when handling food
    b. Avoiding certain foods
    c. Taking food supplements
    d. Proper hand-washing

NCLEX-Style Quiz

Situation One

Mr. N. has complained about fever, diarrhea, vomiting, and cramps on three separate occasions. He admits to the following behaviors: eating peanut butter directly out of the jar; storing and drinking milk at room temperature; eating two hard-cooked eggs each day, and cutting his fruits and vegetables in very small pieces before eating.

1. As the nurse, you would most likely suspect which of the following behaviors to be related to Mr. N.'s physical complaints?
   a. Eating peanut butter directly out of the jar
   b. Storing and drinking milk at room temperature
   c. Eating eggs
   d. Cutting and eating his produce in small pieces

2. Mr. N.'s behavior, however, may be related to which other behavior or situation?
   a. Bacteria in the peanut butter
   b. Storing his hard-cooked eggs at room temperature
   c. Not cleaning his produce sufficiently
   d. All of the above

Situation Two

3. When taking the history of a patient with a gastrointestinal upset, the nurse should document:
   a. All the food consumed during the past 36 hours
   b. Any eating establishment patronized during the previous 3 days
   c. The patient's immunization status
   d. The frequency of urination

Situation Three

4. If a jar or can of food shows signs of spoilage, the person should:
   a. Boil the food before eating.
   b. Discard the food item.
   c. Skim off the top of the food in the can and discard.
   d. Taste the food.

BIBLIOGRAPHY

American Institute for Cancer Research. Newsletter 28: Summer 1990.

Atkins, HA (ed): When seafood sickness strikes. Emergency Medicine, June 15, 1990.

Benenson, AS (ed): American Public Health Department: Control of Communicable Diseases in Man, ed 15. American Public Health Association, Washington, DC, 1990.

Christian, JL and Gregor, JL: Nutrition For Living. Benjamin-Cummings Publishing, Redwood City, CA, 1991.

Department of Health and Human Services: unpublished memorandum. Public Health Services: Center for Disease Control. Questions and Answers about Salmonella. Atlanta, June 8, 1990.

Food and Drug Administration Office of Public Affairs: Eating Defensively: Food Safety Advice for Persons with AIDS. September 1989. (Distributed by National AIDS Information Clearinghouse. Call 1-800-458-5231.)

Food Marketing Institute: Trends: Consumer Attitudes and the Supermarket. Food Marketing Institute, Washington, DC, 1990.

Goldblatt, BI (ed): Report of salmonella contamination exaggerated. Environmental Nutrition 13:6, 1990.

Graven, R: Meals, Microbes, and You: A Sanitation Program for Food Service Personnel. Cornell University, Ithaca, NY.

Hui, YH: Human Nutrition and Diet Therapy. Wadsworth Health Education Service, Monterey, CA, 1983.

Lefferts, LY and Schmidt, S: Mold: The fungus among us. Nutrition Action. Center for Science in the Public Interest, Washington DC, 1991.

Morris, GK: Salmonella Enteritidis: Assessment and Risk. Nutrition Close-Up. Egg Nutrition Center, Washington, DC, September 1990.

Owen, AL: The impact of future foods on nutrition and health. J Am Diet Assoc 90:1217, 1990.

Penner, KP: Contaminated raw seafood. Nutrition and the MD 16 (6), 1990.

Ritchie, HD: Agriculture on the stand: Are modern production practices safe? Michigan State University, 1990. Unpublished paper.

Robinson, CH and Weigley, ES: Basic Nutrition and Diet Therapy. Macmillan, New York, 1989.

Food Service, Nutritional Care, and Nutrient Delivery in the Healthcare Facility

Key Terms

As a study aid, each key term is followed by the page number where the term is defined in the chapter. Terms that appear in **boldface** or <u>underscored</u> in the chapter text are located in the glossary.

Food Services, Nutritional Care, and Nutrient Delivery in the Healthcare Facility

Learning Objectives

After completing this chapter, the student should be able to:

1. Identify three routes used to deliver nutrients to patients, and potential complications with two of these routes.
2. Discuss the kinds of commercial formulas available for oral and tube feedings.
3. Discuss why it is important to carefully control the concentration, rate, and volume of a formula delivered to a patient.
4. List at least five reasons for the high incidence of malnutrition in institutionalized patients and the interventions nurses can use to combat malnutrition.
5. Describe suggested procedures for administering medications through tube feedings.

ood services in healthcare facilities have two major functions: the preparation and physical delivery of meals to patients, and the nutritional care of patients. The nutritional care of patients includes three areas:

1. Assessing the patient's need for nutrients
2. Monitoring the patient's nutrient intake
3. Counseling the patient about nutritional needs

Quality nutritional care saves both the patient and society not only health-care dollars but also preventable hardship.

FOOD SERVICE IN INSTITUTIONS

All nurses need to become familiar with some aspects of the food service in the organizations where they are employed. Specific duties of nurses are often related to meal distribution systems and meal service patterns.

Meal Distribution Systems

A food service can be either centralized or decentralized. In a centralized service, patient trays are assembled in the kitchen and delivered to the patient units. In a decentralized service, food is sent in bulk to the patient areas. Individual trays are then assembled on the patient units.

Many institutions have a central dining room for patients. This is most common in long-term care facilities, rehabilitation centers, and psychiatric hospitals. Patients who, for medical reasons, cannot come to the dining room have their trays delivered to their rooms. There are many benefits to a congregate meal site. Menu items can usually be more attractively displayed and served in a more homelike atmosphere in a dining room. This increases the acceptability of the food to the patient. In addition, patients can interact with each other during mealtime and the eating experience becomes more enjoyable. This also increases food acceptance. For these reasons, the use of room trays when a congregate dining room is available is discouraged.

Food acceptance record—A checklist that indicates food items accepted or rejected by the patient.

Healthcare workers also benefit when patients consume their meals in a common setting. The charting of a **food acceptance record** is less time-consuming. The food acceptance record refers to an easily kept checklist that indicates food items eaten or refused at each meal (Table 13–1). Many institutions also use mealtimes to dispense medications more efficiently. In this situation, care must be taken not to administer the types of medications that should not be taken with food (Chapter 14).

Meal Service Patterns

Most institutions serve not only three meals to patients each day but also several between-meal feedings. Feedings between meals are available for patients in need of extra nutrients, those who desire extra food, or those unable to consume sufficient kilocalories at the regular mealtimes. It is important for nurses to become familiar with the times meals are served to patients.

The dietary and nursing departments need to coordinate their respective schedules so patients receive their food while it is hot and attractive.

The administration of medications sometimes must also be coordinated with meal delivery schedules. Scheduling the patient for diagnostic tests, blood work, and educational sessions should be coordinated with the meal service schedule. <u>Diagnostic</u> means pertaining to scientific and skillful methods to establish the cause and nature of a sick person's disease.

NUTRITIONAL CARE SERVICES

Institutions vary in the types of nutritional services available to patients. A larger teaching hospital or medical center frequently has nutrition professionals who specialize in the treatment of a particular type of patient. For example, a critical care dietitian has special training to assess, plan, implement, and counsel patients in high-risk stages of trauma, disease, and processes involving nutritional support. In this situation other healthcare workers can rely on the critical care dietitian to provide technical support. At the other end of the spectrum, in a small community hospital or a long-term care facility, a dietitian may be present only on a part-time basis or as a consultant. Thus, other healthcare workers must plan to make the best use of the dietitian's services when he or she is available. In this situation the nursing staff needs to assume more responsibility for the nutritional care of patients.

Assessment, Monitoring, and Counseling

Nutritional care is a joint responsibility of both the dietary and nursing departments. Assessing, monitoring, and counseling activities are usually done in collaboration.

Assessment

Some dietary departments screen patients for nutritional problems upon admission. Those patients who are found to be at a nutritional risk have a complete nutritional assessment, which usually includes the following:

1. Height, weight, and weight history
2. Laboratory test values
3. Food intake information
4. Potential food-drug interactions
5. Mastication and swallowing ability
6. Patient's ability to feed himself or herself
7. Bowel and bladder function
8. Presence of <u>pressure ulcers</u>
9. Food allergies and intolerances
10. Any other factors affecting nutritional status, such as food preferences, cultural and religious beliefs about food
11. Determination of body composition
12. Severe burns, trauma, infection, or other physiological stress that increases nutrient needs and is likely to prolong hospital stay

In some healthcare facilities, nurses are responsible for screening patients for nutritional problems. If the nurse finds a patient at a nutritional risk, she or he should make a referral to the dietitian.

All residents in long-term care facilities are required to have a nutri-

TABLE 13-1 *Typical Food Aceptance Record Used in a Long-Term Care Facility*

FOOD ACCEPTANCE RECORD

MONTH/YEAR _____ PATIENT'S NAME _____ ROOM NUMBER _____

DIET _____ SUPPLEMENTS _____

CODE:
½	refused ½ of meal/item
¾	refused ¾ of item/meal
R	refused all of item/meal

M — meat/protein
L — milk
V — vegetable
F — fruit/dessert
S — salad

Sp — soup
P — potato/starch
C — cereal
B — bread
E — egg

Day	BREAKFAST						LUNCH								DINNER								SUPPLEMENT		
	All	E	L	F	C	B	All	M	L	V	F	P	B	S	SP	All	M	L	V	F	P	B	S	SP	AM	PM	HS*
1																											
2																											
3																											
4																											
5																											
6																											
7																											
8																											
9																											
10																											

11			
12			
13			
14			
15			
16			
17			
18			
19			
20			
21			
22			
23			
24			
25			
26			
27			
28			
29			
30			
31			

*HS is Latin for hour of sleep; means give at bedtime or around 8:00 PM.

tional assessment performed by a registered dietitian. After the initial nutritional assessment is completed, patients at a nutritional risk should be identified. The care plan should reflect nutritional problems identified during the assessment.

Monitoring

All patients should be reassessed or monitored at appropriate intervals. Some patients in hospital intensive care units require continuous monitoring. Other patients require reassessment daily.

The patient care conference will be the most productive if all healthcare workers come prepared. Prior to the conference, information on the nutritional care of the patient should be gathered including:

1. The patient's initial nutritional assessment
2. The patient's present body weight and weight history
3. A record of the patient's recent food acceptances
4. Any changes in the patient's medical condition
5. The patient's diet order

With the above information, most changes in the patient's nutritional status can be easily identified. For example, whether the patient has been losing weight can be determined by comparing his or her weight at admission with his or her present body weight. A review of the patient's food acceptance record, if available, can verify whether such a weight loss is likely a result of poor food intake.

Those patients determined to be at a nutritional risk because of poor food intake should be treated. Treatment may include a nutritional supplement, between-meal feedings, a change in diet, or a change in feeding status. For example, perhaps a patient's condition has deteriorated to the point where he or she has a self-care deficit in feeding. In this case, the patient's feeding status would need to be changed from self-feed to feed. Monitoring the patient's weight, laboratory values, and food intake is an important part of delivering quality nutritional care.

Counseling

All patients should be evaluated for nutritional counseling. The assumption that a patient is not expected to be discharged and therefore is not entitled to education is unjustified. Educating the patient about nutritional concerns helps the patient assume responsibility for his or her own care, thus promoting self-esteem and a sense of worth.

Diet Manuals

Current accreditation standards require all institutions to have a diet manual available to all healthcare workers. The diet manual defines all diets used in the facility and includes information about the food service operation. Many healthcare workers are surprised to learn that a soft diet may vary slightly from one institution to another. For example, one soft diet may allow lettuce, whereas another does not. This is because a diet manual is approved and developed jointly by all healthcare professionals in a facility. Regional food preferences and the unique training of the facility's medical staff and other professionals influence the choice of food items allowed and avoided on special diets.

Usually, the administrative dietitian is responsible for initiating the selection of a diet manual or for writing the manual. Most aspects of the nutritional care given to patients are covered in such a manual, including nutritional supplements stocked by the pharmacy, purchasing, and/or dietary departments; dietary preparation for diagnostic procedures; kilocalorie count procedures; meal service delivery schedules; patient educational services; a listing of foods allowed, restricted, and avoided on the various diets; and nursing procedures to follow when transmitting a diet order. When preparing the manual, the dietitian usually consults with other department heads and members of the medical staff. After the manual is written, it must be approved by the facility administrator and the medical staff. Physicians are usually requested to follow the manual when prescribing diets for patients. The medical staff, nursing department, and other professionals in the hospital can and do influence the nutritional care given to patients by participating in the diet manual approval process.

Diet Orders

The physician is responsible for ordering a diet for the patient. Just as you cannot administer a medication to a patient without a medication order, you cannot legally choose a diet for a patient without a physician's order. One of the functions of the diet manual is to define a diet. The diet manual is the first place to look when patients request food items that are not being served to them. As defined in the diet manual, perhaps the food items is restricted or not allowed on the patient's prescribed diet.

SPECIAL DIETS   The purpose of a special or modified diet is to restore or maintain a patient's nutritional status. This can be accomplished by modifying one or more of the following aspects of the diet:

1. Basic nutrients such as calcium, iron, sodium, potassium, and so forth may be increased, decreased, or eliminated
2. Kilocalories may be either restricted or increased
3. Texture or consistency of foods may be altered, for example, only clear liquids may be served
4. Seasonings such as pepper may be restricted or eliminated

All modified diets are variations of the general diet, since the patient still needs all the essential nutrients. For this reason, each modified diet must be carefully planned to provide each of the essential nutrients or a documented reason why one or more essential nutrients are not provided.

Much confusion results when the terminology in the diet order is not the same as the terminology in the diet manual. For example, a low-salt diet may not be the same as a low-sodium diet as defined in the diet manual. Physicians may persist in ordering a low-salt or low-sodium diet even though the diet manual requests that all sodium-restricted diets be ordered in units of sodium such as 2-gram sodium or 4-gram sodium. Many facilities have eliminated this confusion by defining a low-sodium and low-salt diet in the diet manual. Expect the definitions for both low-salt and low-sodium diets to differ markedly from one facility to another. Other vague diet orders are *salt-*

free, diabetic, regular diabetic, low-fat, fat-free, and *as tolerated*. The nursing or dietetic staff should clarify all vague diet orders with the physician before the patient is served. All healthcare workers should become familiar with the terminology in the facility's diet manual.

Diet manuals are not usually designed to be used directly for patient instruction. Much of the information in the diet manual is directed to physicians and other healthcare workers to assist in the implementation of special diets. For example, the diet manual describes indications and contraindications for use of a particular diet. An **indication** is the circumstance that indicates when the diet should be used. A **contraindication** describes circumstances when the diet should not be used. The diet manual also lists nutrients deficient in a particular diet. This type of information may alarm and confuse some patients.

Indication—A circumstance that indicates when a treatment should or can be used.

Contraindication—Any circumstance indicating that a treatment should not be given.

COMMON DIET ORDERS   Some of the common diet orders are *clear liquid, full liquid, soft*, and *general* or *regular*. A clear liquid diet is any transparent liquid that can be poured at room temperature. Gelatin, some juices, broth, tea, and coffee are clear liquids. A clear liquid diet is nutritionally inadequate. A full liquid diet is any liquid that can be poured at room temperature. Milk, custard, thinned hot cereals, all fruit juices, ice cream, and all items allowed on the clear liquid diet are allowed on most full liquid diets. The major difference between a clear liquid and a full liquid diet is that the latter contains milk and milk products (Table 13–2).

Soft diets vary greatly from one facility to another. For example, a mechanical soft diet is ordered when the patient has only a few or no teeth (edentulous). A soft diet is ordered following surgery when easily digested foods are required. A facility that specializes in treating patients with eye, ear, nose, and throat disorders may have many types of soft diets. A pureed diet consists of foods soft enough to be mashed easily in the mouth and safely swallowed. Table 13–3 lists recommended foods on a pureed, mechanical soft, and a soft diet. A general or regular diet means that the patient is on an unrestricted diet.

TABLE 13–2 *Composition of Liquid Diets*

Diet	Protein (Grams)	Fat (Grams)	Carbohydrate (Grams)	Sodium (Milliequivalents)	Potassium (Milliequivalents)	Kilocalories
Clear liquid	5	trace	70–95	65	20	375+
Clear liquid with three 6-ounce servings of Citrotein	30	1	140–165	80	30	750+
Full liquid	50	55	205	110	65	1500

SOURCE: Adapted from Pemberton, CM, et al: Mayo Clinic Diet Manual: A Handbook of Dietary Practice, ed 6. BC Decker, Philadelphia, 1988, p 47.

TABLE 13–3 *Consistency Modifications—Recommended Foods*

Food Group	Pureed Diet	Mechanical Soft Diet	Soft Diet
Soups	Broth; bouillon; strained or blenderized cream soup	Broth; bouillon; strained or blenderized cream soup	Broth; bouillon; cream soup
Beverages	All	All	All
Meat	Strained or pureed meat or poultry; cheese used in cooking	Ground, moist meats, or poultry; flaked fish; eggs; cottage cheese; cheese; creamy peanut butter; soft casseroles	Moist, tender meat, fish, or poultry; eggs, cottage cheese; mild flavored cheese; creamy peanut butter; soft casseroles
Fat	Butter; margarine; cream; oil; gravy	Butter; margarine; cream; oil; gravy; salad dressing	Butter; margarine; cream; oil; gravy; crisp bacon; avocado; salad dressing
Milk	Milk; milk beverages; yogurt without fruit, nuts, or seeds; cocoa	Milk, milk beverages, yogurt without seeds or nuts; cocoa	Milk; milk beverages; yogurt without seeds or nuts; cocoa
Starch	Cooked, refined cereal; mashed potatoes	Cooked or refined ready-to-eat cereal; potatoes; rice; pasta; white, refined wheat, light rye bread or rolls; graham crackers as tolerated	Cooked or ready-to-eat cereal; potatoes; rice; pasta; white, refined wheat, light rye or graham bread, rolls, or crackers
Vegetables	Strained or pureed; juice	Soft, cooked, without hulls or tough skin as in peas and corn; juice	Soft, cooked, vegetables; limit strongly flavored vegetables and whole-kernel corn, lettuce and tomatoes
Fruit	Strained or pureed; juice	Cooked or canned fruit without seeds or skins; banana; juice	Cooked or canned fruit; banana; citrus fruit without membrane; melon; juice
Desserts	Gelatin; sherbet; ice cream without nuts or fruit; custard; pudding; fruit ice; Popsicle	Gelatin; sherbet; ice cream without nuts or fruit; custard; pudding; fruit ice; Popsicle	Gelatin; sherbet; ice cream without nuts; custard; pudding; cake; cookies without nuts or coconut; fruit ice; Popsicle
Sweets	Sugar; honey; jelly; candy; flavorings	Sugar; honey; jelly; candy; flavorings	Sugar; honey; jelly; candy; flavorings
Miscellaneous	Seasonings; condiments	Seasonings; condiments	Seasonings; condiments

SOURCE: From Pemberton, CM, et al: Mayo Clinic Diet Manual: A Handbook of Dietary Practice, ed 6. BC Decker, Philadelphia, 1988, p 49, with permission.

Diets for Diagnostic Procedures

Many diagnostic procedures that require dietary preparation are performed in hospitals. There are dozens of diagnostic procedures, and of course not every procedure will be discussed in this text. Instead we will concentrate on why it is important to follow the facility's diet manual when preparing a patient for a procedure.

POOR PATIENT PREPARATION A poor dietary preparation can force a patient to have an expensive procedure repeated or postponed. For example, Figure 13–1 shows two colon roentgenograms, or x-ray studies. Figure 13–1 (A) is a roentgenogram from a poorly prepared patient. Feces in the colon would block the view of structures within the colon. Figure 13–1 (B) shows the colon of a well-prepared patient. There is an absence of fecal material and the entire length of the colon can be visualized.

Some roentgenograms are not only expensive but also uncomfortable. The patient must have the procedure repeated if necessary bodily structures cannot be visualized. Although the specific dietary preparation for x-ray studies of the colon may vary from one facility to another, dietary preparations usually includes some similarities. The patient should be instructed not to eat or drink anything after midnight on the day of the imaging study. In addition, the patient may need to follow a clear liquid diet for 12 to 48 hours prior to the procedure.

Many patients have x-rays studies performed as outpatients. The nurse working in a physician's office is usually responsible for dietary instruction prior to these procedures. A reliable diet manual should be consulted before the scheduling of patients for such studies.

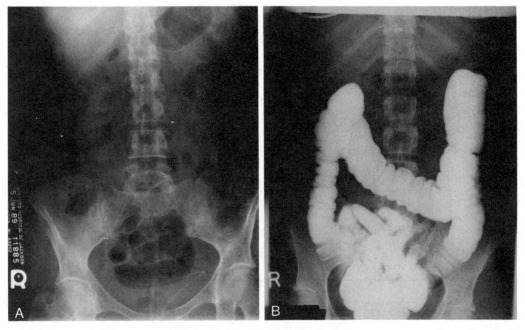

FIGURE 13–1. (*A*) An image of a patient who was poorly prepared for a barium enema. (*B*) An image of a patient who was adequately prepared for a barium enema. (Courtesy of Dr. Russell Tobe.)

MISDIAGNOSIS   A poor dietary preparation can lead to a misdiagnosis. For example, a blood sample for a fasting blood glucose (FBS) test should be drawn on a fasting individual. **Fasting** means that the patient has not had any food or fluid by mouth for at least 8 hours prior to the test. If the patient eats before the procedure, his or her glucose level may be elevated. This may cause a misdiagnosis of diabetes. A misdiagnosis may cause a patient unnecessary anxiety.

Fasting—The state of having had no food or fluid by mouth since midnight the previous evening.

IMPORTANCE OF NUTRITIONAL CARE

Malnutrition associated with both acute and chronic disease is common in hospital settings. Acute means that the illness is characterized by a rapid onset, severe symptoms, and a short course. Chronic means that the illness is characterized by a long duration. The presence and importance of malnutrition has been increasingly recognized over the past 15 to 20 years.

Malnutrition is one of the most common diseases affecting the care of hospitalized patients. According to one study, approximately 40 to 50 percent of all patients whose medical records contained necessary data were considered at nutritional risk (malnourished). Additionally, 75 percent of all patients who were hospitalized for 2 weeks or longer demonstrated a declining nutritional status. Only 10 percent of the hospital patients whose charts contained evidence of a nutritional problem received the appropriate follow-up care (Kamath and associates, 1986). The healthcare community has not done well in identifying or treating malnourished patients in our institutions. Unfortunately, many healthcare workers, including some physicians, still refuse to acknowledge the documented presence of malnutrition in institutions.

Malnutrition is associated with a 25 percent morbidity and a 5 percent mortality. Morbidity is defined as the state of being diseased. Mortality is defined as the death rate. A malnourished patient is thus more likely to be sicker and run a higher risk of death than a well-nourished patient with the same diagnosis. Because malnutrition affects morbidity and mortality, it is also associated with a prolonged hospital stay.

Iatrogenic Malnutrition

The term iatrogenic malnutrition was first used in 1974 (Butterworth and Blackburn, 1975). Iatrogenic malnutrition is a less offensive phrase than induced malnutrition by a physician or an institution. Routine hospital practices such as extended periods of food or nutrient deprivation due to treatments or diagnostic tests that interfere with the patient's meal schedule or cause a lack of appetite are related to the high prevalence of malnutrition. Drug therapy may also affect a patient's appetite. Some drugs cause drowsiness, lethargy, nausea, and anorexia. Problems related directly to an illness, such as pain, unconsciousness, paralysis, vomiting, and diarrhea can also interfere with eating.

Many undesirable practices that can affect the nutritional health of institutionalized patients were identified in 1974 (Butterworth and Blackburn, 1975). Today many institutions have written policies and procedures for both nurses and dietitians to follow to minimize the likelihood of iatrogenic malnutrition. Clinical Application 13–1 discusses several undesirable practices of healthcare workers and the duties that both dietitians and nurses should perform to combat institutional malnutrition.

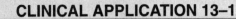

CLINICAL APPLICATION 13–1
Undesirable Practices Affecting Hospitalized Patients and Methods to Combat Iatrogenic Malnutrition

Some practices performed by healthcare professionals are undesirable. Many of these practices can affect the nutritional health of hospitalized patients. The result may be iatrogenic malnutrition. However, undesirable practices can be avoided and methods have been established for dietitians and nurses to combat institutionally induced malnutrition.

UNDESIRABLE PRACTICES PERFORMED BY HEALTHCARE PROFESSIONALS

1. Failure to record actual height and weight of patients
2. Diffusion of the responsibility for patient care, that is, among nurses, physicians, dietitians, and other healthcare workers
3. Prolonged intravenous feedings of glucose and saline (saline is a mixture of salt and distilled water and is considered isotonic in the body)
4. Failure to observe and document patients' food intake
5. Withholding meals because of diagnostic tests
6. Administering tube feedings in inadequate amounts, of uncertain composition, and under unsanitary conditions
7. Ignorance of the composition of vitamin mixtures and other nutritional products by all healthcare team members
8. Failure to recognize increased nutritional needs due to injury or illness
9. Failure to ascertain whether the patient is optimally nourished before surgery and failure to provide inadequate nutritional support after surgery
10. Failure to appreciate the role of nutrition in the prevention of and recovery from infection, with an unwarranted reliance on antibiotics
11. Lack of communication among physicians, nurses, and dietitians
12. Delay of nutritional support until a patient is in an advanced state of depletion, which is irreversible

METHODS FOR DIETITIANS AND NURSES TO COMBAT IATROGENIC MALNUTRITION

Duties to be completed by the dietitian:

- Description of recent food consumption patterns, eating habits, and meal composition (diet history)
- Circumstances of food purchase, storage, and preparation in the home (diet history)
- Estimate of daily average kilocaloric consumption (assessment)

Box continued on next page.

CLINICAL APPLICATION 13–1 *(Continued)*
Undesirable Practices Affecting Hospitalized Patients and Methods to Combat Iatrogenic Malnutrition

- Estimate of energy expenditure—for example, low, average, or high level of physical activity) (assessment)
- Estimate of possible nutrient deficiencies, based on suspected imbalances (assessment)
- Food tray viewed (monitoring)

  Duties to be completed by the nursing staff:

- While hospitalized, documentation of actual food consumption, including any provided by nonhospital sources (monitoring)
- Estimate of fluid intake (monitoring)
- Estimate of stool frequency, urinary losses, losses by suction tube, drainage, and so forth (monitoring)
- Behavior patterns, vomiting, unusual comments patients make about food (assessment and monitoring)
- Careful recording of weight at regular intervals (monitoring)

Adapted from Butterworth and Blackburn, 1975, p 8.

METHODS OF NUTRIENT DELIVERY

Nutrients can be delivered to the patient orally in foods or supplements, by a tube feeding, or parenterally through veins. An **enteral tube feeding** means the feeding of an appropriate formula or liquid via a tube to a patient's gastrointestinal tract. A **parenteral feeding** designates any route other than the gastrointestinal tract, such as intravenous (IV), meaning through the veins.

Enteral tube feeding—The feeding of a formula by tube into the gastrointestinal tract.

Oral Delivery

Parenteral feeding—Feeding administered by any route other than the gastrointestinal tract.

Most institutionalized patients are fed orally. All of the factors mentioned throughout this text influence whether or not the food items served are actually consumed by the patient. Whenever possible, the patient should be encouraged to eat foods, not only as an optimal way to obtain nutrients but also because it is beneficial for the patient to continue to experience the normal psychologic and physical pleasure associated with eating.

The Menu

An institution's menu can be selective or nonselective. A selective menu is similar to a restaurant menu in that patients can choose the specific menu items that appeal to them. Everyone has food likes and dislikes. What appeals to one patient may not appeal to another. Patients eat best when they fill out their menu, or a close significant other does so for them. Figure 13–2 illustrates a healthcare worker assisting a patient in filling out his menu.

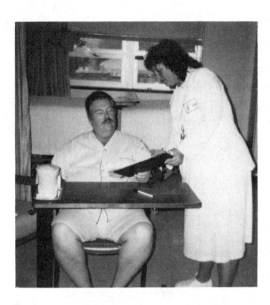

FIGURE 13–2. A hospital employee assisting a patient in filling out his menu.

Marking the menu is one way in which a patient can participate daily in care planning.

Some institutions do not have a selective menu. Only one menu is prepared and served to all patients. A nonselective menu is less expensive to serve than a selective menu.

Eating Environment

Healthcare workers need to create as pleasant an environment as possible immediately before and during mealtime. The room should be checked for objectionable odors, sounds, and sights. Obviously, a full bedside commode or an emesis basin filled with sputum or vomitus discourages eating. The patient should be prepared to eat when the tray arrives. Cleaning the patient's hands and face facilitates enthusiasm about eating. The patient's bedside table should be cleared of all miscellaneous items so that the table can be used for the patient's tray. Because all food loses temperature quickly, unnecessary delays in serving the tray should be avoided. The patient should be properly positioned to eat. This includes elevating the head of the bed (if condition permits) and positioning the bedside table to the correct height.

Some patients may find the odor of food offensive. For these patients it is best for the nurse not to uncover the food items directly in front of them, so as to minimize the risk of nausea.

Feeders versus Self-Feeders

Some patients must be fed. Food should be offered to feeders in bite-size portions and in the order that the patient prefers. The temperature of all hot liquids should be checked against the inside of the nurse's wrist before these items are offered to the patient. Patients should not be rushed during feeding. Talking with the patient while feeding makes mealtime more pleasant and signals to the patient that he or she is not rushed. Sitting while feeding the patient also indicates a willingness to spend time with the patient. Sitting also helps the patient relax.

In a long-term care facility, it is important that a patient's ability to feed himself or herself be reevaluated at regular intervals. Any patient's condition can change, and healthcare workers need to constantly be aware of any changes in the patient's condition.

Assisting the Handicapped Patient

A patient with a handicap may require either total or partial assistance with eating. Partial assistance may include opening milk cartons and plastic bags containing condiments and eating utensils, buttering the bread, and cutting the meat. Blind patients may be able to feed themselves once they are told where the food is placed on the plate. Relating food placement to the numbers on a clock may be helpful.

Some patients can feed themselves but they may be very slow, clumsy, and messy. A towel under the chin may assist in cleanup. Offering hot beverages in small amounts may minimize the likelihood of an accident.

Sometimes the type of food offered to patients may influence whether or not they can feed themselves. The consistency of food offered to the patient is one example. A thin liquid may cause some patients to choke. A thicker substance such as yogurt may be better tolerated. Finger foods such as French fries or hard-cooked eggs are better accepted by some handicapped people. The handicapped patient's food tolerances and preferences are best learned by observation and simply by asking the patient what he or she can tolerate.

Healthcare workers should encourage patients to remain as independent as possible in all the activities of daily living, including eating. If a patient cannot feed himself or herself, an evaluation should be made. Some patients' inability to feed themselves may be related to neuromuscular disabilities. Many special eating devices have been developed to assist these patients. The occupational therapist has had special training in the selection and fitting of such eating devices.

Supplemental Feedings

Many patients are unable to consume sufficient kilocalories and/or nutrients because of anorexia or an increased need. The first step with this type of patient is to offer additional foods at or between meals. Any between-meal feedings must adhere to the patient's diet order. A kilocalorie count should be started for poor eaters; Kilocalorie counts are one method to monitor the effectiveness of nutritional care. If the patient will not accept the supplemental feedings, another treatment approach may need to be implemented.

Liquid supplementation is often useful because liquids are better accepted than solids by many patients. Many debilitated patients seem to feel less full after drinking a beverage than after eating a comparable number of kilocalories and nutrients in foods. Liquid supplements can include milk, milk shakes, and instant breakfast drinks. Many different commercially prepared liquid formulas are available. Four different types of supplements are used as oral feedings: modular supplements, intact or "polymeric" formulas, elemental or "predigested" formulas, and disease-specific formulas.

Modular supplement—A nutritional supplement that contains a limited number of nutrients, usually only one.

MODULAR SUPPLEMENTS   A **modular supplement** contains only one nutrient. These are designed for patients who require the addition of only one nutrient. You were already introduced to one type of modular supplement in the chapter on carbohydrates. Moducal, Nutrisource CHO, Polycose, and Sumacal are supplements produced by different manufacturers that contain only carbohydrate. Another type of modular supplement, medium-chain triglycerides, was introduced in the chapter on fats. Medium-chain triglycerides supply only one form of lipid. Microlipid is another example of a of lipid supplement. Modular supplements for protein also exist. Examples include Pro Mod, Propac, Pro-Mix and Casec. Modular supplements are available in a liquid or powder form. Modular supplements may be added to foods, other types of oral supplements, or tube feedings.

Intact or "polymeric" formula—An oral or enteral feeding that contains all the essential nutrients in a specified volume.

INTACT OR "POLYMERIC" FORMULAS   An **intact or "polymeric" formula** is used when the GI tract is functional and the patient needs all of the essential nutrients in a specified volume. There are dozens of these products on the market. A complete supplement should always be used when the sole source of nutrition is the formula. Ensure, Sustacal, Resource, and Meritene are examples of complete nutritional supplements. Some complete nutritional supplements are also designed as tube feedings. The consistency and flavor of a feeding designed to be tube-fed will probably not be acceptable to the patient when fed orally.

Intact formulas differ from one another. Some contain lactose and some do not. Some provide fiber. The product may be a powder for reconstitution, a liquid, or a pudding. It may be flavored or unflavored. The percent of kilocalories derived from carbohydrates, fats, and proteins may be different. The source of the carbohydrate, fat and protein may be derived from various sources. For example, the protein source in Meritene is concentrated skimmed milk, while the protein source in Ensure is sodium and calcium caseinates and a soy-protein isolate. For many reasons the source of any of the three energy nutrients may be important. For example, Meritene is not a good supplement to use for a patient with a lactose intolerance. Citrotein is a clear liquid polymeric formula.

Commercial supplements should be used only after the patient's requirements for nutrients have been assessed. Unfortunately, this is not always practiced. Some healthcare workers still think that if some is good, more is better and therefore encourage the patient to consume greater amounts of oral supplement. Excess nutrients, however, are rarely beneficial. Not only do patients become frustrated because they cannot consume all of the supplement served to them, but to do so may be medically harmful. Many organs in the human body are in a stress situation in the poorly nourished patient. Why subject the patient's kidneys or liver to unnecessary work if the nutrients cannot be used efficiently? Clinical Calculation 13–1 demonstrates a suggested procedure to follow when determining the volume of an oral supplement to serve to a patient.

Elemental or "predigested" formula—Formula that contains either partially or totally predigested nutrients.

ELEMENTAL OR "PREDIGESTED" FORMULAS   Another group of oral supplements includes **elemental or "predigested" formulas.** Examples of elemental or predigested formulas include Flexical, Vital, and Vivonex. The nutrients in these formulas are easier to digest or partially digested. For example, maltrodextrins, corn syrup solids, oligosaccharides, and glucose polymers are rapidly hydrolyzed by maltase and oligosaccharidases, which are apt to be present in higher concentrations than lactase.

Protein is either partially or totally predigested. Partially predigested protein (small peptides) offer an advantage over totally predigested protein (single amino acids). Peptides and free amino acids do not inhibit each other's transport, so that absorption of nitrogen is actually improved by the inclusion of small peptides. Easier-to-digest fats include medium-chain triglycerides. Partially digested fats include mono- and diglycerides.

Predigested formulas contain little lactose and residue and may be given orally or through a tube. These formulas are very expensive and are designed only for use with patients with limited gastrointestinal function and/or metabolic disorders. They are less palatable than intact feedings, so patient acceptance is sometimes a problem when they are administered orally.

DISEASE-SPECIFIC FORMULAS   The last group of oral supplements includes those designed for patients with specific metabolic problems. For example, special formulas are available for patients with liver and kidney disorders. These special formulas are discussed in subsequent chapters.

Oral supplements are also used extensively to wean patients from both tube and parenteral feedings. Once a patient ceases to consume foods orally, a transition period is always necessary to wean the patient back to oral feedings.

Enteral Tube Feeding

Tube feedings are the second way nutrients can be delivered to patients. Some medical conditions may render oral feeding impossible, insufficient, or impractical. Table 13–4 lists several common conditions in which a tube feeding is indicated.

Tube feedings, like oral supplements, can be made from table foods or purchased commercially prepared. If money is tight and the patient has no impairment of digestion and absorption, he or she can be taught to prepare a tube feeding from table foods prior to discharge. Home-prepared tube feedings are less expensive than commercially prepared feedings but more prone

TABLE 13–4 *Conditions Indicating a Tube Feeding**

Condition	Examples
Patient has mechanical difficulties that make chewing and/or swallowing impossible or difficult	Obstruction of the esophagus, weakness or nausea, mouth sores, throat inflammation
Patient has an intestinal disease and cannot digest or absorb food adequately	Malabsorption syndromes
Patient refuses to eat or cannot eat	Anorexia nervosa, senile dementia
Patient is unable to consume a sufficient amount of food because of clinical condition	Coma, serious infections, trauma victims, patients with large kilocalorie requirements

*Other conditions will be discussed in subsequent chapters.

to contamination. Many of the commercial products described under the previous section can be used in the tube-fed patient.

Use the Gut and Make It Work

The gut should always be used to the extent possible. Oral supplements should be considered before tube feeding; tube feeding should always be considered before intravenous feeding. Tube feeding is safer, cheaper, and more physiologic than an intravenous feeding (Feldman, 1988); in other words, it mimics normal feeding conditions. Nutrients should be supplied intact as opposed to predigested if the patient has normal digestion. **Intact nutrients** are nutrients that are not predigested. With intact nutrients the body must keep producing all the secretions and enzymes necessary for digestion. This forces the gut to function.

Intact nutrients— Nutrients that have not been predigested

Tube Placement

Tubes can enter the body either through the nose or by a surgically made opening. The most common tube insertion method is through the nose. If the patient is fully alert during the procedure, he or she can assist in passing the tube by swallowing. A nasogastric (NG) tube runs from the nose to the stomach. A nasoduodenal (ND) tube runs from the nose to the duodenum. A nasojejunal (NJ) tube runs from the nose to the jejunum. These types of tubes are designed for short-term use only because of patient discomfort and tissue irritation.

When a tube is needed long-term or cannot be inserted into the nose, esophagus, or stomach because of an obstruction, an **ostomy,** or surgically formed opening, is created. An esophagostomy is a surgical opening into the esophagus through which a feeding tube is passed. A gastrostomy is a surgical opening in the stomach through which a feeding tube is passed. A jejunostomy is a surgical opening in the jejunum through which a tube is passed.

Ostomy—A surgically formed opening

Each tube location has advantages and disadvantages. One advantage of a feeding ostomy located in the intestines is that the patient is the least likely to regurgitate the feeding. Regurgitate means to cause to flow backward. Regurgitation is more likely when a feeding is administered to patients through a nasogastric tube, esophagostomy, or gastrostomy. During regurgitation the feeding backs up. If the feeding backs up into the patient's lungs, a lung infection can develop. When a patient has inhaled fluids regurgitated from the stomach, he or she may develop aspiration pneumonia. Aspiration is the state whereby a substance has been drawn into the nose, throat, or lungs. Aspiration pneumonia can be a fatal complication of a tube feeding (or improper oral feeding). Another advantage of a jejunostomy is that it bypasses any existing esophageal or gastric outlet obstruction.

Contamination

Unfortunately, tube feedings provide an excellent environment for the growth of microorganisms. When a tube feeding becomes contaminated with bacteria, the patient receiving the feeding may become ill and may suffer from gastrointestinal problems such as nausea, vomiting, or diarrhea. For this reason, many hospitals and nursing homes use only commercially prepared tube feedings (as opposed to those prepared in-house from table foods). Commercial feedings are packaged under sterile conditions. Most hospitals do not have a sterile area in their dietary departments. Even commercially prepared formulas can become contaminated if they are not handled safely after opening.

To eliminate contamination, first check the can for the correct product, flavor, expiration date, and signs of contamination such as swelling. If the can is swollen, notify your supervisor. Do not administer a feeding from a damaged can. Other cans in the same shipment should be checked for contamination.

Good personal hygiene is important. The following recommendations will reduce the possibility of contamination:

- Always wash your hands before opening the can.
- Wash the top of the can carefully before opening.
- Shake the can well before opening.
- If a can opener is needed, be sure it is clean.
- Transfer the formula into a clean container.
- Use sterile, bottled, or boiled water to dilute formula (if indicated).
- Label any remaining formula carefully with the patient's name, room number, the date the formula was opened, amount in the container, name of the product, and other pertinent information. Other information may include whether the formula is diluted or contains medications, vitamins, or other additives.
- Store the formula in the refrigerator in a covered container. When a new supply of formula is received, place it in the rear of the storage area so that the older formula is used first.
- Once opened, most formulas should be discarded after 24 hours.

Administration

Tube feedings can be administered either continuously, intermittently, or by bolus.

CONTINUOUS FEEDING Many professionals feel that a **continuous feeding** is preferable. A continuous feeding is always recommended for formulas delivered directly into the small intestine. One recommended rate is 30 to 50 milliliters per hour, increasing daily by 25 milliliters per hour to the rate necessary to provide energy needs (Feldman, 1988). This gradual increase in the formula's volume gives the patient's gastrointestinal tract a chance to adjust to the formula. This will assist in the prevention of many complications seen in tube-fed patients. Safety precautions for continuous feedings include (1) flushing the tube with water every 4 to 6 hours; and (2) allowing no more than a 4-hour hang time for each bag of formula. This will assist in preventing contamination and bacterial growth.

Continuous feeding—Delivery of a tube feeding on an ongoing basis.

Figure 13–3 illustrates some of the equipment used to deliver a specific volume and rate of a formula to a patient. An infusion pump is necessary for precise control of a continuous feeding.

INTERMITTENT FEEDING An **intermittent feeding** means giving a 4- to 6-hour volume of feeding solution over 20 to 30 minutes. Patients tolerate intermittent feedings much better than bolus feedings because these feedings more closely approximate normal eating behavior. The tube needs

Intermittent feeding—Giving a 4- to 6-hour volume of a tube feeding over 20 to 30 minutes.

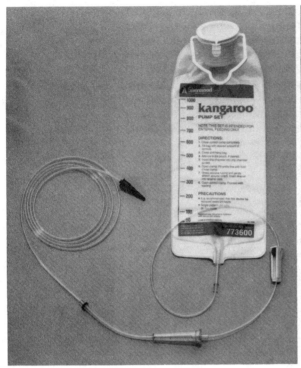
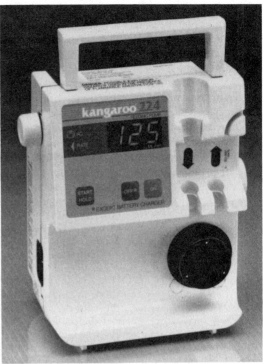

FIGURE 13–3. Equipment used to deliver a specific volume and rate of a formula to a patient. (*A*) This is a pump set. The nurse would pour the formula in the top of the bag. (*B*) This is a feeding or infusion pump (necessary for a continuous feeding). The flow rate of the formula is maintained with this device. (Photographs were provided courtesy of Sherwood Medical, St Louis, MO. Kangaroo is a registered trademark.)

to be flushed after each feeding to minimize bacterial growth and prevent contamination.

Bolus feeding— Giving a 4- to 6-hour volume of a tube feeding within a few minutes.

BOLUS FEEDING   A **bolus feeding** means giving a 4- to 6-hour volume of feeding solution within a few minutes. A patient is thus fed only four to six times per day. Feedings given by this method are frequently poorly tolerated, with patients complaining of abdominal discomfort, nausea, fullness, and cramping. Some patients, however, can tolerate bolus feedings after they have had a period of adjustment to the tube feeding. Bolus feedings are usually poorly tolerated for feedings that enter the intestines. The adjustment period should follow the procedure described above, that is, the volume of feeding is slowly increased. Patients on bolus feedings should be instructed not to recline for at least 2 hours following the feeding (Feldman, 1988). Tubes should be irrigated (flushed) after each bolus feeding to prevent contamination. Irrigation means flushing water through the tube or cavity.

Potential Complications

Many of the complications seen in the tube-fed patient have already been discussed. Complications fall into three categories: mechanical, gastrointestinal, and metabolic. Many of the metabolic complications are discussed later in this chapter and in subsequent chapters. Table 13–5 reviews the mechanical and gastrointestinal complications of tube-fed patients and lists prevention strategies.

Osmolality

The osmolality of a solution is based on the number of dissolved particles in the solution. The greater the number of particles, the higher the osmolality (see Chapter 9).

TABLE 13–5 *Common Mechanical and Gastrointestinal Complications of Tube-Fed Patients and Prevention Strategies*

Complication	Prevention Strategy
Mechanical	
Tube irritation	Consider using a smaller or softer tube
	Lubricate the tube before insertion
Tube obstruction	Flush tube after use
	Do not mix medications with the formula
	Use liquid medications if available
	Crush other medications thoroughly
	Use an infusion pump to maintain a constant flow (Fig. 13–3)
Aspiration and regurgitation	Elevate head of patient's bed greater than or equal to 30 degrees at all times
	Discontinue feedings at least 30 to 60 minutes before treatments where head must be lowered (e.g., chest percussion)
	If the patient has an endotracheal tube in place, keep the cuff inflated during feedings
Tube displacement	Replace tube and obtain physician's order to confirm with x-ray imaging
Gastrointestinal	
Cramping, distention, bloating, gas pains, nausea, vomiting, diarrhea*	Initiate and increase amount of formula gradually
	Bring formula to room temperature before feeding
	Change to a lactose-free formula
	Decrease fat content of formula
	Administer drug therapy as ordered, e.g., Lactinex, kaolin-pectin, Lomotil
	Change to formula with a lower osmolality
	Change to formula with a different fiber content
	Practice good personal hygiene when handling any feeding product
	Evaluate diarrhea-causing medications the patient may be receiving (e.g., antibiotics, digitalis)

*The most commonly cited complication of tube feeding is diarrhea.

At a given concentration, the smaller the particle size, the greater the number of particles present. Oral supplements and tube feedings with a high osmolality draw body fluid into the bowel, resulting in a fluid imbalance. The symptoms are diarrhea, nausea, and flushing. The osmolality of normal body fluids is approximately 300 milliosmoles per kilogram. Predigested nutrients have a higher osmolality than intact nutrients. An isotonic feeding has an osmolality of 300 milliosmoles, the same osmotic pressure as body fluids. Table 13–6 lists the osmolality of selected formulas.

There is a great variation from one individual to another in sensitivity to the osmolality of oral supplements and tube feedings. All patients need a period of adjustment to a formula with a high osmolality. The majority of patients are able to develop a tolerance to a high-osmolality formula. Some patients, however, are more likely to develop symptoms of an intolerance. These include debilitated patients, patients with gastrointestinal disorders, preoperative and postoperative patients, gastrostomy and jejunostomy patients, and patients whose gastrointestinal tract has not been challenged by food for a significant period of time.

Administration of Medications to a Tube-Fed Patient

All healthcare workers should be aware of potential drug-food interactions so that proper steps can be taken to minimize or avoid complications (see Chapter 14). Clinical Application 13–2 discusses suggested procedures for administering medications through feeding tubes. Medications can be physically incompatible with the tube feeding. This may be related to changes in the feeding's viscosity (thickness), or flow characteristics. Some medications may also cause the feeding to separate, granulate, or coagulate.

Monitoring the Tube-Fed Patient

The tube-fed patient requires special monitoring. The purpose of the monitoring is to check for tolerance to the feeding and to determine if the nutritional status of the patient is declining, stable, or improving (Quality Assurance Committee of the American Dietetic Association, 1984). The categories of factors that should be monitored include physical factors, intake factors, and laboratory data. Clinical Application 13–3 discusses factors that should be routinely monitored in each of these categories.

TABLE 13–6 *Osmolality of Selected Formulas*

Formula	Milliosmoles*	Description
Stresstein	910	Elemental formula
Vivonex HN	810	Elemental formula
Ensure	450	Intact or polymeric
Isocal	300	Intact or polymeric

*Please note the wide range in osmolality of the various formulas.

CLINICAL APPLICATION 13–2

Procedures for Administering Medications through Feeding Tubes

Procedures for the administration of medications through feeding tubes may vary slightly from one institution or facility to another. The following suggested procedures, however, are common in most facilities:

1. If possible, administer drugs in liquid form.
2. If the drug is not available in liquid form, consult with the pharmacist; he or she may be able to procure a liquid form or similar drug provided by the American Society of Hospital Pharmacists in Pediatric Extemporaneous Formulation List of the manufacturer's suggestions.
3. Exercise caution when calculating equivalent liquid doses. Many liquid dosage forms are intended for pediatric use and the dose of the drug must be adjusted appropriately for adults.
4. Administer crushed tablets only when no other alternatives are available.
5. If crushed tablets are administered, crush the tablet to a fine powder and mix with water. Do not crush any tablet on the list of oral drugs that should not be crushed or drugs with enteric coatings. Do not crush drugs with a sustained-release action. If in doubt, do not hesitate to consult with the pharmacist.
6. Administer each drug separately. Do not mix all the medications for one dosing time. Flush with at least 5 milliliters (one teaspoonful) of water between each medication.
7. Flush the tube with at least 30 milliliters of water before giving the medication and before restarting the tube feeding.
8. To avoid causing gastric irritation and diarrhea, drugs that are hypertonic or irritating to the cells that line the gastrointestinal tract, such as potassium chloride, should be diluted in at least 30 milliliters of water prior to administration.
9. If the medication is ordered to be added to the feeding, observe the feeding after the addition for any reaction or precipitation. Shake the solution thoroughly. Label the feeding with at least the name and amount of the drug added, the time, date, and your initials.
10. Drugs usually administered with meals to avoid gastric irritation, such as indomethacin, should also be diluted with water prior to administration.
11. Sustained- or slow-release formulations of drugs that are used for once-daily dosing may need to have divided dosing schedules when administered in liquid form.

Adapted from Wright, 1986, p. 33.

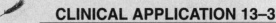

CLINICAL APPLICATION 13–3

Physical and Intake Factors and Laboratory Data to Monitor in the Patient Receiving Nutritional Support

Patients who are receiving nutritional support such as tube feeding require special monitoring. This is done (1) to check for tolerance to the feeding and (2) to determine the effect of the feeding. Many physical factors and intake factors are routinely monitored; certain laboratory data are monitored as well.

Physical factors to routinely monitor include:

- A change in gastrointestinal tract function
- Abdominal discomfort or gas
- Stool consistency, frequency, odor, and color (when the onset of diarrhea occurs without a formula change, consider medication rather than feeding as probable cause; potential formula factors include rapid administration, cold feedings, fat malabsorption, lactase deficiency, protein malnutrition, bacterial contamination, or high osmolality). Constipation may be caused by dehydration, impaction, and/or obstruction (Feldman, 1988).
- Gastric retention, that is, formula remains in the stomach (formula has too high an osmolality) (Feldman, 1988)
- Weight changes (should not exceed ¼ to ½ pound per day)
- Intake and output
- Temperature
- Patient's physical condition
- Psychological impact of the feeding

Intake factors to routinely monitor include:

- Volume ordered
- Volume actually administered
- Adequacy of intake compared to needs (kilocalorie/protein count)

Laboratory data to monitor include:

- Urinary glucose/serum glucose
- Serum electrolytes
- Calcium-to-phosphorus ratio
- CBC with differential
- Liver function tests
- Urinary urea nitrogen (if available)
- Transferrin (if available)
- Retinol-binding protein
- Skin testing (to assess immunocompetence)
- BUN/creatinine
- Serum albumin
- Cholesterol/triglycerides (should be tested at least 6 hours after lipid infusion has stopped)

Adapted from The Quality Assurance Committee of the American Dietetic Association, 1984, p. 89 with permission.

Metabolic, fluid, and electrolyte complications can occur during enteral nutritional support. Adequate monitoring of the patient on an enteral feeding is not merely cost-effective but critical to ensure successful therapy.

Home Enteral Nutrition

Many patients on tube feedings are being discharged from hospitals and nursing homes. Most hospitals and nursing homes that discharge patients on home enteral nutrition (HEN) have a **nutrition support service.** The delivery of effective nutritional support requires a team effort. Team members usually include the physician, pharmacist, nurse clinician, dietitian, and social worker. Team functions vary from one facility to another. Members of nutrition support teams are responsible for the assessment and monitoring of inpatients, for patient education, and for the instruction of patients discharged on home enteral nutrition. Some nutrition support service team members also arrange for patient follow-up in outpatient clinics.

Nutrition support service—A team service that assesses, monitors, and counsels patients on enteral and parenteral feedings.

Parenteral Nutrition

Parenteral nutrition is the third way nutrients can be delivered to the patient. Nutrients are delivered to the patient through the veins (intravenously) in parenteral nutrition. **Peripheral parenteral nutrition (PPN)** means to fed the patient via a vein away from the center of the body. In **total parenteral nutrition** (TPN) the patient is fed via a central vein. TPN and PPN can be used to provide partial or total daily nutritional requirements. Patients who cannot or should not be fed through the gastrointestinal tract are some of the candidates for TPN and PPN.

Peripheral parenteral nutrition (PPN)—An intravenous feeding via a vein away from the center of the body.

Total parenteral nutrition (TPN)—An intravenous feeding via a central vein that provides total nutrition.

Peripheral Parenteral Nutrition

Intravenous (IV) feedings are routine in most healthcare institutions. IV solutions usually contain water, dextrose, electrolytes, and occasionally other nutrients. IV solutions are used to maintain fluid, electrolyte, and acid-base balance. Intravenous solutions do contain kilocalories. Clinical Calculation 13–2 describes how to calculate the kilocalorie content of an intravenous solution.

Amino acids and fat can be supplied peripherally. To prevent ketosis, intravenous lipid emulsions should contribute no more than 60 percent of the total kilocalories provided (McCoy, 1991). Dextrose concentrations are limited to approximately 10 percent since peripheral veins are unable to withstand concentrations greater than 900 milliosmoles per kilogram (Moore, 1993). Thus, PPN has often failed to provide adequate kilocalories and other nutrients for repair and replacement of losses. PPN has been used to supplement a partially successful enteral nutrition program.

A new system for PPN (called all-in-one or three-in-one) has been developed that allows a higher osmotic load (1200 to 1350 milliosmoles per liter to be delivered peripherally. Lipids, amino acids, and dextrose are all incorporated in one container. Tolerance of this higher osmotic admixture in peripheral veins might be attributed to the buffering and dilution effects of intravenous fats in combination with the higher pH of the amino acid solutions and the addition of heparin to the admixture (Hoheim, 1990).

The ratio of nonprotein to protein kilocalories is important in peripheral feedings. Please see Chapter 22 for a discussion of this topic.

Total Parenteral Nutrition

When nutrients are infused into a central vein, parenteral nutrition is often referred to as TPN or hyperalimentation. Hyperalimentation is actually a misnomer because it implies that the solution exceeds nutritional requirements. The superior vena cava is one of the largest-diameter veins in the human body and is often used for TPN. Total parenteral nutrition can deliver greater nutrient loads because the blood flow in the superior vena cava rapidly dilutes these solutions 1000-fold (Feldman, 1988). Concentrations for both dextrose and amino acids are determined by the patient's needs.

For example, 2500 milliliters of a 25 percent dextrose solution with 3.5 percent amino acids would provide 625 grams of dextrose and about 87 grams of amino acids. This would provide about 375 kilocalories from amino acids and 2500 kilocalories from carbohydrate. Please note that the standard values of 4 kilocalories per gram for both carbohydrate and protein are not used when calculating kilocalories provided via hyperalimentation. Kilocalories are calculated using the values of 4.3 kilocalories per gram of amino acids provided and 3.4 kilocalories per gram of carbohydrate provided (Quality Assurance Committee of the American Dietetic Association, 1984).

INSERTION AND CARE OF TPN LINE   The physician inserts the TPN line usually through the subclavian vein and into the superior vena cava (Fig. 13–4). It can be inserted at the patient's bedside following strict aseptic technique. The TPN solution is a sterile mixture of glucose, amino acids, vitamins, and minerals. The pharmacist usually prepares the TPN solution. Lipids are usually administered to the patient in a separate solution. Vitamins B_{12}, K, and folic acid are given to the patient separately.

Total parenteral nutrition has both advantages and disadvantages. Central TPN should not be carried out without experienced personnel and proper facilities. One disadvantage of TPN is that it takes a highly trained staff to provide safe administration and close monitoring. This makes the therapy expensive. The TPN nurse is responsible for assessing, monitoring, and educating the patient destined for home TPN. The clinical dietitian on the TPN team usually has an advanced degree and special training. The dietitian is responsible for constant nutrition assessment, monitoring, interpretation of data, and calculating formula needs with the physician.

MONITORING   Careful administration of the TPN solution is important. Most reputable institutions have a strict protocol that must be followed by all healthcare professionals. A protocol is a description of steps to be followed when performing a procedure. Protocols vary widely from one institution to another. Most TPN protocols include the following: a slow start, a strict schedule, close monitoring, instructions for increasing the volume, maintenance of a constant rate, and instructions on a slow withdrawal. The solution may require adjustment. This can be done by increasing or decreasing any or all of the nutrients. Both careful monitoring of the patient's response to TPN and taking corrective measures when needed are essential for safe administration of these solutions.

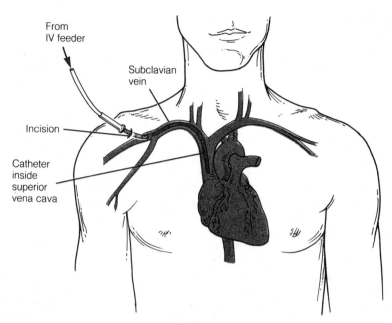

FIGURE 13–4. TPN line placement via subclavian vein to superior vena cava. (With permission from Williams, SR: Essentials of Nutrition and Diet Therapy, ed. 5, Times Mirror/Mosby College Publishing, St Louis, MO, 1990.)

Many metabolic complications are possible with TPN. Rapid shifts of potassium, phosphorus, and magnesium intracellularly result in a lowering of their concentrations in the serum. The TPN solution may need to be altered if there is a drop in the serum values of these electrolytes. Providing glucose in excess of kilocaloric needs can result in several problems, including carbon dioxide retention with respiratory difficulty. Liver function test results will become abnormal after an excess glucose load. Excess glucose may lead to hyperlipidemia and fatty deposits in the liver. The avoidance of metabolic complications directly related to a glucose overload is one reason TPN patients need to be monitored closely. These complications can be avoided by providing only an appropriate and not an excessive amount of kilocalories. In addition, an initial slow infusion at low concentrations prevents complications.

TRANSITION AND COMBINATION FEEDINGS   Patients need a transition period from TPN to oral feedings. Some physicians prefer to wean patients from TPN by using tube feeding. Other physicians prefer to avoid the tube and wean patients orally. In the latter case, as the patient's oral intake increases, the TPN solution is gradually withdrawn. Expect the patient who has been on TPN for a significant period of time to experience some difficulty with oral feedings. One of the problems with TPN is that the gut does not have to work during its administration. Consequently the gut will have undergone some negative structural cellular changes during TPN. Oral foods should be offered slowly during the weaning process. Some physicians avoid this problem by allowing some patients to consume a clear liquid or light diet while on TPN, if their condition permits.

HOME PARENTERAL NUTRITION   Increasingly, patients are being discharged on TPN. Patients need adequate follow-up by either the hospital or a community home agency.

Summary

The nutritional care of patients is a joint responsibility of both the dietary and nursing departments. All nurses who work in institutions need to know not only how meals are distributed to patients but also current meal service schedules. This will have an impact on the administration of medications and the scheduling of patients for procedures. Nutritional care includes three areas: assessing the patient's need for nutrients, monitoring nutrient intake, and counseling patients about nutritional needs.

Nutrients can be delivered to patients orally, via tube feeding, and/or parenterally. One principle is followed when selecting a feeding route: if the gut works, use the gut to maximum capability. Every means should be attempted to assist patients to eat orally and independently. Oral feedings should be considered before tube feeding. Tube feeding should be considered before intravenous feeding. Intravenous feeding can be delivered peripherally or through the superior vena cava. Patients on either tube feedings or intravenous feedings need to be closely monitored.

A case study and a sample plan of care appear below. Both are designed to show you how the information you have studied in this chapter can be used in nursing practice.

CASE STUDY 13–1

P. was brought in to the emergency room by ambulance with his mother. The mother stated her son was hit by a car while riding his bike. P. is 11 years old, 4 feet 11 inches tall, and weighs 89 pounds. The patient's mother stated her son was well prior to the accident. In the emergency room it was observed that both his eyes were surrounded by contusions, his throat and the left side of his face were swollen. Communication at first with the patient was minimal because it was painful for him to speak. An intravenous solution of D_5W was started in the emergency room. He was also shown to have a fractured femur (long bone in the thigh). Surgery was required to reset the bone. The physician determined that traction would be necessary. Traction is the process of drawing the body by weights into alignment. P. is expected to require traction, and thus hospitalization, for 3 to 5 weeks.

Five days later, P. is still having problems swallowing. He has not progressed beyond sips of clear liquids. The kilocalorie count showed an average daily intake of 395 kilocalories, with only 8 grams of protein for the past 3 days. P. appears to be in pain when he swallows and has choked twice on larger sips of the clear liquids. The patient speaks only in single words or short sentences. It is still painful for him to talk. The swelling in his esophagus has decreased enough to allow the insertion of a small silicone feeding tube. The physician has ordered a nasogastric feeding tube with Enrich. The order reads:

Day 1	Continuous drip	50 milliliters per hour	1/2 strength
Day 2	Continuous drip	50 milliliters per hour	3/4 strength
Day 3	Continuous drip	50 milliliters per hour	full strength
Day 4	Continuous drip	84 milliliters per hour	full strength

Enrich contains 1.1 kilocalories per milliliter and 39.7 grams of protein per 1000 milliliters. P. may have ice chips and small amounts of clear liquids in addition to the tube feeding as desired. The physician stated, "The patient will remain on a tube feeding until he can consume his kilocalorie requirement orally. This patient requires adequate nutrition to enable the femur to heal properly." P. is not expected to be discharged on a home enteral tube feeding. His prognosis is good and he is expected to make a full recovery.

The physician inserted the nasogastric tube himself because of the swelling in the esophagus and the danger of a perforation. As the nurse, you assisted at the patient's bedside. The patient held your hand tightly as the tube was inserted. He had a worried look on his face, increased facial perspiration, and increased pulse/respirations during the procedure.

NURSING CARE PLAN FOR P.

Assessment

Subjective: Patient held hand tightly during nasogastric tube insertion and appeared worried, apprehensive, and jittery.

Objective: Patient is a trauma victim who showed increased perspiration and increased pulse/respirations during the tube insertion procedure.

Nursing Diagnosis

Fear: Patient fear related to enteral nutrition therapy and situational crisis as evidenced by facial tension during tube insertion and increased pulse/respirations and perspiration.

Desired Outcome/Evaluation Criteria

1. The patient will state he needs the food in the tube feeding to heal his leg until he is eating better.

Nursing Actions/Interventions with Rationales in Italics

1a. Explain enteral nutrition therapy procedures as performed. *A tube feeding is unfamiliar to most patients. Knowledge about the procedure may relax the patient.*

1b. As the patient's condition permits, be available to the patient for listening and talking. Encourage the patient to acknowledge and express feelings. *The patient needs to vent his feelings about both the tube feeding and the situational crisis (the accident).*

STUDY AIDS

Chapter Review Questions

1. Modular formula feedings:
   a. Always have a low osmolality
   b. Are designed for patients with malabsorption
   c. Contain a limited number of nutrients
   d. Are always predigested

2. The best way the nurse can effectively combat iatrogenic malnutrition is by:
   a. Estimating the patient's energy expenditure
   b. Carefully recording weight at regular intervals
   c. Ordering a predigested supplement for all poor eaters
   d. Encouraging patients to clean their plates

3. A(n) _____ provides all of the essential nutrients in a specified volume.
   a. Intact or polymeric formula
   b. Modular feeding
   c. Intravenous feeding

4. Careful administration of total parenteral nutrition does *not* include:
   a. A slow start
   b. Close monitoring
   c. Abrupt withdrawal
   d. A strict schedule

5. Potential tube-feeding complications do *not* include:
   a. Refusal due to lack of palatability
   b. Overfeeding
   c. Diarrhea, nausea, and vomiting
   d. Aspiration and regurgitation

6. A diet manual usually contains all of the following except one. Identify the *exception*.
   a. Meal service delivery schedules
   b. Food items restricted and allowed on special diets
   c. Nursing procedures for transmitting a diet order to the dietary department
   d. Patient diet instruction sheets

7. Too rapid an infusion of TPN is *not* related to:
   a. Hyperlipoproteinemia
   b. Respiratory difficulty
   c. Fatty deposit in the liver
   d. Cancer

8. Diarrhea in the tube-fed patient is most likely to be caused by the following:
   a. A continuous infusion feeding
   b. A bolus feeding
   c. A fluid deficit
   d. Insufficient kilocalories

9. Total parenteral nutrition is the same as:
   a. Oral modular feedings
   b. Enteral feedings
   c. A tube feeding
   d. Hyperalimentation

10. Which of the following is *not* a recommended procedure for administering medications through a tube feeding?
    a. Mix all the medications together, crush thoroughly, mix with water, and add to the formula.
    b. If at all possible, use medications in the liquid form.
    c. Flush the tube with at least 30 milliliters of water prior to giving the medication and before resuming the tube-feeding formula.
    d. If a medication is ordered to be added to the formula, observe the feeding after the addition for any reaction or precipitation.

NCLEX-Style Quiz

Situation One

Mr. J., 58 years old, visits his physician with a complaint of abdominal pain. He is scheduled for a diagnostic work-up, which will include a barium enema (x-ray study of his colon).

1. The nurse prior to this procedure should instruct the patient to:
    a. Eat a large breakfast on the day of the examination, such as orange juice, cereal, toast, scrambled eggs, and milk.
    b. Drink ample fluids on the morning of the examination, including at least 12 ounces of juice, 1 cup of gelatin, and broth.
    c. Take nothing orally after midnight on the day of exam and consume only gelatin, clear broth, tea, coffee, and grape, apple, or cranberry juice on the day before the exam.
    d. Drink milk, juices, and coffee and eat only strained cream soups, ice cream, and gelatin on the day before the exam and take nothing orally after midnight.

Situation Two

Ms. L. has a jejunostomy. She was discharged from the hospital last week after receiving instructions on home care from the nutrition support service.

2. The local pharmacy is out of the Vivonex formula she has been instructed to use. As the nurse, you recommend that:
    a. She substitute Ensure
    b. She substitute Polycose
    c. She contact the Nutrition Support Service for instructions
    d. She substitute an intact or polymeric formula

Situation Three

Mr. W. has been receiving a tube feeding of Ensure via nasogastric tube for 3 weeks via a bolus infusion. He has just started to have loose stools (300 milliliters each × 6 today).

3. You should first suspect the following to be responsible for the diarrhea:
    a. A new medication added to his treatment plan
    b. Bacterial contamination
    c. Intolerance to the bolus delivery method
    d. Lactose intolerance

Situation Four

Mr. L. has been a resident of the nursing home for the past 12 months. During the past month he has lost 2 pounds and his food acceptance has been poor (less than 50 percent of the total amount served). He has been on a general diet. As the nurse you should first recommend:

    a. A tube feeding
    b. TPN
    c. More frequent oral feedings
    d. PPN

CLINICAL CALCULATION 13–1

How Much Oral Supplement Is Indicated?

1. Place patient on a kilocalorie count.
2. Calculate patient's kilocalorie allowance.
3. Select an appropriate oral supplement for the patient. Some hospitals allow patients to taste several supplements and choose the one most palatable to them.
4. Determine the difference between the patient's recorded food intake and kilocalorie allowance.
5. Determine the kilocaloric concentration of the formula. This can be done by referring to either the appropriate table in the diet manual or the supplement's label. Usually formulas are between 1.0 to 2.0 kilocalories per milliliter.
6. Determine how many milliliters of formula are needed to meet the patient's kilocalorie allowance.
7. Divide the total milliliters needed by the number of feedings to be offered.
8. Calculate the patient's protein allowance (0.8 grams per kilogram).
9. Check to make sure that the patient's protein allowance will be met by the combination of recorded protein intake and volume to be provided in the supplement. Also check to make sure that the patient will not be receiving more than twice the RDA for protein.

Example:

1. Assume that the patient ate 550 kilocalories.
2. Assume that the patient is a woman who weighs 60 kilograms, is 55 years of age, and is 5 feet 6 inches tall. (Review Chapter 2 if necessary to calculate kilocalorie allowance; the 30 kilocalories per kilograms was taken from Table 8–4.)

    Patient needs approximately 30 kilocalories per kilogram

    Kilocalories = 30 kilocalories per kilogram × 60 kilograms

    Kilocalories allowance = 1800 kilocalories

3. Assume that the patient has tasted several supplements and prefers Sustacal Liquid.

Box continued on next page.

CLINICAL CALCULATION 13–1 *(Continued)*

How Much Oral Supplement Is Indicated?

4. The patient's kilocalorie allowance is 1800 kilocalories.

> The patient ate 550 kilocalories.
> The difference is 1250 kilocalories.

5. Sustacal Liquid contains 1.0 kilocalories per milliliter (information obtained from the product's label).
6. The patient needs 1250 milliliters of Sustacal Liquid.

$$\frac{1250 \text{ kilocalories}}{1 \text{ kilocalorie per milliliter}} = 1250 \text{ milliliters}$$

7. The patient stated she would prefer to drink this feeding six times per day—some on each tray and at three between-meal feedings.

$$\frac{1250 \text{ milliliters}}{6 \text{ feedings}} = 210 \text{ milliliters per feeding*}$$

8. Assume from the patient's recorded food intake that she is eating about 10 grams of protein per day. A woman weighing 60 kilograms has a protein allowance of 0.8 grams per kilogram.

$$60 \text{ kilograms} \times 0.8 \text{ grams per kilogram} = 48 \text{ grams of protein}$$

Subtract the 10 grams eaten from trays -10

The supplement should provide at least 38 grams of protein and no more than 96 grams (48 × 2) of protein.†

9. Sustacal Liquid contains 61 grams of protein per 1000 milliliters or 0.061 grams per milliliter.

$$1250 \text{ milliliters} \times 0.061 \text{ grams per milliliter} = 76.25 \text{ grams of protein}$$

The patient's protein allowance will more than be met by 1250 milliliters of Sustacal Liquid.

---

*This product is available is both quarts and 240-milliliter units. Some institutions stock only 240-milliliter units and may prefer to dispense this feeding in 240-milliliter units. In this situation, divide 240 milliliters into 1250 milliliters. The patient would need only 5.2 feedings per day. This would be offered to the patient in four feedings of 240 milliliters for a total of 960 milliliters and one feeding of 290 milliliters to equal the 1250 milliliters.

†It is important that the feeding not provide more than twice the patient's protein allowance. In this case, 48 × 2 = 96 grams. As the patient is eating about 10 grams of protein per day and will consume about 76 grams more in the supplement, her total protein intake would be approximately 86 grams per day. This amount does not exceed twice her RDA for protein and is therefore acceptable.

CLINICAL CALCULATION 13–2

Calculation of Kilocalories in IV Solutions

D_5W means 5 percent dextrose in water. The subscript following the D tells you the percent of dextrose in the solution. Other common concentrations of sugar and water are $D_{10}W$ and $D_{50}W$.

A 5 percent concentration of dextrose means 100 milliliters of water contains 5 grams of dextrose. A 10 percent concentration of dextrose means 100 milliliters of water contains 10 grams of dextrose. A 50 percent concentration of dextrose means 100 milliliters of water contains 50 grams of dextrose. A simple proportion should be used to calculate the amount of kilocalories in a any given volume of a solution.

The formula is:

$$\frac{\text{percent of concentration}}{100 \text{ milliliters}} \quad \text{as} \quad \frac{x \text{ grams of dextrose}}{\substack{\text{volume of solution} \\ \text{patient received}}}$$

For example, a patient has received 2000 milliliters of D_5W:

$$\frac{5 \text{ grams of dextrose}}{100 \text{ milliliters}} \quad \text{as} \quad \frac{x \text{ grams of dextrose}}{2000 \text{ milliliters}}$$

Proportions are solved by cross-multiplication and division: (5 grams × 2000 milliliters) divided by 100 milliliters = 100 grams of dextrose. One gram of carbohydrate given intravenously provides 3.4 kilocalories; thus 100 grams × 3.4 kilocalories per gram = 340 kilocalories.

BIBLIOGRAPHY

American Osteopathic Association: AOA Fact Sheet. American Osteopathic Association, Chicago, 1990.

Butterworth, CE: The skeleton in the hospital closet. Nutrition Today 9:8, 1975.

Butterworth, CE and Blackburn, GL: Hospital malnutrition and how to assess the nutritional status of a patient. Nutrition Today 10:8, 1975.

Cerra, FB: Pocket Manual of Surgical Nutrition. CV Mosby, St Louis, 1984.

Edes, TE, Walk, BE, and Austin, JL: Diarrhea in tube-fed patients: Feeding formula not necessarily the cause. Am J Med 88:91, 1990.

Feinstein, PJ: Healthcare Economics. John Wiley & Sons, New York, 1983.

Feldman, EB: Essentials of Clinical Nutrition. FA Davis, Philadelphia, 1988.

Hoheim, TA, et al: Clinical experience with three-in-one admixtures administered peripherally. Nutrition in Clinical Practice 5:118, 1990.

Hopkins, JL (ed): QRC Advisor: Managing Hospital Quality, Risk, and Cost. Aspen Publications, Volume 4 Number 7. May, 1988.

Hui, YH: Human Nutrition and Diet Therapy. Wadsworth Health Sciences, Monterey, CA, 1983.

Kamath, SK, Lawyer, M, Smith, AE, and Olson, R: Hospital Malnutrition: A 33 hospital screening study. J AM Dietc Assoc 86: 2, 203, 1986.

McCoy BL: TPN in the pediatric patient. Support line, Dietitians in Nutritional Support 12:5, 1991.

Metheny, N, Eisenberg, P, and McSweeney, M: Effect of feeding tube properties and 3 irrigants on clogging rates. Nursing Research 37(3):165, 1988.

Michigan Department of Public Health: Feeding the Aged. G-24N, May 1966.

Moore, MC: Pocket Guide to Nutrition and Diet Therapy. CV Mosby, St Louis, 1993.

Norwich-Eaton Pharmaceuticals: Care and Handling of Enteral Products. Norwich, NY, 1983.

Pagana, KD and Pagana, TJ: Diagnostic Testing and Nursing Implications. CV Mosby, St Louis, 1992.

Poleman, CM and Capra, CL: Nutrition: Shackelton's Essentials and Diet Therapy, ed 5. WB Saunders, Philadelphia, 1984.

Robinson, CH and Weigley, ES: Basic Nutrition and Diet Therapy, ed 6. Macmillan, New York, 1989.

Rohde, Cl and Baun, TM: Home Enteral/Parenteral Nutrition Therapy: A Practitioner's Guide American Dietetic Association, Chicago, 1986.

Stanfield, P: Nutrition and Diet Therapy: Self-Instructional Modules. Jones & Bartlett, Boston/Monterey, 1986.

The Quality Assurance Committee of the American Dietetic Association: Suggested Guidelines for Nutrition Management of the Critically Ill Patient. American Dietetic Association, Chicago, 1984.

West, CW and Suitor, MF: Nutrition: Principles and Issues in Health Promotion. JB Lippincott, Philadelphia, 1984.

Whitney, EN, Cataldo, CB, and Rolfes, SR: Understanding Normal and Clinical Nutrition, ed 3. West, St Paul, 1991.

Williams, SR: Essentials of Nutrition and Diet Therapy, ed 5. Times Mirror/Mosby College Publishing, St Louis, 1990.

Wright, B: Enteral feeding tubes as drug delivery systems. Nutr Supp Serv 6:33, 1986.

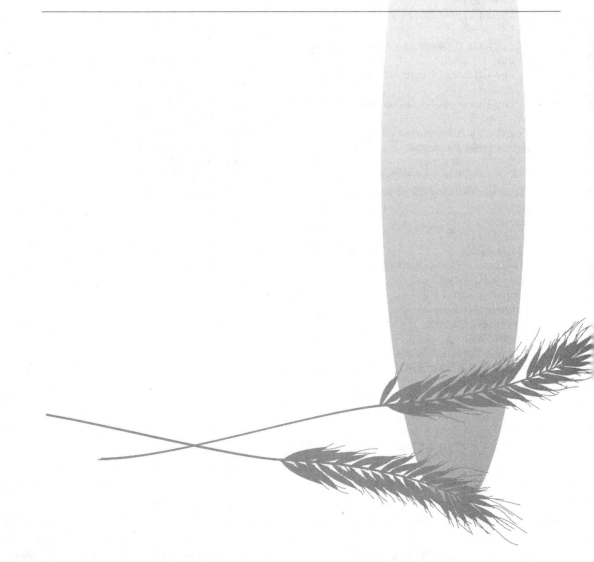

Unit Three
Clinical
Nutrition

Chapter Outline

Key Terms

As a study aid, each key term is followed by the page number where the term is defined in the chapter. Terms that appear in **boldface** or <u>underscored</u> in the chapter text are located in the glossary.

Food, Nutrient, and Drug Interactions

Learning Objectives

After completing this chapter, the student should be able to:

1. Explain the importance of proper scheduling of medications in relation to food intake.
2. Identify two groups of patients likely to experience food-drug interactions.
3. Recognize the effects of various foods and beverages on drug action.
4. Describe four ways in which nutrients and drugs can interact and give an example of each.
5. Discuss one food-drug interaction that is potentially life-threatening and design nursing interventions to avoid this possibility.
6. Relate sodium-water balance to the effects of lithium.

*T*his chapter explains and gives examples of the different ways in which drugs interact with foods (including beverages); nutrients (including nutrient formulas and supplements); and the nonnutrient components of foods. In no sense is the discussion exhaustive. Refer to pharmaceutical references when administering medications.

A drug is a substance other than food intended to affect the structure or function of the body. As used in the text, the term "drug" includes alcohol and both prescription and over-the-counter drugs. As is the practice in most hospitals, we use the **generic name** of the drug.

THE EFFECTS OF DRUGS ON NUTRITIONAL STATUS

Generic name— The name given to the drug by the original developer; usually the same as the official name given to it by the Food and Drug Administration.

Any person taking a drug risks potentially harmful effects from food and drug interactions. Nutritional status can be affected because these interactions can alter (1) food intake, (2) the absorption of nutrients or drugs, (3) the metabolism of nutrients or drugs, and (4) the excretion of nutrients or drugs. Some known interactions are considered clinically desirable and result in the control of a disease process. For example, by restricting a patient's dietary vitamin K, the effect of warfarin (an anticoagulant) is prolonged. However, many effects resulting from food and drug interactions are undesirable. These include nutritional deficiencies, growth retardation in children, loss of disease control, and acute toxic reactions. Some persons, especially the elderly, are at higher risk than others for suffering unwanted effects.

Identifying Patients at High Risk

Persons at highest risk for food and drug interactions are those who (1) take many drugs, including alcohol, (2) require long-term drug therapy, or (3) have poor or marginal nutrition. These and other risk-increasing factors are listed in Clinical Application 14–1. The elderly are particularly vulnerable because they are more likely to have several of the risk factors mentioned in the Clinical Application (Fig. 14–1). They are also more prone to such interactions as a result of self-medication, noncompliance, and changes in their nutritional-status needs associated with aging. Clinical Application 14–2 lists factors that should trigger investigation of the patient's risk of drug-nutrient interactions. Both drug and food intake may need to be modified, especially in the elderly, to minimize food and drug interactions that may adversely affect nutritional status.

Minimizing Food and Drug Interactions

Known adverse outcomes of food and drug interactions can be offset by changes in either drug dosage or diet or changes in both. Because drugs often increase or decrease the absorption of nutrients, it may be necessary to change (1) the route of administration, (2) the dose of a drug, (3) the time interval between doses, and/or (4) whether or not the drug is administered with food. For example, therapeutic drug levels may not be achieved or may take longer to build if less drug is absorbed due to an interaction with food. This could prolong a disease or prevent its cure. Dosage adjustments often will minimize such effects.

CLINICAL APPLICATION 14–1

Factors Increasing the Risk of Drug-Nutrient Interactions

The risk of a drug-nutrient interaction is increased if a patient:
- *Is malnourished*
- *Consumes alcohol*
- *Takes a high-potency vitamin or mineral supplement*
- *Is receiving many drugs*

or if the patient's drugs:
- *Are given with meals*
- *Are instilled into a feeding tube*
- *Are prescribed long-term to control chronic disease*
- *Are known to cause malabsorption or have antinutrient effects*

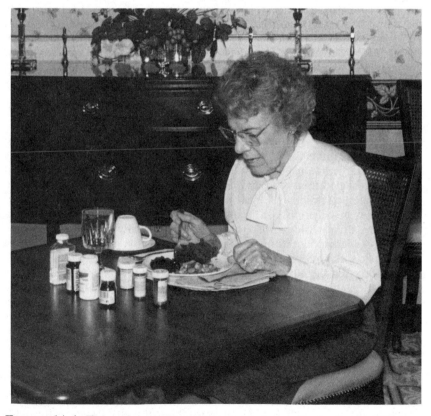

FIGURE 14–1. This woman displays several risk factors for drug-nutrient interactions. She is elderly, is on a multiple drug regimen, and takes some of her medications with a meal.

CLINICAL APPLICATION 14–2

Screening Patients at Risk of Drug-Nutrient Interactions

Further nutritional assessment may be in order if the patient:

1. Relates a recent weight change
2. Abuses alcohol
3. Consumes a modified diet, including one characterized by significant changes in protein content
4. Takes medication with meals
5. Suffers a loss of disease control after a medication or diet change
6. Displays laboratory values indicating nutrient depletion
7. Receives medications known to interfere with nutrition

Certain foods or nutrients (including supplements) may be (1) added to the diet, (2) deleted from the diet, or (3) required in increased or reduced amounts in order to counterbalance adverse nutrient-drug interactions. For example, protein inhibits the absorption of phenytoin, an anticonvulsant drug, whereas carbohydrate increases its absorption. Depending on the desired therapeutic effect, dietary intake of protein and/or carbohydrate may need to be modified.

Professional and Clinical Resources

Food and drug interactions can be complex, especially if the patient is on a multiple-drug regimen or is at high risk for other reasons. Having a sound knowledge of potential food and drug interactions is an important function of healthcare professionals. Physicians, nutritionists, pharmacists, and nurses have a joint responsibility in being aware of and controlling such interactions. The clinical pharmacist can be a valuable ally of the nurse when scheduling medications for optimal effect. Likewise, the clinical dietitian may be asked to assess a patient's risk for food-drug interactions. A good reference library on the clinical unit is also helpful in providing information.

Food and drug interactions can occur at every stage of the nutritive process. Drugs may affect food and nutrients, and food, in turn, may affect drugs.

THE EFFECTS OF DRUGS ON FOODS AND NUTRIENTS

A number of drugs have a variety of effects on foods and nutrients: (1) drugs can affect food intake; (2) drugs can alter the absorption of nutrients through both luminal and mucosal effects; (3) the metabolism of nutrients can be affected by drugs; and (4) drugs can increase or decrease the excretion of certain nutrients.

The Effects of Drugs on Food Intake

Even before food is ingested, drugs can affect food intake. Several drugs increase or decrease appetite, interfere with the senses of taste and smell, and cause gastric irritation. Food is sometimes used to temper these and other side effects of drugs.

Decreased Appetite

CNS stimulants, including dextroamphetamine and methylphenidate, both used in the treatment of narcolepsy or the management of attention deficit disorder (ADD), have the effect of depressing the desire for food. One of the side effects of these stimulants in children is slowed growth. Dextroamphetamine is more likely to interfere with growth than methylphenidate.

Antineoplastics, drugs or agents that prevent the development, growth, or proliferation of malignant cells, are notorious for causing a loss of appetite (anorexia). Loss of appetite is further increased by other side effects including severe nausea, vomiting, and **stomatitis.** Examples of such antineoplastic drugs are bleomycin, plicamycin, and vincristine.

Poor appetite can also result from drugs that cause a dry mouth. Many antihistamines, including brompheniramine and diphenhydramine, decrease saliva output.

Nursing considerations regarding drugs that decrease appetite concern assessment and interventions. When assessing a patient with a weight-loss history or a patient taking drugs known to cause food and drug interactions, nurses should review the patient's drug regimen. Both physician-prescribed and self-prescribed drugs and nutritional supplements are pertinent to include.

Antineoplastic— A drug or other agent that prevents the development, growth, or proliferation of malignant cells.

Stomatitis—An inflammation of the mouth.

Increased Appetite

Some antidepressants may promote appetite and lead to marked weight gain. One such drug, bupropion, can either increase or decrease appetite. Another antidepressant, doxepin, increases the appetite.

Medroxyprogesterone, a female hormone used as an oral contraceptive and in cyclic hormone therapy after menopause, also increases appetite. This hormone occurs naturally in the second half of the menstrual cycle and in pregnancy (to support the growth requirements of the mother and fetus). To minimize its effects, several nursing interventions might be appropriate: increasing the fiber content of the patient's diet and encouraging the patient to drink 6 to 8 glasses of water daily, eat slowly, and chew food thoroughly.

Changes in Taste or Smell

The senses of taste and smell influence the response to foods. Some drugs alter the perception of these senses; thus foods and beverages can taste bitter, metallic, or unpleasant. This usually leads to a decreased appetite, but some individuals will try to get rid of the taste sensation by eating constantly.

Acetylsalicylic acid (ASA), more commonly known as aspirin, is a drug used to control pain or to reduce fever. Currently, it is also being taken in small daily doses to decrease the risk of heart attacks. One gram of ASA, about three adult-dose tablets, increases the taste perception of bitterness.

An anti-infective reserved for tuberculosis and other serious infections, streptomycin, is excreted in the saliva. One result is a metallic or bitter taste even when the drug is administered by intramuscular injection.

Lithium carbonate, an antimanic drug, causes a strange, unpleasant taste sensation. Other common side effects of this drug related to nutritional intake are dry mouth, anorexia, nausea, vomiting, and diarrhea. Lithium carbonate also has serious interactions with a person's fluid and electrolyte balance (discussed later in the chapter).

Penicillamine, a drug given for heavy metal poisoning or for <u>Wilson's disease,</u> causes a loss of taste and smell. This is because penicillamine may induce zinc deficiency.

Nursing interventions that may help a patient with taste changes include providing good oral hygiene before meals and avoiding bitter foods in favor of the other taste sensations—sweet, sour, or salty.

Gastric Irritation

Drugs that cause gastric irritation are often taken with food to reduce this side effect. Chronic use of aspirin can lead to gastric bleeding and anemia. Taking aspirin with food, milk, crackers, or a full glass of water reduces the likelihood of stomach irritation.

The Effects of Drugs on Nutrient Absorption

Drugs can affect the absorption of nutrients in several ways. Drug-induced alterations in absorption are categorized according to two general mechanisms of action: the luminal effect or the mucosal effect.

Luminal Effects

Luminal effect— Drug-induced changes within the intestine that affect the absorption of nutrients or drugs without altering the intestine itself.

The **luminal effect** refers to drug-induced changes within the intestine that affect the absorption of nutrients or drugs without altering the intestine itself. These drug-induced changes may affect peristalsis, pH, or the formation of complexes.

PERISTALSIS Laxatives may interfere with the absorption of both nutrients and other drugs because they stimulate peristalsis and thus cause a rapid transit time of intestinal contents. Long-term use may result in physical dependence and electrolyte imbalances. Two laxatives, bisacodyl and phenolphthalein (common ingredients in over-the-counter preparations), interfere with the uptake of glucose, water, calcium, sodium, and potassium.

Other drugs may slow peristalsis and thus cause a slow transit time. The long-term use of either docusate sodium, a stool softener, or chlorpromazine, an antipsychotic drug, results in the increased absorption of cholesterol. However, increasing serum cholesterol is not a desirable effect in most patients.

CHANGES IN PH The absorption of weakly acidic drugs takes place in the stomach. The absorption of neutral and alkaline drugs takes place in the small intestine. Drug-induced changes in the pH of these sites influence the absorption of both nutrients and drugs. For example, an acid pH is necessary for folic acid absorption. It is also required for intrinsic factor to combine with vitamin B_{12} (extrinsic factor) for the absorption of vitamin B_{12}. Because long-term antacid or potassium chloride therapy neutralizes gastric acidity, the result is a decrease in the absorption of both folic acid and vitamin B_{12}. Antacids and potassium also decrease the absorption of iron. This is because the conversion of ferric iron to ferrous iron, which is the more absorbable form, requires an acid medium also.

FORMATION OF COMPLEXES Sometimes, foods or nutrients bind with or form complexes with drugs. This combining can increase, decrease, or prevent the absorption of one or the other.

Cholestyramine, a lipid-lowering agent, binds with bile salts, which increases the excretion of cholesterol. Unfortunately, it may also bind with the fat-soluble vitamins A, D, and K. These vitamins are then excreted along with the cholesterol. Because vitamin K is not stored in the body in significant amounts, cholestyramine therapy can lead to hemorrhage and a deficiency of prothrombin (blood-clotting factor II). However, water-soluble forms of these vitamins are available for patients who need them. Cholestyramine also interferes with the absorption of folic acid, vitamin B_{12}, calcium, and iron.

Mineral oil, a lubricant, is sometimes used as a laxative. Taking mineral oil long-term on a daily basis is undesirable. The fat-soluble vitamins (A, D, E, and K) dissolve in the indigestible oil and are excreted; calcium and phosphorus are excreted too. Children and elderly adults with relaxed cardiac sphincters are at risk for aspiration pneumonia if the mineral oil is regurgitated.

Mucosal Effects

The luminal effects we have just discussed take place within the gastrointestinal tract but do not affect the tissues or organs. In contrast, **mucosal effects** are drug-induced changes that affect the absorption of nutrients or drugs by damaging or altering tissue structures. Mucosal effects include decreased digestive enzymes, damaged intestinal mucosa, and inhibited transport mechanisms.

Mucosal effect—Drug-induced changes within the intestine that affect the absorption of drugs or nutrients by damaging or altering the tissues.

DECREASED DIGESTIVE ENZYMES Hundreds of enzymes are involved in digestion. Many drugs, including alcohol, can destroy the structural integrity of digestive organs by damaging tissues. This usually results in decreased enzyme production, which in turn leads to poor absorption.

Long-term alcohol consumption damages the pancreas, decreasing enzyme production. Thus the breakdown of amino acids and fats, which is mostly governed by the action of pancreatic enzymes, is slowed or insufficiently completed. The result is reduced or poor absorption of amino acids and fats.

DAMAGED INTESTINAL MUCOSA A number of drugs contribute to the malabsorption of drugs by their damaging effect on the intestinal mucosa. Some drugs produce general malabsorption; other drugs are more specific and decrease the absorption of only certain nutrients.

Alcohol abuse causes several changes in the intestinal mucosa that lead to the malabsorption of many nutrients. Most commonly affected are thiamin and magnesium, but folic acid, niacin, and pyridoxine also may be malabsorbed.

Because neomycin, an anti-infective, inhibits protein synthesis in bacteria, it is sometimes used to reduce the bacterial count in the bowel before intestinal surgery. Changes produced in the intestinal mucosa by neomycin lead to the decreased absorption of fat; vitamins A, D, and K; folic acid; and vitamin B_{12}. This malabsorption is not likely to cause problems when the drug use is short-term.

Gastrointestinal tract cells, because of their short service life and rapid turnover, are killed by many antineoplastic drugs, such as methotrexate. Consequently methotrexate administration results in the malabsorption of vitamin B_{12}, folic acid, and calcium.

Colchicine, an antigout drug, also inhibits the absorption of vitamin B_{12}, folic acid, and calcium. In addition, colchicine reduces the absorption of fat, lactose, and carotene.

INHIBITED TRANSPORT MECHANISMS   Several nutrients have to be helped across the intestinal membrane to the bloodstream. A number of drugs impair the absorption of nutrients through their effects on the transport mechanism. For example, the sedative/hypnotic drug glutethimide impairs the transport of calcium.

Para-aminosalicylate, an antitubercular drug, is administered for a prolonged period (1 to 2 years) to be effective. This drug interferes with the uptake and transport of vitamin B_{12} across the mucosal wall. When taking a patient history, then, the nurse should gather any pertinent data, not just data concerning *recent* changes in a patient's life or health.

Phenytoin, a drug used to control epileptic seizures or heart rhythm irregularities, decreases folic acid levels by inhibiting the intestinal enzymes necessary for its absorption. Reduced folic acid absorption also occurs with sulfasalazine, an anti-inflammatory agent used to treat ulcerative colitis. The decrease in absorption is due to the inhibited transport of folic acid.

The Effects of Drugs on Nutrient Metabolism

Many drugs alter the metabolism of nutrients. Just a few examples are presented here. Therapeutic use of naturally occurring hormones can radically alter the body's use of the energy nutrients. Drugs can disrupt vitamin metabolism by a variety of mechanisms.

Acceleration of Catabolism

Corticosteroids are hormones produced by the adrenal gland. Pharmaceutical doses of these drugs are given for their anti-inflammatory effects. The side effects of the drug produce signs and symptoms like those of the disease called Cushing's syndrome, which results from oversecretion of corticosteroids. The metabolism of all the energy nutrients is affected. Corticosteroids stimulate the conversion of fat and protein to glucose. Hyperglycemia results, or preexisting diabetes is worsened. Corticosteroids increase the catabolism of the matrix of the bone, inhibit the osteoblasts from building new bone, and prevent the liver from processing vitamin D. When this lack of vitamin D results in insufficient calcium being absorbed by the intestine, parathyroid hormone causes withdrawal of calcium from the bones, and osteoporosis is the consequence. Similar protein wasting affects the skin and skeletal muscle, producing easy bruising and weakness. Corticosteroids also cause a redistribution of fat deposits to the trunk, the back of the neck, and the face so that the person eventually develops a "moon face" and "buffalo hump."

Interference with Vitamin Metabolism

Although vitamins have specific and singular functions in the body, several mechanisms can interfere with their proper metabolism. The same vitamin may be affected by different drugs at various phases of its metabolism.

Anti-infectives, especially tetracycline, destroy intestinal bacteria, which synthesize vitamin K. Sometimes buttermilk or yogurt is effective in replacing the intestinal bacteria.

The molecular structure of warfarin, an anticoagulant drug, resembles that of vitamin K. Warfarin achieves its therapeutic effect by "fooling" the liver into using it in place of vitamin K to manufacture prothrombin. Warfarin also interferes with the synthesis of clotting factors VII, IX, and X. Eating large amounts of food high in vitamin K during anticoagulant therapy with warfarin decreases or may even negate the desired effect of the drug. Patients should not stop eating foods containing vitamin K, but they should avoid wide swings in the amounts eaten. A problem might arise if they eat a lot of green leafy vegetables one day and none for several days.

Methotrexate, an antineoplastic agent, is an antagonist of folic acid. It successfully destroys cancer cells because they, too, require folic acid for DNA replication. In the process, normal body cells' efforts to divide are thwarted.

Both the antitubercular drug isoniazid and the antiparkinson agent levodopa form a complex with pyridoxine. The kidney then excretes this complex in the urine rather than returning it to the bloodstream. The interaction can move in the opposite direction, also. The amount of pyridoxine in a normal diet creates no problem. Supplemental pyridoxine may be added to a levodopa regimen to correct a deficiency. However, this will decrease the effectiveness of levodopa.

An anticonvulsant, phenytoin, interferes with the liver's processing of vitamin D. Patients receiving long-term therapy need an estimated 15 to 25 micrograms of vitamin D daily to prevent rickets or osteomalacia.

The Effects of Drugs on Nutrient Excretion

Drugs usually cause excessive excretion, rather than retention, of nutrients. Drugs can act on the excretion of nutrients in four ways: they can (1) compete with nutrients for binding sites, (2) form chemical bonds with the nutrient, (3) deplete the nutrient supply in the body's tissues, and (4) interfere with the kidneys' reabsorption of the nutrient back into the bloodstream.

Competition for Binding Sites

Many drugs circulate in the bloodstream attached to plasma proteins. These plasma proteins serve a similar function in relation to some nutrients. The plasma protein and its hitchhiker drug or nutrient form a large particle. Sometimes there are too few binding sites for all the drug or nutrient. When that happens, excess drug or nutrient accumulates as free, small particles in the bloodstream. The kidney is likely to excrete these small particles rather than to restore them to the bloodstream. One common drug that interferes in this manner with a nutrient is acetylsalicylic acid, or aspirin. It displaces folic acid from its plasma protein. The kidney then excretes the folic acid in the urine.

TABLE 14–1 *The Effects of Drugs on Nutrients*

Drug Group	Drug	Effects/Action on Nutrient	Mechanism of Action
		ALTERATION IN FOOD INTAKE	
Analgesic	Acetylsalicylic acid	Decreases appetite	Altered taste; gastric irritation
Antineoplastic	Bleomycin, plicamycin, vincristine	Decreases appetite	Side effects: anorexia, nausea, vomiting, and stomatitis
Antihistamine	Brompheneramine, diphenhydramine	Decreases appetite	Side effect: dry mouth
Antidepressant	Bupropion	Increases/decreases appetite	Side effects
CNS stimulant	Dextroamphetamine, methylphenidate	Decreases appetite	Depressed desire for food
Antidepressant	Doxepin	Increases appetite	Side effect
Antimanic	Lithium carbonate	Decreases appetite	Altered taste; side effects: dry mouth, anorexia, nausea, and vomiting
Hormone	Medroxyprogesterone	Increases appetite	Effect of hormone
Chelating agent	Penicillamine	Decreases appetite/overeating	Altered taste and smell
Anti-infective	Streptomycin	Decreases appetite/overeating	Altered taste
		ALTERATION IN NUTRIENT ABSORPTION	
Alcohol	Alcohol (ethanol)	Decreases absorption of amino acids, fat, thiamin, folic acid, niacin, magnesium, and pyridoxine	Decreased enzyme production, damaged intestinal mucosa
Antacid; electrolyte	Antacids; potassium therapy	Decreases absorption of folic acid, vitamin B_{12}, and iron	Changes in pH
Laxative	Bisacodyl, phenolphthalein	Interferes with uptake of glucose, potassium, calcium, sodium, and water	Altered peristalsis

Drug class	Drug	Alteration in nutrient metabolism	Mechanism
Lipid-lowering agent	Cholestyramine	Interferes with absorption of vitamins A, D, K, B$_{12}$, folic acid, and calcium	Formation of complexes
Antigout agent	Colchicine	Malabsorption of vitamin B$_{12}$, folic acid, calcium; reduces absorption of fat, lactose, and carotene	Damaged intestinal mucosa
Stool softener	Docusate sodium	Increases absorption of cholesterol	Altered peristalsis
Sedative/hypnotic	Glutethamide	Leads to calcium deficiency	Impaired transport mechanism
Antineoplastic	Methotrexate	Decreases absorption of vitamin B$_{12}$, folic acid, and calcium	Damaged intestinal mucosa
Laxative—lubricant	Mineral oil	Decreases absorption of vitamins A, D, E, and K, calcium, and phosphorus	Formation of complexes
Anti-infective	Neomycin	Decreases absorption of fat, fat-soluble vitamins, vitamin B$_{12}$, lactose, iron, sucrose, sodium, potassium, calcium	Damaged intestinal mucosa
Antitubercular	Para-aminosalicylate	Reduces absorption of vitamin B$_{12}$	Inhibited transport mechanism
Anticonvulsant	Phenytoin	Reduces absorption of folic acid	Inhibited intestinal enzymes
Anti-inflammatory	Sulfasalazine	Reduces absorption of folic acid, iron	Inhibited transport mechanism

ALTERATION IN NUTRIENT METABOLISM

Drug class	Drug	Alteration in nutrient metabolism	Mechanism
Alcohol	Alcohol (ethanol)	Amino acids poorly utilized	Damaged intestinal mucosa
Anticonvulsant	Anticonvulsants	Folic acid and vitamin D deficiency	Impeded conversion of vitamin D to intermediate form
Anti-infective	Anti-infectives	Decreased vitamin K synthesis	Destruction of intestinal bacteria
Corticosteroid	Corticosteroids	Decreases glucose tolerance; produces tissue wasting, "moon face," and "buffalo hump"	Glyconeogenesis; protein catabolism; mobilization of fats

TABLE 14–1 *The Effects of Drugs on Nutrients (Continued)*

Drug Group	Drug	Effects/Action on Nutrient	Mechanism of Action
Hormones in oral contraceptives	Estrogen/progestogen	Folic acid, vitamin B_6, and vitamin B_{12} deficiencies; increased serum lipid levels	Multiple mechanisms
Antitubercular; antiparkinson	isoniazid; levodopa	Pyridoxine deficiency	Increased urinary excretion
Antineoplastic	Methotrexate	Folic acid deficiency	Destruction of GI tract cells
Anticoagulant	Warfarin	Depletes vitamin K	Interference with synthesis of clotting factors
ALTERATION IN NUTRIENT EXCRETION			
Analgesic	Acetylsalicylic acid	Increases excretion of folic acid	Competition for binding sites
Alcohol	Alcohol (ethanol)	Increases excretion of folic acid	Depletion of nutrient supply
Diuretic	Furosemide	Increases excretion of sodium, potassium, and calcium	Interference with reabsorption by kidneys
Chelating agent	Penicillimine	Increases excretion of metals, esp. zinc and copper	Formation of chemical bonds
Glucocorticoid	Prednisone	Increases excretion of vitamin C	Depletion of nutrient supply

Formation of Chemical Bonds

To combat heavy metal poisoning, an antidote drug that combines chemically with the metal is administered. The drug plus the metal then is excreted harmlessly. As with many treatments, the drug is not specific and will combine with nutrients as well as the noxious heavy metal. An example of this type of interaction involves penicillamine. It forms a stable bond with zinc, copper, and other metals, causing excessive excretion, thus possibly leading to deficiencies.

Depletion of Nutrient in Tissues

As part of its overall catabolic effect, the anti-inflammatory glucocorticoid prednisone depletes tissues of ascorbic acid. The ascorbic acid accumulates in the blood and is excreted. Because ascorbic acid is necessary for the healing of wounds, one side effect of prednisone and other corticosteroids is poor wound healing.

When alcohol is present, folic acid leaks from the liver into the bloodstream. Its fate from there is excessive excretion in the urine, leading to folic acid deficiency.

Interference with Reabsorption by Kidney

Many diuretic agents prevent normal reabsorption of sodium into the bloodstream within the kidney. This increases the amount of sodium excreted by the kidney into the urine. Along with the sodium, water is also excreted. Often the drug is not specific enough to dispose of sodium alone. Many diuretics also cause loss of potassium. Sometimes the patient must take pharmacologic doses of potassium chloride to prevent hypokalemia. One diuretic, furosemide, produces calcium loss in addition to potassium loss by the same mechanism.

Table 14–1 summarizes the effects of drugs on foods and nutrients.

THE EFFECTS OF FOODS AND NUTRIENTS ON DRUGS

Foods and nutrients can decrease, delay, or increase the absorption of drugs. They can also cause alterations in drug metabolism.

The Effects of Foods on Drug Absorption

In some cases the interaction of food with a drug can be used to therapeutic advantage. In other situations, knowledge of interactions will aid the health-care team to schedule meals and medication doses to the best advantage of the patient.

Decreased or Delayed Absorption

Food, nonnutrient components of foods, or nutrients in food may decrease or delay the absorption of drugs. This may often be used to advantage. For example, food delays the absorption of cortisone, a glucocorticoid used as an anti-inflammatory drug. Taking cortisone with food produces a more consistent blood level of the drug. Other factors, such as a drug's susceptibility to acid degradation or its ability to form insoluble complexes, also influence whether a drug is administered with food or between meals.

Food in the stomach, acidic fruit or vegetable juices, and carbonated beverages increase gastric acidity. Anti-infectives particularly susceptible to acid degradation are penicillin G, cloxacillin, and ampicillin. An acid medium breaks down these drugs, producing a less effective blood level. To diminish such acid degradation, these anti-infectives are administered between meals.

Enteric-coated— Type of drug preparation designed to dissolve in the intestine rather than in the stomach.

Drugs formulated to dissolve in the intestine rather than in the stomach are **enteric-coated;** an acid-resistant shell covers the active ingredient (see Fig. 14–2). The stomach normally is acid and the duodenum alkaline. Milk raises the pH of the stomach, making it more alkaline. Taking enteric-coated drugs with milk, then, will allow the coating to dissolve early and therefore will decrease the action of the drug. One of these drugs is erythromycin, an anti-infective. It should not be taken with milk. Alcohol and hot beverages can also cause premature erosion of the enteric-coating on drugs.

Tetracycline, an anti-infective, combines with the salts of iron, magnesium, aluminum, and calcium to form insoluble compounds. This decreases the absorption of the drug. For this reason, tetracycline should not be administered within 1 to 3 hours of iron supplements or iron-containing foods (red meat, egg yolks), milk or other dairy products, or antacids containing magnesium, aluminum, and/or calcium.

Amino acids compete for absorption with levodopa, a drug used in the management of Parkinson's disease. Separating the dose from high-protein intake by 3 hours improves absorption. Protein also delays the action of phenytoin (an anticonvulsant) and inhibits the absorption of theophylline, a bronchodilator used to treat asthma.

Other foods that affect the absorption of drugs: (1) A high-fiber meal decreases the absorption of digoxin, a drug used to treat congestive heart failure. (2) The pectin in apples and jelly reduces the absorption of acetaminophen, an analgesic.

Increased Absorption

Foods and nutrients may also increase or facilitate the absorption of drugs. Some drugs are affected in one or more ways by one or more nutrients. Lev-

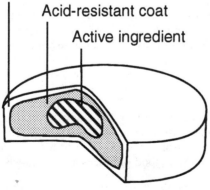

Color coat
Acid-resistant coat
Active ingredient

FIGURE 14–2. Diagram of an enteric-coated tablet. Substances that penetrate the acid-resistant coating defeat the purpose of this type of tablet. (From Clayton, BD and Stock, YN, p 56, with permission.)

odopa, the drug used in the management of Parkinson's disease, has a second interaction with food. Whereas protein delays the absorption of levodopa, carbohydrate facilitates it. Giving levodopa with carbohydrate-rich snacks improves the absorption of the drug. Similarly, protein delays the anticonvulsant action of phenytoin, but the presence of carbohydrate increases the absorption. Protein inhibits the absorption of theophylline (a bronchodilator), but carbohydrate accelerates its absorption. A high-carbohydrate, low-protein diet decreased the number of wheezing spells suffered by asthmatic children receiving theophylline (Feldman, 1980).

Fatty foods enhance the absorption of griseofulvin, an antifungal drug. For a person on a low-fat diet, the drug can be administered either in a **micronized** form or in a low-fat suspension. The pharmacist can suspend the drug in a small amount of corn oil.

Micronize—To pulverize a substance into very tiny particles.

The Effects of Foods on Drug Metabolism

Foods can alter the metabolism of drugs. One metabolic food-drug interaction can be life-threatening.

Monoamine Oxidase Inhibitors

This class of drugs includes antidepressants and an antihypertensive. The antidepressants are isocarboxazid, phenelzine, and tranylcypromine. The **monoamine oxidase inhibitor** used to treat hypertension is pargyline hydrochloride. The usual abbreviation for this group is MAO inhibitor.

Monoamine oxidase (MAO) inhibitor—A class of antidepressant drugs that may have critical interactions with foods.

MECHANISM OF DRUG ACTION   These drugs prevent the breakdown of tyramine and dopamine, chemicals necessary for proper functioning of the nervous system. The drugs' therapeutic effect is to increase the concentration of epinephrine, norepinephrine, serotonin, and dopamine in the central nervous system, thus counteracting depression.

In the peripheral nervous system the MAO inhibitors also prevent the release of norepinephrine that builds up in the nerves. The stores of norepinephrine become especially high in the nerves that regulate the size of blood vessels. The result is a decreased ability to constrict peripheral blood vessels. The vasodilation thus produced leads to hypotension. To compound the situation, the drugs also inhibit the body's normal response to a low blood pressure, an increased heart rate. Thus the individual displays the unusual combination of hypotension and bradycardia.

EFFECT OF FOODS ON MAO INHIBITORS   Some foods contain **tyramine,** a metabolic intermediate product in the conversion of the amino acid tyrosine to epinephrine. Foods containing degraded protein, such as aged cheese, are high in tyramine. When a patient on MAO inhibitors consumes foods or beverages high in tyramine, the drugs prevent the normal breakdown of tyramine. As a consequence, the tyramine oversupply leads to excessive epinephrine, producing hypertension. Sometimes the blood pressure is severely elevated, which can cause intracranial hemorrhage (stroke).

Tyramine—A monoamine present in various foods that will provoke a hypertensive crisis in persons taking MAO inhibitors.

As in many situations, an individual's response to tyramine varies. Several factors interact to determine the severity of reaction: (1) the amount of tyramine ingested, (2) the dose of the MAO inhibitor, (3) patient susceptibility, and (4) the time between the drug dose and tyramine-containing meal.

TYRAMINE-RICH FOODS Many foods contain enough tyramine to create problems for the person receiving MAO inhibitors. These include foods and beverages such as cheese, beer, and chianti wine, in which aging is used to enhance flavor. The amount of tyramine varies even in different samples of a particular food. Table 14–2 lists tyramine-containing foods. Since this interaction can be life-threatening, the best advice to give a patient is to avoid all foods capable of causing problems, even though a small amount of the food, or a given batch of a product, might be safe.

Effects of Other Nutrients

Certain nutrients increase the amount of a drug in the bloodstream, thus increasing or decreasing the risk of toxicity. For example, fat displaces the antianxiety drug diazepam from **protein binding sites,** thus increasing the amount of unbound drug circulating in the bloodstream. This increased serum concentration leads to increased activity of the drug.

Protein binding sites—Various sites in the body tissues to which drugs may become attached, rendering the drug temporarily inactive.

TABLE 14–2 *Tyramine-Containing Foods*

Foods	To Avoid	To Use Moderately
Breads and cereals	None	None
Fruit and Vegetables	Avocados Bananas Figs Broad (fava) beans Chinese pea pods Eggplant Italian flat beans Mixed Chinese vegetables	
Dairy	Aged cheese (brick, blue, brie, cheddar, Camembert, Swiss, Romano, Roquefort, mozzarella, Parmesan, provolone) Yogurt	Gouda cheese Processed American cheese
Meat and fish	Any canned meat Beef or chicken liver Sausage (bologna, salami, pepperoni, summer) Fish (caviar, dried fish, salt herring)	
Beverages	Ale, beer, sherry, red and white wines	Coffee, colas, hot chocolate (1–3 cups per day)
Other	Chocolate, bouillon and other protein extracts, meat tenderizer, soy sauce, yeast concentrates	

TABLE 14–3 *The Effects of Foods on Drugs*

Effect	Type of Food/Nutrient	Action on Drug
Decrease in absorption	Amino acids in proteins	Inhibit absorption of levodopa
	Calcium in dairy products	Combines with tetracycline to impair absorption
	High-fiber meal	Decreases absorption of digoxin
	Milk, alcohol, hot beverages	Cause premature erosion enteric-coatings
	Pectin in jelly, apples	Reduces absorption of acetaminophen
Increase in absorption	Carbohydrate	Enhances absorption of levodopa
	Fatty foods	Enhance absorption of griseofulvin
Altered metabolism	Caffeine	Enhances effect of theophylline
	Fat	Enhances activity of diazepam
	Tyramine-containing foods	May cause hypertensive crisis when combined with MAO inhibitors
	Vitamin E	Protects premature infants from oxygen toxicity

Correct potassium levels are necessary for adequate muscle function, including that of the heart. Hypokalemia, low serum potassium, increases the risk of toxicity from digitalis.

Premature infants have immature respiratory systems. Even though they need oxygen to survive, the oxygen often becomes toxic to them. Vitamin E protects these infants from bronchopulmonary dysplasia due to oxygen toxicity.

Although not a nutrient, caffeine is part of a person's oral intake. It should be included as part of the dietary assessment. Caffeine increases the effect of both theophylline and stimulant drugs. Table 14–3 summarizes the effects of foods and nutrients on drugs.

THE BODY'S HOMEOSTATIC MECHANISMS AFFECT DRUG EXCRETION

In addition to nutritional status, the status of both acid-base balance and fluid and electrolyte balance affect the excretion of drugs. To consider either acid-base balance or fluid and electrolyte balance in isolation risks oversimplifying the body's functions. Keep in mind that the functions of these two regulatory systems are interwoven as you read about each separate topic.

Acid-Base Balance

Rather than thinking of the kidney as the manufacturer of urine, picture it as the gatekeeper of the bloodstream. The contents of the urine reflect the metabolic state of the body. The end products of the foods consumed and the drugs we take make the urine either more acid or more alkaline. Freshly voided urine usually has an acid pH, averaging about 6.0.

Alkaline Urine

Drinking large amounts of citrus juices or consuming a vegetarian diet causes the urine to become alkaline. When the body is producing alkaline urine, the kidney will take longer to excrete alkaline drugs. Higher levels of the drugs will remain in the bloodstream for a longer period. Examples of alkaline drugs are the cardiac antidysrhythmic quinidine; the tricyclic antidepressant imipramine; and the amphetamine stimulants. If the patient's metabolism causes an alkaline urine, these drugs will give more pronounced and prolonged effects. Patients treated with these drugs should neither change the amounts of citrus juice they consume nor become vegetarians without consulting the physician.

The opposite effect occurs when a person's metabolism produces alkaline urine and the drugs are acidic. The kidney excretes acidic drugs faster than usual if the urine is alkaline. One acidic drug that should spring to mind immediately is acetylsalicylic acid. Another acidic drug is the barbiturate commonly used as an anticonvulsant, phenobarbital. The kidney will discard either of these drugs faster than normal if the patient is producing an alkaline urine.

Acid Urine

Large doses of ascorbic acid (vitamin C) make the urine more acidic. Vitamin C is sometimes given specifically for the purpose of acidifying the urine. For example, a urinary pH of 5.5 or less is necessary for the urinary anti-infective drug methenamine to be effective. In an acid urine, the drug becomes ammonia and formaldehyde, both bactericidal chemicals.

Sulfonamides are another class of drugs given for urinary tract infections. One of the possible side effects of sulfonamides is crystalluria, crystallization of the drug in the urinary tract. Although some drugs crystallize more readily than others, this class of drugs is more likely to crystallize in concentrated or acid urine. For this reason, patients should be instructed to drink ample fluid. It may also be necessary to deliberately alkalinize the urine to prevent crystallization. Table 14–4 summarizes the effects of acid-base balance on the excretion of drugs.

Fluid and Electrolyte Balance

Fluid and electrolyte status also influences the effects of drugs. An increase or decrease in sodium, the mineral most closely associated with water balance, can affect the excretion of certain drugs. Imported licorice may cause serious imbalances in fluid and electrolyte status.

TABLE 14–4 *Effects of Urinary pH on Drugs*

	Alkaline Urine	Acid Urine
Increased excretion	Acetylsalicylic acid Phenobarbital	Amphetamines Imipramine Quinidine
Decreased excretion	Amphetamines Imipramine Quinidine	Acetylsalicylic acid Phenobarbital
Necessary for adequate effect	Sulfonamides	Methenamine

Sodium, Fluids, and Lithium Carbonate

Both sodium intake and increased fluid intake affect the antimanic drug lithium carbonate. This drug is absorbed, distributed, and excreted alongside of sodium. Therefore, decreased sodium intake with decreased fluid intake may lead to lithium retention and overmedication. Conversely, increased sodium intake and increased fluid intake increase the excretion of lithium and decrease the antimanic effect. Because of this important interaction, patients taking lithium are taught to monitor the concentration or specific gravity of their urine.

Licorice

A flavoring agent, licorice, when taken to excess, can cause hypokalemia, sodium and water retention, hypertension, and alkalosis. This is an action of natural licorice only. It is imported into this country. The licorice commonly manufactured in the United States contains artificial flavoring and does not produce these ill effects. Imported licorice, however, may cause problems for patients on low-sodium diets or potassium-wasting diuretics.

RESPONSIBILITIES OF HEALTHCARE PROFESSIONALS

This chapter has only touched the surface of the subject of food and drug interactions. For every drug selected for discussion, many others were omitted. We have included commonly prescribed drugs and those with significant interactions with foods. In addition, we have discussed various modes of food and drug interactions. The healthcare professional needs to constantly review and update his or her knowledge of such interactions.

Summary

Persons at highest risk for food-drug interactions are those who (1) take many drugs, including alcohol, (2) require long-term drug therapy, or (3) have poor or marginal nutrition. Food-drug interactions can affect (1) food intake, (2) absorption of nutrients or drugs, (3) metabolism of nutrients or drugs, and (4) excretion of nutrients or drugs.

Medications influence food intake. They can decrease or increase appetite, cause taste changes, or provoke gastric irritation.

Foods and drugs can interfere with the absorption of each other. More often than not, the interaction of nutrients and drugs produces decreased absorption of one or the other, or both.

In addition to interactions involving intake and absorption, foods and drugs can affect one another's metabolism. Two important nutrient-drug interactions are those of tyramine-containing foods with MAO inhibitors and of sodium and water with lithium carbonate.

Foods and drugs interact during excretion of waste products also. At special risk are patients in unstable acid-base or fluid and electrolyte balance or those with alterations in serum proteins.

A case study and a sample plan of care appear below. Both are designed to show you how the information you have studied in this chapter can be used in nursing practice.

CASE STUDY 14–1

Mrs. S., a 72-year-old patient, is being seen by the home health nurse to reaffirm her suitability for independent living. She has a history of congestive heart failure for which she has been successfully treated with digoxin 0.125 milligrams daily for the past 6 months. Mrs. S. takes the tablet with her usual breakfast of orange juice and tea.

Recently she has had difficulty with constipation. Obtaining information on bowel hygiene on her own, she decided to improve her nutritional intake by adding a high-fiber cereal to her breakfast.

After 1 week, her constipation has been relieved, but she now is becoming fatigued easily. When climbing a flight of stairs she finds it necessary to rest twice en route.

The nurse asked Mrs. S. to weigh herself. Mrs. S. reported she had gained 5 pounds in 2 weeks. Based on the above data and her observations, the home health nurse prepared a nursing care plan. The portion of it pertinent to food and drug interactions appears below.

NURSING CARE PLAN FOR MRS. S.

Assessment:

Subjective
　Easily fatigued
　Short of breath < 1 flight of stairs
　History of constipation, relieved by addition of high-fiber cereal to diet
　Medications—digoxin, 0.125 mg daily in morning with breakfast.
Objective: Alert, oriented, cooperative. Vital signs normal except pulse 90 beats per minute. Weight gain—5 pounds over 2 weeks.

Nursing Diagnosis
　Health maintenance, altered: related to food-drug interaction as evidenced by beginning signs of heart failure.

Desired Outcome/Evaluation Criteria

Patient will revise medication or meal schedule immediately to maximize effectiveness of digoxin.

Nursing Actions/Intervention with Rationale in Italics

Teach patient to separate digoxin dose from high-fiber foods. *High-fiber foods decrease the absorption of digitalis preparations.*

STUDY AIDS

Chapter Review Questions

1. Which of the following patients would be at greatest risk for food-drug interaction?
   a. A 50-year-old man with no current disease
   b. A 75-year-old woman with several chronic diseases requiring medication
   c. A 12-year-old within normal limits on the height and weight chart
   d. A 25-year-old pregnant woman

2. Which of the following are ways in which food and drugs interact?
   a. Drugs may affect food intake.
   b. Either may affect the absorption of the other.
   c. Certain foods and drugs specifically interfere with the metabolism of the other.
   d. Nutrients and drugs can increase or decrease the rate of excretion of one another.
   e. All of the above are true.

3. Which of the following medications has been known to increase appetite?
   a. Dextroamphetamine
   b. Medroxyprogesterone
   c. Methotrexate
   d. Phenytoin

4. For which of the following reasons is it recommended that levodopa be taken with carbohydrate-rich snacks but separated from any high-protein meal by 3 hours?
   a. Glucose from the carbohydrate aids in the distribution of the drug.
   b. Carbohydrate causes the release of insulin, which is necessary for the absorption of levodopa.
   c. Amino acids compete with levodopa for absorption.
   d. Levodopa is likely to sensitize the person to various proteins.

5. Which of the following is the best reason to recommend taking anti-infectives between meals?
   a. Many anti-infectives are degraded by an acid medium, and food stimulates secretion of gastric acid.
   b. Since nausea and vomiting are common side effects, taking the drug on an empty stomach would produce less vomitus.
   c. Food competes with the drug for absorption from the large intestine.
   d. Anti-infectives combine with many foods to produce toxic compounds.

6. Which of the following foods should not be taken within 2 to 3 hours of tetracycline?
   a. Eggs and poultry
   b. Red meats and fatty fish
   c. Dried fruits and coconut
   d. Milk and cheese

7. Phenytoin inhibits intestinal enzymes necessary for _____ absorption.
   a. Ascorbic acid
   b. Vitamin K
   c. Folic acid
   d. Potassium

8. Persons taking monoamine oxidase inhibitors must avoid foods containing:
   a. Tyramine
   b. Histamine
   c. Phenylalanine
   d. Alcohol

9. The side effects of "moon face" and "buffalo hump" that occur during corticosteroid therapy are related to the drug's interference with body _____ distribution.
   a. Glycogen
   b. Muscle tissue
   c. Sodium
   d. Fat

10. Individuals taking the anticoagulant warfarin must be counseled to avoid wide swings in amounts consumed of:
    a. Green leafy vegetables
    b. Vegetable oils
    c. Whole-grain cereals and breads
    d. Dried fruits

NCLEX-Style Quiz

Situation One

Mr. A. S. is being admitted to your long-term care facility. He is a 45-year-old post-trauma patient. The motor vehicle accident in which he became paralyzed also killed his wife and daughter. The accident occurred 6 months ago. In the meantime he has been treated at a rehabilitation center, but his depression interfered with his progress. After many trials of various antidepressants, he is now receiving phenelzine. The following questions relate to his care.

1. Although most long-term care facilities do not take vital signs every day on every patient, Mr. A. S. should have his _____ monitored at least daily as long as he is taking phenelzine.
   a. Temperature
   b. Pulse
   c. Respirations
   d. Blood pressure

2. To ensure that everyone caring for Mr. A. S. is alerted to potential complications related to his drug therapy, the nurse begins a nursing care plan. Which of the following nursing diagnoses best states this problem as described by the data?
   a. Coping, ineffective individual: related to deaths of family members as evidenced by need for antidepressant therapy
   b. Potential vascular impairment related to inappropriate diet combined with phenelzine therapy
   c. Knowledge deficit related to potential food-drug interaction between tyramine-containing foods and monoamine oxidase inhibitor
   d. Bowel elimination, altered: related to paraplegia as evidenced by incontinence

3. Which of the following statements would be an appropriate outcome criterion for Mr. A. S.?
   a. Patient will participate in one social activity within 2 weeks.
   b. Patient will list foods he must avoid by the end of the first week in the long-term care facility.

   c. Patient will not consume foods that interact with his drugs as long as the antidepressant therapy is continued.

   d. Patient will increase the high-fiber foods in his diet by 50 percent within 3 weeks of admission to the long-term care facility.

4. Close attention to Mr. A. S.'s diet is essential. Which of the following foods will he have to avoid completely?

   a. Baked beans, dates, and roast beef

   b. Sugar, molasses, and maple syrup

   c. Bologna, cheddar cheese, and wine

   d. Green beans, whole-wheat bread, and oranges

5. When teaching the nursing assistants about the dietary restrictions needed by Mr. A. S., the nurse should be sure the nursing assistants understand that:

   a. The potential complication can be life-threatening.

   b. Mr. A. S. is to be kept unaware of the complication.

   c. As time goes on, the forbidden foods can be added to the diet slowly, one at a time.

   d. If Mr. A. S. does not cooperate in his dietary care, his paralysis is likely to worsen.

CHARTING TIPS 14–1

  ✓ Be sure to document the patient's knowledge at the start of your teaching.

  ✓ Indicate evidence, such as verbalization or recitation, that indicates patient understood your teaching.

  ✓ Whenever possible, give the patient a choice. If the patient makes a choice, chart the decision as the patient's.

BIBLIOGRAPHY

Collins, JL and Lutz, RJ: In vitro study of simultaneous infusion of incompatible drugs in multilumen catheters. Heart Lung 20:271, 1991.

Clayton, BD and Stock, YN: Basic Pharmacology for Nurses, ed 9. CV Mosby, St Louis, 1989.

Deglin, JH and Vallerand, AH: Davis's Drug Guide For Nurses, ed 3. FA Davis, Philadelphia, 1993.

Feldman, CH: Effect of dietary protein and carbohydrate on theophylline metabolism in children. Pediatrics 66:956, 1980.

Hui, YH: Human Nutrition and Diet Therapy. Wadsworth, Monterey, CA, 1983.

Kuhn, MM: Pharmacotherapeutics: A Nursing Process Approach, ed 2. FA Davis, Philadelphia, 1991.

Loeb, S: Nurse's Handbook of Drug Therapy. Springhouse, Springhouse, PA, 1993.

Pemberton, CM, et al: Mayo Clinic Diet Manual, ed 6. BC Decker, Philadelphia, 1987.

Roe, DA: Diet and Drug Interactions. Van Nostrand Reinhold, New York, 1989.

Shlafer, M and Marieb, EN: The Nurse, Pharmacology, and Drug Therapy. Addison-Wesley, Redwood City, CA, 1989.

Skidmore-Roth, L: Mosby's Nursing Drug Reference. CV Mosby Year Book, St Louis, 1992.

Swonger, HK and Matejski, MP: Nursing Pharmacology, ed 2. JB Lippincott, Philadelphia, 1991.

Whitney, EB, Cataldo, CB, and Rolfes, SR: Understanding Normal and Clinical Nutrition, ed 3. West, St Paul, 1991.

Williams, SR: Nutrition and Diet Therapy, ed 6. Times Mirror/Mosby College Publishing, St Louis, 1989.

Chapter Outline

Key Terms

As a study aid, each key term is followed by the page number where the term is defined in the chapter. Terms that appear in **boldface** or <u>underscored</u> in the chapter text are located in the glossary.

Weight Control

After completing this chapter, the student should be able to:

1. Discuss the effects of weight loss on the body.
2. Identify the medical, psychological, and social problems associated with too much and too little body fat.
3. Describe the healthy way to lose weight.
4. Discuss the dangers of inappropriate weight loss.
5. Describe the symptoms commonly exhibited by a patient with anorexia nervosa and/or bulimia.

*W*eight control is a problem for many people. As a society, we are very concerned with physical appearance. In a recent government survey, it was found that 46 percent of the women and 27 percent of the men questioned were attempting to lose weight. In 1989, 1.78 billion was spent on commercial weight-loss programs and 5.49 billion on hospital or medical-center-affiliated programs (Environmental Nutrition, 1990). The intent of this chapter is to help the student understand the basic principles of weight control on both a personal and professional level. Many of us need assistance in weight control.

ENERGY IMBALANCE

Energy imbalance—Situation in which kilocalories eaten do not equal the number used for energy.

Energy imbalance results when the number of kilocalories eaten does not equal the number used for energy. An individual can determine whether food intake is meeting energy needs by monitoring his or her weight. If more kilocalories are eaten than are used by the body, weight gain will occur. If fewer kilocalories are eaten than are used by the body (and protein intake is adequate), weight loss will occur. Monitoring body weight to assess energy imbalance is especially useful when one healthcare provider follows the progress of a patient for an extended time.

Basic Principles

There are two basic principles of energy imbalance. First, it takes a specific number of kilocalories to gain or lose a pound of body fat. Second, the body stores energy and uses stored energy in a highly specific manner.

The Five-Hundred Rule

One pound of body fat contains approximately 3500 kilocalories. To lose 1 pound of body fat per week, the individual must eat 500 kilocalories fewer per day than his body expends for 7 days (3500 kilocalories divided by 7 days). To gain 1 pound of body fat per week, the individual must eat 500 kilocalories more per day for 7 days than his body expends. The gain or loss of body fat need not occur during the course of a week; the kilocalorie surplus or deficit may occur over a month or year. The principle is the same. The total number of kilocalories required to gain or lose a pound of body fat is 3500.

Body Fat Stores

Obesity—Excessive amount of fat on the body; obesity for women is a fat content greater than 33 percent; obesity for men is a fat content greater than 25 percent.

Excess kilocalories are stored as body fat in adipose tissue. The human body is able to store adipose fat tissue in unlimited amounts. This can lead to **obesity**. During a kilocalorie deficit, the body will first seek the energy necessary to sustain body functions in glycogen stores which are limited. When a kilocalorie deficit occurs for longer than about 1 day, the body will seek the energy necessary to sustain its functions in *both* body fat stores (adipose tissue) and body protein stores (organ and muscle mass).

THE OVERLY FAT PATIENT

Many health experts consider the number of overly fat people in our society to be excessive. There are many social, psychological, and health consequences for the overly fat patient. At the same time, the entire scientific community struggles with how to define and diagnose overly fat patients. How a patient is diagnosed often determines which treatment approach is indicated.

Diagnosing the Overly Fat Patient

Diagnosing the patient as underweight, normal weight, mildly obese, moderately obese, or severely obese is often necessary. How the patient is classified often determines whether treatment is indicated and the kind of treatment that is appropriate. However, classifying the overly fat patient is often difficult for the healthcare professional. This is due in part to (1) the lack of universally accepted definitions and (2) the widespread use of several different methods of diagnosis.

One major problem in diagnosing the overly fat patient is that there is no universally accepted definition for the following words: overweight, mildly obese, moderately obese, and severely obese. This is why most authors define these terms at the beginning of each book or article on weight control that they publish. This text defines these terms and includes a discussion on three of the methods used to diagnose patients: percent healthy body weight, body mass index, and percent body fat. This section begins with a discussion of height/weight tables because these tables are used to calculate percent healthy body weight.

Height/Weight Tables

Height/weight tables have been used to diagnosis the overly fat patient for years. Insurance companies developed the first height/weight table in 1908. Its original purpose was to determine insurance rates based on life expectancy studies. The medical community subsequently adopted this and similar tables for clinical use. In 1942 and 1943, the Metropolitan Life Insurance Company introduced the term "ideal body weight" and called its table "Ideal Weights for Men and Women." Nutrition researchers use the term "ideal" when reference is made to this height/weight table. The assumption of this table is that a stable body weight throughout the life cycle has a health benefit. The Desirable Weight for Height Table was introduced in 1959. The assumption of this table is that maintaining a lower-than-average weight has a health benefit. Nutrition researchers use the term "desirable" when reference is made to this height/weight table. The authors of this text have avoided the use of the terms "ideal" or "desirable" because these terms refer to specific height/weight tables (each of which are based on different assumptions of what constitutes a healthy body weight).

The height/weight table found in Appendix B is the 1983 Metropolitan Height and Weight Table, which was developed so as not to be labeled with any term denoting a value judgment.

The assumption of this table is that a modest increase in weight (2 to 13 pounds) throughout adulthood does not result in a decreased life expectancy. Thus, the weights in the 1983 table are about 2 to 13 pounds heavier than those in the 1959 Table in each sex, frame size, and height category.

Much controversy exists concerning which height/weight table best meets the health needs of the population. In fact, many other organizations and researchers have developed their own height/weight tables because of a dissatisfaction with the Metropolitan Life Insurance Company's tables. It is important to realize that the height/weight tables of the Metropolitan Life Insurance Company are based on mortality or death rates. The weights presented are not necessarily the weights at which any individual is the healthiest, performs his or her job optimally, or even looks his or her best. Height/weight tables cannot replace a thorough physical assessment, an accurate diet history, information about exercise patterns, or measurement of a patient's body fat content.

Percent Healthy Body Weight

Descriptive words such as underweight, normal weight, mildly obese, and so forth are often expressed in terms of percent healthy body weight (HBW). Healthy body weight may vary depending on which height/weight table is used. This text uses the 1983 Metropolitan Height and Weight Table. **Overweight** is often used to mean 10 to 20 percent above HBW. **Obese** is often used to mean more than 20 percent above HBW. The obese patient may be classified further as:

> *Mildly obese*—20 to 40 percent overweight or 120 to 140 percent HBW
> *Moderately obese*—41 to 100 percent overweight or 141 to 200 percent HBW
> *Severely obese*—Greater than 100 percent overweight or 200 percent + HBW (Stunkard, 1984)

Overweight—10 to 20 percent above healthy body weight; 110 to 120 percent healthy body weight.

Obese—more than 20 percent above healthy body weight

Body Mass Index

A patient's body mass index (BMI) is his or her body weight in kilograms divided by height in meters squared. BMI can be determined without doing any calculations by using a chart called a <u>nomogram.</u> A nomogram is a chart that shows a relationship between numerical values. Figure 15–1 is a nomogram used to determine BMI. Note that the left side of the chart is labeled "weight" and the right side is labeled "height." To determine your BMI, place a ruler between your body weight (without clothes) on the left to your height (without shoes) on the right. Your body mass index is at the point where the line crosses the middle column.

A BMI of 20 to 25 kilograms per meters squared is normal. Overweight patients will have a BMI of 25 to 30 kilograms per meters squared. The severely overweight patient will have a BMI of above 40 kilograms per meters squared. The massively overweight patient will have a BMI greater than 40 kilograms per meters squared (National Research Council, 1989).

Percent Body Fat

Although a HBW expressed as a percent over 120 or a BMI in excess of 30 kilograms per meters squared may alert the healthcare worker that the patient may be overly fat, this is not always foolproof. Two examples are discussed to illustrate this concept.

First let us consider the 5-foot 4-inch woman with shoes (1-inch heels) who has a medium frame size and was weighed wearing indoor clothing. According to the 1983 Metropolitan Height and Weight Table for Adults (see Appendix B) she should weigh between 124 and 138 pounds. Let us review the calculation of HBW: if we subtract 124 pounds from 138 pounds, the difference would be 14 pounds; if we divide 14 pounds by 2 pounds, the

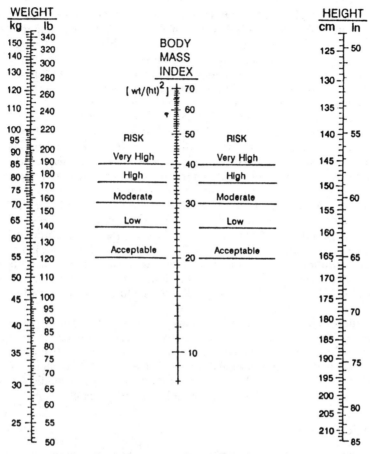

FIGURE 15–1. Nomogram for Determining Body Mass Index (National Research Council: Diet and Health 1989)

answer would be 7 pounds; if we add 7 pounds to 124 pounds, the sum would be 131 pounds. Thus 131 pounds is this patient's theoretical HBW. Suppose this patient weighed 131 pounds. Her HBW would be 100 percent. Can we automatically conclude that this patient is not obese? The answer is no. The optimal body fat content for females is 18 to 22 percent. A more accurate definition of obesity for females is a body fat content of greater than 33 percent. A person at her HBW is metabolically obese if her body fat content exceeds 33 percent. The woman in the preceding example may have all of the health risks of obesity even at 100 percent HBW if her body fat content exceeds 33 percent.

Second, let us consider a 5-foot 9-inch man with shoes (1-inch heels) who has a medium frame and was weighed wearing indoor clothing. According to the same table used above, this individual should weigh between 148 and 160 pounds. The same process can be used to derive his HBW. First, subtract 148 pounds from 160 pounds; the answer is 12 pounds. Next divide 12 pounds by 2 pounds; the answer is 6 pounds. When you add 6 pounds to 148 pounds, you have calculated his HBW, which is 154 pounds. Suppose this patient weighed 205 pounds. Dividing 154 pounds into 205 pounds would equal 133 percent. Can we automatically classify this patient as moderately obese? The answer is no. This patient may have a body fat content of only 15 percent. Remember, the optimal fat content for men is 15 to 19 percent. The individual described above would most likely be a trained athlete and the excess weight would be the result of increased muscle mass. A fat content in excess of 25 percent is considered obese for males.

The need to determine a patient's percent body fat should be apparent by now. At least half of the body fat is located just beneath the skin. Therefore, the measurement of skinfold thickness is the most commonly used technique to estimate a person's body fat content. In this chapter, the four-site measurement technique to determine percent body fat is discussed. This technique requires a minimum of calculations.

The worksheet in Clinical Calculation 15–1 can be used to assist in calculating a patient's percent body fat using skin calipers. A total of 12 measurements should be taken at four different sites. The three numbers obtained at each site are averaged to give a value of one number per site. All of these numbers are added and compared with the number on a standard table to determine the patient's percent body fat. This Body Fat and Skinfolds table is located in Appendix I. This procedure takes time and requires accurate measurements.

Other techniques to estimate body fat involve the use of tissue x-ray studies, ultrasound, electrical conductivity, electrical impedance, computed tomographic scans, and magnetic resonance imaging scans. (Committee on Diet and Health of the National Research Council, 1989). Many of these techniques to measure body fat are practiced only at major medical centers, because the technology to perform them is still in its infancy.

Prevalence

Prevalence means the total number of cases of a specific disease in an existing population at a certain time. One in four Americans may be classified as either overweight or obese. The prevalence of excess body weight is thus 25 percent (Table 15–1). Very few persons are classified as severely obese. Most of the people with excess body weight are mildly obese.

TABLE 15–1 *Classification and Percent Healthy Body Weight for a Reference Woman of 5 Feet 4 Inches*

Classification	Percent of Total Obese 5-Foot 4-Inch Population	HBW	Reference 5-Foot 4-Inch Woman (Medium Frame)*
Normal weight	None	95–105 percent	124–138 pounds
Mildly obese	90 percent	120–140 percent	157–196 pounds
Moderately obese	9 percent	140–200 percent	183–262 pounds
Severely obese	0.5 percent	200 percent +	>262 pounds

*Weight in pounds with indoor clothing weighing 3 pounds; shoes with 1-inch heels.

The development of excess body weight is strongly influenced by age and sex and by economic, racial, and ethnic factors. Females, especially black females; females below the poverty level; male Mexican-Americans; and older persons are the most likely to be overweight or obese.

Many experts are concerned about the prevalence of obesity in the nation's children. Obesity ranges from 10 to 12 percent in children of preschool age through adolescence (Ginsberg-Fellner, 1981). Asian children have the lowest incidence of obesity. <u>Incidence</u> is defined as the frequency of occurrence of any event or condition over time and in relation to the population in which it occurs. Native Americans have the highest incidence of obesity. After you read this chapter, read Clinical Application 15–6, which discusses tips for weight control in young children.

The prevalence of overly fat persons in the population is increasing. In 1960 to 1962 approximately 27.3 percent of the white female adult population was overweight. This compares to 27.5 percent in 1976 to 1980. Although a 0.2 percent increase may not appear very high, other racial groups are also experiencing an increase in the prevalence of obesity. For the adult black female population during the same period, the prevalence of overweight has increased from 47.3 percent to 49.5 percent. (Presently, almost one half of the adult female black population are overweight) This same trend has been observed in both black and white males. The population is becoming heavier.

Consequences of Obesity

Obese persons suffer socially, psychologically, and medically. The distribution of body fat affects a person's susceptibly to medical problems.

Social

The social consequences of obesity are connected to cultural expectations and the documented prejudice many obese people experience.

CULTURAL EXPECTATIONS   Culture, in this context, refers to the convictions of a given people during a given period. Currently, many Americans are preoccupied with leanness. Leanness means being attractive and desirable. Fatness means being unattractive and undesirable. Yet, what is and has been considered attractive has changed over time. Leanness has not always been the preferred body build. During one period, the overly fat body was considered the most attractive. Carrying excess weight meant that the person was well-to-do; he or she could afford to overeat. Many experts feel that members of our society are slowly changing their perception of what is attractive. For example, the female with well-developed muscles is considered more attractive to many than her lean, not-as-muscular counterpart. The increased numbers of female body builders demonstrate this attitudinal change.

In the United States the obese patient has been under intense pressure to lose weight. In an effort to be attractive, many obese patients try to lose weight. Over time, most people who lose weight regain the weight they have lost. When the reduced-weight obese person regains the weight lost, he or she often gains an additional few pounds over and above the original weight. Thus, a self-defeating cycle begins, which is described later in this chapter.

PREJUDICE DOCUMENTED   Several classic studies show that obese persons are the objects of prejudice and unfair discrimination. For example, obese students were accepted at lower rates than normal-weight students into higher ranking prestigious colleges, even though they did not differ in qualifications or total number applying (Canning and Mayer, 1966). Healthcare workers should try to understand their own feelings about fatness, obesity, and obese persons. All too often, healthcare workers insult obese patients without even being aware of it. Patients benefit when healthcare workers are sensitive to their psychological needs. Above all else, the nurse should treat the obese patient with respect, kindness, and patience.

Psychological

The science of the mind and mental processes is known as psychology. Obesity can be associated with a range of psychological problems. In this section we discuss one aspect of the psychological consequences of obesity—body image disturbances. Other psychological aspects of obesity are discussed in a later section.

BODY IMAGE DISTURBANCES   Body image is defined as the mental picture a person has of himself or herself. It is one's thoughts or feelings of physical self. A disturbed body image can manifest itself in two ways. First, people with distorted body images are dissatisfied with their bodies. Chronic complaints, demands for extra attention, and frequent negative statements made by patients about the way they look may be signs of an underlying body image disturbance. Second, persons with distorted body images frequently do not view their bodies realistically. For example, obese persons may view themselves as having certain body parts larger than they actually are. Later in this chapter the patient with anorexia nervosa is discussed. People with anorexia nervosa frequently have body image disturbances: very thin patients who have this condition frequently view themselves as overweight.

Body image disturbance is not found in emotionally healthy obese individuals (Stunkard and Mendelson, 1967). Body image disturbance is most common in young women of the middle and upper-middle classes who have been obese since childhood, who have a generalized neurotic disturbance, and whose parents and peers criticized them for their obesity (Stunkard and Burt, 1967; Stunkard and Mendelson, 1961).

Medical

Obesity is considered a major health problem in the United States. Excessive body weight has been associated with both a decreased life expectancy and nonfatal disease risks.

LIFE EXPECTANCY   The relationship between life expectancy and severe obesity is clear: the severely obese patient has a shorter life expectancy than his or her lean counterpart. Less clear is the relationship of overweight, mild obesity, and moderate obesity to life expectancy. Some researchers are questioning whether these patients do have a shorter life expectancy. This is one reason for the current controversy over whether the medical community should be encouraging all overweight patients to lose weight.

DISEASE RISK   Obesity is connected to many chronic diseases. Obesity is strongly linked to heart disease as well as high blood pressure, high cholesterol levels, and noninsulin-dependent diabetes (National Institute of Health Consensus Development Panel on the Health Implications of Obesity, 1985). Obesity is also associated with gallbladder disease fatty liver, lung function impairment, endocrine abnormalities, childbearing and childbirth complications, trauma to the weight-bearing joints, excessive protein in the urine, and increased hemoglobin concentration (Bray, 1985). Overweight men have higher rates for colorectal and prostate cancer; overweight women have higher rates for cancer of the ovary and of the breast (National Research Council, 1989).

The distribution of body fat affects risks. Abdominal obesity is more dangerous than gluteal-femoral obesity (Bjorntorp, 1986). **Abdominal obesity** means that the excess weight is between the patient's chest and pelvis. The patient with abdominal obesity is said to be shaped like an apple. Patients with abdominal obesity are especially vulnerable to the nonfatal risks associated with excessive body weight. **Gluteal-femoral obesity** means that the excess weight is around the patient's buttocks, hips, and thighs. The patients with gluteal-femoral obesity is said to be shaped like a pear. Patients with gluteal-femoral obesity are not as susceptible to the nonfatal risks associated with excessive body fat.

The treatment of obesity is an important means of controlling major chronic and degenerative diseases. For example, in some noninsulin-dependent diabetics, weight loss will lower blood glucose levels.

Abdominal obesity—Excess body fat located between an individual's chest and pelvis.

Gluteal-femoral obesity—Excess body fat centered around an individual's buttocks, hips, and thighs.

Theories about Obesity

Theories about obesity are plentiful (Box 15–1). The truth may be that any one of these theories may be accurate for a specific patient but that none is true for everyone.

Obesity may actually consist of a group of diseases. If this is the case, there may be more than one cause for the development and maintenance of body fat content. Keep these theories in mind when counseling the patient who is overly fat or underweight. Experts believe strongly that body fat content is primarily metabolic in origin. This means that some individuals are genetically prone to obesity or extreme thinness.

Effects of Weight Loss on the Body

Weight loss affects body composition. The health benefits of weight loss are all related to a loss of body fat, not a loss of lean body mass.

Loss of Fat versus Loss of Water and Protein

Most people, especially the mildly and moderately obese, can lose only about 2 pounds of body fat a week by eating less. Any weight loss beyond that is probably due to loss of water and/or lean muscle tissue (Strand, 1990). There is always some loss of body protein along with body fat during weight loss. The loss of body protein from reduced food intake alone is greater than the loss of body protein from a combination of reduced food intake and regular exercise. Also, the greater the rate of weight loss, the more organ and muscle mass is lost. For example, Table 15–2 considers the patient who loses 13 pounds of body weight over a 2-week period by diet alone.

BOX 15–1

Frequently Asked Questions about Theories of Obesity

Can a malfunctioning hypothalamus cause weight gain?

Appetite and satiety are regulated by a part of the brain called the hypothalamus. Satiety is the feeling of satisfaction after eating. Appetite refers to the pleasant sensation based on previous experience that causes a person to seek food for the purpose of eating. Hunger is the sensation caused by a lack of food, characterized by a dull or acute pain at or around the lower part of the chest. A malfunctioning hypothalamus could cause an individual to receive incorrect hunger signals, thus stimulating continued eating, and as a result gain weight. Appetite, satiety, and hunger may be incorrectly processed by a malfunctioning hypothalamus.

Is obesity the result of poor metabolism?

Some obese individuals actually require fewer kilocalories for normal body functions than do lean individuals. Some obese individuals use kilocalories very efficiently.

What is the function of brown fat, and how does it affect obesity?

Brown fat, a special type of fat cell, accounts for less than 1 percent of total body weight. The function of brown fat is to burn kilocalories and release the energy as heat. Energy released as heat is not stored as body fat. Some obese people may have defective brown fat or less brown fat then lean people.

What is the set point theory?

The set point theory argues that each individual has a unique, relatively stable, adult body weight that is the result of several biological factors. The obese person may have a higher set point than his or her lean counterpart.

Why should the number of fat cells in the body influence weight?

Obese individuals have many more fat cells than do their lean counterparts. A kilocalorie deficit can reduce the fat in each cell but cannot break down the entire cell. Once manufactured, a fat cell exists until death. Empty fat cells pressure the reduced obese person to fill the depleted cells. The reduced obese person must learn to constantly ignore internal hunger signals. Although obese individuals are able to do this for a short period, long-term adaptation to hunger pains is difficult.

Are there any enzymes in the metabolic chain that contribute toward obesity?

Lipoprotein lipase is an enzyme that is involved in the uptake of fatty acids for the manufacture of fat in individual fat cells. Research has shown that the activity of this enzyme increases during weight reduction. This action makes the fat cell even more efficient in synthesizing fats.

Box continued on next page.

BOX 15–1 *(Continued)*

Frequently Asked Questions about Theories of Obesity

References

Bennett, W and Gurin, J: The Dieter's Dilemma. Basic Books, New York, 1982.
Bray, GA: Brown tissue and metabolic obesity. Nutrition Today 17:23, 1982.
National Dairy Council: Weight Management: A Summary of Current Theory and Practice. National Dairy Council, Rosemont, 1985.
Mayer, J: Overweight: Causes, Cost, and Control. Prentice-Hall, Englewood Cliffs, NJ, 1968.

Variation with the Severity of Obesity

The amount of lean body mass an individual loses during weight reduction also depends on the degree of severity of his or her obesity (Van Itallie, 1988). Severely obese patients can tolerate very low-calorie diets better than the moderately obese patient. By tolerate, we mean that they conserve body protein during weight loss. This means mildly and moderately obese individuals are at a higher risk of becoming protein-depleted during rapid weight loss. Rapid weight loss (0.5 to 1.0 pounds per day), if sustained for many

---

TABLE 15–2 *Example of the Yo-Yo Effect—Weight Loss and Regain*

Patient Information	Weight		
	Before Dieting	After Dieting for 2 Weeks	After Regain
Body weight (pounds)	217	204	217
Body fat (pounds)	70	66	79
Percent body fat	32.2 percent	32.3 percent	36 percent
Lean body mass lost		2.5 pounds muscle and organ mass	
		6.5 pounds water	
		4 pounds fat	
		13 total pounds*	

*Does not take into account that most people regain more weight than they originally lost.

Fat and lean body mass are inversely proportional. As one goes up, the other goes down. Water composition is directly proportional to lean body mass. About 72–73 percent of lean body mass is water. Over a 12-week period on the diet, about 15 pounds of muscle and organ mass (not including water) may be lost.

weeks, is associated with an excessive loss of lean body mass and protein depletion of the heart (Van Itallie, 1988). Malnutrition of the heart muscle can lead to sudden death. As individuals lose more and more fat during weight loss, their ability to conserve lean body mass decreases. Thus, the length of time an individual diets as well as his or her beginning total body fat content has an impact on the amount of lean body mass lost.

Success Rates for Weight Loss

Weight cycling and the type of diet eaten by the individual attempting weight loss can influence the success rate.

Weight Cycling

The individual who loses weight rapidly has a difficult time keeping the lost weight off. This is because original weight loss is a combination of fat and lean body mass. Because it takes fewer kilocalories to support fat than protein tissue, weight regain occurs. Any weight regained is usually all body fat. When a patient gains and losses weight repeatedly, the net result is called the yo-yo effect, also known as weight cycling (Fig. 15-2).

Self-prescribed Fad Diets

Many kinds of fad diets have come and gone. Typically, such diets limit the person to a few specific foods or food combinations.

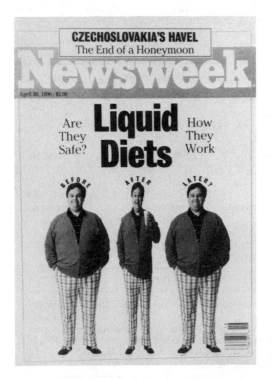

FIGURE 15–2. Illustrative Example Weight Cycling. (from the cover of *Newsweek* magazine 4/30/90), Newsweek Inc. All rights reserved. Reprinted with permission, Marty Ames, staff photographer.)

For example, one common fad diet recommends the consumption of a high-fat diet. Carbohydrates are restricted. This diet does not meet the recommendations of The American Heart Association, the American Cancer Society, and the American Dietetic Association and may be harmful. High fat intake has been associated with many chronic and degenerative diseases. Another example of a fad diet is the grapefruit diet, on which the individual is allowed only grapefruit. Such a diet is not nutritionally balanced and cannot possibly lead to a lifelong change in eating behaviors.

Treatment of the Overly Fat Patient

The fact that an individual is obese by any standard does not automatically make him or her a suitable candidate for treatment. The following sections of the chapter describe the screening of patients for weight reduction and the various treatments available.

Screening

How do health professionals decide whom to treat and whom not to treat? Not all patients should be encouraged to lose weight. Repeated gaining and losing of weight is harmful. Inappropriate weight-loss methods, including repeated crash diets, can have damaging effects on physical health and psychological well-being (Foster, 1988; Van Itallie, 1984; Wadden and Stunkard, 1985).

Screening patients is part of responsible weight-loss programs. Such screening usually includes the following (Petermarck, 1989):

1. Is weight loss indicated for this patient? Is the patient internally motivated to lose weight? The basic motivation to undergo treatment must originate from the patient.
2. What level of health supervision is necessary? Are patients screened for psychosocial conditions that would make weight loss inappropriate? Are patients at medical risk, requiring a physician's care?
3. What factors in the patient's history and lifestyle are relevant to the weight-loss program? For example, a weight-loss program that is costly may not be affordable for the low-income patient.

The best candidates for weight reduction are those who express the desire to change their total lifestyle. The patient must be motivated enough to agree to participate in a routine exercise program, follow a low-kilocalorie diet, and change lifelong food behaviors. A significant time investment on the patient's part is also necessary. The capacity to succeed is best demonstrated by deeds rather than words (Van Itallie, 1988). For example, will the patient attend all program sessions and self-monitor his or her food intake?

In addition, the best candidates for weight reduction are not currently under stress. Stressful life events such as a recent divorce, the death of a significant other, or a change in living situation or job status decrease the chances of success.

MOTIVATION   Most individuals associate weight loss with being more attractive. The association between weight loss and wellness is a secondary consideration. The health benefits of weight loss are related to a loss of body fat, however, and not to a loss of lean body mass. The individual who loses a large amount of lean body mass as opposed to body fat derives minimal health benefits from weight loss.

Setting Realistic Goals

Nurses can assist patients in setting realistic goals for weight reduction. Many times the patient has an unrealistic weight-loss goal. For example, the weight-reduction diet may be planned to allow for a loss of 1 pound per week, but the patient may expect to lose 5 pounds per week. The female patient may expect to lose enough weight to be able eventually to wear a size 5 dress, even though this is not a realistic expectation for a patient who has a large frame.

VALUE OF WEIGHT MAINTENANCE All overweight patients should be educated to stop gaining weight. A valuable service is provided by healthcare workers when they teach patients how to prevent weight gain. Clinical Application 15–1 may be of assistance when counseling the patient on weight maintenance.

The Triangle: Diet, Behavior Modification, and Exercise

Sound weight-control programs include nutrition education, instruction on behavior modification, and an exercise program. The best programs offer a lifelong support component. Recognition by both the nutrition counselor and the patient that it is far easier for the patient to lose excess body fat than to keep the lost fat off is important for a good long-term patient outcome.

Dietary Treatment

Weight-reduction diets can be divided into two types: the so-called very low-calorie diets. And the low-kilocalorie diets. Clinical Application 15–2 lists three guidelines for both patients and nurses to evaluate a low-kilocalorie, weigh-reduction diet.

Very low-calorie diet (VLCD)—Diet that contains less than 800 kilocalories per day.

VERY LOW-CALORIE DIETS Very low-calorie diets (VLCD) contain approximately 400 to 800 kilocalories per day. A VLCD diet may include only very lean meat and vitamin and mineral supplements. A beverage form of the diet is also widely used. Weight loss on these diets is dramatic. The typical man loses about 6.6 pounds per week. The typical woman loses about 4.4 pound per week.

This is not exclusively fat loss. Significant amounts of water and lean body mass are also lost. This is the key reason why mild and moderately obese patients should avoid VLCD. Grossly obese individuals not only have increased body fat but also increased lean body tissue compared with smaller individuals. Thus they can afford to lose more lean body mass than their less obese counterparts. <u>Cardiac arrhythmia</u> or irregular heart action (heartbeat), has occurred suddenly and without warning in mildly and moderately obese individuals who have followed drastic weight-reduction regimens.

An important feature of VLCDs is that in addition to the diet, patients should receive a program of physical exercise and behavior modification in order to develop long-lasting lifestyle changes that could ensure mainte-

CLINICAL APPLICATION 15–1
Prevention and Control of Excess Body Fat

Weight maintenance is the key to weight control. How can we as healthcare workers help our patients to achieve and maintain a healthy body weight?

First, we know it takes more kilocalories to support body protein content than body fat content. Healthcare workers should encourage patients to exercise more to increase their body protein content. Many experts feel that our society's increasingly sedentary lifestyle may be responsible for the increasing prevalence of obesity.

Second, fat is fattening. Here are some reasons to avoid dietary fat:

1. The patient gets more usable kilocalories from fat (Pawlak, 1989). Teaspoon for teaspoon, fat contains more kilocalories than either carbohydrate or protein. Dietary fat is fattening. So if a patient must overeat, encourage him or her not to overeat foods containing fat. Exchanges that include fat are the meat, fat, and some milk lists.
2. When eaten in excess, fat kilocalories are rapidly and effortlessly stored in fat cells (Pawlak, 1989). There is very little energy cost to convert fat in food to body fat. Carbohydrates in food must be converted to fat before carbohydrate can be stored in fat cells. This conversion requires an expenditure of kilocalories. Kilocalories used to convert carbohydrate in food to body fat are not stored as body fat.
3. The fat cell strongly resists release of its stored fat (Pawlak, 1989). Once a fat cell has been manufactured, there is no evidence that it can ever be broken down; it exists until death. According to one theory, fat cells "like" to store a certain amount of fat. When dieting, a person can reduce the amount of fat in each fat cell but not break down the cell completely. Some researchers believe that an empty fat cell sends a message to the reduced-obese person's brain to eat. The reduced-obese/overweight person must learn to cope with a message constantly coming from the brain to eat. This is another reason why it is very difficult for a patient to keep weight off permanently. Prevention of weight gain is the easiest way to maintain a reasonable body weight.

Third, a low-fiber intake may predispose a patient to obesity. Fiber has a high satiety value. Satiety is the feeling of satisfaction after eating. Obesity is uncommon among the populations of countries where a high proportion of dietary kilocalories is consumed as starchy vegetables nearly undepleted of their natural fiber content (Van Itallie, 1978). Educating patients to eat the recommended six to eleven servings of starch and five to nine servings of fruits and vegetables may help patients achieve satiety. Many starches, fruits, and vegetables contain appreciable amounts of fiber.

To summarize, the health care worker can educate patients to (1) exercise more, (2) eat less fat, and (3) eat more fiber.

CLINICAL APPLICATION 15–2

Guidelines for a Healthy Weight-Reduction Diet for the
Overly Fat Patient

Any healthy weight-reduction diet should meet the following
guidelines:

1. It should contain at least 1200 kilocalories.
2. It should not exclude any of the five major food groups.
3. The rate of weight loss should be between 1 and 2 pounds per
   week.

---

nance of the weight loss achieved. Patients on VLCD programs should be
closely monitored by a medically supervised healthcare team. The team usually includes a physician, a dietitian, an exercise trainer, a nurse, and a
behavioral therapist (Scheingart, 1989).

Low-Kilocalorie Diets

The most common tool used for teaching patients how to eat in order to lose
weight is the American Diabetic and Dietetic Association's Exchange Lists.
The ADA Exchange lists are located in Appendix H.

Nutritional counselors should encourage patients to make major behavioral changes in their eating habits slowly. The goal in weight-reduction
counseling is to help the patient make permanent lifestyle changes. The
current recommendation is that patients should be encouraged to change
only one to two negative food behaviors at a time. For example, if the nutrition counselor recommends that the patient substitute skimmed milk for
whole milk, it is not wise to simultaneously discourage the use of sweets.
The goal is to encourage *permanent* changes in eating behavior, so the patient
needs time to make the necessary adjustments. With this in mind, perhaps it
is best to review one exchange list at a time with some patients. Priority
should be given to eliminating foods in the fat, milk, and meat lists that are
high in fat and in which the patient overindulges.

The average woman will lose weight on a 1200-kilocalorie diet. Larger
women and most men will lose weight on a 1500-kilocalorie diet. Clinical
Application 15–3 identifies several reasons why exchange lists continue to be
so widely used for weight reduction.

Exercise

Exercise plays a critical role in the loss and maintenance of body weight.
Exercise is important for increased energy expenditure, maintenance of lean
body mass, and as part of a total change in lifestyle. For the greatest benefit,
the exercise chosen should involve movement that increases the heart rate
and is acceptable to the patient. Walking, running, swimming, and bicycling
are all good forms of exercise. The recommended exercise should be done at

---

CLINICAL APPLICATION 15-3
Advantages of Using Exchange Lists in Weight Reduction

Exchange lists in weight reduction are perhaps the best tool used to teach healthful eating behaviors. The use of exchange lists is still encouraged because:

1. The distribution of carbohydrate, fat, and protein can be calculated to conform to the Dietary Recommendations of the National Research Council, the American Heart Association, and the American Cancer Society. For example, if the patient is eating too much total fat, exchange lists can be used to discuss alternatives available to the patient to decrease his or her fat intake.
2. Exchange lists can be used to teach patients appropriate portion sizes and food preparation methods.
3. Exchange lists can be adopted to accommodate the needs of patients who require modifications in their intake of sodium, fat, protein, cholesterol, saturated fat, potassium, fluid, and phosphorus.
4. This method of dietary control can be used to teach meal spacing and meal frequency.
5. Two versions of the diet are available. The main version requires a 10th-grade reading level. A simplified version, available from the American Dietetic Association, requires only an 8th-grade reading level.
6. Exchange lists in several different languages are available from the American Dietetic Association.
7. Exchange lists are used by most hospitals and healthcare organizations throughout the country, so familiarity with them is widespread.
8. Increasingly, cookbooks and frozen food items are being labeled with the number of exchanges in a recommended serving. Many fast-food restaurants have the exchange value of their menu items available on customer request.
9. This tool encourages a wide variety of foods from each of the major food groups so that weight-reduction diets are likely to be balanced.
10. The cultural food preferences of most individuals can be accommodated with exchange lists. Most food items can have their exchange value calculated.
11. Once the patient learns the exchange system, his or her changing kilocaloric requirements can easily be adjusted according to need.
12. The rate of weight loss can be controlled with this system, so the patient does not lose weight too rapidly (with too high a loss of lean body mass).

---

least three times per week. Daily exercise maximizes weight loss. If daily exercise is done, it is best to change the activity every other day. For example, a patient may swim 3 days a week and walk a mile on the other 4 days of the week.

The exercise should last at least 30 minutes. Longer than 30 minutes is preferable. A 30-minute exercise period may need to be approached gradually by some patients. Each exercise period should include a warm-up and a cool-down period in which exercise is done at a slower pace.

To identify those individuals at a major heart disease risk, all patients should be screened by a physician before exercise recommendations are made. Patients with known heart, lung, or metabolic disease should have a physician-supervised stress test before to beginning an exercise program.

When following an exercise program, fluid intake should be adequate. Individuals should drink water before, during, and after exercise. Close attention to thirst should be given to prevent dehydration. The thirst mechanism may not be adequate to prevent dehydration in many elderly persons and in individuals involved in heavy exercise during hot weather (Petersmarck, 1989). Such persons need to be taught to drink water even if they are not thirsty.

Behavior Modification

Permanent weight loss can only result from a permanent change in eating and exercise behaviors. The behavioral strategies most commonly applied in weight-reduction programs include self-monitoring, stimulus control, slowed-down eating, a reward system, and cognitive behavior modification. Table 15–3 lists specific techniques used to help patients modify their behaviors.

SELF-MONITORING Patients keep their own food records, track their body weights, and record exercise completed during self-monitoring. Many patients come to regard self-monitoring of their food intake as the single most helpful strategy in a weight-reduction program (Foreyt, 1990, unpublished lecture). Recording of food intake seems to work best when patients know they must turn in the records to their nutritional counselor.

Requiring patients to monitor their weight is also a helpful behavioral strategy. When patients are gaining weight they tend to avoid scales and mirrors. Requiring patients to weigh themselves helps to keep them on their eating plan. Patients should also be asked to record what exercise is completed in a notebook. Again, the notebook should be reviewed regularly in the training program (Foreyt, 1990, unpublished lecture).

STIMULUS CONTROL Stimulus-control strategies are designed to help patients rearrange their lifestyle to reduce the chances of inappropriate eating habits (Foreyt, 1990, unpublished lecture). Patients are taught to examine their behaviors to determine which ones may trigger them to eat inappropriately. For example, a truck driver may eat two doughnuts every morning for breakfast because he or she drives by the bakery on the way to work. The nutritional counselor may recommend that this patient take a different route to work in order to reduce the probability of his or her buying doughnuts.

SLOWED-DOWN EATING Some obese people eat very rapidly. It takes approximately 20 minutes from the time food has been eaten for the brain to receive the message that food has been consumed. An individual can consume many extra kilocalories in 20 minutes. Obese patients are frequently taught a number of behavioral techniques to slow down their eating.

TABLE 15–3 *Weight Control: Behavior Modification Techniques*

Self-Monitoring
- Keep a food diary and record all food intake.
- Keep a weekly graph of weight change.
- Keep an exercise diary.

Stimulus Control
- At home, limit all food intake to one specific place.
- Plan food intake for each day.
- Rearrange your schedule to avoid inappropriate eating.
- Sit down at a table while eating.
- At a party, sit a distance from snack foods, eat before you go, and substitute lower kilocalorie drinks for alcohol.
- Decide beforehand what you will order at a restaurant.
- Save or reschedule everyday activities for times when you are hungry.
- Avoid boredom; keep a list of activities on the refrigerator.

Slowed-Down Eating
- Drink a glass of water before each meal. Drink sips of water between bites of food.
- Swallow food before putting more food on the utensil.
- Try to be the last one to finish eating.
- Pause for a minute during your meal and attempt to increase the number of pauses.

Reward Yourself
- Chart your progress.
- Make an agreement with yourself or a significant other for a meaningful reward.

Cognitive Strategies
- View exercise as a means of controlling hunger.
- Practice relaxation techniques.
- Image yourself ordering a side salad, diet dressing, low-fat milk, and a small hamburger at a fast-food restaurant.

REWARD SYSTEM   Many patients respond better to any type of suggested behavioral change when they are working for specific rewards. In one program, for example, whenever a patient performs a desirable behavior he or she earns tokens. The tokens are redeemable at the hospital's gift shop for merchandise.

COGNITIVE STRATEGIES   Many weight-reduction programs include cognitive strategies. Cognitive means pertaining to the act of knowing. The goal of cognitive strategies is to increase the patient's knowledge of his eating behaviors so that he or she may develop skills to cope with negative behaviors. Teaching the patient to relax is one type of cognitive strategy. The use of imagery is another form of cognitive strategy. Imagery strategy involves asking patients to imagine themselves coping successfully with anxiety-arousing events.

Social Support Systems

Obesity is a chronic ailment. Since there are no known cures that significantly reduce obesity for most patients, a program should always include long-term continuing evaluation.

TABLE 15–4 *A Comparison of Weight-Loss Programs*

Program*	Approach	Expected Weight Loss	Staff
Diet Center	Five-phase program, frequent individual counseling, behavior modification, weekly group education on nutrition, food selection and exercise. *Conditioning*—prepares dieters for weight reduction. *Reducing*—Women: 945 calories, Men: 1300 calories. Private counseling 6 days a week. Individuals make transition from usual eating habits to moderate calorie diet which includes lean meats, whole grains, fresh fruit and vegetables. *Sta*b*lite*—Women: 1465 calories, Men: 1725 calories. As dieters approach weight goals, variety of foods introduced; private counseling 2–3 times a week. *Maintenance phase*—Women and men: 1465–2125 calories, weekly consultations, nutritional eating habits established. *Image One Series*—a 24-lesson series of weekly classes and 10-part video series covering nutrition, behavior modification, self-direction, relaxation, stress management, meal selection and preparation and 3 levels of exercise.	Women: 2½–3½ pounds per week. Men: 3–5 pounds per week	Nonprofessional counselors who have lost weight on the program. Program is developed by a full-time medical director, 4 staff registered dietitians at headquarters and medical consultants. Centers encouraged to organize local medical advisory boards, although figures are not available as to the number of local boards.
Health Management Resources	A 3-phase program in which clients consume liquid diet supplement, a multivitamin-mineral supplement and/or HMR entrées. *Weight loss*—clients consume liquid supplement providing 520–800 calories or liquid supplement and 2 entrées (9 varieties) for a total of 800–1000 calories per day.	2–5 pounds per week	Doctors, nurses, group leader is usually a registered dietitian, psychologist or other healthcare professional. Long-term intensive training provided for all staff.

Length	Availability & Headquarters	Cost	Comments
Conditioning—2 days. *Reducing*—Until weight loss is achieved. *Sta*b*lite I and II*—Up to 9 weeks. *Maintenance*—Up to 1 year after reaching desired weight. *Image One*—Weekly through all phases.	2000 centers in US, Canada, England, Australia, Singapore, Bermuda, and Guam. Headquartered in Pittsburgh, PA.	Varies. Determined by amount of weight to lose. Average cost for person to lose 30 pounds including the five phases is $650–$700. Fees include conditioning, reducing, Sta*b*lite (9 weeks), maintenance (1 year), and weekly Image One classes.	Not medically supervised, though individuals with preexisting medical conditions or those wishing to lose more than 50 pounds must have a physical examination, with additional examination. Diet consists of self-selected and prepared foods, although 75 Diet Center products are available for purchase. Calcium sources restricted during conditioning and Sta*b*lite phases. Question the need for Diet Center soy supplement and StaLite Nutrition Bar and restriction of starches to 2–3 servings per week. Program suitable for individuals who wish to prepare own meals and who require frequent individual counseling
Three phases: *Weight loss*—10–16 weeks. *Refeeding*—2–6 weeks. *Maintenance*—6–18 months.	Affiliated with hospitals, medical schools, medical centers, and corporations. Over 600 centers in the US. Headquartered in Boston, MA.	Varies among locations. Maintenance is $55 per month. Both options include medical screening and behavioral education classes. Medically monitored program is $115 per week, including	Medically supervised supplement program recommended for individuals 20 percent above ideal body weight or at least 30 pounds above ideal body weight. Clients taking liquid supplements only may experience unpleasant side effects such as

TABLE 15–4 *A Comparison of Weight-Loss Programs (Continued)*

Program*	Approach	Expected Weight Loss	Staff
	Refeeding—gradual decrease in supplement or entrées, increase in food calories; calorie level determined individually. Intensive behavior and nutrition education. Medically supervised or unsupervised options both include medical screening. Emphasizes lifestyle changes such as reducing dietary fat, increasing physical activity, and balancing food and exercise. Staff is on call on a 24-hour basis for support or medical emergencies.		
Jenny Craig International Weight Loss Centers	Personal counseling and group classes focus on behavior modification, nutrition and exercise. Multi-vitamin/mineral supplement is taken. Clients required to purchase most of their food at centers. Modified diet with meal plans. Women: 1000 calories. Men and adolescents: 1200 to 1400 calories. Menus are 60 percent carbohydrate, 20 percent protein, 20 percent fat, 2000–3000 milligrams sodium, 100–150 milligrams cholesterol. Clients may prepare own foods 2 days a week when half of desired weight is lost.	1½–2½ pounds per week.	Counselors receive 48 hours of initial training, attend monthly continuing education class. Many are former clients, though it's not a prerequisite. Program designed by staff dietitian, psychologist, and consulting doctors.
Nutri/System	Nonmedically supervised. Nutritional instruction, computer analysis, diet supervision, behavior modification, exercise and weight maintenance. *Reducing Phase*—until weight loss is achieved. *Maintenance*—clients consume Nutri/System foods 2 days per week and	1½–2 pounds per week.	Behavior counselors have backgrounds in nursing, psychology, or education. Nutri/System certified nutritional specialists have degrees in food, nutrition, or dietetics. Headquarters staff include a doctor, a psychologist, a

Length	Availability & Headquarters	Cost	Comments
		supplements and/ or entrées. Medically unsupervised program is $90 per week.	constipation or dry skin. Both options require use of HMR products, a serious commitment, and temporary lifestyle change.
Varies, depending upon the time it takes to reach desired weight. *Permanent Stabilization Program*—one year maintenance includes monthly modification classes, clients return to selecting and preparing own foods.	More than 500 centers in US, Australia and New Zealand. Headquartered in Del Mar, CA.	$1000–$1225 for 17 weeks diet and food. Offers seasonal promotions. Permanent Stabilization Program is $99 per year. Audiotapes at an additional charge of $75.10.	Medically unsupervised, although clients with preexisting health problems are required to get physician approval. Requires temporary change in lifestyle. May appeal to individuals seeking a structured weight reduction program which initially involves a minimum of food preparation.
Reducing Phase: Varies. *Maintenance:* 1 year.	Centers in US, Canada, Australia, and U.K.	Program fee varies according to region, amount of weight to be lost and special promotions. Food cost for 3 meals per day is $54–$66 weekly. Financial incentives include refund of 25	For anyone over 18 years who desires to lose 5–100 pounds. Adolescents (14–17 years) and individuals with preexisting medical problems require physician approval. Dependency on program foods requires temporary

TABLE 15–4 *A Comparison of Weight-Loss Programs (Continued)*

Program*	Approach	Expected Weight Loss	Staff
	prepare own meals 5 days per week. Classes focus on food selection, food preparation and meal planning. Food purchased at centers provides between 1100 and 1500 calories, depending on individual's requirements. 60 percent of calories from carbohydrates, 15 percent fat, 25 percent protein, less than 2500 milligrams sodium and a minimum of 20 grams fiber per day.		nutritionist and 8 registered dietitians.
Optifast	Medically supervised three-phase, hospital- or clinic-based program includes taking a very low-calorie liquid diet formula. Intense behavior modification, psychological group support, nutrition education, exercise and weekly medical monitoring (physician visits and laboratory tests as needed). *Medical Screening*—(1200 calories solid food). Physical examination, laboratory tests, and psychological and nutritional assessments. *Supplemental Fasting Phase*—patients consume Optifast 70 or Optifast 800 five times daily, which provides between 420 and 800 calories. *Refeeding Phase*—reintroduction of foods. *Stabilization Phase*—1200 calories, supplement discontinued. *Encore Program*—optional, non-medically supervised maintenance program. Optifiber, a psyllium-based product has been recently introduced to mix with liquid supplements to relieve constipation or diarrhea associated with very low-calorie diets. One packet provides 3 grams soluble fiber.	2–5 pounds per week or 1–2 percent of body weight each week.	Dietitians, doctors, and psychologists at most locations.

Length	Availability & Headquarters	Cost	Comments
		percent of program cost after 6 months of successful maintenance.	change in lifestyle. May appeal to individuals seeking a structured weight-reduction program. Strong emphasis on company products.
Medical Screening—1 week. *Supplemented Fasting Phase*—12 weeks. *Refeeding Phase*—6 weeks. *Stabilization Phase*—7 weeks. *Encore Program*—6 months.	600 hospitals and medical institutions in the US, 30 in Canada. Headquartered in Minneapolis, MN	Varies among centers, approximately $3000 for 26-week program. Encore maintenance program approximately $500.	For individuals 30 percent or 50 pounds above ideal body weight. Requires serious commitment and temporary lifestyle changes. Certain activities are restricted such as swimming alone, horseback riding, or sitting in a whirlpool or steam bath. Potassium supplements may be necessary. Potential for unpleasant side effects such as bad breath, temporary dizziness, skin dryness, diarrhea or constipation.

TABLE 15–4 *A Comparison of Weight-Loss Programs (Continued)*

Program*	Approach	Expected Weight Loss	Staff
Optitrim	A medically supervised, three- or four-phase program, developed by Sandoz Nutrition, which involves intense nutrition education, behavior modification, liquid supplement and shelf stable *OptiEntree* meals, and exercise. *Phase I*—950 calories: Optitrim supplement 3 times a day and 1 prepackaged meal offering 275 calories. *Transitional Phase*—1100 calories, self-prepared foods. *Maintenance*—calorie level determined by counseling dietitian. *Encore*—6-month optional maintenance phase.	2 pounds per week.	Dietitian, clinical sociologists. Medical monitoring.
Overeaters Anonymous	Nonprofit support group, members admit to a compulsive eating problem believed to be physical, emotional, and spiritual. Members participate in weekly meetings, retreats, and annual conventions. Follows Alcoholics Anonymous 12-step program to correct behavior. No diet plans or nutrition counseling. Encourages members who seek such counseling to consult qualified professionals.	No projections are made.	Nonprofessional members conduct activities.
Registered Dietitians in Private Practice	Dietitian designs individual diet program according to client's lifestyle and caloric needs. Individual or group counseling may include sessions on nutrition, food preparation and recipe modification, behavior modification, and exercise.	Varies on an individual basis.	Registered dietitian. May be associated with doctors, psychologists or exercise physiologist.

Length	Availability & Headquarters	Cost	Comments
Phase I—8 weeks. *Transitional phase*—4 weeks. *Maintenance*—4 weeks. *Encore*—6 months. Total: 40 weeks.	180 hospital-affiliated programs. Headquartered in Minneapolis, MN.	$1800 for food and 18-week program.	For individuals 20–30 percent or 20–50 pounds above ideal body weight. Requires physician referral or examination. Less intensive than the Optifast program.
No limit.	10,500 chapters in 60 countries. Headquartered in Torrance, Ca.	No membership fees.	Noncommercial, does not sell or promote products. Lack of professional guidance and inconsistency in programs among chapters. Although OA does not incorporate weight-loss programs, group support may benefit individuals with compulsive overeating behavior.
Varies on an individual basis.	Nationally. Professional organization, The American Dietetic Association, Chicago, IL.	Usually hourly rates that vary according to region and services offered, ranging from $40–$125 an hour.	Offers individualized, personalized approach to weight loss. To contact a registered dietitian in private practice, consult the Yellow Pages or the local state dietetic association.

TABLE 15–4 *A Comparison of Weight-Loss Programs (Continued)*

Program*	Approach	Expected Weight Loss	Staff
Take Off Pounds Sensibly (TOPS)	International nonprofit support group of 320,000. Helps overweight individuals to attain and maintain physician-prescribed weight goals through support and fellowship. Independent chapters hold weekly meetings and activities to achieve goals. Regularly holds recognition programs, retreats, and annual convention. KOPS—"Keep Off Pounds Sensibly" is an honor society of members who maintain weight loss for 3 months.	No projections made.	Volunteer leaders elected by chapter members annually, assisted by regional directors and coordinators.
Weight Watchers International, Inc.	Nonmedically supervised program that incorporates diet, exercise, behavior modification, and group support. Food Plan—Women: 1000 calories increasing to 1200 calories by the fifth week. Fifteen percent to 20 percent protein, 50–60 percent carbohydrate, 20–30 percent fat, 2000 milligrams sodium, and 250 milligrams cholesterol. Based on a variety of foods adaptable to each individual's lifestyle. Frozen entrées and desserts available for purchase in supermarkets. Maintenance plan reinforces healthy behavior.	1–2 pounds per week.	Weekly meetings conducted by trained nonprofessional group leader who has successfully lost and maintained weight within 2 pounds. Program developed by staff dietitians and medical, exercise, and psychological consultants.

*Programs are listed alphabetically.

Length	Availability & Headquarters	Cost	Comments
No limit.	12,000 chapters in US, Canada, and more than 20 other countries. Headquartered in Milwaukee, WI.	Annual membership US—$16 first 2 years, $14 thereafter.	Noncommercial, does not sell or promote products. Lack of professional guidance, inconsistency in programs among chapters, although economically appealing means of group support following a physician-prescribed weight loss program.
Average 10 weeks.	25,000 meetings held weekly in 24 countries. Headquartered in Jericho, NY.	Registration fee: $20, $7 to $8 weekly meeting fee. At Work Program: fee determined by individual corporations. Members may attend meetings with no charge if they maintain weight loss within 2 pounds.	Designed for individuals 10 years or older who want to lose 10–40 pounds. Encourages members to seek physician approval before beginning program. Members have the flexibility of preparing their own meals or purchasing Weight Watchers products when following individual food plans.

Source: Adapted from Environmental Nutrition Newsletter, December 1990, pp. 4–5, with permission. Environmental Nutrition, Inc., 2112 Broadway, New York, NY 10023.

Psychotherapy

Obesity can be associated with a range of psychological problems. Some individuals have unresolved psychological problems that present insurmountable barriers to success in weight loss. In such cases, where the full benefit of the nutrition and exercise components of weight loss cannot be realized, mental health treatment should occur before or concurrently with weight-loss treatment (Petersmarck, 1989).

All patients enrolled in a weight-loss program should be helped to understand biological/genetic factors that contribute to obesity. Such an understanding not only minimizes guilt and depression but also allows him or her to learn to accept responsibility for variables over which control *can* be achieved (such as food types, meal size, activity level). Nurses should try to help patients appreciate the limitations of weight loss.

Dieting can lead to depression in susceptible persons. In fact, kilocalorie restriction has been known to bring on suicidal behavior (Petersmark, 1989). The stress of kilocaloric restriction can also interfere with treatment of a chronic psychological disorder. Conversely, a number of psychological conditions can affect eating. For all of these reasons, a mental health professional should be part of any weight-reduction program.

Comparison of Weight-Loss Programs

Table 15–4 compares several weight-loss programs. Clearly, no one type of program is appropriate for all overly fat individuals. The expected rate of weight loss, unpleasant side effects, and program costs should all be considered objectively by nurses before referring any patient to a program.

Other Treatment Approaches

Many drastic methods to lose weight have been and continue to be tried. Various types of surgical procedures, jaw wiring, acupuncture, and medications have all been used to promote weight loss.

SURGERY Many different surgical procedures have been and are being used to treat obesity. The removal of fat tissue through a vacuum hose is called lipectomy. This procedure is done more for cosmetic reasons than for weight control. A jejunoileal bypass involves the removal of a part of the small intestine. Patients lose weight after this procedure because they cannot absorb all the food they eat. This places these patient's at a nutritional risk. All gastric (stomach) procedures either route food around (bypass) or through only part of the stomach (reduction). Diagrams of **gastric stapling** and **gastric bypass**, two common procedures, are shown in Figure 15–3. When the stomach is smaller or reduced, only a limited amount of food can be consumed at one feeding. This induces weight loss from reduced kilocalorie intake (Sims, May, 1985). Clinical Application 15–4 discusses problems patients often encounter after gastric surgery for weight reduction. Clinical Application 15–5 suggests general guidelines for these patients to follow.

The results that can be expected from gastric surgery procedures should always be spelled out to patients. No permanent effects can be promised, and having the surgery does not mean that afterward the patient can overeat indefinitely without weight gain. Ninety percent of weight loss occurs in the

Gastric stapling—A surgical procedure on the stomach to induce weight loss by reducing the size of the stomach; also known as gastroplasty.

Gastric bypass—A surgical procedure that routes food around the stomach.

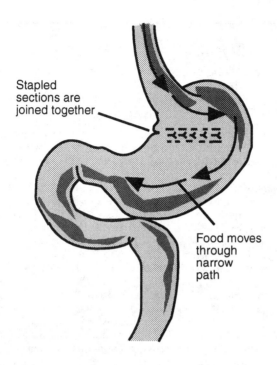

Stapled sections are joined together

Food moves through narrow path

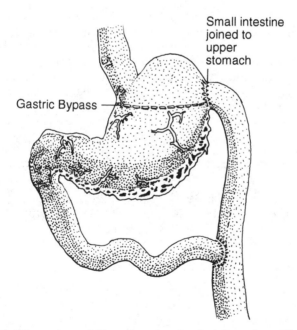

Small intestine joined to upper stomach

Gastric Bypass

FIGURE 15–3. Illustrations of Two Common Surgical Procedures Used to Treat Obesity (A) Gastric Stapling (B) Gastric Bypass

---

CLINICAL APPLICATION 15–4

Complications of Gastric Oplasty and Gastric Bypass

There are many potential complications of gastric surgery for weight reduction. These include:

1. *Nausea, vomiting, bloating, and/or heartburn:* These signs and symptoms can be caused by overeating, not chewing food well, eating too quickly, drinking cold or carbonated beverages, using drinking straws, or eating gassy foods.
2. *Staple disruption (for gastric stapling procedures):* The result of loosened staples is that a larger intake of food is necessary before satiety can be achieved. Excessive food intake or vomiting can cause the staples to become disrupted.
3. *Obstruction:* An obstruction is the blockage of a structure. In this case, a blockage can occur close to the area stapled. A frequent cause of obstruction is poorly chewed food. The result is stomach pain, nausea, and vomiting.
4. *Dumping syndrome:* Intake of concentrated sweets and large quantities of fluids cause quick dumping of food into the small intestine. Abdominal fullness, nausea, diarrhea 15 minutes after eating, warmth, weakness, fainting, racing pulse, and cold sweats are symptoms of this syndrome.

---

first year, and patients often begin to gain again in the second and third years. Only a minority achieve a weight as low as 125 percent of HBW. The procedure should be viewed as a tool to be used in conjunction with behavioral training—the small pouch helps patients in learning to reduce the amount consumed and in slowing down their intake. After the first year, due to stretching of the pouch or intestinal adaptation, much of the effect of the surgery can be overridden.

CLINICAL APPLICATION 15–5

Guidelines for the Patient following Gastric Surgery for Weight Reduction

The patient who has had gastric surgery for weight reduction may find the following general guidelines helpful:

1. Eat three to six small meals per day.
2. Eat slowly.
3. Chew food thoroughly.
4. Eat very small quantities.
5. Stop eating when full.
6. Drink most fluids between meals.
7. Select a balanced diet.
8. Take a multivitamin-multimineral supplement.
9. Exercise regularly.

CLINICAL APPLICATION 15–6
Tips for Weight Control in Young Children

Obesity in young children is frequently genetic in origin. The effect of this genetic disorder can be minimized by sound health habits. Following is a list of health habits that should be encouraged in young overweight children:

1. The degree of obesity is directly related to the number of hours the child spends watching television. The more hours spent watching television, the heavier the child. For this reason, viewing time should be restricted to no more than 2 hours per day.
2. The degree of obesity is directly related to the amount of physical activity the child performs. The more physical activity, the leaner the child. Thus the child should be encouraged to engage in all forms of physical activity. Examples of appropriate activity for very young children include ballet lessons, tricycle or bicycle riding, walking daily with another family member, swimming lessons, and sledding. Try to cultivate the enjoyment of year-round athletic activities in the child (Fig. 15–4).
3. The length of time the child spends chewing food may decrease the number of kilocalories the child spontaneously eats. Always serve fresh fruits and vegetables with every meal, including breakfast. Examples of low-kilocalorie snacks that require chewing include cut-up apples, peaches, pears, carrots, cucumbers, and green peppers.
4. Fat is the most concentrated source of calories. Try to limit the child's fat intake. Foods that contain fat include all

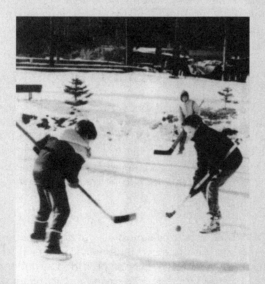

FIGURE 15–4. Young boys who engage in year-round sports activities are better able to maintain their weights

Box continued on next page

CLINICAL APPLICATION 15–6 *(Continued)*
Tips for Weight Control in Young Children

meat, fish, and poultry. It is best to restrict both the amount and kind of meat, fish, and poultry eaten by the overly fat child. The amount of meat a child should eat is frequently calculated by the dietitian. Some dairy products also are high in fat. The child should be encouraged to consume nonfat dairy products such as skimmed milk, partly skimmed cheeses, diet cheeses, and nonfat yogurt. Other sources of fat include salad dressings, margarine, nuts, seeds, oil, bacon, avocado, cream cheese, and sour cream.

5. The child should be taught to be aware of what he or she eats. Teach the child to recite after each meal what he or she has eaten.

6. Try to encourage the child to eat slowly. For example, serve a hot soup at the beginning of a meal. The child will have to wait for the soup to cool before it can be consumed.

7. Try not to make the child feel guilty about his or her weight problem. Again, recent research has shown that massive obesity in children is partly genetic. The child is *not* totally responsible for his or her present body weight. Try to be kind, patient, and considerate but firm.

Jaw wiring, acupuncture, and medications have also been used to promote weight loss. Jaw wiring prohibits the consumption of food. This procedure had a poor long-term outcome because once the wires are removed, patients return to their former eating behaviors and the lost weight is regained. The role of medication in the treatment of obesity remains controversial (Van Itallie, 1988). Drug therapy may decrease with the success of behavior therapy in promoting lasting lifestyle changes.

PATIENTS WITH REDUCED BODY MASS

The patient with a reduced body mass is as difficult, if not more difficult, to treat than the overly fat patient. A patient with a low body fat content usually has a loss of lean body mass as well; that this is functioning tissue gives clinicians concern. Body fat has some important roles in insulation and protection of body organs, and women cease to ovulate and menstruate when the percent of body fat falls below a certain level.

Classification

Methods similar to those used to diagnosis the overly fat patient can be used to diagnosis the patient with reduced body mass. A person whose weight is more than 15 percent below HBW may be classified as underweight. A man with a body fat content of less than 15 percent and a woman with a body fat content of less than 18 percent may be classified as having a reduced body mass. A BMI less than 20 kilograms per meter squared may indicate that the patient has a reduced body mass.

Consequences

Long-term follow-up of studies indicates that extreme leanness is associated with increased mortality and decreased life expectancy. The causes of mortality are different from those associated with excess weight, however (National Research Council, 1989). The excessively lean person is almost twice as likely to succumb to respiratory diseases such as tuberculosis. In addition, these patients have a greater difficulty maintaining body temperature during cold weather. Infections and disturbances of the gastrointestinal tract are more likely in the underweight person.

Causes

A person may be underweight by virtue of genetics or because of a long-term or recent weight loss. As part of the nutrition screening process, a healthcare worker should ask the patient about any change in body weight. A good question is, "Have you experienced any unintentional weight loss?" If the patient responds yes, it is important to determine the time frame of the weight loss. On the other hand, a response such as "I have always been lean" may indicate that the patient's leanness is genetic. Sometimes this assumption may be erroneous.

Rapid Loss Increases Risk

The greater the rate of loss, the more the patient is at a nutritional risk. <u>Rate</u> means loss per unit of time. For example, a 20-pound weight loss in 2 weeks is a large rate of loss. Such a patient has lost a large amount of lean body mass. On the other hand, a 20-pound weight loss over 20 weeks could be attributed mostly to a loss of body fat with a minimal loss of lean body mass. If the patient began with surplus body fat stores, a loss of 20 pounds may not place this patient at a high nutritional risk. If the patient had a reduced body mass, even a slow weight loss may place him or her at a nutritional risk.

Not all changes in body weight are caused by insufficient kilocalorie intake. For example, a patient may lose several pounds of body weight over the course of 1 day as a result of diuretic therapy. The weight loss in this situation would be due to water loss, not body fat or protein loss.

One method to determine whether a patient is eating enough food is to monitor his or her food intake. Kilocalorie intake is monitored by visually recording actual food consumption and calculating the kilocalories eaten.

Eating Disorders

Eating disorders may be caused by psychological factors, resulting in nutritional problems. Many experts are concerned about the prevalence of anorexia nervosa and bulimia.

Anorexia Nervosa

Anorexia nervosa is a medical condition resulting from self-imposed starvation. Symptoms include:

1. Loss of 20 to 40 percent of usual body weight (UBW); refer to Clinical Calculation 15–2 to calculate UBW

Anorexia nervosa—A mental disorder characterized by a 25 percent or greater loss of usual body weight, an intense fear of becoming obese, and self-starvation.

2. Decreased resting energy expenditure (REE)
3. **Amenorrhea,** or the cessation of menstruation
4. Constipation
5. Hair loss
6. Abnormal sleeping patterns
7. Preoccupation with food
8. Body image disturbance
9. Denial of problem
10. Intake of only 500 to 800 kilocalories per day
11. Slow eating
12. Increased physical activity
13. Social isolation
14. Intense fear of becoming obese

This disorder may be life-threatening. Although found primarily in adolescent girls and young women, approximately 4 to 6 percent of the cases are men (National Research Council, 1989). The patient may resort to a variety of devices to lose weight, including starvation, vomiting, and laxative use.

Bulimia

Bulimia is much more common than anorexia nervosa, especially during adolescence and young adulthood (Halmi, et al, 1981). The prevalence of bulimia has been found to be as high as 13 percent in a college population. Bulimics binge and purge. <u>Binging</u> involves the consumption of as much as 5000 to 20,000 kilocalories per day. <u>Purging</u> is the intentional clearing of food out of the system by vomiting and/or using enemas, laxatives, and diuretics.

Treatment

There are many approaches to treatment of eating disorders, including behavioral therapy, family therapy, and group therapy. It is important to help the patient discover the reason he or she chooses to eat, not eat, binge, or purge. Some of these patients are admitted to the hospital for treatment. Careful recording of kilocalories consumed is indicated. Sometimes nurses are asked to sit with these patients and watch them eat. These patients may attempt to hide food in their clothes, mouth, bedding, or anywhere else they can find. It is sometimes necessary for the nurse to accompany these patients to the bathroom. Patients with eating disorders have been known to flush their food down the toilet. For these reasons, daily weights are often ordered by physicians for such patients.

Summary

Energy imbalance results from a malfunction of homeostatic mechanisms. The reason an individual eats more or fewer kilocalories than needed to maintain a stable body weight is not known. The overly fat individual has eaten more kilocalories than he or she has used. The individual with a reduced body mass has eaten fewer kilocalories than he or she has used. One quarter of the US population is overly fat. The prevalence of individuals with excess body fat is increasing. Many experts attribute this to our increasingly sedentary society. At the same time, the prevalence of eating disorders such as anorexia nervosa and bulimia is also high. Many Americans are more concerned with their appearance than with their health. The nurse needs to help the patient focus on the health benefits of weight control.

Americans are willing to spend substantial amounts of money in the hopes of improving their appearance. Over the long term, however, the pursuit of the perfect body frequently has a negative impact on one's health. Repeatedly following crash diets can have serious psychological and medical consequences.

Permanent weight loss can occur only when the individual makes a commitment to change his or her total lifestyle. Exercise; a well-balanced, low-kilocalorie diet; and behavior modification are all necessary parts of a sound weight-reduction program. Surgical interventions, acupuncture, and medications are also used to promote weight loss.

A case study and a sample plan of care appear below. Both are designed to show how the information you have studied in this chapter can be used in nursing practice.

CASE STUDY 15–1

R., admitted to the hospital for an evaluation of her weight loss, is 14 years old, is 5 feet 2 inches tall, weighs 80 pounds, and has a medium frame. She is 64 percent of her healthy body weight. R.'s mother stated "My daughter is melting away to nothing. R. routinely runs every morning before school. She takes a 4-hour nap after school and is awake most of the night. She rarely eats with the family and will not go out to eat with us, although she talks about food constantly. Her beautiful hair looks terrible. She has not had a period in 6 months. I can hear her vomiting in the bathroom during the night." The patient's only complaint is constipation. She denies she has any other problems. According to the patient's medical history, her weight 1 year ago was 115 pounds (HBW = 98 percent) and her assessment revealed a small frame.

NURSING CARE PLAN FOR R.

Assessment

Subjective:
  Patient stated during admission that "I need to lose weight." Per patient's mother, patient has been vomiting.

Objective:
  Weight 1 year ago 115 pounds and HBW 98 percent. Adm. weight 80 pounds and HBW 64 percent. Cessation of menstruation.

Nursing Diagnosis
  Nutrition, altered: related to self-starvation as evidenced by patient's admitted desire to lose weight and a HBW of 68 percent.

Desired Outcome/Evaluation Criteria
  1. Patient will state "I need to gain weight."
  2. Patient will cease losing weight for 2 weeks.
  3. Patient will gain 1 pound per week after weight loss has ceased until she attains her usual body weight.

Nursing Actions/Interventions with Rationale in Italics

1. Educate patient on the dangers of continued weight loss. *The patient must be made to realize that continued weight loss is life-threatening.*
2. Weigh patient daily (in her underwear). *Body weight for this patient would be a reliable indicator of energy balance, as the patient is not edematous.*
3. Record food intake. *In tallying the patient's daily kilocalorie count, the dietitian will need to include the kilocalories obtained from the food the nurse gives the patient.*
4. Offer small quantities of food every 2 hours. *Anorexia nervosa patients frequently have diminished appetite, and small feedings are usually better tolerated.*
5. Reinforce the nutritional care plan prescribed by the physician and planned by the dietitian. This may require the support of Psychological Services. *Given the complexity of the problem, a team approach is indicated for patients with eating disorders. Psychological services may be indicated because patients of this type are often resistant to increased food intake.*

STUDY AIDS

Chapter Review Questions

1. Which of the following statements is true?
   a. Generally speaking, given two individuals of similar height, weight, and activity, the individual with the lowest body fat content will have the lowest resting energy expenditure.
   b. Exercise during weight loss will increase the amount of lean body mass lost.
   c. Generally speaking, given a man and a woman of similar height, weight, and activity, the woman will have a higher kilocalorie requirement than the man.
   d. Following a crash diet will often lower an individual's lean body mass and decrease his or her resting energy expenditure.

2. To lose 2 pounds of body fat per week, an individual must eat _____ fewer kilocalories than used each day for 7 days.
   a. 1000
   b. 1500
   c. 2000
   d. 2500

3. The following statement is true about the overly fat patient's risk of nonfatal disease:
   a. Patients with excessive fat in the gluteal-femoral area are the most susceptible to the risk of nonfatal disease
   b. Obese patients will develop diabetes
   c. Concentration of excessive adipose tissue in the abdomen increases the risk of nonfatal disease
   d. All obese patients are equally susceptible to nonfatal disease risks

4. A very rapid rate of weight loss (1 pound per day) in the mildly obese (Select the best response):
   a. Usually encourages permanent changes in behavior
   b. May lead to sudden death in some patients
   c. Will preserve lean body mass
   d. Fosters long-term weight maintenance

5. A stable body weight can best be achieved by:
   a. Eating a balanced diet with the recommended amount of fiber
   b. Eating a diet with a fat content not in excess of 30 percent of total kilocalories
   c. Incorporating routine exercise into the activities of daily living
   d. All of the above

6. The severely obese patient:
   a. Has a decreased life expectancy
   b. Is at an increased risk for infections and tuberculosis
   c. Will always have noninsulin-dependent diabetes
   d. Is the poorest choice for a "very low-calorie" weight-reduction program

7. Which of the following statements is true?
   a. A patient at 100 percent HBW is never overly fat.
   b. A normal BMI is 20 to 25 kilograms per meter squared.
   c. The obese female has a body fat content in excess of 22 percent.
   d. The healthiest range of body fat for males is 25 to 30 percent.

8. The excessively lean person is almost twice as likely to succumb to _____.
   a. Gallbladder disease

b. Diabetes
c. Heart disease
d. Respiratory disease

9. A patient with reduced body mass_____.
   a. has an increased resting energy expenditure
   b. frequently complains of constipation
   c. is not likely to have a body image disturbance
   d. typically seeks the company of others

10. Any healthy weight-reduction diet should meet all of the following guidelines except one. Please select the *exception.*
    a. It should contain at least 1200 kilocalories.
    b. It should exclude all fats.
    c. It should include all of the major food groups.
    d. The rate of weight loss should be between 1 and 2 pounds per week.

NCLEX-Style Quiz

Situation One

Mrs. R. is a 40-year-old mother of three. She has arthritis in both knees. She weighs 165 pounds, has a medium frame, and is 5 feet 3 inches tall. Her HBW is thus 128 percent. Her body fat content is 34 percent. Her physician has told her to lose weight, as this would help reduce her knee pain. According to Mrs. R. she never thought she was overweight until she was 24 years old. At this time, her weight started increasing. When she weighed 140 pounds, she started to diet. One time she lost a total of 25 pounds, which she promptly regained plus an additional 5 pounds. The patient described four additional weight cycles. Mrs. R. claims she cannot exercise because "it is too painful on my knees." She has tried every conceivable type of diet. Mrs. R. states that for the past year, no matter how little she eats, she cannot lose weight even on a 1200-kilocalorie diet.

1. The best initial approach to help this patient would be:
   a. To help her understand the biological/genetic factors that contributed to her obesity
   b. To encourage a further reduction in food intake
   c. To encourage exercise, no matter how painful it is
   d. To encourage the patient to try a very low-calorie diet

2. The above patient:
   a. Apparently knows a great deal about low-kilocalorie foods, because she has successfully lost weight before
   b. Knows very little about foods, because she always regained the weight she lost
   c. Lacks motivation, because she has an inability to follow through with the appropriate behavior
   d. Should be discouraged from further attempts to control her weight

3. This patient may benefit by self-monitoring her behavior. The nurse could teach this concept by:
   a. Encouraging the patient to eat only in one location
   b. Avoiding situations that lead to inappropriate eating
   c. Requesting the patient to keep daily food records
   d. Having the patient imagine herself responding appropriately to difficult situations

4. This patient may benefit by all except one of the following. Identify the *exception:*
   a. Limiting her intake of lean meats
   b. Increasing her intake of whole grains
   c. Restricting all foods from the bread, cereal, rice, and pasta group
   d. Replacing fruit juices with fresh fruits

CLINICAL CALCULATION 15–1

Calculating Body Fat Content Using the Four-Site Technique

Worksheet for calculating percent body fat using skin calipers

Skinfold Measurements	1	2	3	=	Total	÷ 3 =	Average
Biceps	__ +	__ +	__	=	____		_____
Triceps	__ +	__ +	__	=	____		_____
Subscapular	__ +	__ +	__	=	____		_____
Suprailiac	__ +	__ +	__	=	____		_____

Total value of the average of four sites: _____

Procedure to calculate percent body fat using skin calipers in adults

1. Take skinfold measurements directly on the skin, not through clothing.
2. Pick up and hold the skinfold with one hand while measuring it with calipers held by the other hand.
3. Take three measurements at each of the four sites. Then average the three measurements of each skinfold to arrive at a final figure.
   - Biceps—measure the muscle belly of the biceps. This will generally be a point on the straightened arm just opposite the nipple.
   - Triceps—
   - Subscapular—measure on the back just under the shoulder blade.
   - Supraillac—measure approximately 1 inch above the hip bone.
4. Add the averages of all skinfold sites to arrive at a total skinfold measurement.
5. To determe the percent body fat, compare the total measurement with the values in the appropriate Body Fat and Skinfolds table located in Appendix G.

(Adapted, courtesy of Jan Wohgulmuth, PT, Director of Physical Therapy at Doctor's Hospital)

CLINICAL CALCULATION 15–2
Percent Usual Body Weight

The healthcare worker can calculate the patient's percent usual body weight (UBW). The formula is:

$$\frac{\text{present weight}}{\text{usual weight}} \times 100$$

A 5 percent weight loss over a month may not be significant. However, 5 percent weight loss over a week may be significant. The kilocalorie deficit may be related to a recent change in medication, an underlying but as yet undiagnosed condition, a recent change in living situation, or not taking the time to eat.

BIBLIOGRAPHY

Bennett, W and Gurin, J: The Dieter's Dilemma. Basic Books, New York, 1982.

Bjorntorp, P: Fat cells and obesity. In Brownell, KD and Foreyt, JP (eds): Handbook of Eating Disorders: Physiology, Psychology, and Treatment of Obesity, Anorexia, and Bulimia. Basic Books, New York, 1986.

Bray, GA: Brown tissue and metabolic obesity. Nutrition Today 17:23, 1982.

Bray, GA: Complications of obesity. Ann Int Med 103:1052, 1985.

Canning, H and Mayer, J: Obesity: Its possible effect on college acceptance. N Engl J Med 275:1172, 1966.

Crisp, AH: Treatment and outcome in anorexia nervosa. In Goodstein, RK (ed): Eating and Weight Disorders: Advances in Treatment and Research. Springer, New York 1983.

Environmental Nutrition: Winning at the Weight Loss Game: Choosing the Right Program. Environmental Nutrition Newsletter, December 1990.

Foreyt, JP: Unpublished lecture, Spring Michigan Dietetic Association Conference, Michigan State University, East Lansing, 1990.

Foster, G, et al: Resting energy expenditure, body composition, and excess weight in the obese. Metabolism 37:467, 1988.

Ginsburg-Feller, F: Growth of adipose tissue in infants, children, and adolescents: Variations in growth disorders. Int J Obes 5: 1981.

Grubbs, L: The critical role of exercise in weight control. Nurse Practitioner 18:4, 1993

Guthrie, H: Introductory Nutrition, ed 6. St Louis, CV Mosby, 1986.

Halmi, KA, Falk, JR, and Schwartz, E: Binge-eating and vomiting: A survey of a college population. Psychol Med 11:697, 1981.

Harrison JE: Metabolic bone disease. In Jeejeebhoy, KN (ed): Current Therapy in Nutrition. Decker, Toronto, Canada, 1988.

Larkin, JC and Pines, HA: No fat persons need apply: Experimental studies of the overweight stereotype and hiring preference. Sociology of Work and Occupations 6:312, 1979.

Mayer, J: Overweight: Causes, Cost and Control. Prentice-Hall, Englewood Cliffs, NJ, 1968.

National Dairy Council: Weight Management: A Summary of Current Theory and Practice. National Dairy Council, Rosemont, Illinois, 1985.

National Institute of Health Consensus Development Panel: Health Implications of Obesity. Ann Intern Med, 103:1073, 1985.

National Research Council: Diet and Health Implications for Reducing Chronic Disease Risk. Report of the Committee and Diet and Health, Food and Nutrition Board, Commission on Life Sciences. National Academy Press, Washington, DC, 1989

A losing formula: The liquid diet craze. Newsweek, April 30, 1990.

Pawlak, L: Life Without Diets. Communications Marketing Incorporated, Palm Springs, CA 1989.

Petersmark, KA: Toward Safe Weight Loss. Michigan Health Council, East Lansing, MI, 1989.

Pyle, RL, Mitchell, JE, and Eckert, ED: Bulimia: A report of 34 cases. J Clin Psychiatry 42:60, 1981.

Rock, CL and Coulson, AC: Evaluation of weight loss programs. Nutrition and the MD 15:2, 1989

Roe, DA and Eickwork, KR: Relationships between obesity and associated health factors with unemployment among low income women. J Am Med Wom Assoc 31:193, 1976.

Romsos, DR: Efficiency of energy retention in genetically obese animals and in dietary-induced thermogenesis. Fed Proc 40:2524, 1981.

Scheingart, DE: Unpublished material, 1989.

Sims, EA: Why, oh why can't they lose weight? Nutrition and the MD 11:1, 1985.

Stern, JS and Lowney, P: Obesity: The role of physical activity. In Brownell, KD and Foreyt, JP (eds): Handbook of Eating Disorders: Physiology, Psychology, and Treatment of Obesity, Anorexia, and Bulimia. Basic Books, New York, 1986

Strand, G: Some Basic Facts About Losing Weight. Insights, March 1990.

Stunkard, AJ and Burt, V: Obesity and body image II. Age on onset of disturbances in the body image. Am J Psych 123:1443, 1967.

Stunkard, AJ and Mendelson, M: Disturbances in body image of some obese persons. J Am Diet Assoc 38:328, 1961.

Van Itallie, TB: Fiber and obesity. Am J Clin Nutr 31:S252, 1978.

Van Itallie, T and Yang, M: Cardiac dysfunction in obese dieters: A potential complication of rapid weight loss. Am J Clin Nutr 39:695, 1984.

Van Itallie, TB: Obesity. In Jeejeebhoy KN (ed): Current Therapy in Nutrition. BC Decker, Toronto, Canada, 1988.

Wadden, T and Stunkard, A: Social and psychological consequences of obesity. Ann Int Med 103:1062, 1985.

Weigley, ES: Average? Ideal? Desirable? A brief overview of height-weight tables in the United States. J Am Diet Assoc 4:84.

Chapter Outline

Key Terms

As a study aid, each key term is followed by the page number where the term is defined in the chapter. Terms that appear in **boldface** or <u>underscored</u> in the chapter text are located in the glossary.

Diet in Diabetes Mellitus and Hypoglycemia

Learning Objectives

After completing this chapter, the student should be able to:

1. Define and classify diabetes mellitus and describe the treatment for each type.
2. Discuss the goals of nutritional care for persons with diabetes mellitus.
3. List nutritional guidelines for illness, exercise, delayed meals, alcohol, hypoglycemic episodes, vitamin/mineral supplementation, and eating out for people with diabetes.
4. Describe dietary treatment for reactive hypoglycemia as compared to diabetes mellitus.

his chapter discusses two diseases associated with insulin secretion and/or resistance to insulin accompanied by characteristic long-term complications. Diabetes mellitus is caused by the low secretion and/or use of insulin. Hypoglycemia is caused by excessive secretion of insulin. Diabetes mellitus has been diagnosed in approximately 6 million people in the United States, and an additional 4 to 5 million individuals are believed to have undiagnosed diabetes. Each year about 500,000 new cases are diagnosed (National Research Council, 1989). Nationally, diabetes is the fourth leading cause of death. Hypoglycemia is much rarer than diabetes mellitus. Nutrition is integral to the management of diabetes. This chapter provides an introduction to the importance of nutrition in both diabetes and hypoglycemia.

DEFINITION AND CLASSIFICATION

Hyperglycemia— An elevated level of glucose in the blood; fasting value above 110 or 120 milligrams per deciliter, depending on technique used

Diabetes is a disorder characterized by the passage of sweet urine, excessive urine production, thirst, excessive hunger, and in some cases, weight loss. Records from the ancient Greeks described this condition as early as the first century AD. Diabetes mellitus can be defined as a group of disorders with a common characteristic of hyperglycemia. **Hyperglycemia** means an elevated level of glucose in the blood. Definitions and classifications for the various subclasses of diabetes mellitus have been standardized (Guthrie, 1988). The following sections define and classify the major types of diabetes.

Definition

Insulin-dependent diabetes mellitus (IDDM)—Type I diabetes; persons with this disorder must take insulin to survive.

Diabetes is diagnosed and defined by laboratory analysis. Multiple tests of a patient's blood sugar level are necessary before the diagnosis can be established. Fasting glucose levels of at least 140 milligrams per deciliter on more than one occasion are required for diagnosis in nonpregnant adults. Refer to Clinical Application 16–1 for an explanation of other tests used for diabetes.

Classification

Noninsulin-dependent diabetes mellitus (NIDDM)—Type II diabetes; although some persons with this disorder take insulin, it is not necessary for their survival.

There are two major forms of diabetes: **insulin-dependent diabetes mellitus** (IDDM) and **noninsulin-dependent diabetes mellitus** (NIDDM). The World Health Organization (WHO) has further classified diabetes into three additional categories: secondary diabetes, impaired glucose tolerance (IGT), and gestational diabetes.

Insulin-Dependent Diabetes Mellitus

Ketoacidosis— Acidosis due to an excess of ketone bodies.

Hypoglycemia— An abnormally low level of glucose in the blood.

IDDM is also called type I diabetes. Patients with this disorder cannot survive without daily doses of insulin because their blood glucose levels vary significantly from the norm. These variations in blood glucose levels make these patients prone to two conditions. The first condition is **ketoacidosis**. The signs of ketoacidosis are hyperglycemia and excessive ketones. More is said about ketoacidosis later in this chapter. The second condition is **hypoglycemia,** or a low blood glucose level. IDDM can occur at any age, although its usual onset is during childhood. Five to ten percent of the peo-

CLINICAL APPLICATION 16–1
Laboratory Tests for Diabetes

Several types of biochemical tests are discussed below: fasting blood sugar, glucose tolerance test, urine tests, and glycolated hemoglobin.

FASTING BLOOD SUGAR

A measurement of a fasting blood sugar (FBS) is performed routinely on most diabetic patients. In preparation, the patient should be instructed not to eat or drink for 12 hours before the test. Water is the exception, as it will not interfere with test results. If the patient usually takes insulin or a hypoglycemic agent, the medication should not be taken or given until the blood test is done. Normal FBS should be 70 to 110 milligrams per deciliter. A finding of 140 milligrams per deciliter on two occasions is diagnostic of diabetes mellitus.

GLUCOSE TOLERANCE TEST

In the glucose tolerance test, a measured amount of glucose is given orally or intravenously after a fasting blood sugar sample has been drawn. Blood samples are then drawn at specified intervals. The patient's ability to process glucose can be evaluated by this means. A blood glucose value above or equal to 200 milligrams per deciliter at 2 hours and at least one other sample at less than 2 hours are required for the diagnosis in nonpregnant adults. A normal 2-hour blood sample would have an upper level of 140 milligrams per deciliter. Values between 140 and 200 milligrams per deciliter are indicative of impaired glucose tolerance.

Patients may need to discontinue certain drugs for 3 days prior to the test. Also, a high-carbohydrate diet should be followed for the same period. A high-carbohydrate diet is defined as 300 grams of carbohydrate per day. The patient should be given written instructions explaining the pretest dietary requirements. An inadequate diet prior to the glucose tolerance test may diminish carbohydrate tolerance and cause high glucose levels, creating a false-positive result. During the test, the patient should not be permitted to have anything by mouth except water. Tobacco, coffee, and tea can all alter the test results.

URINE TESTS

For most people, when blood glucose reaches 180 to 200 milligrams per 100 milliliter, the kidneys begin to spill glucose into the urine. This point of spillage is called the renal threshold. At one time, this test was assumed to reflect the glucose content of the blood. We now know that the renal threshold varies from individual to individual. The renal threshold may also change in a given individual with decreasing kidney function. Although urine tests still are used as screening tests, they are less reliable than the blood glucose tests now available for home use

Box continued on next page.

CLINICAL APPLICATION 16–1 *(Continued)*
Laboratory Tests for Diabetes

URINE ACETONE

As a consequence of the body's inability to metabolize glucose, fat is partially broken down for energy. The intermediate products of fat breakdown are ketone bodies. These ketone bodies build up in the blood because the quantity of fat being catabolized exceeds the body's capacity to process these intermediate products effectively. As this occurs, ketone bodies begin to spill into the urine. One of the ketone bodies is acetone, which can be measured in the urine. The presence of acetone in the urine is called ketonuria. Ketonuria is a sign that the diabetes is out of control. Patients are often taught to test for urinary ketones if their blood glucose level exceeds 240 milligrams per deciliter. When a patient exhibits ketonuria, the physician should be consulted for changes in the diet prescription or insulin dosage.

GLYCOSYLATED HEMOGLOBIN

Glucose attaches to the hemoglobin molecule in a one-way reaction throughout the 120-day life of the red blood cell. In a high-glucose environment, a greater percentage of the hemoglobin is glycosylated. This blood test is performed on a random blood sample; the patient does not have to fast. The result is not influenced by exercise or diabetic drugs.

Because the glycosylated hemoglobin value reflects the average blood glucose level for the preceding 2 to 3 months, it is a good test of the effectiveness of long-term therapy. A patient cannot follow the prescribed regimen for just a few days prior to a doctor's visit and claim otherwise. Glycosylated hemoglobin will be 4 to 7 percent of the total hemoglobin in persons without diabetes. Patients with diabetes will have greater than 7 percent of their hemoglobin glycosylated.

---

ple with diabetes have IDDM. The onset of this disorder is usually abrupt, and the condition is difficult to control.

Noninsulin-Dependent Diabetes Mellitus (NIDDM)

NIDDM is also called type II diabetes. Persons with NIDDM are not insulin dependent or prone to ketoacidosis. However, some of them do use insulin because of persistent hyperglycemia. Patients with this condition can manufacture some insulin but do not make a sufficient amount or cannot use insulin efficiently. Typically, the noninsulin-dependent diabetic patient develops his or her condition after age 40. Most of these patients are obese, and weight reduction usually improves their ability to process glucose. About 90 to 95 percent of all people with diabetes in the United States have NIDDM. The prevalence of NIDDM is markedly increased among native Americans, African Americans, and Hispanics. The onset of this disorder is gradual. The condition is fairly stable and usually easier to control than IDDM. Table 16–1 summarizes the differences between IDDM and NIDDM.

TABLE 16–1 *Insulin Dependent and Noninsulin-Dependent Diabetes Mellitus*

	IDDM	NIDDM
Cause	Beta cells damaged	Tissues resist insulin
Most Common Age at Onset	Under 20 years	Over 40 years
Body Build	Thin, underweight	Obese
Cornerstone of Treatment	Insulin injections	Weight loss
Diet Modification	Balanced intake every 4 to 5 hours	3 meals per day; balance of each not crucial

Secondary Diabetes

Most diabetes results from a primary failure of insulin production and/or use, but diabetes can occur as a result of a variety of disorders including pancreatitis, surgical removal of the pancreas, Cushing's disease, pharmacologic doses of glucocorticoids (e.g., prednisone) or other hormones or drugs. The term **secondary diabetes** is used when one of these disorders is responsible for the hyperglycemia. The diabetes may be resolved if the cause is alleviated. If the cause is not correctable, secondary diabetes is treated similarly to other forms of diabetes.

Impaired Glucose Tolerance

Impaired glucose tolerance (IGT) is the term used for patients who do not meet the criteria for diabetes as defined by the WHO. These patients have fasting plasma glucose levels of less than 140 milligrams per deciliter or 2-hour tolerance plasma glucose values between 140 and 200 milligrams per deciliter, and intervening oral tolerance test plasma glucose values greater than 200 milligrams per **deciliter.** IGT may represent a step in the development of IDDM or NIDDM. In fact, 25 percent of the patients with IGT later develop diabetes mellitus.

Gestational Diabetes

Gestational diabetes (GDM) is the term used when glucose intolerance is discovered or develops during pregnancy. Women who are diagnosed as diabetic before pregnancy are not classified as having gestational diabetes. Clinical Application 16–2 discusses diabetes mellitus in pregnancy. Gestational diabetes is diagnosed slightly differently than other forms of diabetes. After an oral glucose load, diagnosis of gestational diabetes is made if two plasma values equal or exceed the following (Pastors, 1992):

Fasting: 105 milligrams per deciliter
1 hour: 190 milligrams per deciliter
2 hours: 165 milligrams per deciliter
3 hours: 145 milligrams per deciliter

Women who have had gestational diabetes are at an increased risk for developing NIDDM as they mature.

Secondary diabetes—A World Health Organization (WHO) classification for diabetes when the hyperglycemia occurs as a result of a second disorder.

Impaired glucose tolerance (IGT)—A type of classification for hyperglycemia; for persons who have a glucose intolerance but do not meet the criteria for having diabetes.

Deciliter—100 milliliters or 100 cubic centimeters.

Gestational diabetes (GDM)—Hyperglycemia related to the increased metabolic demands of pregnancy.
Glucagon—A

CLINICAL APPLICATION 16-2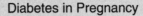

Diabetes in Pregnancy

Pregnancy raises blood insulin levels in all women. It is an adaptive mechanism. Early in pregnancy, the woman's body cells store energy. Later, the woman's tissues become insulin resistant so that the fetus can draw on energy stores when the woman is fasting.

When the pregnant woman has or develops hyperglycemia, the high blood glucose level stimulates the fetus to produce more insulin of its own. This happens because the mother's high blood glucose crosses the placenta but her insulin does not. Then the fetus produces more insulin, which increases fat deposition. Diabetic and prediabetic women have large babies for this reason.

Perinatal mortality of infants born to diabetic women is more than 200 per 1000 live births. Ketosis in early pregnancy can produce congenital malformations, central nervous system disorders, and low intelligence. With strict control of the diabetes, however, 97 percent of the fetuses survive, compared with 98 to 99 percent born to women without diabetes.

Insulin resistance is greater in the morning in pregnant women. For this reason, usually only 10 to 15 percent of the total kilocalories from carbohydrate are usually planned into the breakfast meal plan. There is a heightened tendency for maternal ketosis during fasting, and the possible adverse effects of ketones on the fetus suggest that periods of fasting during pregnancy should be avoided. A bedtime snack that contains at least 15 percent of the total kilocalories from carbohydrate is recommended to minimize an accelerated production of ketones, which has been known to occur during sleeping. Patients should also be reminded not to skip meals.

PREGNANT WOMEN WITH NONINSULIN-DEPENDENT DIABETES MELLITUS

Nutritional regulation is central to management of NIDDM in pregnant women. During pregnancy the most commonly recommended kilocaloric distribution is: 40 to 45 percent carbohydrate, 20 to 25 percent protein, and 30 to 40 percent fat. This is not the same kilocaloric distribution commonly used in nonpregnant diabetic individuals.

The treatment goal is to prevent hyperglycemia, defined as fasting plasma concentrations of 70 to 90 milligrams per deciliter and 2-hour postprandial plasma glucose levels of less than 140 milligrams per deciliter. Some medical experts believe that this goal is too rigid because hypoglycemia during early pregnancy may be teratogenic. Ter-atogenic refers to the development of abnormal structures in an embryo, resulting in a severely deformed fetus. Hypoglycemic agents have been shown to cause significant risk to the fetus. In most instances, women are advised to discontinue use of hypoglycemic agents before conception. If medication is necessary to control hyperglycemia, insulin is safer for the fetus.

THE EXTENT OF DIABETES MELLITUS

Estimates of the number of persons with diabetes mellitus range from 5 to 7 percent of the US population. Diabetes is more common in older people, affecting 15 percent of those over age 50. More women have diabetes than men. Obesity increases the risk of NIDDM. In general, people with NIDDM have fewer years of schooling, are less likely to be employed, and have lower family incomes than the general population (National Research Council, 1989).

NORMAL NUTRIENT METABOLISM

To understand diabetes mellitus, it is necessary to know about the pancreas, the organ that produces insulin. It is also important to know the cellular sources of glucose, the normal blood glucose curve, and the functions of insulin and other hormones, all of which are discussed in the following sections of this chapter.

Anatomy of the Pancreas

The pancreas is a gland that lies outside the true abdominal cavity behind the stomach. It has both exocrine and endocrine secretions. The exocrine functions of the pancreas (discussed in Chapter 5) include the flow of enzymes into the intestine via ducts. Endocrine secretions (hormones) flow directly into the bloodstream.

Clusters of cells in the pancreas called the <u>islets of Langerhans</u> produce three hormones. These islets contain three types of cells: alpha, beta, and delta. The alpha cells produce **glucagon,** the beta cells produce insulin, and the delta cells produce **somatostatin** (Fig. 16–1). Special sensors at junctions of the three types of cells monitor levels of blood glucose and stimulate the release of the appropriate hormone.

Glucagon—A hormone secreted by the alpha cells of the islets of Langerhans; it increases the concentration of glucose in the blood.

Functions of Insulin

Insulin is the only hormone that lowers blood glucose. A person normally secretes insulin in response to an elevated blood glucose level. Insulin decreases blood glucose by accelerating its movement from the blood into cells. As glucose enters the cells, it may be metabolized to yield energy, may be stored as glycogen, or may be converted to fat (Table 16–2). The ultimate fate of glucose once inside the cell depends on body need and the amount of glucose that enters the cell. The cells' energy needs will be met first. If cells have available glucose over and above immediate energy needs, the excess glucose is stored as glycogen. Insulin stimulates the storage of glucose as glycogen. Once the glycogen stores are filled to capacity, any remaining glucose is converted to fat.

Somatostatin—A hormone produced by the delta cells of the islets of Langerhans; it inhibits both the release of insulin and glucagon production.

Insulin influences the metabolism of both protein and fat. Insulin stimulates entry of amino acids into cells and enhances protein formation. It also enhances fat storage in adipose tissue and indirectly inhibits the breakdown of fat for energy. If the body has ample glucose available for energy, protein and fat need not be broken down to meet energy needs.

Insulin levels go up and down in the blood. Normally, blood insulin levels increase as the blood glucose level increases. A high level of insulin in

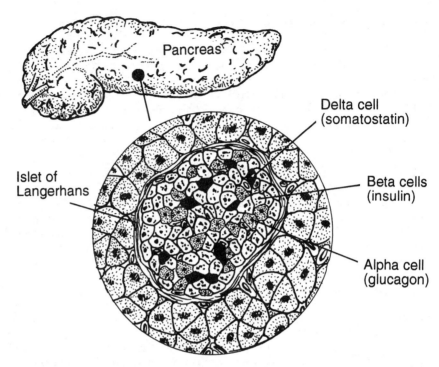

FIGURE 16–1. A view of the pancreas and an enlarged islet of Langerhans. Alpha cells secrete glucagon, beta cells secrete insulin, and delta cells secrete somatostatin. (From Williams, SR: Nutrition and Diet Therapy, ed 6. CV Mosby, St. Louis, 1989, p 817, with permission.)

the blood signals the cells not to break down stores for energy (Table 16–3). An anabolic or building state exists when metabolism is normal and glucose and insulin levels are high. Insulin levels decrease as the blood sugar level decreases. A low level of insulin in the blood indirectly signals the body to begin to break down body stores for glucose. A catabolic or breaking-down state exists when metabolism is normal and glucose and insulin levels are low. Figure 16–2 illustrates glucose use by the cells.

TABLE 16–2 *Metabolic Activities Promoted by Insulin*

Activity	Name of Metabolic Pathway
Movement of glucose into cells	None
Energy production from glucose	Glycolysis
Manufacture of glycogen	Glycogenesis
Fat formation from carbohydrate and protein	Lipogenesis

Note: "Genesis" means building up.

TABLE 16–3 *Metabolic Activities Inhibited by a High Level of Insulin*

Activity	Name of Metabolic Pathway
Manufacture of glucose from noncarbohydrate sources, e.g., glycerol and amino acids	Gluconeogensis
Release of glucose from glycogen	Glycogenolysis
Breakdown of fat from adipose tissue	Lipolysis

Note: "Lysis" means breaking down.

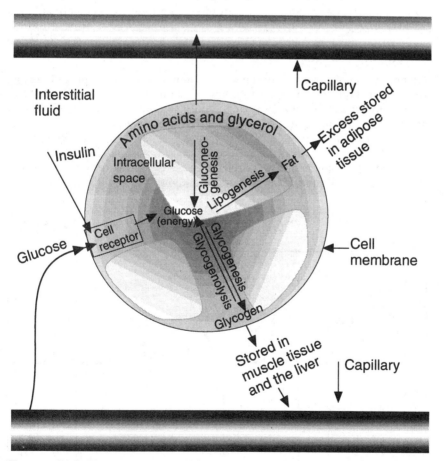

FIGURE 16–2. Insulin is necessary for glucose to gain entry into a cell. Once inside the cell, glucose can meet several fates. Glucose can be burned as energy, stored as glycogen, or stored as fat. In the event that the cell lacks sufficient glucose for energy needs, glycogen, or the glycerol portion of a fat molecule or some amino acids can be broken down into glucose.

Other Hormones

Glucagon and somatostatin assist in coordinating the storage and mobilization of the energy nutrients. Glucagon increases blood glucose levels and stimulates the breakdown of body protein and fat stores. Somatostatin acts locally within the islets of Langerhans to depress the secretion of both insulin and glucagon (Guyton, 1986). Evidence has shown these hormones may not be at optimal levels in some diabetic patients.

Cellular Sources of Glucose

The cells obtain glucose from food eaten and internal glucose stores. All of the carbohydrate eaten, about 50 percent of the protein eaten, and about 10 percent of the fat eaten will enter the blood as glucose. The internal body stores that can be converted to glucose are glycogen, some protein, and the glycerol portion of triglycerides. Body fat is stored as triglycerides in adipose tissue. To understand diabetes it is necessary to know how the body coordinates all internal and external sources of glucose to maintain a normal blood glucose range.

Blood Glucose Curve

Given the vital need for every cell to have an uninterrupted supply of energy, the human body has evolved to allow an uninterrupted energy supply to reach cells without continuous eating. A normal blood glucose range is usually about 70 to 110 milligrams per deciliter. (Some laboratories assign a normal blood glucose range of 80 to 120 milligrams per deciliter. The difference is due to the type of equipment the laboratory uses, not the glucose content of the blood.) The blood glucose level increases in the fed state and decreases in the fasting state. Figure 16–3 illustrates the normal blood glucose curve.

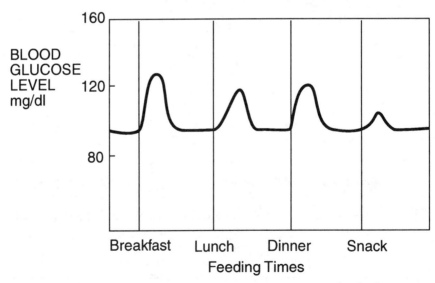

FIGURE 16–3. A person's blood glucose level normally goes up after food consumption and then down between feedings.

CAUSES OF DIABETES

The causes of diabetes include genetic factors, lifestyle, and viral infections. Although these causes are explained separately for the sake of clarity, in reality they are often interconnected.

Genetic Factors

Some of the susceptibility to diabetes is genetic. Researchers have discovered that people with IDDM have certain genes associated with their immune response. These particular genes are often found in children with IDDM. However, not everyone with these genes displays clinical diabetes. Before diabetes becomes apparent, this genetic susceptibility is often triggered by the individual's lifestyle or other environmental factors. These factors cause a series of events that result in damage and/or destruction to the pancreatic beta cells. Inheritance is even more prominent in the development of NIDDM than in IDDM, as the next section describes.

Insulin Resistance

A person may be genetically susceptible to **insulin resistance.** Insulin resistance occurs when both the patient's glucose and blood insulin levels are elevated. Insulin may not be released at the right times and/or be unable to assist the movement of glucose into the cells because of a lack of receptor sites. Before glucose can enter the cells, the insulin must first attach itself to specific receptor sites on the cells' outer surfaces. Persons with type II diabetes may lack enough receptor sites, have faulty receptor sites, or have postreceptor defects. Excess body weight seems to be related to a decrease in the number of receptor sites (Pastors, 1992). NIDDM is often associated with insulin resistance.

Insulin resistance—A disorder characterized by elevated glucose and insulin levels; thought to be related to a lack of insulin receptors.

Lifestyle

Excessive body fat, inactivity, and stress are risk factors for diabetes. Up to 90 percent of noninsulin-dependent diabetic patients are overly fat. A loss of body fat alone is sometimes sufficient to balance the insulin produced with a modified food intake. Inactivity is a risk factor that predisposes one to diabetes. Sometimes emotional or physical stress is the stimulus that causes the hyperglycemia. The body's stress response involves the release of epinephrine from the adrenal glands. One action of epinephrine is to raise the blood sugar level so the person has energy for "fight or flight." Healthy lifestyle behaviors are particularly important for the prevention of diabetes in genetically susceptible patients.

Viral Infections

Links have been noted between viral epidemics and the onset of diabetes. During the late fall and winter months, a disproportionate number of cases of IDDM diabetes are diagnosed. Since these seasons also are associated with peak occurrence of childhood viral diseases, the possibility exists of a causal connection between viral epidemics and the onset of IDDM.

Antibodies to islet cells have been found in some people with diabetes. This lends credence to the concept of IDDM as an autoimmune process, in

Autoimmune disease—A disorder in which the body produces an immunological response against itself.

which the body destroys its own beta cells. In **autoimmune diseases,** the body cannot recognize its own cells but rather treats them as foreign invaders. The event that provokes this process usually is a viral infection. Both islet cell antibodies (ICAs) and anti-insulin antibodies (AIAs) have been found to be elevated in patients with IDDM. These elevated antibodies may be detected in about 90 percent of patients prior to the diagnosis of diabetes (Guthrie, 1988).

SIGNS AND SYMPTOMS OF DIABETES

Polyuria—Excessive urination.
Polydipsia—Excessive thirst.
Polyphagia—Excessive hunger.

The classic triad of signs and symptoms includes **polyuria,** or increased urination; **polydipsia,** or increased thirst; and **polyphagia,** or increased appetite. The triad is most commonly seen in IDDM. The following section describes these and other signs and symptoms commonly seen in persons with diabetes.

Classic Triad

Glycosuria — abnormally high amount of glucose in the urine.

In diabetes, glucose cannot optimally move from the intravascular space across a cell membrane into the intracellular space. This is why the diabetic person's blood glucose level remains elevated after eating. Under normal circumstances, the blood glucose level does not increase excessively because excess glucose undergoes glycolysis and is readily converted to adipose tissue or stored as glycogen inside the cell. As the glucose-rich blood circulates through the kidneys, these organs reabsorb all of the glucose of which they are capable. After this point is reached, glucose enters the urine. **Glycosuria** means an abnormally high amount of glucose in the urine. As the glucose exits the body in the urine, water is pulled out also as a result of the osmotic effect of glucose. This results in polyuria, or a large urine output. The large loss of water causes excessive thirst, polydipsia, and prompts the person to drink fluids.

When glucose is not available for energy inside the cells, the body will begin to break down protein and fat for energy. In untreated IDDM, the body's cells are starving. These starving cells send a message to the brain to turn on the person's appetite. The person responds by eating to satisfy the craving for food. The third symptom or sign of diabetes is polyphagia, an abnormal increase in appetite. Polyphagia, polyuria, and polydipsia are the three classic signs or symptoms reported or seen in patients with diabetes.

Other Signs and Symptoms

The abnormal carbohydrate metabolism of diabetes and its effects on the body's tissues cause other problems. Poor wound healing and weight loss occur. Weight loss is more commonly seen in patients with IDDM than in patients with NIDDM. Blurred vision is common in both type I and type II diabetes. Fatigue is frequently seen in these patients. In women, the glucosuria predisposes the patient to vaginitis, caused by yeast. Men may complain of impotence.

COMPLICATIONS

The complications of diabetes mellitus are both acute and chronic. Acute complications require immediate care. Chronic complications include diseases of the eye, kidneys, heart, and nervous system. Chronic complications are responsible for the increased death rate among diabetics and the diminished quality of life that many of these patients experience.

Acute Clinical Situations

Three acute complications are seen in diabetic patients: ketoacidosis, hyperglycemic hyperosmolar nonketotic syndrome, and hypoglycemia.

Ketoacidosis

Individuals with IDDM who experience a profound insulin deficiency may progress to the condition of ketoacidosis. The three main precipitating factors in ketoacidosis are: a decreased or missed dose of insulin, an illness or infection, or uncontrolled disease in a previously undiagnosed person. Ketoacidosis is a complex life-threatening condition demanding emergency treatment. The predominant clinical manifestations of dehydration, acidosis, and electrolyte imbalances and general principles of treatment will be discussed.

DEHYDRATION   Without insulin, glucose cannot be transferred across the cell membranes into the cells. A greatly increased number of glucose molecules (300 to 800 mg/dl) in the blood exert an osmotic effect, causing water to move from within the cells to the intravascular space, producing cellular dehydration. The body excretes the water and the glucose in the urine, along with electrolytes, producing polyuria.

ACIDOSIS   Unaware that the problem is not lack of glucose, but lack of insulin, the body proceeds to increase blood glucose by mobilizing protein and fat from the tissues to be converted to glucose by the liver. As the human body can use only the glycerol portion of the triglyceride molecule for glucose, the fatty acid portion is processed into ketones. Normally the ketones are metabolized and excreted as carbon dioxide and water. Under conditions of ketoacidosis, however, the body cannot metabolize this overload of ketones rapidly enough to maintain homeostasis, thus the patient displays excessive ketones in the blood (ketonemia) and spills ketones in the urine (ketonuria). Acetone is one of the ketone bodies for which urine is tested. The ketone bodies are acid, thus the term, ketoacidosis.

Several homeostatic mechanisms can be initiated by the body as it attempts to correct the acidosis. It decreases the level of carbonic acid in the blood by increasing the excretion of carbon dioxide through involuntary deep, rapid breaths called Kussmaul respirations. The lungs can also excrete the volatile acetone, giving the patient's breath a fruity odor. The kidney increases the hydrogen ion content or acidity of the urine it excretes. Buffering of hydrogen can occur in the cells, also, where it displaces potassium to the extracellular fluid.

ELECTROLYTE IMBALANCES   Patients with severe ketoacidosis may excrete 6.5 liters of fluid and 400 to 500 milliequivalents of sodium, potassium, and chloride in 24 hours. A fluid loss of 15 percent of body weight is not unusual. Most critical in the treatment of electrolyte imbalances in diabetic ketoacidosis is the body's level of potassium. As the cells are being catabolized for fuel, the intracellular potassium is transferred to the intravascular space. Serum potassium levels can be low, normal, or elevated in the person with ketoacidosis, depending upon the body's current coping mechanism. Regardless of the serum concentrations of potassium and sodium, the pathological process of diabetic ketoacidosis depletes these electrolytes. Either hypokalemia or hyperkalemia can lead to cardiac arrhythmias and must be carefully managed in the patient with ketoacidosis.

TREATMENT   Patients with severe diabetic ketoacidosis are critically ill. Serum electrolyte levels change dramatically once treatment commences. Intensive care is necessary to provide the careful monitoring and frequent adjustments in therapy required as the fluids and electrolytes are being replaced. Intravenous regular insulin will permit the use of carbohydrate for energy and will halt the body's excessive use of fat, which has produced the ketone bodies. Insulin drives glucose back into the cells. Potassium is essential to this process. It, too, moves from the intravascular space to the intracellular space, necessitating frequent measurement of the serum levels of both glucose and potassium. When the patient recovers, identification of the precipitating factor for the ketoacidosis and education focused on preventing additional occurrences is essential.

Hyperglycemic Hyperosmolar Nonketotic Syndrome

The four signs of **hyperglycemic hyperosmolar nonketotic syndrome** (HHKS) are blood glucose level greater than 600 milligrams per deciliter, absence of or slight ketosis, plasma hyperosmolality, and profound dehydration. This life-threatening emergency is usually seen in the elderly or undiagnosed people with NIDDM. HHKS is like DKA except that the insulin deficiency is not as severe, so increased **lipolysis** does not occur. Because these patients do not have symptoms of vomiting, nausea, and acidosis brought on by severe ketosis as do patients with type I diabetes, they often do not seek prompt medical help. Their blood sugar levels are higher and their dehydration more severe than is seen in ketoacidosis.

In these patients, prolonged osmotic diuresis and dehydration secondary to hyperglycemia lead to decreased renal blood flow and allow the blood glucose to reach very high levels. Medications that cause an increase in blood glucose levels, chronic disease, and infection may contribute to this condition. Treatment includes correction of the electrolyte imbalance, hyperglycemia, and dehydration.

Lipolysis— Catabolism of adipose tissue.

Hypoglycemia

In both IDDM and NIDDM (treated with any medications) the person can develop hypoglycemia. Hypoglycemia may be caused by too much insulin (accidental or deliberate); too little food intake; a delayed meal; excessive exercise; alcohol (especially in the fasting state); and/or medications such as oral hypoglycemic agents. Symptoms include confusion, headache, double vision, rapid heartbeat, sweating, hunger, seizure, and coma. The immediate treatment goal is to increase the blood glucose level as rapidly as possible. Hypoglycemia usually can be prevented by educating patients about the signs and symptoms, causes, and treatment of hypoglycemia. Patients should be advised to carry a source of carbohydrate with them at all times. In the event that a meal is delayed (preplanned or not preplanned) by ½ hour or more, a snack should be consumed. At least one significant other (a family member or friend of the patient) should be instructed about hypoglycemia and how to measure blood glucose levels (see Self-Monitoring of Blood Glucose, below). The family member or friend should also be instructed on what to do in case the patient becomes unconscious, including the proper techniques for injecting glucagon or for squeezing a commercial glucose gel into the patient's mouth where it can be absorbed through the mucous membranes. Patients taking insulin should always wear an identification badge or bracelet (medical alert) to advise bystanders or emergency medical personnel of the fact that they take insulin. Patients should be warned that the symptoms of hypoglycemia may change over time because of a diminished production of epinephrine, which commonly occurs in IDDM. Frequent monitoring of blood glucose levels should be encouraged in anticipation of this situation.

Chronic Complications

Patients with both IDDM and NIDDM of sufficient duration are vulnerable to serious complications involving the eyes, kidneys, and nervous system. Diabetic **retinopathy** is a disorder that involves the retina. Diabetes is a leading cause of blindness and of visual loss in the adult US population (Guthrie, 1988). The blurred vision reported by these patients is related to retinopathy. These patients are also at a higher risk for cataracts.

Retinopathy— Any disorder of the retina; diabetes is a leading cause of both visual loss and blindness in the adult population in the United States.

Diabetic **neuropathy** is the most common complication of diabetes mellitus. Patients may complain of a lack of sensation in their extremities. They may puncture, cut, or burn their feet and not feel any pain. A wound may become infected and heal poorly. Gangrene, or tissue death, may follow. The treatment for gangrene is amputation. Neuropathy can affect gastric or intestinal motility, erectile function, bladder function, cardiac function, and vascular tone (Nathan, 1993). **Gastroparesis** may occur and alter the absorption of meals, which makes glycemic control problematic. Heart disease is more common in these patients. Chapter 17 discusses heart disease in greater detail.

Neuropathy— Any disease of the

Gastroparesis— Partial paralysis of the stomach.

Diabetic **nephropathy,** or kidney disease, is the most common complication in diabetic patients. Chapter 18 is devoted to kidney disease. Tragically, many patients with diabetes do not take the threat of chronic complications seriously until much damage has occurred.

Nephropathy—A kidney disease characterized by inflammation and degenerative lesions.

TREATMENT

The current medical goal is to *normalize* the blood glucose throughout the day, which goes far beyond what has been clinical practice in the past. A normal blood glucose level is 60 to 120 milligrams per deciliter before a meal and less than 140 milligrams per deciliter 2 hours after a meal. Realistic target levels for individuals with diabetes treated intensively are 70 to 140 milligrams per deciliter before meals; less than 180 milligrams per deciliter 2 hours after meals; and glycosylated hemoglobin within 1 percent of normal. A recent study known as the Diabetes Control and Complications Trial demonstrated that intensive control of blood glucose levels delays the onset and slows the progression of diabetic retinopathy, nephropathy, and neuropathy with IDDM (Diabetic Control and Complications Trial Research Group, 1993).

According to this study's preliminary results, people with type I diabetes who followed a tightly controlled regimen, compared with those who followed a standard regimen, showed reductions of about:

- 76 percent in progression of diabetic retinopathy
- 50 percent in rates of diabetic nephropathy
- 60 percent in rates of neuropathy

A tightly controlled regimen is not without problems, however (increased incidence of insulin-induced hypoglycemic episodes, more demands on the patient, and interference in normal lifestyle).

All healthcare workers should assist the general population in the early detection of diabetes and prevention of complications. As Figure 16–4 emphasizes, the three cornerstones of diabetic treatment after diagnosis are physical activity, medication, and diet. Self-monitoring of blood glucose levels enables the patient to assess how each of these factors interact. Blood glucose monitoring, physical activity, medication, and diet are discussed below.

Self-Monitoring of Blood Glucose

Many individuals monitor their own blood glucose levels with a device called a blood glucose meter. This procedure is called self-monitoring of blood glucose (SMBG). Individual response to medication, diet, and exercise can be determined with this advanced technology. SMBG can be performed in 1 to 2 minutes using a single drop of blood. The patient obtains the drop of blood from a finger with either a lancet or a spring-loaded device. The blood sample is placed in the meter, and the test results are available in just a minute or two. The patient can then adjust insulin dose and food and exercise behaviors accordingly. Many experts consider SMBG to be the most important development in diabetes management since the discovery of insulin.

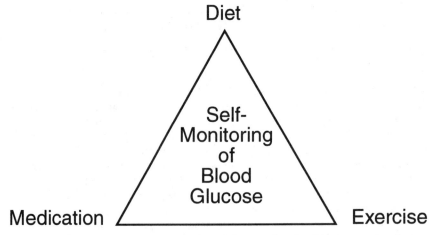

FIGURE 16–4. Diet, medication, and exercise are the three cornerstones of treatment for diabetes. Each of these cornerstones has an influence on blood glucose levels. An individual can identify how each of these cornerstones impacts his or her blood glucose level by self-monitoring of blood glucose.

SMBG has allowed diabetic patients to try normalizing their blood glucose levels throughout the day. Healthcare workers need to carefully teach patients how to use this technology. Continual reassessment of the patient's technique and blood glucose records are necessary to guide treatment decisions. To evaluate the need for changes in diet or medications, monitoring should be done at least twice a day. Four times a day for 3 days each week is preferable for patients who are stable. If near-normalization of blood glucose is the treatment goal, SMBG must be done four to eight times daily (before and 2 hours after each meal and/or snack). During acute illness, more frequent self-monitoring is indicated.

Physical Activity

The intensity and duration of physical activity influences blood glucose levels. Exercise recommendations are universally accepted for NIDDM but more controversial for IDDM. For this reason, we discuss exercise for each type of diabetes separately.

Exercise and Noninsulin-Dependent Diabetes Mellitus

Exercise is an important tool in managing type II diabetes. Physical activity increases the number and binding capacity of insulin receptors, assists in lowering blood glucose levels in NIDDM, and reduces insulin requirements in persons who use insulin. Improved blood lipid levels occur in some patients who engage in regular exercise. This helps delay or prevent the heart disease complications often seen in these patients. Exercise assists in weight control and improves flexibility and muscle strength.

Exercise and Insulin-Dependent Diabetes Mellitus

Exercise for IDDM receives a mixed endorsement from many medical experts. Exercise changes insulin requirements sometimes in unpredictable ways—and sometimes more than 24 hours after the exercise. Retinopathy, neuropathy, and renal disease may worsen in some patients with IDDM who exercise. Blood pressure may also become elevated. Yet most healthcare professionals encourage patients to live as normally as possible, including participating in sports if desired. General guidelines for those patients who do exercise include:

- Know how to prevent hypoglycemia.
- Avoid exercise if the blood glucose is more than 240 milligrams per deciliter or if ketones are present.
- Wear a diabetes ID badge or bracelet during exercise.

Medications

Two types of medications are used with diabetic patients: insulin and oral hypoglycemic agents. Patients with IDDM (type I) require insulin. Patients with NIDDM (type II) may not require any medication or may need to have an oral hypoglycemic agent or insulin prescribed. Frequently, patients with type II diabetes are able to discontinue the medication after a loss of body fat.

Insulin

The four sources of insulin are beef, pork, biosynthetic human, and semisynthetic human. Human insulin is made by converting pork insulin to the human amino-acid sequence (semisynthetic), or manufactured by recombinant-DNA technology (biosynthetic). Human insulin (Humulin) produces fewer allergic reactions. Human insulin is also the drug of choice by vegetarians. Insulin cannot be taken orally because the gastrointestinal tract enzymes would digest it before absorption. Insulin must be administered by needle either <u>subcutaneously</u> (beneath the skin) or intravenously (IV). Only regular insulin is given IV. The substances used to delay absorption of intermediate- and long-acting insulins are not designed for IV administration. Regular insulin is usually administered IV only for the severely hyperglycemic patient.

Insulin can also be administrated with an insulin pump. These pumps are designed to provide a small inflow of insulin continuously and large inflows before eating, thus mimicking normal insulin secretion.

Medications are described according to the onset, peak, and duration of action. Insulin is categorized as rapid-acting, intermediate-acting, or long-acting. Table 16–4 lists the times of onset, peak, and duration of insulin. Variation in duration makes it possible to inject insulin in a pattern that is as close as possible to normal insulin activity. Ideally, the medication is planned around the diet, not vice-versa. Most experts know that it is far easier to change a medication than a food behavior.

Oral Hypoglycemic Agents

Oral hypoglycemic agents lower blood glucose levels in noninsulin-dependent diabetics. These drugs stimulate insulin release from the pancreatic beta cells and reduce glucose output from the liver. Recently, oral agents and insulin have been used successfully simultaneously to treat type I diabetes. Commonly prescribed oral hypoglycemic agents include glipizide, glyburide, and tolazamide.

TABLE 16–4 *Times of Onset, Peak, and Duration of Action for Rapid-Acting, Intermediate-Acting, and Long-Acting Insulin*

Insulin	Time in Hours		
	Onset	Peak	Duration
Rapid-acting			
Regular intravenously	0.17–0.5	0.25–0.5	0.5–1
Regular subcutaneously	0.5–1	2–4	5–7
Intermediate-acting			
Lente subcutaneously	1–3	8–12	18–28
NPH subcutaneously	3–4	8–12	18–28
Long-acting			
Ultralente subcutaneously	4–6	18–24	36

Nutritional Management

Diabetes is directly related to how the body uses food. Nutrition is an essential component of management for all persons with diabetes. Patients report improved health, better control over body weight, improved control of blood glucose and lipid levels, and improved use of insulin when they adhere to dietary recommendations. The goals of nutritional care for the person with diabetes are related to the control and prevention of complications. This involves the promotion of normal nutrition and dietary manipulation to control blood glucose and lipid levels. The person with diabetes needs specific meal-planning guidelines to meet these goals. The following sections of the text describe these goals.

Goals of Nutritional Care

There are eight nutritional goals to remember when counseling the individual with diabetes:

1. To attain and maintain normal blood glucose levels
2. To attain and maintain near-normal blood lipid levels, including cholesterol, triglyceride, high-density lipoprotein (HDL), low-density lipoprotein (LDL), and very-low-density lipoprotein (VLDL) levels; see Chapter 17
3. To determine an appropriate meal plan based on the person's lifestyle and eating behaviors as determined by food intake information such as diet history or food records
4. To attain and maintain a healthy body weight. A person's healthy body weight is not always identical to the weight shown on any particular height/weight table. Although in some cases a greater, more desirable weight loss is necessary, sometimes a loss of only 5 to 10 pounds helps the patient maintain normal blood glucose levels. A greater weight loss may not be realistic or achievable for some patients. It is important to help patients succeed. Success is not usually realized by setting unrealistic weight goals.
5. To maintain a normal growth rate in children
6. To attain and maintain optimal nutrition during pregnancy and lactation
7. To facilitate consistency in the timing of meals and snacks, so as to prevent wide swings in blood glucose levels for individuals on insulin
8. To improve wellness through good nutrition

The medications prescribed and the type of diabetes the individual has determine goal priority. A high priority for the person taking insulin is to facilitate consistency in the timing of meals and snacks to prevent wide swings in blood glucose. This requires coordination among exercise, insulin, and food intake. A high priority for the individual with type II diabetes is a loss of body fat. The amount of body fat a person should be encouraged to lose is determined on an individual basis.

Meal Spacing

Meal spacing is more crucial in IDDM than in NIDDM. A consistent timing of meals assists in the stabilization of blood glucose levels in IDDM. These persons should be instructed to eat before their serum insulin level peaks. Meals are usually evenly spaced throughout the day to avoid hypoglycemic episodes. Eating soon after the injection of insulin is essential. The noon and evening meals are usually planned to establish evenly spaced intervals. An evening snack is usually indicated. This snack assists in the prevention of late-night and early-morning hypoglycemic episodes. Individuals who work nights or afternoons usually need some assistance in planning their meal spacing. Meal spacing is not as crucial for NIDDM.

Meal Planning Systems

No single meal planning system works in every situation. The person's educational level may prohibit some systems from being used. This book has used the American Diabetic and Dietetic Food *Exchange Lists* to teach both food composition and menu planning. This system of meal planning is the most frequently used tool for teaching nutrition to diabetic patients. Yet, research has shown that an individual needs to have at least an eighth-grade reading level to understand this system. The American Dietetic and Diabetes Associations also publish an excellent tool called *Healthy Food Choices* for use by persons who have a lower reading level or who do not care to invest the time and energy into learning a more complicated meal planning system.

Some people benefit the most from a set of preplanned menus. These people just want to be told what to eat and will follow through with appropriate food behaviors when given several days or weeks of menus. Sample menus should be written only after the healthcare worker has some understanding of the patient's normal eating patterns. Some people have greater success at losing body fat by counting either grams of fat or kilocalories eaten. Many diabetic persons who are more highly educated use "The High Carbohydrate Fiber (HCF)" (Anderson, 1984) approach to plan their meals. The true test to evaluate the effectiveness of any meal planning system is to monitor the patient's lipid and glucose levels and body weight.

Nutritional Recommendations

The diabetic diet is simply a healthy, well-balanced diet that follows the Dietary Guidelines for Healthy Americans (United States Department of Agriculture, 1992). Recommendations for the distribution of the energy nutrients are important for some people with diabetes. Because many individuals with diabetes frequently ask questions about both alcohol and vitamin and mineral supplementation, these subjects are discussed below.

Dietary Guidelines

The Dietary Guidelines for Healthy Americans were written with the intent to help reduce the risk from chronic disease in the general population. Almost all the risk factors for heart and circulatory diseases for the general population are more prevalent in the diabetic population (Guthrie, 1988). The sodium, fiber, alcohol, fat, protein, and carbohydrate intake of these patients should at least be planned to meet the Dietary Guidelines for Healthy Americans. It is especially important for diabetics to know these guidelines and follow them to reduce their risk of developing the chronic complications of diabetes.

Distribution of Energy Nutrients

The distribution of energy nutrients refers to the percentage of total kilocalories that should be derived from carbohydrate, fat, and protein, respectively. Distribution of energy nutrients also refers to the division of carbohydrate, fat, and protein among the day's feedings. Clinical Calculation 16–1 shows how the percentage of energy nutrients is converted into grams of carbohydrate, fat, and protein and distributed throughout the day's feedings. Also included in distribution of energy nutrients is the amount of carbohydrate that should be derived from simple versus complex carbohydrates. The distribution of the kilocalories from fat also needs to take into account the respective fat kilocalories to be derived from saturated, monounsaturated, and polyunsaturated fats.

CARBOHYDRATE Fifty-five to 60 percent of the kilocalories may be derived from carbohydrate. Some experts recommend that up to 70 percent of kilocalories be provided in the form of complex carbohydrate. The actual amount is dependent on the impact on blood glucose and lipid levels, as well as individual eating patterns. Usually the percentage of kilocalories derived from carbohydrate is determined individually.

Generally, emphasis is placed on the substitution of carbohydrates with fiber for carbohydrates with simple sugars. The individual's fiber intake may need to be increased to a total of 40 to 50 grams per day or 25 grams per 1000 kilocalories. A high fiber intake assists in delaying the absorption of sugars from the gastrointestinal tract, and this helps to modulate blood glucose levels.

Historically, people with diabetes were told never to consume simple sugars unless they had symptoms of hypoglycemia. Meal plans are now slightly more liberal because recent research has shown that blood glucose levels are not always worsened by the inclusion of sugars in the diet. The use of small amounts of simple sugars such as table sugar and honey may be acceptable but is dependent on metabolic and weight control (Guthrie, 1988). Therefore, some patients may have simple sugars planned (sparingly) into their diet. However, many foods that contain sugar are also high in fat. High-fat foods are not indicated for persons with diabetes, especially for those who need to lose weight. Also, sugar should not displace more nutritious foods in the diet. See Clinical Application 16–3 for a discussion on the glycemic index of food, a new concept in meal planning.

PROTEIN Because persons with diabetes are at an increased risk of kidney disease, it is important that protein be eaten in moderate amounts. The patient should always receive at least the RDA for protein, which is 0.8 grams per kilogram body weight. This is usually in the range of 12 to 20 percent of total kilocalories.

FAT The American Diabetes Association recommends that total fat be less than 30 percent of total kilocalories. Note that this is similar to the Dietary Guidelines for Healthy Americans. Ten percent of fat should come from polyunsaturated fat, 10 percent from saturated fat, and 10 percent from monounsaturated fat. In addition, cholesterol should ideally be kept under 300 milligrams per day.

Special Foods

There is a list of free foods that contain less than 20 kilocalories per serving (see Appendix H). Some of the food items on the free food list may be eaten

---

CLINICAL APPLICATION 16–3
Glycemic Index

Different food sources that contain equal amounts of carbohydrate have been found not to have an equal impact on blood glucose levels. The glycemic index of food attempts to classify foods according to their impact on blood glucose. The higher the glycemic index value, the higher the blood glucose would be expected to rise after ingestion of the food.

Foods high in water-soluble fiber, in the raw state, high in binders, and eaten as part of a mixed meal reduce the glycemic response. Dairy products, pasta, dried peas, and legumes are examples of foods with a low glycemic index. Potatoes, some cereals, and bread are examples of foods with a high glycemic index.

Food is usually eaten as mixed nutrient sources. For example, spaghetti is usually eaten with tomato sauce or as part of a meal. Because a mixed meal tends to dilute the glycemic index of any one of the meal's constituents, the glycemic index is rarely taught in clinical practice. However, some highly motivated and well-educated people with diabetes are beginning to use information about the glycemic index of foods to assist in meal planning. Thus it is important to understand this concept. The following table compares effects of foods based on equal amounts of carbohydrate, not serving sizes or energy content. By convention, white bread is assigned a value of 100.

Food	Glycemic index
Glucose	138
Potato, russet, baked	135
Cornflakes	119
White bread	100
White table sugar (sucrose)	86
Rice	83
Banana	79
All-Bran cereal	73
Spaghetti	66
Dried peas	56
Apple	53
Ice cream	52
Milk	49
Honey (fructose)	30

---

in whatever quantity desired. Some are free in that they are not counted as exchanges but are restricted to two or three servings per day.

There is no need for the person with diabetes to purchase dietetic foods. Fruits packed in water or natural fruit juice are generally less expensive than those labeled dietetic. Some dietetic foods are for low-sodium diets and may contain significant amounts of sugar. The astute shopper reads product labels.

Sugar substitutes such as saccharin, cyclamates, and aspartame are used extensively by people with diabetes. There has been some concern about possible side effects from sugar substitutes. To date, most evidence associating saccharin and cyclamate with chronic disease relates to bladder cancer. Studies completed thus far have been unable to link the use of artificial sweeteners by a particular individual to bladder cancer in that same person.

Alcohol

The dietary guideline on the use of alcohol, "alcohol should be used in moderation only," applies especially to persons with diabetes. Moderation is defined as not more than 2 ounces at a time and no more than twice a week. One ounce of alcohol is equal to 1.5 ounces of distilled liquor, 4 ounces of wine, or 12 ounces of beer (Guthrie, 1988). Clinical Application 16–4 provides additional information on alcoholic drinks. In addition, alcohol should not be consumed on an empty stomach because to do so may cause hypo-

---

 CLINICAL APPLICATION 16–4

Alcoholic Beverages and Diabetes

All drinks are not equal to the diabetic. The person with diabetes should avoid drinks containing excessive kilocalories. This means avoiding drinks with fruit juices or sugar as well as knowing which alcoholic beverages are high in kilocalories. Whiskey, gin, vodka, and rum have no appreciable carbohydrate and therefore are low in kilocalories. Listed below are the carbohydrate and kilocaloric contents of several alcoholic beverages in the amounts usually considered "one drink."

Beverage	Kilocalories	Grams Carbohydrate
Crème de menthe, 1.5 fluid ounces	186	21
Sweet dessert wine, 4 fluid ounces	181	14
Beer, 12 fluid ounces regular	146	13
Beer, 12 fluid ounces light	100	5
Dry red wine, 3.5 fluid ounces	74	2
Rosé wine, 3.5 fluid ounces	73	2
White wine, 3.5 fluid ounces	70	1
Gin, 1.5 fluid ounces, 80 proof	97	<0.1
Rum, 1.5 fluid ounces, 80 proof	97	<0.1
Vodka, 1.5 fluid ounces, 80 proof	97	<0.1
Whiskey, 1.5 fluid ounces, 80 proof	97	<0.1

glycemia: alcohol inhibits the release of glucose from glycogen in the liver. This effect can be seen with as little as 2 or 3 ounces of alcohol. Alcohol use can contribute to poor weight control. For individuals attempting to lose weight, alcohol, when used at all, should be substituted for fat in the meal plan.

For these reasons, the use of alcohol should be restricted to people with well-controlled diabetes. A well-controlled individual does not have wide swings in blood sugar levels and has near-normal lipid levels.

Vitamin and Mineral Supplementation

There is no evidence to support the need for vitamin and mineral supplementation in persons with diabetes. Individuals on very low-calorie diets (less than 800 kilocalories) or pregnant women may need a vitamin and mineral supplement. Any disease condition that normally affects the ingestion, digestion, absorption, metabolism, and excretion of nutrients may require a supplement as it would for the person without diabetes.

SPECIAL CONSIDERATIONS

Persons with diabetes frequently ask questions about nutritional problems related to acute illness, exercise, eating out, and delayed meals. The following sections of this chapter discuss these nutrition-related problems.

Nutrition During Acute Illness Episodes

Acute illness affects everyone, including the diabetic person. Colds and flu-like symptoms can be fatal for some people with diabetes unless precautions are taken. Secretion of both glucagon and epinephrine increases during illness and contributes to an increase in blood glucose levels. This in turn may lead to a loss of glucose, fluid, and electrolytes. Dehydration, electrolyte depletion, and a loss of nutrients may follow. Acute illnesses can lead to DKA in IDDM and to HHKS in NIDDM.

Dehydration is more rapid if the electrolytes and fluids are not replaced. Vomiting, diarrhea, and fever all represent fluid loss. During acute illness the individual should be instructed to monitor his or her blood glucose level every 4 to 6 hours until the symptoms subside. Urine ketone levels should be checked if the blood glucose level is in excess of 240 milligrams per deciliter. Generally, if the blood glucose level exceeds 240 milligrams per deciliter for longer than 24 hours, the physician should be informed immediately. Some physicians may provide their patients with slightly different instructions. Care must be taken not to confuse the patient.

The risk of dehydration is reduced by an increase of fluids. Patients who are vomiting or nauseated and are unable to tolerate regular food should drink liquids that contain carbohydrate and/or electrolytes (Table 16–5). A general guideline is that approximately 15 grams of carbohydrate should be consumed every 1 to 2 hours. Some patients have an individually calculated sick-day menu based on the carbohydrate content of their regular diet.

Other meal-planning tips that may prove helpful during periods of acute illness include (1) increasing water intake even for patients who can eat regular food; (2) eating smaller, more frequent feedings; and (3) eating soft, easily digested foods.

TABLE 16–5 *Easily Consumed Carbohydrate-Containing Foods for "Sick Days"*

Food	Amount	Grams of Carbohydrate
Regular cola	½ cup	13
Ginger ale	¾ cup	16
Milk	1 cup	12
Apple juice	⅓ cup	15
Grape juice	⅓ cup	15
Orange juice	½ cup	15
Pineapple juice	⅓ cup	15
Prune juice	⅓ cup	15
Regular gelatin	½ cup	20
Sherbet	½ cup	30
Broth*	Any	0
Tomato juice*	½ cup	5

*High in sodium.

Exercise Precautions

As exercise recommendations differ for NIDDM and IDDM, dietary recommendations differ also.

Exercise Precautions for Patients with Noninsulin-Dependent Diabetes Mellitus

A planned exercise program is an essential part of the treatment plan for NIDDM. The meal plan should include adequate kilocalories for routine exercise. Although a daily regular exercise program is preferable, this is not always feasible. For example, some people may play tennis or golf only once a week. Some people may expend many kilocalories in holiday shopping for hours at a time by walking and carrying heavy packages.

Exercise Precautions for Patients with Insulin-Dependent Diabetes Mellitus

People with type I diabetes who do exercise and type II patients who engage in nonroutine exercise should monitor their blood glucose levels before, during, and after exercise. If the blood glucose level is greater than 100 milligrams per deciliter, there is usually no need for additional food if the planned exercise is of short duration and low intensity. Exercise of long duration and high intensity will generally require more kilocalories. An additional 15 to 30 grams of carbohydrate-containing food should be ingested for every 30 to 60 minutes of exercise (Franz, 1987). Good choices for snack foods include fruit, starch, and milk exchanges. Exercise is best done 60 to 90 minutes after meals when the blood glucose level is highest.

Eating Out and Fast Foods

The best advice for persons with diabetes who enjoy eating out is that they know their meal-planning system and order small. For example, a small hamburger at McDonald's with a side salad, diet dressing, and a glass of skimmed milk are equal to:

2 starch exchanges	(hamburger bun)
1 meat exchange	(from the hamburger patty)
1 vegetable exchange	(from the salad)
1 fat	(from the hamburger patty)
1 skimmed milk	(milk exchange)

The individual can always mix 4 ounces of orange juice with diet soft drinks for a fruit punch drink if he or she needs a fruit exchange.

Delayed Meals

When meals are delayed as a result of an unavoidable situation, persons on insulin may experience a hypoglycemic reaction. If the patient is self-monitoring his or her blood glucose, at the first sign or symptom of hypoglycemia, he or she should measure the blood glucose level. If the blood glucose level is less than 60 milligrams per deciliter, 15 grams of carbohydrate should be consumed. Fifteen grams of carbohydrate is equal to two to three glucose tablets, 6 to 10 lifesaver candies, or 4 to 6 ounces of juice. Fifteen minutes later, he or she should measure the blood glucose a second time. This is called the 15-15 rule. The process may need to be performed a second time to achieve a blood glucose level of between 80 and 120 milligrams per deciliter (or 70 to 110 milligrams per deciliter; check laboratory's normal range). Treat with 15 grams of carbohydrate, wait 15 minutes, and retest. If the reaction is not resolved, treat again. A physician should be consulted if this self-treatment approach is ineffective in normalizing the patient's blood glucose level.

By carrying an extra package of saltines in a purse, briefcase, or car, these persons may avoid a hypoglycemic episode. Persons with diabetes should always have immediate access to a sugar-containing food such as hard candy, a lump of sugar, or a tube of concentrated glucose in case they feel the symptoms of hypoglycemia, or their glucose is low as determined by SMBG.

TEACHING SELF-CARE

Persons with diabetes ultimately treat themselves. The better educated the individual is about diabetes, the better the likelihood of his or her avoiding the acute and chronic complications of this disease (see Charting Tips 16–1). Figure 16-5 illustrates a healthcare worker teaching a patient about self-care. Many public health departments, hospitals, and clinics hold classes for patients with diabetes. Initially, these persons need to learn survival skills. The healthcare worker often has to repeat instructions several times before the patient understands the survival skills being taught. Because of the genetic predisposition toward diabetes, many newly diagnosed patients have relatives who have suffered from the acute and chronic complications

CHARTING TIPS 16–1

Nurses traditionally chart in detail the procedures they perform for the patient. Nurses also teach the patient while performing such procedures. Often, though, nurses do not chart the teaching in detail:

✓ Try to record the content taught, as well as objective evidence that the patient has learned the material. For instance, if the dietitian instructs a patient on an ADA diet, the nurse might later ask the patient to recall what the dietitian said.

✓ If recall is charted in some detail, as "Could classify milk products correctly," the dietitian would know what areas of teaching to review.

✓ Should it be needed at a later date, the record would testify that instruction had been received.

of diabetes. Hearing about such complications firsthand often creates fear in newly diagnosed patients. They need time to accept their condition. Occasionally, it may take as long as a full year before patients can grasp the principles of self-care. This is especially difficult for children (see Clinical Application 16–5).

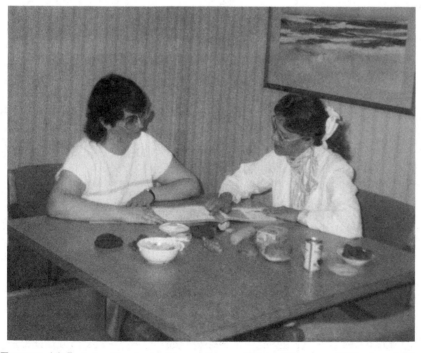

FIGURE 16–5. A healthcare worker teaching self-care. The use of life-size plastic food models assists in teaching meal planning.

CLINICAL APPLICATION 16–5
Children with Diabetes

Kilocalorie allowances are based on a person's weight. As a rough estimate, a 1-year-old child needs 1000 kilocalories per day. For older children, 100 kilocalories per year of age are added to the daily intake.

All the growth changes that occur in other children also take place in diabetic children. Because their activity may vary markedly from one day to the next, managing this metabolic disease is an ongoing challenge.

Diabetic children must eat every few hours. They also benefit from being served regular meals that contain the same foods that are being eaten by the rest of the family. The diabetic diet exemplifies good nutritional practices, and other family members could profit from it as well as the child with diabetes.

Parents should avoid labeling foods "good" or "bad." Certain cakes and cookies are listed on the Exchange Lists for occasional use. A diabetic child is permitted to have a birthday cake. Parents and older children should work with the dietitian to keep the meals interesting. Recipes are available that adapt popular "in" foods for diabetic use.

Because IDDM is a lifetime condition, we need to do whatever we can to teach the child self-management. To this end, experiences such as a camp for diabetic children can be very valuable. The child learns how others have coped and picks up some tips on managing the disease, while having fun outdoors.

HYPOGLYCEMIA

Hypoglycemia, caused by increased endogenous insulin production (hyperinsulinism), is much rarer than diabetes mellitus. Hyperinsulinism is most likely caused by islet cell tumors or, less often, by reactive hypoglycemia. Hypoglycemia that occurs 1 to 3 hours after a meal and resolves spontaneously with the ingestion of carbohydrate is often termed "reactive hypoglycemia."

The dietary management of reactive hypoglycemia consists of avoiding simple carbohydrates and sometimes taking small, frequent feedings. The meal plans for diabetes offer a reasonable guide to meal planning. Table 16–6 is a 1-day meal plan for this type of diet.

The dietary treatment for hypoglycemia caused by an islet cell tumor is food given at frequent intervals in amounts necessary to prevent symptoms. Sugar is not avoided in these patients, as it may be particularly useful for the rapid correction of symptoms. In fact, some reports have indicated as much as 1000 grams of glucose administered each 24 hours are occasionally indicated to counteract a tremendous production of insulin (Guyton, 1986).

Summary

Diabetes and hypoglycemia are both caused by either an undersecretion or oversecretion of insulin, respectively. Diabetes is actually a group

TABLE 16–6 *Sample Meal Plan for Hypoglycemic Diet*

Exchange Group	Sample Menu
Morning	
1 fruit	½ cup unsweetened orange juice
1 starch	¾ cup whole-grain cereal
1 meat	1 ounce low-fat cheese
½ skimmed milk	½ cup skimmed milk
Free	Decaffeinated coffee
Mid-morning	
1 meat	1 tablespoon peanut butter
1 starch	4 whole-grain crackers
Noon	
Chef's salad	
2–4 meat	2–4 ounces of lean meat
1 vegetable	Lettuce, tomatoes, and
1 fat	Dressing
1 fruit	1 small piece of fresh fruit
1 skimmed milk	1 cup skimmed milk
1 starch	2 breadsticks (4 × ½ inches)
Mid-afternoon	
1 meat	1 ounce low-fat cheese
1 starch	4 whole-grain crackers
Evening	
2–4 meat	2–4 ounces lean meat
1 starch	½ cup potato or pasta
1 vegetable	½ cup vegetable
1 fat	Lettuce salad with dressing
1 fruit	1 piece of fresh fruit
Free	Decaffeinated coffee or tea
Bedtime	
1 starch and 1 meat	½ sandwich (1 slice whole-grain bread and 1 ounce of lean meat)
1 vegetable	Fresh vegetables
Free	Decaffeinated beverage

of disorders with a common sign of hyperglycemia. There are two major types of diabetes: insulin-dependent diabetes mellitus (IDDM) and non-insulin-dependent diabetes mellitus (NIDDM). Impaired glucose tolerance, secondary diabetes, and gestational diabetes are recently named new categories of this disease. Persons with diabetes suffer from both acute and chronic complications. Treatment involves medication, diet, and exercise. Nutrition is a fundamental part of treatment. Hypoglycemia, a much rarer condition than diabetes, is also treated with dietary manipulation.

A case study and a sample plan of care appear below. Both are designed to show you how the information you have studied in this chapter can be used in nursing practice.

CASE STUDY 16-1

Mrs. S., a 45-year-old black woman, admitted to the hospital with medical diagnoses of NIDDM and cellulitis of the left leg. Her admitting height was 5 feet 5 inches and weight 200 pounds. Wrist measurement shows Mrs. S. has a large frame. Vital signs were temperature 98.6°F, pulse 70 beats per minute, respirations 16 per minute, and blood pressure 160/95.

Mrs. S. reported a gradual increase in her weight since her third child was born 20 years ago. That baby weighed 12 pounds. Two previous pregnancies produced infants weighing 10 and 11 pounds.

None of the children live at home. Mrs. S. lives with her husband, who works fairly regularly as a construction laborer. She has been seasonally employed as a hotel maid at a nearby resort. Health insurance coverage is sporadic. They have a new insurance policy now.

Mrs. S. is the oldest of six children. Her father died of a heart attack at age 60. Her mother died of a stroke at age 62 following 15 years of treatment for diabetes mellitus. The sister who is closest to Mrs. S. in age developed diabetes mellitus 3 years ago and is being treated with oral medication. Their youngest sister was diagnosed as an insulin-dependent diabetic at age 18 following an episode of mumps.

Mrs. S. reports a good appetite and a fluid intake of about 3 quarts per day. Her favorite beverage is iced tea with sugar and lemon. She does most of the grocery shopping and cooking.

Mrs. S. hit her left ankle with the screen door about 2 months ago. The resulting sore has not healed but has gotten worse. Mrs. S. knows that a sore that does not heal is a sign of cancer, which is why she sought medical attention. The ankle now has an open lesion 5 centimeters in diameter over the lateral ankle bone. The entire foot is swollen to twice the size of the right foot. The bandage over the sore had greenish-yellow drainage on it.

A random blood glucose test in the doctor's office 3 hours after her last meal was 400 milligrams per deciliter. Her urine glucose was negative for ketones. Before she left the office, the physician told Ms. S she had noninsulin-dependent diabetes mellitus.

The physician prescribed the following care for Mrs. S:

- Bed rest with L leg elevated
- Beside commode
- 1200-kilocalorie ADA diet
- Multivitamin, one capsule, daily
- Culture and sensitivity of drainage from left leg
- Cefuroxime, 250 milligrams, orally every 12 hours
- Warm, moist dressing to ulcer left leg four times per day
- Fasting blood sugar (FBS), electrolytes in AM

The admitting nurse constructed the following Nursing Care Plan for Mrs. S.

NURSING CARE PLAN

Assessment

Subjective:
  Family history of diabetes mellitus
  Large appetite
  Large fluid intake
  Delay in seeking medical attention

Objective:
  Obesity (HBW 134 percent)
  Newly diagnosed NIDDM
  Possible hypertension (only one reading given)
  Open lesion 5 centimeter diameter over left lateral ankle; purulent
    discharge

Nursing Diagnosis

  Health maintenance, altered: related to inappropriate self-care as evi-
    denced by delay in seeking medical attention

Desired Outcomes/Evaluation Criteria

  Patient will verbalize self-care measures related to NIDDM by hospi-
    tal discharge.
  Patient will verbalize willingness to continue nursing/medical regimen
    after discharge.

Nursing Actions/Interventions with Rationale in Italics

  1. Refer to dietitian for instruction on 1200-kilocalorie ADA diet. *The
     cornerstone of treatment of NIDDM is weight loss. Although any weight loss
     will help, to reach a healthy weight, Mrs. S. needs to lose 51 pounds. A dietit-
     ian's expertise is needed.*
  2. Refer to social worker for sources of medical attention when unin-
     sured. *Social workers are most familiar with community resources.*
  3. Teach principles of wound care, including effect of high blood sugar
     on infection. *If Mrs. S. understands that high blood sugar feeds the bacteria
     causing the infection, she may be more willing to work hard to control the dia-
     betes.*
  4. Reinforce dietitian's instruction.
     a. Have Mrs. S. state the Dietary Guidelines and the reason why they
        are important. *Knowledge usually precedes behavior change.*
     b. Have Mrs. S. identify Free Food Exchanges such as lettuce,
        spinach, and diet beverages.
        *Short periods of instruction are most effective; frequent review of the mate-
        rial will help the patient master it.*
  5. Remind physician to discuss exercise regimen when the blood sugar
     is under control. *Mrs. S. needs a prescribed exercise program suited to her
     level of conditioning.*

STUDY AIDS

Chapter Review Questions

1. The nurse can assume a patient has _____ diabetes if insulin is prescribed:
   a. Type I
   b. Type I or type II
   c. Endocrine
   d. Primary

2. The following statement is true:
   a. Acute illness lowers blood glucose levels.
   b. Fluid and electrolyte replacement is essential during episodes of acute illness in all persons with diabetes.
   c. Persons with diabetes who have an acute illness require a vitamin and mineral supplement.
   d. Persons with diabetes should never eat forms of simple sugar.

3. Insulin levels:
   a. Are stable in the blood
   b. Remain unchanged during exercise
   c. Decrease as the blood glucose level decreases
   d. Decrease after food consumption

4. Dietary guidelines for people with diabetes include:
   a. Drink alcohol in moderation.
   b. Consume no more than 2000 milligrams of sodium each day.
   c. Restrict fat intake to less than 30 percent of total kilocalories.
   d. Consume at least 100 grams of fiber each day.

5. Dietary fiber:
   a. Modulates the absorption of carbohydrate from the gut
   b. Stimulates lipolysis
   c. Inhibits glycogenesis
   d. Stimulates gluconeogenesis and inhibits glycogenolysis

6. To decrease the risk of heart disease, people with diabetes should:
   a. Avoid all dietary cholesterol.
   b. Restrict dietary cholesterol to less than 500 milligrams per day.
   c. Avoid all forms of saturated fat.
   d. Restrict dietary cholesterol to less than 300 milligrams per day and total fat intake to less than 30 percent of total kilocalories.

7. People with diabetes should eat at least the following amount of daily protein:
   a. 0.1 grams per kilogram
   b. 0.5 grams per kilogram
   c. 0.8 grams per kilogram
   d. 1.2 grams per kilogram

8. Individuals with NIDDM are encouraged to have a planned exercise program because physical activity:
   a. Increases the number of insulin receptors on cell membranes
   b. Stimulates the storage of glycogen
   c. Increases the low-density lipoproteins
   d. Stimulates the pancreas to release insulin

9. For most patients, the cornerstone of treatment of NIDDM is:
   a. Stress management
   b. Weight loss
   c. Strict adherence to five planned meals per day
   d. Hypoglycemic drugs

10. The diet for reactive hypoglycemia includes the following features:
    a. Small, frequent meals with restricted simple sugar
    b. Three meals with ample simple sugars and high in complex carbohydrate
    c. Four to six small meals that are high in fat
    d. Three high-carbohydrate meals that are moderate in fat

NCLEX-Style Quiz

Situation One

Ms. N., a 14-year-old white girl, has been an insulin-dependent diabetic for 1 year. Her blood sugar levels have been stable on an intermediate-acting insulin and a 2700-kilocalorie ADA diet. She is now being seen in the doctor's office for routine follow-up. The nurse is reviewing Ms. N.'s knowledge of self-care.

1. Ms. N's meal pattern calls for four milk exchanges. Recommending one of the following foods as preferable to the other three would demonstrate that the nurse understands both Ms. N.'s physiological needs and the complications of diabetes. Which is the preferable food?
   a. 2 percent milk
   b. Fruited yogurt
   c. Skimmed milk
   d. Whole milk

2. To assess Ms. N.'s knowledge, the nurse asks Ms. N. how she would handle a day when she could not eat solid foods. Which of the following answers would show Ms. N.'s understanding of the usual procedure?
   a. She would skip her insulin that day.
   b. She would call the doctor after missing one meal.
   c. She would replace the carbohydrates in the meal plan with liquids containing equal amounts of carbohydrate.
   d. She would take half her usual insulin dose and double her usual fluid intake.

3. Ms. N. plays volleyball for her high school team. She usually is moderately active during practices and games. SMBG records indicate a daily glucose level of between 120 and 140 milligrams per deciliter prior to the time she usually plays volleyball. Which of the following behaviors are appropriate for her before playing?
   a. No additional food is indicated.
   b. Increase her intake by one starch exchange.
   c. Increase her intake by one milk exchange.
   d. Increase her intake by one vegetable exchange and fat exchange.

4. The nurse asks Ms. N. what she carries to treat hypoglycemia. Which of the following is preferred?
   a. Dietetic candy
   b. A small box of raisins
   c. Sugar substitute
   d. Two large sugar cubes

5. Ms. N. says she is getting tired of pricking her finger several times a day. She asks the nurse why she cannot manage her diabetes using urine testing as her grandmother does. Which of the following responses by the nurse would be most appropriate?
   a. "The urine test is more accurate in older people."
   b. "The point at which sugar is spilled in the urine varies even for one individual. Therefore, the blood test is more accurate."
   c. "Urine tests are more costly."
   d. "The blood test is the newest thing. Your grandmother's doctor must be old-fashioned."

CLINICAL CALCULATION 16–1

How to Distribute the Energy Nutrients and Calculate a Diabetic Diet Using the Exchange System

The physician or dietitian usually determines the appropriate food intake for each patient. All the energy nutrients are involved in diabetes and thus are controlled in the diet. The diet prescription may be written simply as "1800 ADA diet." This means an 1800-kilocalorie diet using the American Dietetic Association distribution. These standards are 55 to 60 percent of the kilocalories from carbohydrate, 12 to 20 percent from protein, and 25 to 30 percent from fat. If the physician wants a different distribution, the prescription could specify the percentages desired, as "1500 kcal diabetic diet (60% CHO, 15% protein, 25% fat)."

In the following example, an 1800-kilocalorie diet is being converted to 55 percent carbohydrate, 20 percent protein, and 25 percent fat.

$$1800 \text{ kilocalorie} \times .55 = 990 \text{ kilocalorie} \div 4 \text{ kilocalorie per gram}$$
$$= 248 \text{ grams carbohydrate}$$

$$1800 \text{ kilocalorie} \times .20 = 360 \text{ kilocalorie} \div 4 \text{ kilocalorie per gram}$$
$$= 90 \text{ grams protein}$$

$$1800 \text{ kilocalorie} \times .25 = 450 \text{ kilocalorie} \div 9 \text{ kilocalorie per gram}$$
$$= 50 \text{ grams fat}$$

In the following example, 248 grams of carbohydrate, 90 grams of protein, and 50 grams of fat are converted to a ⅕, ⅖, ⅕, and ⅕ distribution. Each fraction represents one meal: thus ⅕ of the energy nutrients are to be provided each at breakfast, supper, and the evening snack; ⅖ of the energy nutrients are to be provided at the noon meal. Please note: ⅕ equals 20 percent and ⅖ represents 40 percent.

248 grams of carbohydrate × .20 = 50 grams × 3 meals = 150

248 grams of carbohydrate × .40 = 99 grams × 1 meal = 99
                                                        249

90 grams of protein × .20 = 18 grams × 3 meals = 54

90 grams of protein × .40 = 36 grams × 1 meal = 36
                                                  90

Because only a small percentage of dietary fat enters the bloodstream as glucose, normally fat is not calculated into the distribution. Lunch (⅖ distribution) would contain about 99 grams of carbohydrate and 36 grams of protein. Each of the other meals (⅕ distribution) would contain about 50 grams of carbohydrate and 18 grams of protein.

Box continued on next page.

CLINICAL CALCULATION 16–1 *(Continued)*

How to distribute the Energy Nutrients and Calculate a Diabetic Diet Using the Exchange System

The next step is to determine the number of exchanges to be provided from each of the six exchange groups. There is no exact method used to determine this step. Usually the patient is consulted to determine the amount of nonfat milk, fruits, vegetables, and so forth that he or she would be willing to consume. An effort should be made to calculate the diet with at least the recommended servings given in the Food Pyramid guide. Many healthcare workers determine the amount of nonfat milk, fruits, and vegetables to be provided first. This is followed by the grams of carbohydrate to be contributed by these groups. The remaining carbohydrate is then allocated to the starch group.

The protein is determined by first calculating the amount previously provided by nonfat milk, vegetables, and starches; the remaining protein is then allocated to meat exchanges. The fat is determined by first calculating the amount previously provided by the meat exchanges; the remaining fat is then allocated to fat exchanges. The calculations and meal plan for our sample 1800 kilocalories with 55 percent carbohydrate, 20 percent protein, and 25 percent fat with a ⅕, ⅖, ⅕, and ⅕ distribution appear in Table 16–7.

TABLE 16–7 *Sample 1800–Kilocalorie Diabetic Diet**

DIVISION OF ENERGY NUTRIENTS AND EXCHANGES

Exchange List	Number of Daily Exchanges	Protein (90 g)	Fat (50 g)	Carbohydrate (218 g)	Breakfast	Lunch	Dinner	HS
Skimmed milk	2	16	0	24	½	1		½
Starch	11	33	0	165	2	4	3	2
Fruit	3	0	0	45	1	1	0	1
Vegetable	3	6	0	15	0	2	1	0
Meat	5	35	25	0	1	2	1	1
Fat	5	0	25	0	1	1	2	1

MEAL PLAN AND SAMPLE MENUS

Meal Plan	Sample Menu 1	Sample Menu 2
Breakfast		
½ skimmed milk	½ cup skimmed milk	½ cup skimmed milk
2 starch	2 slices of toast	1 cup of oatmeal
1 fruit	½ cup orange juice	½ banana
1 meat	¼ cup low-cholesterol egg substitute	1 low-fat sausage link
1 fat	1 teaspoonful margarine	2 pecans
Lunch		
1 skimmed milk	1 cup skimmed milk	1 cup skimmed milk
4 starch	1⅓ cup brown rice	2 slices of bread†
		1 cup broth-type vegetable soup and 3 ginger snaps
1 fruit	1 apple	½ cup pineapple juice
2 vegetable	1 cup green beans	½ cup asparagus and 1 cup raw carrots
2 meat	2 ounces, stir-fried chicken	2 slices low-fat cheese†
1 fat	1 teaspoonful oil	1 teaspoonful margarine†
Dinner		
3 starch	1 large baked potato	¼ pizza, thin crust and 2 bread sticks (4 × ½ inch)
1 vegetable	½ cup broccoli‡	Sliced tomato
Free vegetable	Lettuce salad	Lettuce salad
1 meat	1 ounce ground beef‡	(on pizza)
2 fat	2 tablespoon sour cream‡	(on pizza)
	1 tablespoon French dressing	1 tablespoon Italian dressing
Free	Coffee	Diet soft drink
HS		
½ skim milk	½ cup skimmed milk	½ cup skimmed milk
2 starch	1½ ounces pretzels	6 cups hot-air popped popcorn
1 fruit	15 grapes	1 peach
1 meat	1 ounce low-fat cheese stick	1 tablespoon Parmesan cheese
1 fat	2 walnuts	1 tablespoon diet margarine

*The calculations and meal plan based on 55 percent carbohydrate, 20 percent protein, and 25 percent fat with a ⅕, ⅖, ⅕, and ⅕ distribution.

†Cheese sandwich.

‡Potato toppings.

BIBLIOGRAPHY

American Dietetic Association: Manual of Clinical Dietetics, ed 4. American Dietetic Association, Chicago. 1992.

Anderson, JW: Nutrition Management of Metabolic Conditions. HCF Diabetes Research Foundation, Inc., Lexington, KY, 1986.

Black, JM and Matassarin-Jacobs: Luckmann and Sorenson's Medical-Surgical Nursing, ed 4. WB Saunders, Philadelphia, 1993.

Bullock, BL and Rosendahl, PP: Pathophysiology, ed 3. JB Lippincott, Philadelphia, 1992.

Diabetes Control and Complications Trial Research Group: The effect of intensive treatment of diabetes on the development and progression of long-term complications in insulin-dependent diabetes mellitus. New Engl J Med 329: 977-986, 1993.

Franz, MJ: Exercise and the management of diabetes mellitus. J Am Diet Assoc 87:872, 1987.

Guthrie, AW, Hinnen, D and De Shelter, E (eds): Diabetes Education: A Core Curriculum for Health Professionals: American Association of Diabetes Educators, Alexandria, VA, 1988, p 2.

Guyton, AC: Textbook of Medical Physiology. ed 7 WB Saunders, Philadelphia, 1986, p 932.

Nathan, DM: Long-term complications of diabetes mellitus: New Engl J Med 328:1676, 1993.

National Research Council, Committee on Diet and Health, Food and Nutrition Board, Commission on Life Sciences: Diet and Health. National Academy Press, Washington, DC, 1989.

Pastors, JG: Nutritional Care of Diabetes: Nutrition Dimension, San Marcos, 1992, p 7.

Pemberton, CM, et al: Mayo Clinic Diet Manual, ed 6. BC Decker, Philadelphia, 1988.

Smeltzer, SC and Bare, BG: Brunner and Suddarth's Textbook of Medical-Surgical Nursing, ed. 7. JB Lippincott, Philadelphia, 1992.

United States Department of Agriculture, Human Nutrition Information Service: The Food Guide. Home and Garden Bulletin Number 252, Hyattsville, MD, 1992.

Chapter Outline

Key Terms

As a study aid, each key term is followed by the page number where the term is defined in the chapter. Terms that appear in **boldface** or <u>underscored</u> in the chapter text are located in the glossary.

Diet in Cardiovascular Disease

After completing this chapter, the student should be able to:

1. Discuss the relationship of fat, cholesterol, and sodium intakes to the development of cardiovascular disease.
2. Distinguish between type II and type IV hyperlipoproteinemias as to aggravating factors and dietary modifications.
3. Identify strategies likely to reduce the risk of cardiovascular disease.
4. Describe the traditional 2-gram sodium diet.
5. List several flavorings and seasonings that can be substituted for salt on a sodium-restricted diet.

*T*he cardiovascular system includes not only the heart and blood vessels but the blood-forming organs as well. This chapter discusses common diseases of the heart and blood vessels that can be influenced by diet modification. Conditions resulting from faulty blood forming are included in other chapters. Iron-deficiency anemia was discussed in Chapters 7 and 10. Pernicious anemia was addressed in Chapter 6. Nutritional care of the leukemia patient is included in Chapter 20.

OCCURRENCE OF CARDIOVASCULAR DISEASE

Atherosclerosis—A form of arteriosclerosis characterized by the deposit of fatty material inside the arteries; ninth leading cause of death and major factor contributing to heart disease.

Diseases of the cardiovascular system are 3 of the 10 most common causes of death in the United States. Coronary heart disease is by far the most frequent cause of death: 318 per 100,000 people. Cerebrovascular disease ranks third, with 62 deaths per 100,000 people. **Atherosclerosis,** hardening of the arteries, ranks ninth, with 9 deaths per 100,000 people.

One million persons suffer heart attacks in the United States every year—more than 2700 every day. Every year in the United States 636,000 people die from heart attacks. Cardiovascular disease occurs 10 times more frequently in this country than in Japan. Later you will learn some of the reasons suggested for this great difference.

Every year, one-half million persons in the United States suffer a **cerebrovascular accident (CVA),** also known as a stroke.

Cerebrovascular accident (CVA)—An abnormal condition in which the brain's blood vessels are occluded by an embolus or hemorrhage, resulting in damaged brain tissue.

Contributing to both heart attacks and stroke is **hypertension,** or high blood pressure. Estimates of the adult population afflicted with hypertension vary from 20 to 33 percent. One reason for this wide range is the existence of many undiagnosed cases of hypertension. Hypertension can exist without signs or symptoms. For this reason, blood pressure checks are a good idea (Fig. 17–1).

UNDERLYING PATHOLOGY

Hypertension—Blood pressure above normal, usually more than 140/90 on three successive occasions.

Two major pathological conditions contribute to cardiovascular disease. One is atherosclerosis, the most common form of **arteriosclerosis.** The second is hypertension.

Atherosclerosis

Arteriosclerosis—A group of cardiovascular diseases characterized by the thickening, hardening, and loss of elasticity of the arterial walls.

Although the symptoms of atherosclerosis may not appear until middle or old age, the process is proceeding in all of us, because it accompanies aging. Even healthy young soldiers who died from other causes showed evidence of atherosclerosis on autopsy. The rate is decreasing. In the 1950s, 77 percent of the American soldiers killed in Korea had atherosclerotic changes compared with 45 percent of those killed in Vietnam.

In atherosclerosis, fatty deposits of cholesterol, fat, or other substances accumulate inside the artery. Initially, the deposited material, or plaque, is soft, but later it becomes fibrosed, that is, hard. This disease process interferes with the pumping of blood through the artery in two ways: (1) The deposits gradually make the opening smaller and smaller, and (2) the fibrosis makes it progressively harder for the artery to constrict or dilate in response to the tissues' needs for oxygenated blood (Fig. 17–2). When the lumen, or

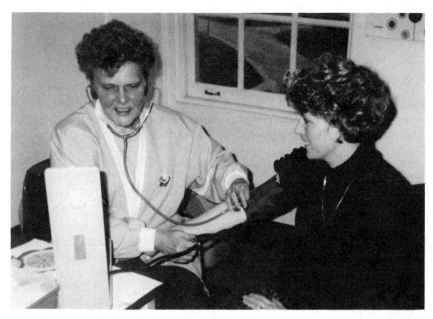

FIGURE 17–1. Hypertension is a silent killer. Even children occasionally are hypertensive. Routine blood pressure monitoring whenever a patient visits a clinic is a good idea.

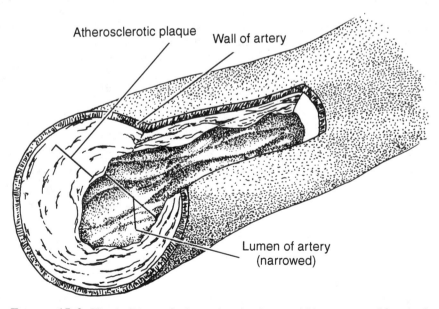

FIGURE 17–2. The build-up of atherosclerotic plaque within an artery. Note both the narrowed diameter and the roughness within the lumen. (From Scanlon and Sanders, p 288, with permission.)

opening through the artery, is 70 percent blocked by atherosclerotic plaque, the person is likely to show symptoms.

Hypertension

Blood pressure—Force exerted against the walls of blood vessels by the pumping action of the heart.

Blood pressure is the force exerted against the walls of the arteries by the pumping action of the heart. It is reported in two numbers, such as 120/80. The top number is the pressure during a heartbeat (contraction). It is called the **systolic pressure.** The bottom number is the pressure between beats (relaxation). It is called the **diastolic pressure.** Both numbers are reported in millimeters of mercury.

Systolic pressure—Pressure exerted against the arteries when the heart contracts; the upper number of the blood pressure reading.

Diagnosis of Hypertension

A condition in which the blood pressure is higher than normal is hypertension. A measurement of 140/90 or higher is accepted as hypertensive. Several readings are taken on different days to eliminate the possibility of excitement or nervousness causing a transient hypertension. Hypertension is classified as mild, moderate, severe, borderline isolated systolic, or isolated systolic (Table 17–1).

Diastolic pressure—Pressure exerted against the arteries between heartbeats, the lower number of a blood pressure reading.

Types of Hypertension

Depending on the cause of the hypertension, it is labeled primary or secondary. About 90 percent of hypertensive patients have primary or essential hypertension. There is no single, clear-cut cause for this high blood pressure.

Secondary hypertension occurs in response to another event or disease process in the body, such as pregnancy-induced hypertension. Birth control pills that contain progesterone stimulate the production of renin, which results in an elevation in blood pressure. The combined intake of monoamine oxidase (MAO) inhibitors and tyramine-rich foods or beverages can also cause hypertension. Secondary hypertension can result from diseases of the kidney, adrenal glands, or nervous system as well.

TABLE 17–1 *Classification of Hypertension*

Category	Systolic mm Hg	Diastolic mm Hg
Normal	< 130	< 85
High normal	130–139	85–89
Hypertension		
Stage 1 (mild)	140–159	90–99
Stage 2 (moderate)	160–179	100–109
Stage 3 (severe)	180–209	110–119
Stage 4 (very severe)	≥ 210	≥ 120

Positive Feedback Cycle

Many cardiovascular conditions have interlocking causative factors. The interaction between atherosclerosis and hypertension is a **positive feedback cycle.** The presence of the second condition worsens the first. Atherosclerosis narrows the lumen of the arteries, and the smaller opening increases the blood pressure. Consider what happens when someone puts a finger over the end of the garden hose: the water squirts out with greater force. In the body, high blood pressure forces more lipids into the arterial wall. Fat that is stored in the body also increases blood pressure. Hypertension is aggravated by obesity because the heart has more miles of blood vessels to fill and tissues to supply.

END RESULT OF PATHOLOGY

Most people do not have atherosclerosis *or* hypertension. They probably have both conditions. Although many organs are likely to be damaged by atherosclerosis and hypertension, here we are concerned with the effects on the heart and brain.

Coronary Heart Disease

Coronary heart disease (CHD) results when the coronary arteries that supply the heart muscle with blood become blocked. If the blockage is temporary, owing to increased activity and increased demand for oxygen, the person may display **angina pectoris,** or severe pain and a sense of constriction about the heart. Rest and the administration of vasodilating medications may stave off heart damage. However, if the vessel is blocked by a **thrombus,** a blood clot that develops at the site, or an **embolus,** a circulating mass of undissolved matter, the heart tissues beyond the point of obstruction receive no oxygen or nutrients. When this happens, the person has a **coronary occlusion,** or heart attack. When the blood supply cannot be restored quickly, part of the heart dies. The medical diagnosis then becomes **myocardial infarction (MI).**

Congestive Heart Failure

Congestive heart failure (CHF) occurs when the heart fails to maintain adequate circulation of the blood. CHF results from an injury or a reduction in function of the heart muscle. Causes may be atherosclerosis, hypertension, myocardial infarction, rheumatic fever, or a birth defect. When the heart cannot keep up with the demands on it, a sequence of events sets up another positive feedback cycle.

The right side of the heart collects the blood returning from the body and pumps it to the lungs to be cleared of carbon dioxide and refilled with oxygen. If the right ventricle is failing, usually owing to lung disease, the blood backs up into the veins that empty into the right atrium, and the patient will display the signs of peripheral edema.

The left side of the heart receives the oxygenated blood from the lungs and pumps it out to the body. If the left ventricle is failing, usually following a myocardial infarction, the blood will back up into the lungs. The patient

Coronary heart disease (CHD)— Disease resulting from the decreased flow of blood through the coronary arteries to the heart muscle.

Angina pectoris— Severe pain and sense of constriction about the heart caused by relative lack of oxygen.

Thrombus—A blood clot that obstructs a blood vessel.

Embolus—A circulating mass of undissolved matter in a blood or lymphatic vessel; may be composed of cells, tissues, fat globules, air bubbles, clumps of bacteria, or foreign bodies including pieces of medical devices.

Coronary occlusion—Blockage of one or more branches of the coronary arteries, which supply the heart muscle with oxygen and nutrients.

Myocardial infarction—Area of dead heart muscle; usually the result of coronary occlusion.

Congestive heart failure (CHF)— Condition resulting from failure of the heart to maintain adequate blood circulation; due to complex reactive mechanisms, fluid is retained in the body's tissues.

will display shortness of breath and moist lung sounds and will expectorate a frothy pink sputum.

In addition, if the heart cannot pump enough to maintain blood pressure, the body will implement the renin-angiotensin response (see Chapter 9.) Angiotensin II constricts the blood vessels, raising blood pressure. Aldosterone prompts the kidney to conserve sodium, and with it, water. More fluid fills the blood vessels. The higher blood pressure pushes this fluid out into the interstitial spaces, causing edema.

Obviously, one side of the heart cannot function indefinitely while the other side is failing. Nevertheless, the healthcare worker learns to look for signs of early heart failure in the extremities in right-sided failure or in the lungs in left-sided failure.

Cerebrovascular Accident

When a blood vessel in the brain becomes blocked by atherosclerosis, the tissue supplied by that artery dies. This is the most common cause of cerebrovascular accidents, or strokes. Strokes also can be caused by an embolus or a ruptured blood vessel. Cerebrovascular accidents are usually secondary to atherosclerosis, hypertension, or a combination of both.

RISK FACTORS IN CARDIOVASCULAR DISEASE

Many risk factors are related to cardiovascular disease. Some of them are behaviors that patients can modify. Others are attributes we are given at birth.

Unchangeable Risk Factors

Atherosclerosis and hypertension develop in persons with certain characteristics. The unchangeable risk factors, or qualities we cannot alter, are age, sex, race, and family history.

Age

After age 40, coronary atherosclerosis increases. If hypertension is likely to develop, it usually appears in people at about the age of 50 or 60.

Sex

Sex-change operations notwithstanding, we categorize sex as an unchangeable risk factor. Females have less atherosclerosis and consequent coronary heart disease than males until menopause. After that, the rate becomes the same as men's. Women with diabetes are an exception, as is shown later.

Race

Hypertension is twice as common in blacks as in whites. Many genetic factors contribute to hypertension. The proportionate contributions of genetics and lifestyle have not been determined. One psychosocial factor that affects blood pressure is stress. Stressful situations have been described as those in which the person has little control over events. For some black patients, this theory might partially explain the racial difference in hypertension occurrence. However, whites as well as blacks may feel the stress of helplessness.

Family History

A family history of cardiovascular disease increases a person's risk two to five times. Family history includes both genetic and environmental factors.

An argument for the predominance of genetic susceptibility to cardiovascular disease is obtained from studies of adopted children. Those whose biological parents died of vascular causes were five times as likely to die of vascular disease as children whose adoptive parents died that way. Since the lifestyle of the adoptive parents did not increase risk of cardiovascular disease in the children, genetic susceptibility emerges as a major factor in cardiovascular diseases.

Of special concern are the **hyperlipoproteinemias,** or increased lipoproteins and lipids in the bloodstream (Table 17–2). One of these hyperlipoproteinemias, type 4, is very common and is often associated with noninsulin-dependent diabetes mellitus (NIDDM). Some of the other types are seen less often. Note in the table that all six types have a connection to food intake of fats, carbohydrates, or both. Note also that the blood plasma values vary in each condition. For example, type 1 hyperlipoproteinemia is aggravated by fat, and the chylomicrons (a type of lipoprotein) are elevated because they carry exogenous triglycerides that cannot be broken down. Thus, plasma triglyceride levels are elevated as well. Clinical Application 17–1 offers patient education information on triglycerides.

Hyperlipoproteinemia— Increased lipoproteins and lipids in the blood.

Type 2 hyperlipoproteinemia results from a single gene defect in the cell receptor that binds circulating low-density lipoproteins. Individuals with this defect manifest a rate of coronary heart disease 25 times that of the normal population. In addition, patients with type 2 hyperlipoproteinemia generally develop heart disease 15 years earlier than the rest of the population. Some even suffer heart attacks in infancy and childhood. The average age at death for these patients is 21 years.

TABLE 17–2 *Hyperlipoproteinemias*

Type	Frequency	Aggravated	Increased Plasma Values				
			Lipoprotein			Lipid	
			Chylomicrons	*VLDL*	*LDL*	*Cholesterol*	*Triglycerides*
I	Very rare	Fat	X				X
IIA	Common	Fat			X	X	
IIB	Common	Fat		X	X	X	X
III	Uncommon	Carbohydrate	Remnants			X	X
IV	Very common	Carbohydrate		X			X
V	Rare	Fat and carbohydrate	X	X		X	X

CLINICAL APPLICATION 17–1
National Cholesterol Education Program

The National Institutes of Health held a conference in the fall of 1984 to discuss the growing body of evidence linking an elevated blood cholesterol level to heart disease. Conference participants reviewed the evidence presented and arrived at two important conclusions:

1. There is sufficient scientific evidence that high cholesterol levels cause some forms of heart disease.
2. Lowering cholesterol levels through diet or medications could reduce the incidence of heart attacks and the death rate from heart disease.

It was estimated that 50 percent of the adult population had blood cholesterol levels above 200 milligrams per deciliter.*

The National Cholesterol Education Program (NCEP) was formed to direct a nationwide program for the detection, evaluation, and treatment of high blood cholesterol levels. The NCEP recommends two components be included in the treatment of elevated cholesterol: diet modification and drug therapy. A further recommendation is that drug therapy not be considered until at least 6 months of diet modification have been attempted. The NCEP has divided the diets used to treat an elevated cholesterol into two separate diets called Step 1 and Step 2 (see below). The Step 1 diet guidelines are located in Table 17–4. Typically, the Step 1 diet is reviewed with the patient by the physician's office nurse. If, after following the Step 1 diet (and guidelines) for 3 months, no significant change in cholesterol levels occurs, the patient proceeds to the Step 2 diet and should be seen by a registered dietitian. If no significant change in cholesterol levels occurs after following Step 2 for 3 months, then drug therapy must be considered. Nurses employed in the physician's office should have a working knowledge of the Step 1 diet.

COMPARISON OF THE STEP 1 AND STEP 2 DIETS

	Step 1 Diet Percent Total Kilocalories	Step 2 Diet Percent Total Kilocalories
Total fat	<30	<30
Saturated	<10	<7
Polyunsaturated	<10	<10
Monosaturated	10–15	10–15
Carbohydrate	50–60	50–60
Protein	10–20	10–20
Cholesterol (milligrams/deciliter)	<300 milligrams/day	<200 milligrams/day

Changeable Risk Factors

Unlike age, sex, race, and family history, some risk factors for cardiovascular disease can be modified to some extent. For coronary heart disease, the most important changeable risk factors are cigarette smoking, hypertension, and elevated blood cholesterol. None of these is completely independent of the others. Other factors over which the person can exert some control are NIDDM and intakes of sodium and alcohol.

Cigarette Smoking

The nicotine in cigarette smoke is a vasoconstrictor. Narrowing the blood vessels raises blood pressure. In addition, cigarette smokers exhibit lower levels of high-density lipoproteins even when weight is held constant. The lower a person's high-density lipoprotein levels, the higher the risk of coronary heart disease.

Hypertension

Both cigarette smoking and obesity contribute to hypertension. Moreover, the location of the excess adipose tissue has a particular significance in relation to cardiovascular disease. Abdominal fatness (apple-shape) is related to cardiovascular disease and diabetes more than is gluteal-femoral fatness (pear-shape). For obese people, the key to decreasing blood pressure is weight loss. Even a 10-pound weight loss has been found to lower blood pressure.

Elevated Blood Cholesterol

High blood cholesterol relates most directly to the risk of atherosclerosis. A high blood cholesterol level also is unquestionably linked to coronary heart disease.

RELATIONSHIP TO PATHOLOGICAL CHANGES   A person with a blood cholesterol greater than 250 milligrams per deciliter has triple the risk of atherosclerosis as the person with a lower value. Put the opposite way, for every 1 percent reduction in serum cholesterol achieved, a person decreases his risk of cardiovascular disease by 2 percent. A person with a serum cholesterol level of 269 milligrams per deciliter has twice the risk of coronary artery disease as the person with a reading of less than 210. Even a blood cholesterol level above 200 milligrams per deciliter is associated with increased heart disease.

RELATIONSHIP TO DIET   Cholesterol, manufactured by livers, is present in foods of animal origin. Human beings can manufacture cholesterol, too. Nevertheless, the diet contributes a small but important part of a person's serum cholesterol.

LIPOPROTEINS AS RISK FACTORS   Fats cannot dissolve in water but are bound to proteins for transportation in the bloodstream. These fat-carrying complexes are called lipoproteins. There are four main classes of lipoproteins: **chylomicrons, very low-density lipoproteins** (VLDL), **low-density lipoproteins** (LDL), and **high-density lipoproteins** (HDL). Table 17–3 summarizes the functions and significance of laboratory values of these four lipoproteins.

Chylomicron—A lipoprotein that carries triglycerides after meals.

Very low-density lipoprotein (VLDL)—A plasma protein containing mostly triglycerides with small amounts of cholesterol, phospholipid, and protein; transports triglycerides from the liver to the tissues.

Low-density lipoprotein (LDL)—A plasma protein containing more cholesterol and triglycerides than protein; elevated blood levels are associated with increased risk of heart disease.

High-density lipoproteins (HDL)—A plasma protein which carries fat in the bloodstream to the tissues or to the liver to be excreted; elevated blood levels are associated with a decreased risk of heart disease.

TABLE 17–3 *Functions and Significance of Various Lipoproteins*

Lipoprotein	Normal Value in 12–14- Hour Fasting Specimen	Function	Clinical Significance
Chylomicrons	0	Transport exogenous triglycerides from intestines to blood stream	Present in blood only after a meal
VLDL	13 to 32 percent	Main transporter of endogenous triglyceride	Synthesized by liver and small intestine from free fatty acids, glycerol, and carbohydrate
LDL	38 to 40 percent	Transports cholesterol to body cells	Major form of lipoprotein in atherosclerotic lesions. The higher the LDL level, the greater the risk of coronary heart disease.
HDL	20 to 48 percent	Transports cholesterol from body cells to liver to be excreted	Synthesized by liver and intestines. The higher the HDL level, the lower the risk of CHD; aerobic exercise increases HDL level.

A person's LDL levels parallel the serum cholesterol values. The higher a person's LDL value, the greater the risk of coronary heart disease. The LDLs carry cholesterol to the tissues.

On the other hand, the higher a person's HDL levels, the less the risk of coronary heart disease. The HDLs transport cholesterol from the tissues to the liver to be made into bile and then excreted.

Diabetes Mellitus

Insulin is required to maintain adequate levels of lipoprotein lipase. This enzyme breaks down chylomicrons. When lipoprotein lipase is inadequate owing to diabetes, chylomicrons and VLDL particles accumulate in the blood. After the diabetes is controlled, the lipid levels decrease.

At any given cholesterol level, diabetic persons have two to three times the risk of atherosclerosis as other people. Diabetic women lose the advantage of being female in regard to cardiovascular risk. Regardless of age or estrogen levels, they run the same risk as diabetic men. It is a significant risk. One third of persons with insulin-dependent diabetes mellitus (IDDM) die of coronary heart disease by age 55.

Sodium Intake

Despite the prevalence of atherosclerosis in the United States, not all the world's elderly develop hypertension. This age-related increase in blood pressure is not seen in populations with low sodium intakes.

A person has to be genetically susceptible to a sodium-induced hypertension to develop it. An estimated 9 to 20 percent of the US population is genetically susceptible to essential hypertension. For them, sodium restriction is a wise move.

Epidemiological studies have shown an increase of 12 millimeters of mercury in systolic blood pressure and 7 millimeters of mercury in diastolic pressure for every 100-milliequivalent increase in sodium intake. An increase of 100 milliequivalents of sodium would be about 2300 milligrams. Considering that the average American diet contains 5 grams of sodium, a 2-gram sodium diet should reduce a hypertensive patient's blood pressure by 16/9 points.

For people who are not genetically susceptible, a high sodium intake will not increase blood pressure, at least in the short term. Experts are currently debating whether to recommend sodium restriction for the general populace. At this time, following the Dietary Guidelines to "avoid excess sodium" is wise.

Alcohol Intake

An estimated 30 to 60 percent of alcoholics have hypertension. When hospitalized for detoxification, the average alcoholic's systolic blood pressure decreases by 20 millimeters of mercury. The relationship of alcohol to hypertension is dose related. Moderate doses dilate peripheral vessels, which lowers blood pressure. High doses, more than 2 ounces per day, raise blood pressure. A high intake of alcohol also increases triglyceride levels. In addition, alcohol has been found to induce strokes, even in normotensive patients.

PREVENTION OF CARDIOVASCULAR DISEASE

Because cardiovascular disease causes such a large proportion of deaths in the United States, many of the current Dietary Guidelines (United States Department of Agriculture, 1992) are aimed at reducing the risk of cardiovascular disease. The wise American will decrease consumption of fat, particularly saturated fat; increase intake of fiber and starches; avoid excess salt; and drink alcohol in moderation, if at all.

Prevention of Atherosclerosis

Keys to preventing atherosclerosis include a healthy diet plan and a regular exercise program. General principles are discussed here. Persons at high risk of cardiovascular disease require the services of a healthcare team to aid them in modifying their lifestyle.

Dietary Recommendations

The Dietary Guidelines apply to all healthy American adults. Next we will elaborate on desirable intakes of fat; breads and cereals; fruits and vegetables; meat, fish, and poultry; and sugar in relation to atherosclerosis.

FAT   Fat should not exceed 30 percent of kilocalories; saturated fat should not exceed 10 percent of kilocalories. Two saturated fatty acids, palmitic acid in whole milk and stearic acid in red meat, increase cholesterol levels. For this reason nonfat and low-fat milk products are preferable to whole milk, and low-fat fish and poultry are preferable to fatty meats. Clinical Application 17–1 discusses the Step 1 diet for cholesterol control.

Monounsaturated fats may significantly lower LDL and cholesterol as well as protect against blood clots. Sources of monounsaturated fats include olive, canola, and peanut oils. Vegetable oils, because they are all fat, will contribute toward the total fat kilocalories.

Dietary cholesterol should be limited to 300 milligrams per day. It is more important to control saturated fat intake than cholesterol intake. Reducing saturated fat intake has a greater effect on decreasing blood cholesterol than does reducing dietary cholesterol. Choosing servings of nonfat or low-fat dairy products over regular dairy products can reduce fat intake by as much as 90 percent. See Table 17–4 for guidelines on how to choose foods low in cholesterol and saturated fat. This table reproduces the American Heart Associations Step 1 Diet Guide.

Not all animal fat is equally threatening to one's heart and blood vessels. Eskimos following their traditional diet eat a lot of animal fat; they also have a low rate of coronary heart disease. Many researchers attribute this to the high omega-3 fatty acid content of the fish Eskimos eat. Cold-water ocean fish, some cold-water inland fish, and some other foods contain this substance in varying amounts. It helps to decrease serum triglycerides, while lowering total cholesterol and blood pressure. Eating 3 to 4 ounces of the fish

---

TABLE 17–4 *How to Choose Foods Low in Cholesterol and Saturated Fatty Acids*

Food Group	Recommended	Avoid or Use Sparingly
Meat, Poultry, Fish, Dried Beans and Peas, Nuts, Eggs	Chicken, turkey, fish, shellfish (clams, crab, oysters, scallops), lean red meats, egg whites, specially processed low-fat luncheon meats. Dry beans and peas such as kidney beans, lima beans, vegetarian-style baked beans, pinto beans, lentils, chick peas, split peas, navy beans. Soybean curd (tofu), peanut butter, cholesterol-free egg substitutes.	Duck, goose, heavily marbled meats, luncheon meats, bacon, sausage, ham, frankfurters, organ meats such as heart, kidney, sweetbreads and liver. Egg yolks (limit to three or four per week—including yolks used in cooking).
Vegetables and Fruits (canned, fresh, or frozen)	All varieties.	Avoid if fried or served in cream, butter, or cheese sauces.

TABLE 17–4 *How to Choose Foods Low in Cholesterol and Saturated Fatty Acids (Continued)*

Food Group	Recommended	Avoid or Use Sparingly
Breads and Cereals	Breads made with a minimum of saturated fat, such as whole-wheat, enriched white, French, Italian, oatmeal, rye, pumpernickel, English muffins, pita. Pasta, cereal, rice, melba toast, water crackers, matzos, pretzels, popcorn with unsaturated oil, water bagels.	Pastries, butter rolls, commercial biscuits, muffins, doughnuts, cakes, egg breads, cheese breads, commercial mixes containing dried eggs and whole milk. Many of these products are made with saturated fat (lard, butter, suet, palm oil, coconut oil, hydrogenated vegetable oil, etc.). Check the food labels.
Milk Products	Milk products that are low in saturated fatty acids: skimmed milk and powdered skimmed milk, low-fat products, buttermilk (from skimmed milk), low-fat yogurt, evaporated skimmed milk. Cheeses that are low in saturated fatty acids: low-fat cottage cheese; farmer's, hoop and baker's cheese from skimmed milk; partly skimmed mozzarella and ricotta. Choose the option with the lowest fat content.	Whole milk and whole milk products include: ice cream, cheeses made from whole milk or cream, butter. All creams (sour, half-and-half, whipped).
Fats and Oils	Margarines with no more than 2 grams of saturated fatty acids per tablespoon; Salad dressings and mayonnaise made from unsaturated oils; Vegetable oils—corn, sesame, soybean, sunflower, safflower, canola, olive.	Butter, lard, suet, salt pork, bacon, meat fat, chicken fat, coconut oil, palm and palm kernel oil, completely hydrogenated margarines and shortenings. Peanut oil and vegetable shortening occasionally for flavor.
Desserts, Beverages, Snacks, and Condiments	Fresh, frozen, canned or dried fruit, cocoa or carob powder, fruit ices, sherbet, gelatin, fruit whip, angel food cake, cakes made with unsaturated oils. Vinegar, mustard, herbs, spices.	Coconut, cream products, fried food snacks (potato chips, corn chips, etc.), chocolate pudding, ice cream, and most commercial cakes, pies, cookies and mixes.

Note: New, acceptable versions of standard products are appearing on the market. Be sure to read product labels on any items you are interested in purchasing.

Source: Reproduced with permission from *Culinary Hearts Kitchen Teaching Manual*, 1992. Copyright American Heart Association.

twice a week is effective. Fish that contain omega-3 fatty acids include herring, mackerel, salmon, swordfish, and tuna. Other food sources of omega-3 fatty acids are butternuts, soybeans, and walnuts.

BREADS AND CEREALS   For persons without hyperlipoproteinemia, carbohydrates should provide at least 55 percent of the daily kilocalorie intake. Six or more servings of bread and cereals per day are needed. Soluble fiber helps lower cholesterol by binding with it, thereby preventing its absorption, and then carrying it out of the body in the feces. Examples of soluble fiber sources include legumes, oats, barley, broccoli, apples, and citrus fruits. The substitution of two packages of instant oatmeal for other carbohydrates was shown to lower serum cholesterol levels (Van Horn, 1991).

FRUITS AND VEGETABLES   In addition to the foods just mentioned, the insoluble fiber in fruits and vegetables may prevent absorption of cholesterol by hastening the passage of the food through the intestinal tract. To this end, two servings (½ cup each) of fruits and three servings of vegetables are recommended.

MEAT, FISH, AND POULTRY   Daily intake of 5 to 7 ounces of meat, fish, or poultry is recommended. Because of the fat in meat and poultry, only lean meats should be eaten regularly. Visible fat should be trimmed or drained off before serving (see Fig. 17–3). Meats should be baked, broiled, boiled, or grilled, not fried. Legumes are an excellent substitute for meat and contribute soluble fiber as well.

SUGAR   In persons with elevated triglyceride levels, a high sucrose intake further increases triglyceride levels. For these people, sugar should be limited to decrease the risk of atherosclerosis. For other people, sugar con-

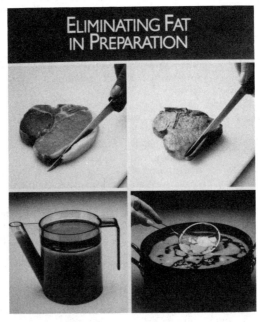

FIGURE 17–3. Selecting lean meat, trimming off visible fat, and skimming fat from meat juices reduce the amount of fat consumed. (From National Live Stock and Meat Board, Chicago, 1990, with permission.)

tributes to obesity, which is itself a risk factor for cardiovascular disease. Almost any recipe can be satisfactorily made using two thirds to three fourths the amount of sugar indicated. Increasing the amounts of vanilla extract and cinnamon will give the impression of sweetness.

Exercise

Exercise helps to control weight. In some studies, body weight was the most important single determinant of cholesterol level. Exercise raises the serum level of HDLs, which carry the cholesterol to the liver for the manufacture of bile, which in turn is excreted in the feces.

Aerobic exercise, that producing an acceptable target heart rate and requiring sustained effort, strengthens the heart and the blood vessels. It changes the proportions of lean and fatty tissue as long as the exercise is continued on a regular basis. If the regimen is abandoned, the proportion of fatty tissue will again increase.

Hypertension Prevention

Because atherosclerosis and hypertension share causative factors, the above strategies to prevent atherosclerosis also are recommended to prevent hypertension. Weight control, exercise, and a low-fat diet all will assist in lowering blood pressure. An estimated 50 percent of hypertensive cases could be prevented by weight control. Consequently, in mild hypertension, diet should receive a 6-week trial before other treatment measures are instituted. As in other lifestyle changes, participation in a dedicated group can provide valuable social support and behavioral reinforcement.

Not all persons with hypertension are salt sensitive, but moderate salt restriction meets the Dietary Guidelines. Whereas the average American consumes 4 to 6 grams of sodium per day, an upper limit of 2.3 grams per day is suggested. Salt can be eliminated from any recipe except one containing yeast. More is said about sodium-restricted diets later in this chapter.

Avoiding tension is an important step for the person with hypertension. Relaxation can be learned through various exercises. Healthy relaxation should be accomplished without the aid of smoking or drinking alcohol. Hypertensive patients should not smoke because of the vasoconstrictive effect of nicotine. Any alcohol consumption should be limited to 1 ounce per day. An exercise program will not only help reduce stress but also aid weight control.

DIETARY MODIFICATIONS IN CARDIOVASCULAR DISEASE

Persons who already have cardiovascular disease will have some of the same modifications to their diets as were discussed under prevention. Other dietary prescriptions are implemented depending on the nature and severity of the disease.

Energy Modifications

For the obese person, achieving weight loss requires exercising, practicing behavior modification techniques, and limiting intake of kilocalories. The important task of losing weight is discussed in detail in Chapter 15.

For the person who is sick, energy intake also must be modified. A person who is expending less energy will require fewer kilocalories. The patient with heart disease needs nutrient-dense meals to aid the healing process without burdening the gastrointestinal or circulatory systems.

Fat Modifications

Depending on the underlying pathology, a patient with cardiovascular disease may be instructed to modify fat to a greater extent than someone without disease. Because of its impact on some hyperlipoproteinemias, carbohydrate intake may be altered as well.

Some Fats Are Beneficial

Some forms of dietary fat are more healthful than others. Monounsaturated and polyunsaturated vegetable oils can help to decrease blood cholesterol levels. Omega-3 fatty acids decrease triglycerides and reduce platelet aggregation while decreasing the synthesis of VLDL. Eating cold-water fish or other food sources of omega-3 fatty acids is preferable to taking capsules because of the risk of hypervitaminosis A and D. Too much of virtually any food, including fish, can produce obesity.

Diet in Hyperlipoproteinemia

Beyond the general recommendations to lower saturated fat consumption, patients with hyperlipoproteinemia need more stringent diets. All of these patients who are overweight are urged to lose the excess weight. You may wish to refer again to Table 17–2 as you read about diet modifications for the different types of hyperlipoproteinemias.

TYPE 1   In this hyperlipoproteinemia, the person is deficient in the enzyme triglyceride lipase. Consequently, triglyceride cannot be broken down. The serum chylomicrons are elevated because they carry the exogenous triglyceride in the bloodstream after meals. To treat this condition, food sources of triglyceride are restricted. Usually a 20- to 30-gram fat diet is prescribed, which generally limits the person to 3 to 4 ounces of lean meat per day. The dietitian devises a dietary pattern in consultation with the patient.

TYPE 2A   The diet in Type 2A hyperlipoproteinemia contains less than 200 milligrams of cholesterol per day. LDL and cholesterol elevations characterize Type 2A hyperlipoproteinemia. Polyunsaturated and monounsaturated fats should outnumber saturated fats by a factor of 1.5 or 2 to 1.

TYPE 2B   In Type 2B hyperlipoproteinemia, the diet is the same as for Type 2A, plus limitation in alcohol and high-carbohydrate foods, especially simple sugars. In Type 2B hyperlipoproteinemia, triglyceride levels are elevated, whereas in Type 2A they are not. Alcohol and carbohydrate stimulate triglyceride production, and therefore are to be restricted. Usually the diet is calculated to provide only 40 percent of the kilocalories from carbohydrate.

TYPE 3   Carbohydrate aggravates Type 3 hyperlipoproteinemia. Here dietary carbohydrate is limited to 35 to 40 percent of kilocalories. Because triglycerides are elevated, alcohol and sugar should be restricted. If cholesterol levels continue to be high after weight loss, dietary cholesterol should be moderately reduced.

TYPE 4   This very common hyperlipoproteinemia also is aggravated by carbohydrate. Therefore only 35 to 40 percent of kilocalories come from carbohydrate. Triglycerides are elevated, so sugar intake should be limited. Alcohol should be consumed at a rate of 1 to 2 ounces per week, if at all.

TYPE 5   Type 5 hyperlipoproteinemia is treated the same as Type 4. In fact, excessive fat and kilocalorie intake can convert a severe Type 4 patient into a Type 5.

Because all hyperlipoproteinemias are not the same, neither are the dietary treatments. For best results, the clinical dietitian should individualize the diet with the patient. Although medications can assist in lowering lipid levels, experts advocate using drug therapy as an adjunct to diet modification, not as a replacement for it. The effect achieved by diet modification and drug therapy together is better than that of either one alone.

Sodium Modifications

Sodium restriction is used in the management of both hypertension and congestive heart failure. It also may be helpful in other edematous patients. Sodium-sensitive individuals benefit from dietary restriction of sodium. Among the persons likely to be sodium sensitive are blacks, persons over 50, patients with chronic renal disease, and persons with hypertensive parents, either one parent or both.

As many as one third of mild hypertensive cases can be controlled with salt restriction. This measure alone should decrease blood pressure by 8 millimeters of mercury. The goal is to limit sodium to 2 grams per day. This intervention may take up to 8 weeks to be effective.

It is difficult to break a habit and establish a new pattern. Fortunately, the desire for salty foods is a learned taste. What is learned can be unlearned. After 3 months on a sodium-restricted diet, most individuals lose their appetite for salt.

Sodium is also restricted for the patient with congestive heart failure. The purpose is to thwart the aldosterone sodium-saving mechanism. Along with diet, many medications assist in relieving the edema.

Sodium-Controlled Diets

The amount of sodium in foods can be calculated, just as kilocalories, fat, protein, carbohydrate, fiber, or any other nutrient can be calculated. Many dietitians will work with a patient to develop an individualized meal plan that stays within the diet prescription. Rather than follow a standard diet, some patients prefer a measured amount of salt to use as they wish every day. When this is done, they must curtail consumption of foods naturally high in sodium, more so than a routine diet prescription would demand.

Preparing a diet containing less than 2 grams of sodium is a difficult task. The 250-, 500-, and 1000-milligram sodium diets typically are prescribed for hospitalized patients or for a short time prior to laboratory tests. Table 17–5 summarizes the traditional sodium-restricted diets, including limitations by food groups.

TABLE 17–5 *Examples of Traditional Restricted-Sodium Meal Plans, Foods Higher, Lower, and Highest in Sodium*

	Meal Plans for Restricted-Sodium Meal Plan			
Food/Item or Group	2 Grams	1 Gram	500 mg	250 mg
Soups	LS*	LS	LS	LS
Milk	2 cups	2 cups	1 cup	LS
Bread	3 slices	3 slices	LS	LS
Cereal	1 serving	LS	LS	LS
Fruits	Free	Free	Free	Free
Egg	1	1	1	1
Meat/Substitutes	6 oz	5 oz	4 oz	4 oz
Vegetables	LS	LS	LS	LS
Desserts	1 serving	LS	LS	LS
Margarine	5 teas	3 teas	3 teas	LS
Condiments	LS	LS	LS	LS

*LS any food on the following lower in sodium list

Foods Higher and Lower in Sodium

Food/Item or Group	Higher in Sodium	Lower in Sodium (LS)
Milk, Yogurt	All milk from animals All yogurt	Commercially made low sodium milk
Cheese	Rinsed cottage cheese	Rinsed cottage cheese
Meat Group	Any fresh or frozen beef, lamb, pork, poultry, fish, and some shellfish Low-sodium peanut butter Dry peas and beans Eggs: 60 mg each	Any fresh or frozen beef, lamb, pork, poultry, fish, and some shellfish Low-sodium peanut butter Dry peas and beans
Bread	Commercially or homemade breads prepared with salt Plain rice and pastas prepared with added salt (small amounts)	Commercially or homemade breads prepared without salt Plain rice and pastas prepared without added salt
Cereal	Most ready-to-eat and cooked cereals	Puffed rice, puffed wheat, shredded wheat; hot cooked cereals without added salt
Fruits/Juices	Most fresh, frozen, and canned fruits All fruit juices	Most fresh, frozen, and canned fruits All fruit juices
Vegetables	Most, fresh, frozen, and low-sodium canned vegetables	Most fresh, frozen, and low-sodium canned vegetables
Desserts	Any commercial or homemade which contain less than 400 mg of sodium	Homemade without added salt
Margarine	Butter or margarine (50 milligrams of sodium per serving)	Low-sodium butter or margarine
Condiments	Low-sodium versions	Low-sodium versions

Foods highest in sodium, listed below, are not usually served on any sodium-restricted diet unless they are calculated into the diet on an individual basis.

TABLE 17–5 *Examples of Traditional Restricted-Sodium Meal Plans, Foods Higher, Lower, and Highest in Sodium (Continued)*

Selected High Sodium Foods (500 milligrams per serving)

Food Item/Group	Amount
Milk:	
Buttermilk	1 cup
Meat/Substitutes:	
Bologna or other lunch meat	1 ounce
Corned beef, cooked	1 ounce
Tuna fish, canned salted	¼ cup
Ham, cooked	1½ ounces
Frankfurter	1
Processed cheese (American)	1 ounce
Cottage cheese	½ cup*
Soup:	
Soup, regular canned	½ cup
Vegetable:	
Tomato or V-8 juice	1 cup
Condiments:	
Salt	¼ teaspoon

*Rinsing with water will reduce the sodium content considerably

Selected High Sodium Foods (200 milligrams per serving)

Meat substitutes:	
Peanut butter, salted	2 tablespoons
Vegetable:	
Sauerkraut	¼ cup
Tomato sauce, regular	2 tablespoons
Fat:	
Bacon	2 slices
Nuts, mixed and salted	2 tablespoons
Olives, small no pits	2
Snack Foods:	
Potato chips	20
Pretzels, thin twisted	2
Condiments:	
Barbecue sauce	1 tablespoon
Catsup	1 tablespoon
Chili sauce	1 tablespoon
Mayonnaise	1 tablespoon
Mustard	1 tablespoon
Salad dressings	1 tablespoon
Tartar sauce	1 tablespoon
Soy sauce	½ teaspoon
Pickle relish	2 tablespoons

Some patients may be permitted foods that are usually excluded from a particular sodium-restricted diet if the dietitian has designed individual patterns for them. For all levels of restriction, highly salted foods are eliminated. The salt content of processed foods is a major concern. For example, 1 cup of dried coconut contains 29 milligrams of sodium if it is unsweetened, compared with 244 milligrams for sweetened. Refer to Box 17-1 for the legal

---

BOX 17–1

Labeling Regulations for Sodium Content Descriptors

The following uniform definitions mean the same for any product on which they appear:

Term	Legal Definition
Free	Less than 5 milligrams of sodium per serving
Salt Free	Must meet the criteria for free
Very Low* Sodium	Less than 35 milligrams of sodium per serving. For meals and main dishes: 35 milligrams or less per 100 grams.
Low* Sodium	Less than 140 milligrams of sodium per serving. Meals and main dishes: 140 milligrams or less per 100 grams.
Reduced or Less	This term means that a nutritionally altered product contains 25 percent less sodium than the regular, or reference, product. However, a reduced claim can't be made on a product if its reference food already meets the requirement for a "low" claim.
Light in sodium or Lightly salted	May be used on food in which the sodium content has been reduced by at least 50 percent compared to an appropriate reference food.
Unsalted or No Added Salt	Must declare "This is not a sodium free food" on information panel if the food is not sodium free.

*Synonyms for low include "little," "few," and "low source of"

---

definitions of labeling terms such as sodium free, low sodium, and very low sodium. Check the serving size listed on labels; sometimes it is incredibly small.

In clinical practice, diet orders such as "no-added-salt diet" or "low-sodium diet" require clarification. Usually, a facility's diet manual defines the terms. A "no-added-salt diet" may be calculated as 4 grams of sodium and a "low-sodium diet" as 2 grams in one facility and at different levels in another. Not only should nurses not use those two terms interchangeably, but they should also alert physicians to local meanings of the terms.

Beverages

The contribution of sodium to drinking water should not be overlooked. The American Heart Association recommends a limit of 20 milligrams of sodium per liter of water as a standard for persons suffering from a heart ailment who require a restricted sodium diet. As much as 42 percent of the nation's water supply exceeds this amount (Korch, 1986). Many municipal water supplies are softened, which can increase the water's sodium content excessively. City water supplies vary from 1.2 milligrams per liter in Seattle to 100 milligrams per liter in Phoenix.

Many households have water softeners in their homes, increase the water's sodium content. Patients who need to adhere to a diet which contains less than 2 grams of sodium may need to use bottled, distilled, deionized, or demineralized water for drinking and cooking.

The sodium content of specialty bottled waters also needs to be considered. "Mineral waters" contain from 8 to 172 milligrams of sodium per liter. A sample of "spring waters" contained from 2 to 60 milligrams of sodium per liter. The advice to "read the label" applies with these products as well.

An additional problem for people who have to restrict sodium is selecting other beverages. Table 17–5, indicated that unlimited use of milk is not an option. Soft drinks also vary in the amount of sodium that they contain (see Table 17–6).

Flavorings and Seasonings

Creative methods of food preparation produce tasty products without adding salt. Table 17–7 lists some of the common flavorings and seasonings permitted in low-sodium diets. Categorization of flavors as "sweet" or "tangy" is a

TABLE 17–6 *Sodium Content of Beverages**

Beverage†	Regular		Diet	
	Sodium (milligrams)	Kilo-calories	Sodium (milligrams)	Kilo-calories
Club soda			75	0
Cola	15	151		
With aspartame			21	2
With saccharin			75	2
Gatorade	39	123		
Ginger ale	25	125	130	4
Koolade	0	150		
With aspartame			0	6
Lemonade	12	150		
Lemon-lime soda	41	149	70	4
Pepper-type	38	151	70	0
Root beer	49	152	170	4

*Serving size is 12 fluid ounces.

†Sodium content may vary, depending on the source of water.

TABLE 17–7 *Sodium-Free Flavorings and Seasonings*

Sweet	Tangy
Allspice	Basil
Almond extract	Bay leaves
Apricot nectar	Caraway seeds
Baking chocolate	Cayenne pepper
Cinnamon	Chives
Coriander	Cloves
Ginger	Curry powder
Lemon extract	Dill weed
Lemon juice	Garlic
Mace	Garlic powder, not salt
Maple extract	Green pepper
Mint	Horseradish
Nutmeg	Marjoram
Orange juice	Mustard powder, not prepared
Peppermint extract	Onion powder, not salt
Pineapple	Onions
Pineapple juice	Oregano
Unsalted pecans	Paprika
Vanilla extract	Parsley
Walnuts	Pepper
Walnut extract	Rosemary
	Sage
	Savory
	Sesame seeds
	Tarragon
	Thyme
	Turmeric

general guideline; experimentation should be encouraged. Cooking meat with nutmeg for example, might give the meat such a different taste that salt would not be missed. Fruit juices can be used as sauces or marinades.

A number of salt substitutes are available. Many of them use potassium instead of sodium. In some cases potassium is inappropriate. Some persons with kidney disease or individuals taking potassium-sparing diuretics are at risk for hyperkalemia. Salt substitutes are not really useful for cooking because they turn bitter.

Over-the-Counter Products

Many toothpastes and mouthwashes contain significant amounts of sodium. Patients should be instructed not to swallow these products. Over-the-counter medications often contain enough sodium to negate all the trouble the patient is taking with the diet. Some classes of drugs requiring caution in this regard are alkalizers, analgesics, antacids, antibiotics, antitussives, laxatives, and sedatives.

Fluid Restrictions

The patient who is retaining fluid may require restriction of fluids. In congestive heart failure, a limitation of 1.5 liters of oral intake in 24 hours is usual, coupled with a 2-gram sodium diet. Depending on the institution, patients who are on restricted fluids receive either a meal tray with no fluids on it or a meal tray containing a measured amount of liquid as allotted to the dietary department. In the first case, the nurses dispense the permitted fluids. In the second case, the nurses also have a designated amount available to administer medications.

Sometimes a patient is unwilling to follow a treatment regimen. Nurses do not have to police such patients as long as they are competent and are not hurting others. Charting Tips 17–1 identifies some of the documentation concerns that should be considered.

Potassium Modifications

Either too much or too little serum potassium can be lethal. Potassium is the major intracellular cation. When muscles contract or impulses are sent along nerves, potassium and sodium exchange places. Potassium leaves the cell and sodium enters. After the muscular contraction or the nerve impulse occurs, these cations return to their original sites, thus becoming available for the next contraction. Either hyperkalemia or hypokalemia can cause muscle weakness and heart irregularities (see Table 17–8).

Because it is a monovalent cation, potassium can be excreted by the kidney when the need for sodium or hydrogen is greater than the need for potassium. With the use of diuretics that are not sodium-specific, potassium is spilled along with the sodium. These are called potassium-wasting diuretics. Often, patients taking these diuretics are encouraged to eat potassium-rich foods or need to take potassium as a medication. Clinical Calculation 17–1 shows how to convert milliequivalents of supplementary potassium to milligrams of dietary potassium. Other diuretics are sodium-specific; they are called potassium-sparing diuretics. Patients taking these diuretics *have no need to increase their intake* of potassium-rich foods.

CHARTING TIPS 17–1

✓ Nurses generally chart a patient's physical progress thoroughly. Often, though, a change in emotional or mental state is omitted in charting for medical/surgical or geriatric patients. Both hypokalemia and hyperkalemia, however, have changes in emotions as symptoms (review Table 17–8).

✓ With the current emphasis on rapid discharge from acute care institutions, assessment of a patient's knowledge and ability to comply with a home care regimen is crucial. Knowledge and ability may be present, but willingness absent. Such information, when documented by quoting the patient, is important to include in the record.

TABLE 17–8 *Signs and Symptoms of Hypokalemia and Hyperkalemia*

	Hypokalemia	Hyperkalemia
General Appearance	Fatigued	Anxious
	Listless	Irritable
	Lethargic	Mental confusion
Cardiovascular/Immune System	Dysrhythmias	Irregular, slow pulse
	Weak, irregular pulse	
Gastrointestinal System	Nausea/vomiting	Abdominal cramps
	Paralytic ileus	Nausea
	Diminished bowel sounds	Diarrhea
Musculoskeletal System	Muscle weakness	Lower extremity weakness
	Leg cramps	
	Decreased muscle tone	
Neurological System	Paresthesias	
	Decreased reflexes	

Normally, since potassium is present in all cells, its intake is adequate if a regular diet is taken. The choices become more complex when a patient is also on a restricted-sodium diet. In general, fruits are high in potassium and low in sodium. A summary of sodium and potassium content of food exchanges appears in Table 17–9.

TABLE 17–9 *Sodium and Potassium Content in Food Exchanges*

Exchange	Amount	Sodium (milligrams)	Potassium (milligrams)	Comments
Starch/ Bread	1 slice regular	150	25	Unsalted available
	1 slice low-sodium	5	40	
Meat	1 ounce	30	80	If unprocessed
Vegetable	½ cup fresh or low-sodium canned	15	120 to 250	
	½ cup regular canned	250	Varies widely	
Fruit	½ banana, 9-inch fresh	0.5	185	If no preservatives added; potassium varies widely
	1 orange, 2½-inch diameter, fresh	1.0	200	
Milk	1 cup	120	370	Whole, 2 percent, skimmed all equal in sodium
Fat	Regular margarine	47	Trace	Unsalted margarines are available

Other Modifications

After a heart attack, the patient is in shock. One adaptive response of the body is to slow gastrointestinal function. Thus the patient should receive nothing by mouth while shock persists. Fluid is given intravenously to maintain fluid balance and to keep an access site open for intravenous medications.

As the patient recovers, the diet progresses from a 1000- to 1200-kilocalorie liquid diet to a soft, "cardiac" diet of small, frequent meals. Large meals can increase the workload of the heart. Food is served at a moderate temperature. Very hot or very cold foods are thought to produce irregular heart rhythms. Iced beverages have been routinely restricted in coronary care units. Recent evidence suggests this is necessary only for an identifiable minority of patients (Kirchhoff, 1990).

Caffeine should be avoided by patients after heart attacks. Normal people have been observed to have serious **arrhythmias** after 9 or more cups of coffee or tea. Persons with histories of abnormal rhythms showed the same effects after 2 cups. The hypertensive patient should use caffeine in moderation because it increases blood pressure.

Arrhythmia— Irregular heartbeat.

For the person in congestive heart failure, the diet order may read "as tolerated." This person's heart is failing. Food should be easily eaten and easily digested. Large meals, which would exert upward pressure on the chest, are undesirable. Liquid formulas can be used to provide nutrients without fullness. An active person confined to bed rest will require fewer kilocalories for resting energy expenditure.

The person who has had a stroke may have chewing or swallowing problems. Often, thicker rather than thinner liquids are easier for a person with swallowing difficulty to manage. In addition, stroke patients may be aphasic and unable to communicate their needs or desires.

Summary

Cardiovascular diseases are responsible for more deaths in the United States than are diseases of any other body system. Some of the causative factors such as age, sex, race, and heredity are beyond a person's control. Other factors such as obesity, cigarette smoking, exercise, dietary lipids, and sodium intake can be modified by a motivated person.

Underlying pathology in cardiovascular diseases involves both atherosclerosis and hypertension. Each reinforces the other in a vicious circle, often leading to coronary heart disease, congestive heart failure, or stroke.

The most important risk factors for coronary heart disease are cigarette smoking, hypertension, and elevated blood cholesterol. Obesity is the most important risk factor for hypertension.

Closely linked to cardiovascular diseases are specific elevations of blood lipids and lipoproteins. The most common hyperlipoproteinemia is type 4. It is aggravated by carbohydrate intake, which must be limited as part of the treatment.

Dietary prevention of cardiovascular disease concentrates on controlling weight, curtailing fat intake, and, for sodium-sensitive persons, restricting sodium. Alcohol increases blood triglycerides and blood pressure, and therefore is ill advised. Of special value in controlling blood lipids are limiting saturated fat intake; exercising aerobically, which increases HDL; and consuming omega-3 fatty acids, which decrease triglycerides.

Dietary modifications after the occurrence of cardiovascular disease follow the same principles as the preventive diets, plus modification of texture and amounts of foods and stimulant intake. Because the total therapeutic plan for the cardiovascular patient may increase the risk of hypokalemia or hyperkalemia, patient education is required.

A case study and a sample plan of care appear below. Both are designed to show you how the information you have studied in this chapter can be used in nursing practice.

CASE STUDY 17–1

Mr. Z. is a 59-year-old white man who was admitted to the acute care hospital with a diagnosis of possible myocardial infarction. Subsequent testing proved Mr. Z. did not have an infarction. His medical diagnoses are myocardial ischemia and type 4 hyperlipoproteinemia. He is being readied for discharge to home.

Mr. Z. is vice president for sales of a large manufacturing company. His business activities involve luncheon and dinner meetings at which alcohol consumption is common. He stated he has "at least one cocktail, usually two" with lunch and with dinner.

The clinical dietitian visited Mr. Z. to instruct him on the diet prescribed by the physician. After the dietitian left, Mr. Z. said to the nurse, "That diet is impossible for my situation. She just doesn't understand the business world. I don't believe there's anything wrong with my heart, anyway. It was just indigestion."

Providing patient care is a dynamic process. Based on the above information, the nurse added the following modifications to Mr. Z's nursing care plan.

NURSING CARE PLAN FOR MR. Z.

Assessment Data
Subjective:
    Reported alcohol intake of 2 to 4 ounces per day
    Perceived incompatibility of prescribed diet with lifestyle
    Stated disbelief in medical diagnosis
Objective: Elevated blood VLDL and triglyceride

Nursing Diagnosis
    Noncompliance: related to denial of illness and negative perception of
        treatment regimen as evidenced by statements to nurse

Desired Outcomes/Evaluation Criteria
    Patient will acknowledge consequences of noncompliant behavior by
        time of hospital discharge.

Nursing Actions/Interventions with Rationales in Italics
    1. Review pathophysiology of hyperlipoproteinemia and atherosclerosis with patient. *Mr. Z. is a competent adult. He is able to make his own choices. Repeating the information on atherosclerosis is an attempt to be sure his choice to reject the treatment regimen is informed.*

2. Analyze with patient the possibility of partial compliance. *Perhaps the many changes required are overwhelming Mr. Z. One or two alterations might be acceptable as a starting point.*
3. Obtain patient's permission to discuss discharge instructions with significant other. *Enlisting a support person might, over time, give Mr. Z. reason to reconsider his decision.*
4. Inform physician of extent of intended noncompliance. *This is a change in the patient's mental condition. It is appropriate to notify the physician and record it on the patient's medical record.*

STUDY AIDS

Chapter Review Questions

1. The underlying pathological processes in cardiovascular disease are:
   a. Atherosclerosis and hypertension
   b. Coronary occlusion and obesity
   c. Diabetes mellitus and cerebrovascular accidents
   d. Kidney failure and congestive heart failure

2. The first action a hypertensive patient should take to lower blood pressure is to:
   a. Restrict fluid to 1500 milliliters per day
   b. Eliminate saturated fat from the diet
   c. Lose weight if necessary
   d. Limit sodium intake to 1 gram per day

3. The carriers of cholesterol to the cells for storage are the
   a. Chylomicrons
   b. High-density lipoproteins
   c. Low-density lipoproteins
   d. Very low-density lipoproteins

4. Monounsaturated fats may help lower blood cholesterol levels. Which of the following are monounsaturated?
   a. Safflower and soybean oils
   b. Canola and peanut oils
   c. Sunflower seed and cottonseed oils
   d. Olive and corn oils

5. Soluble fiber also helps to lower blood cholesterol levels. Which of the following are good sources of soluble fiber?
   a. Broccoli and prunes
   b. Whole-wheat bread and grapes
   c. Green beans and raspberries
   d. Oats and legumes

6. Omega-3 fatty acids contribute to cardiovascular health by lowering triglyceride levels and reducing platelet aggregation. Good sources of these fatty acids are:
   a. Lobster, bass, and oysters
   b. Catfish, shrimp, and clams
   c. Perch, walleye, and pike
   d. Herring, salmon, and tuna

7. Products labeled "very low sodium" must contain less than _____ milligrams of sodium per serving.
   a. 20
   b. 35
   c. 50
   d. 65

8. Which of the following individuals are at increased risk of cardiovascular disease?
   a. Black women over 50 and white men
   b. White women under 40 and black men
   c. Blacks and women with diabetes
   d. White women and low-income blacks

9. The obese person is at increased risk of cardiovascular disease if the excess fat is concentrated in the:
   a. Abdominal area
   b. Hips and thighs
   c. Extremities
   d. Buttocks

10. A high sucrose intake is related to cardiovascular disease because:
    a. Many cardiac patients have a genetic deficiency of sucrase.
    b. A high-sugar diet causes hyperactivity and hypertension.
    c. Excess sugar has to be excreted, causing premature aging of the kidney.
    d. Sucrose stimulates triglyceride production by the body.

NCLEX-Style Quiz

Mr. T. is a 55-year-old black man being seen in a health clinic for hypertension. His blood pressure was 150/102 three months ago when first diagnosed. It has remained below that level but has not returned to normal. Today his blood pressure is 146/100.

Mr. T. is 5 feet 9 inches tall and weighs 173 pounds. He has a medium frame. When first diagnosed, he weighed 178 pounds. A weight-loss diet with no added salt was prescribed, but progress has been slow.

Now the physician is prescribing a 2-gram sodium diet and starting Mr. T. on a mild potassium-wasting diuretic. The clinic nurse is responsible for instructing the patient.

1. The clinic has printed diet instructions. Which of the following selections by the nurse indicates understanding of Mr. T.'s dietary needs?
   a. Low kilocalorie, low sodium, high potassium
   b. High carbohydrate, low fat, low sodium
   c. Low sodium, low potassium, high fiber
   d. High protein, low fat, low sodium

2. Before he or she instructs Mr. T., which of the following actions by the nurse would best assure his compliance with the diet?
   a. Doing a financial analysis to see if Mr. T. can afford the special foods on his new diet
   b. Finding out which favorite foods Mr. T. would have most difficulty giving up
   c. Listing the possible consequences of hypertension if it is not controlled
   d. Asking to see Mrs. T. to instruct her on the preparation of foods for the new diet

3. Which of the following breakfasts would be best for Mr. T.?
   a. Applesauce, raisin bran, 1 percent milk, and a bagel with cream cheese
   b. Canned pears, cornflakes, whole milk, and a cholesterol-free plain doughnut
   c. Cooked prunes, instant oatmeal, 2 percent milk, and raisin toast with margarine
   d. Orange juice, shredded wheat, skimmed milk, and whole-wheat toast with jelly

4. Mr. T. asks about using a salt substitute. Which of the following responses by the nurse is based on correct information?
   a. "You should not use salt substitutes because they are only crutches. You have to retrain your taste buds to reject saltiness."
   b. "Any of the major brands of light salt would be satisfactory."
   c. "Salt substitutes are contraindicated with the medication the doctor is prescribing for you."

d. "If you decide to use a salt substitute, do not use it for cooking because it turns bitter when heated."

5. Mr. T. has agreed to limit his alcohol intake to two drinks per week. He asks the nurse to recommend soft drinks compatible with his diet. Which of the following is the best choice?
a. Diet ginger ale
b. Club soda
c. Diet cola with aspartame
d. Gatorade

CLINICAL CALCULATION 17–1

Converting Milliequivalents of Potassium to Milligrams

Supplementary potassium is recommended for persons who cannot take sufficient dietary potassium. Suppose a patient is taking 20 milliequivalents of potassium three times a day with meals and the physician decides that the patient should get the needed potassium from dietary sources. How many milligrams of potassium would the patient need?

Milligram is a measure of weight. Milliequivalent is a measure of the concentration of electrolytes per volume of solution. The usual amount of solution reported is 1 liter. Dry medications, however, are labeled in milliequivalents also.

In order to convert milliequivalents to milligrams, we have to know the number of milliequivalents, the molecular weight of the substance (in this case potassium), and its valence.

Our problem states that the amount of medicinal potassium the patient is taking is 60 milliequivalents. We need two other values: atomic or molecular weight and valence. The atomic weight for potassium is 39.098. Potassium, like sodium, has a valence of 1.

The formula for converting milliequivalents to milligrams is:

$$milligrams = milliequivalents \times atomic\ weight \times valence$$

Filling in the values we know for this case, we have:

$$X = 60 \times 39.098 \times 1$$

$$X = 2345.9$$

Thus, 60 milliequivalents of potassium equals 2346 milligrams, or 2.346 grams.

BIBLIOGRAPHY

Bousquet, GL: Congestive heart failure: A review of nonpharmacologic therapies. Journal of Cardiovascular Nursing 4(3):35, 1990.

Brunner, LS and Suddarth, DS: Textbook of Medical-Surgical Nursing, ed 7. JB Lippincott, Philadelphia, 1992.

Burke, LE: Dietary management of hyperlipidemia. Journal of Cardiovascular Nursing 5(2):23, 1991.

Burtis, G, Davis, J, and Martin, S: Applied Nutrition and Diet Therapy. WB Saunders, Philadelphia, 1988.

Canobbio, MM: Cardiovascular Disorders. CV Mosby, St. Louis, 1990.

Carroll, KK: Review of clinical studies on cholesterol-lowering response to soy protein. J Am Diet Assoc 91(7):820, 1991.

Cella, JH and Watson, J: Nurse's Manual of Laboratory Tests. FA Davis, Philadelphia, 1989.

Cresanta, JL, et al: Nutrition and cardiovascular disease. In Halpern, SL (ed): Quick Reference to Clinical Nutrition. JB Lippincott, Philadelphia, 1987.

Criqui, MH, et al: Plasma triglyceride level and mortality from coronary heart disease. N Engl J Med 328(17):1220, 1993.

Dunn, FL: Diabetics and hyperlipidemia: An increased risk of atherosclerosis. Medical Management Dynamics 8:3, 1990.

Feldman, EB: Essentials of Clinical Nutrition. FA Davis, Philadelphia, 1988.

Fleury, J: The application of motivational theory to cardiovascular risk reduction. Image 24(3):229, 1992.

Food and Drug Administration: The New Food Label, FDA Backrounder. Department of Health and Human Services, BG 92-40, Washington, DC, 1992.

Freedman, DS, et al: Education, race, and high-density lipoprotein cholesterol among US adults. Am J Public Health 82(7):999, 1992.

Horne, MM, Heitz, UE, and Swearingen, PL: Fluid, Electrolyte, and Acid-Base Balance. Mosby Year Book, St Louis, 1991.

Hunninghake, DB, et al: The efficacy of intensive dietary therapy alone or combined with lovastatin in outpatients with hypercholesterolemia. N Engl J Med 382(17):1213, 1993.

Hunt, SM and Groff, JL: Advanced Nutrition and Human Metabolism. West, St. Paul, 1990.

Joint National Committee on Detection, Evaluation and Treatment of High Blood Pressure. National Institutes of Health, Bethesda, Md, 1992.

Kirchhoff, KT, et al: Electrocardiographic response to ice water ingestion. Heart Lung 19:41, 1990.

Korch, GC: Sodium content of potable water: Dietary significance. J Am Dietc Assoc 86(1): 80, 1986.

Kumanyika, SK and Charleston, JB. Lose weight and win: A church-based weight loss program for blood pressure control among black women. Patient Education and Counseling 19(1):19, 1992.

Kuo, PT, Kostis, JB, and Moreyra, AE: Treatment of hyperlipidemia to prevent development and progression of atherosclerosis. In Halpern, SL (ed): Quick Reference to Clinical Nutrition. JB Lippincott, Philadelphia, 1987.

Lankford, TR and Jacobs-Steward, PM: Foundations of Normal and Therapeutic Nutrition. John Wiley & Sons, New York, 1986.

Moore, MC: Pocket Guide to Nutrition and Diet Therapy, ed 2. CV Mosby, St. Louis, 1993.

Pagana, KD and Pagana, TJ: Mosby's Diagnostic and Laboratory Test Reference. Mosby Year Book, St Louis, 1992.

Pemberton, CM, et al: Mayo Clinic Diet Manual, ed 6. BC Decker, Philadelphia, 1987.

Scanlon, VT and Sanders, T: Essentials of Anatomy and Physiology. FA Davis, Philadelphia, 1991.

Stovsky, B: Nursing interventions for risk factor reduction. Nurs Clin North Am 27(1):257, 1992.

Stoy, DB: Controlling cholesterol with drugs. Am J of Nurs 89:1628, 1990.

United States Bureau of the Census: Statistical Abstract of the United States, ed 110. US Department of Commerce, Washington, DC, 1990.

United States Department of Agriculture, Human Information Service: The Food Guide. Home and Garden Bulletin, No. 252, Hyattsville, MD, 1992.

Van Horn, L, et al: Effects on serum lipids of adding instant oats to usual American diets. Am J Public Health 81(2):183, 1991.

Whitney, EB, Cataldo, CB, and Rolfes, SR: Understanding Normal and Clinical Nutrition, ed 3. West, St Paul, 1991.

Williams, SR: Nutrition and Diet Therapy, ed 6. CV Mosby, St Louis, 1989.

Chapter Eighteen

Diet in Renal Disease

Chapter Outline

Anatomy and Physiology of the Kidneys
  Internal Structure
  Functions
Kidney Disease
  Causes
  Hypertensive Kidney Disease
  Specific Tubular Abnormalities
  Glomerulonephritis
  Nephrotic Syndrome
  Nephrosclerosis
  Progressive Nature of Kidney Failure
Treatment for Renal Disease
  Dialysis
  Kidney Transplant
Nutritional Care of the Renal Patient
  Goals of Nutrition Therapy
  Dietary Components
  National Renal Diet
  Nutrient Guidelines for Adults with
    Renal Disease
  Renal Disease in Children
Kidney Stones
  Causes
  Treatment
Urinary Tract Infections

Key Terms

As a study aid, each key term is followed by the page number where the term is defined in the chapter. Terms that appear in **boldface** or <u>underscored</u> in the chapter text are located in the glossary.

Diet in Renal Disease

After completing this chapter, the student should be able to:

1. Identify the major causes of acute and chronic kidney failure.
2. List the goals of nutritional care for a patient with kidney disease.
3. List the nutrients commonly modified in the dietary treatment of kidney disease.
4. Discuss the relationship among kilocalorie intake, dietary protein utilization, and uremia.
5. Discuss the nutritional care of patients with kidney disease in relation to their medical treatment.

efore one can use diet therapy to treat kidney disease, one must understand the normal function of the kidneys and basic concepts of pathophysiology of renal diseases. (Renal means pertaining to the kidneys.) The nutritional care of patients with renal disease is complex. These patients must frequently learn not just one diet with one to seven nutrients controlled but several different diets as their medical condition changes, and along with it the treatment approach. Failure to follow through with necessary changes in dietary behavior can result in death. One aspect of working with these patients is that inattentiveness to dietary restrictions can be objectively measured in weight changes or changes in the blood chemistry.

This first chapter discusses the internal structure and functions of the kidneys. Common kidney diseases, major forms of treatment available for patients, and dietary treatment for renal disease are then presented. A brief discussion of urinary calculi and urinary tract infections concludes the chapter.

ANATOMY AND PHYSIOLOGY OF THE KIDNEYS

Internal Structure

Nephron—The structural and functional unit of the kidney. There are approximately 1 million nephrons in each kidney.

The functioning unit of the kidney is the **nephron.** Each kidney contains about a million nephrons. Figure 18–1 shows an individual nephron. Each nephron has two main parts. The first part is **Bowman's capsule.** Bowman's capsule is the cup-shaped top of the nephron. Inside Bowman's capsule is a network of blood capillaries called the **glomerulus** (plural, *glomeruli*). The second part of the nephron is the renal tubule. (A *tubule* is a small tube or canal.) The renal tubule is the rope-like portion of the nephron. This rope-like structure ends at the collecting tubule. Several nephrons usually share a single collecting tubule.

Bowman's capsule—Part of the nephron which encloses the glomerulus; functions as a filter in the formation of urine.

Functions

The kidneys assist in the internal regulation of the body by performing the following functions:

Glomerulus—A cluster of capillaries through which blood is delivered for filtration; a part of the nephron.

1. *Filtration.* The kidneys remove the end products of metabolism and substances that have accumulated in the blood in undesirable amounts during the filtration process. Substances removed from the blood include urea, creatinine, uric acid, and urates. Undesirable amounts of chloride, potassium, sodium, and hydrogen ions are also filtered from the blood. The **glomerular filtration rate** (GFR) is the amount of fluid filtered each minute by all the glomeruli of both kidneys and is one index of kidney function. This is normally about 125 milliliters per minute.

Glomerular filtration rate (GFR)—Amount of fluid filtered each minute by all glumeruli; an index of kidney function.

2. *Reabsorption.* Previously filtered substances (e.g., water and sodium) needed by the body are reabsorbed into the blood in the tubules.
3. *Secretion of Ions to Maintain Acid-Base Balance.* Secretion is the process of moving ions from the blood into the urine. Secretion allows for the amount of a particular substance to be excreted in the urine in concentrations greater than the concentration filtered from the plasma in the glomeruli. The kidneys regulate the balance

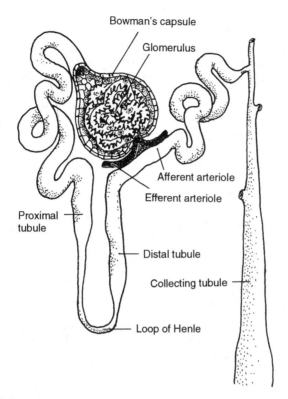

Bowman's capsule

Glomerulus

Afferent arteriole

Efferent arteriole

Proximal tubule

Distal tubule

Collecting tubule

Loop of Henle

FIGURE 18–1. An Individual Nephron. (With permission from Glyys, BA and Wedding, ME: Medical Terminology: A Systems Approach. ed. 2. FA Davis, Philadelphia, 1988.)

between bicarbonate and carbonic acid by the secretion and exchange of hydrogen ions for sodium ions, which are used to form base.

4. *Excretion.* The kidneys eliminate unwanted substances from the body as urine.

5. *Renal Control of Cardiac Output and Systemic Blood Pressure.* The kidneys adapt to changing cardiac output by altering resistance to blood flow both at the beginning of the glomerulus and at the end.

6. *Calcium, Phosphorus, and Vitamin D.* The kidneys produce the active form of vitamin D, calcitriol. Activated vitamin D regulates the absorption of calcium and phosphorus from the intestinal tract and assists in the regulation of calcium and phosphorus levels in the blood.

7. *Erythropoietin.* The kidneys produce a hormone called erythropoietin, which stimulates maturation of red blood cells in bone marrow.

KIDNEY DISEASE

Because the kidneys perform so many different metabolic functions, kidney disease has serious consequences. This section of the text discusses the causes of kidney disease and describes several common kidney disorders.

Causes

Renal disease can be caused by many factors, including trauma, infections, birth defects, medications, chronic disease (e.g., artherosclerosis, diabetes, hypertension), and toxic metal consumption. A physiological stress such as a myocardial infarction or an extensive burn can precipitate renal disease by decreasing the perfusion of the kidney or markedly increasing catabolism. Clinical Application 18–1, which describes the renal response after myocardial infarction, illustrates the effect of reduced renal blood flow. Catabolism causes an increase in nitrogenous products and potassium; these must be excreted, thus overworking the kidneys. There is some evidence that a habitually high intake of dietary protein can cause kidney damage. Renal disease is a feared complication of many pathologies and treatments.

Hypertensive Kidney Disease

High blood pressure can cause vascular or glomerular lesions. A <u>lesion</u> is an area of injured or diseased tissue.

Specific Tubular Abnormalities

A structural problem in the renal tubules may result in abnormal reabsorption or lack of reabsorption of certain substances by the tubules. The effect of a tubular abnormality is that the blood is not effectively cleansed.

Glomerulonephritis

Glomerulonephritis— Inflammation (nephritis) of the glomeruli. May be acute or chronic.

A general term for an inflammation of the kidneys is <u>nephritis.</u> Inflammation of the glomeruli is called **glomerulonephritis,** which can be either acute or chronic. This condition often follows scarlet fever or a streptococcal infection of the respiratory tract. Young children and young adults are often victims. Symptoms include nausea; vomiting; fever; hypertension; blood in the urine,

---

> ### CLINICAL APPLICATION 18–1
> #### Renal Response after a Myocardial Infarction
>
> Immediately after a heart attack or myocardial infarction, blood flow through the <u>systemic circulation</u> is diminished. Systemic circulation refers to the blood flow from the left part of the heart through the aorta and all branches (arteries) to the capillaries of the tissues. Systemic circulation also includes the blood's return to the heart through the veins. Following a heart attack, blood flow to the <u>myocardium,</u> or heart muscle, is decreased, and myocardial function is impaired. Less blood is thus delivered to the tissues. The kidneys sense the decreased cardiac output and try to compensate by reabsorption of additional water. This may lead to a fluid overload and edema. Most patients after a myocardial infarction are on fluid restriction for this reason.

or **hematuria;** a decreased output of urine, or **oliguria;** protein in the urine, or **proteinuria;** and edema. Recovery is usually complete. However, in some patients the disease progresses and becomes chronic. This leads to a progressive loss of kidney function. Some patients develop **anuria,** which is a total lack of urine output; without treatment, this condition is fatal.

Nephrotic Syndrome

The result of a variety of diseases that damage the glomeruli capillary walls is called **nephrotic syndrome.** Signs of nephrotic syndrome include proteinuria, severe edema, low serum protein levels, anemia, and hyperlipoproteinemia. Usually the higher the hyperlipoproteinemia, the greater the proteinuria. The disease is caused by the degenerative changes in the kidneys' capillary walls, which consequently permit the passage of albumin into the glomerular filtrate. Water and sodium are retained. Edema is sometimes so severe that it masks tissue wasting due to the breakdown of tissue protein stores. The degree of malnutrition is hidden until the excess fluid is removed.

Nephrosclerosis

A hardening of the renal arteries is known as nephrosclerosis. This condition is caused by arteriosclerosis and hypertension.

Progressive Nature of Kidney Failure

Kidney disease can be acute or chronic. In acute renal failure, the kidneys stop working entirely or almost entirely. Acute renal failure occurs suddenly and is usually temporary. It can last for a few days or weeks.

Chronic renal failure occurs when progressively more nephrons are destroyed until the kidneys simply cannot perform vital functions. Chronic renal failure occurs over time and is usually irreversible.

As individual nephrons are damaged, the remaining nephrons work harder to maintain metabolic homeostasis. As each functional nephron's workload is increased, the nephron becomes more susceptible to work overload and damage. The normal composition of the blood is altered when the remaining functional nephrons cannot assume any additional workload. Serum levels of blood urea nitrogen (BUN), creatinine, and uric acid become elevated. In some patients, even though the treatment of the underlying condition (e.g., diabetes mellitus or hypertension) is provided, chronic renal disease may lead to **end-stage renal failure.** During end-stage renal failure, most or all of the kidney's ability to produce urine and regulate blood chemistries is severely compromised.

Chronic renal failure often starts with sodium depletion. This occurs when the kidneys lose their ability to reabsorb sodium in the tubule. Symptoms associated with sodium depletion include a reduction of renal blood flow, dehydration, lethargy, decreased glomerular filtration rate, uremia (see below), and patient deterioration. The patient's blood pressure and body weight drop. Urine volume may be increased initially in chronic renal failure. A loss of body fat and protein content is responsible for the weight loss. The patient's serum albumin level may fall as protein is lost in the urine.

As kidney function further deteriorates, some of the above symptoms

Hematuria— Blood in the urine. Urine may be slightly smoky, reddish, or very red.

Oliguria—Diminished amount of urine formation.

Proteinuria— Protein in the urine. May be transient and benign or a symptom of severe renal disease.

Anuria— Absence of urine formation.

Nephrotic syndrome—The result of a variety of diseases that damage the glomeruli capillary wall.

End-stage renal failure—May occur as a result of chronic renal disease. Most or all of the kidney's ability to produce urine and regulate blood composition is severely compromised.

reverse. The kidneys lose the ability to excrete sodium. When this occurs, symptoms include sodium retention, overhydration, edema, hypertension, and congestive heart failure. The body can excrete little or no urine.

The glomerular filtration rate (GFR) gradually declines in chronic renal failure. Most patients with a GFR below 25 milliliters per minute will eventually require either dialysis or transplantation, regardless of the original cause of failure (Ahmed, 1991).

Uremia—Toxic condition associated with renal insufficiency produced by the retention in the blood of nitrogenous substances normally excreted in the kidneys.

If these measures were not implemented, uremia would develop. **Uremia** is the name given to the toxic condition associated with renal insufficiency. Uremia is produced by the retention in the blood of nitrogenous substances normally excreted by the kidneys. The uremic patient manifests many symptoms in virtually every body system as toxic waste products build up in the blood. The patient may complain of fatigue, weakness, and decreased mental ability. The patient's muscles may twitch and cramp. Anorexia, nausea, vomiting, and stomatitis an inflammation of the mouth, may be present. Sometimes patients complain of an unpleasant taste in the mouth. To further complicate matters, gastrointestinal ulcers and bleeding are common. All of these symptoms have a direct effect on the patient's willingness to eat.

Much research is under way to find a way to halt the progression of chronic renal failure. Substantial evidence has accumulated in recent years that restriction of dietary protein and phosphorus can retard the progression of chronic renal failure (Zeller et al, 1991). The idea is to decrease the work of the kidneys and thereby increase the kidneys' productive life span. Dietary intervention is now instituted simultaneously with initial diagnosis.

TREATMENT FOR RENAL DISEASE

Renal functions cannot be assumed by another organ. There is no cure for chronic renal failure. However, many patients can be treated with dialysis (an artificial kidney) and/or a kidney transplant. Artificial kidneys have been used for about 35 years to treat patients with severe kidney failure.

Dialysis—The passage of solute through a membrane; removes toxic materials and maintains fluid, electrolyte, and acid-base balance in cases of impaired kidney function or absence of kidneys.

Dialysis

Dialysis means the passage of solutes through a membrane. Two functions of the kidneys are (1) the removal of waste products and (2) the regulation of fluid and electrolyte balance. By removing waste products from the blood and assisting in the maintenance of fluid balance, dialysis reduces the symptoms of uremia, hypertension, edema, and the risk of congestive heart failure. Dialysis cannot restore the lost hormonal functions of the kidney. In addition, dialysis cannot correct the anemia, which occurs due to a lack of erythropoietin. Some dialysis patients still need treatment for hypertension.

Hemodialysis— A method of providing the function of the kidneys by circulating blood through a machine that contains synthetic semi-permeable membranes.

Hemodialysis

During **hemodialysis,** blood is removed from the patient's artery through a tube, forced to flow over a semipermeable membrane where waste is removed, and then rerouted back into the patient's body through a vein. A solution called the dialysate is placed on one side of the semipermeable membrane while the patient's blood flows on the other side. The dialysate is similar in composition to normal blood plasma. The blood has a higher concentration of urea and electrolytes than the dialysate, so these substances diffuse from the blood. The dialysate also contains glucose, and the more glucose the dialysate contains, the more fluid will move from the blood to the dialysate by osmosis. This process pulls extra fluid from the blood. The composition of the dialysate varies according to the requirements of each patient.

Hemodialysis treatments usually last 4 to 8 hours and are administered three times per week. Some patients are taught to perform their own dialysis treatments at home. Dialysis is not as effective as normal kidney function because blood cleansing occurs only when patients are attached to artificial kidneys. Normal kidneys clear the blood 24 hours a day 7 days a week.

Peritoneal Dialysis

The peritoneum is the lining of the abdominal cavity. During peritoneal dialysis, the dialysate is placed directly into the patient's abdomen. The dialysate enters the body through a permanent catheter placed in the abdominal cavity. The peritoneum thus functions as the semipermeable membrane.

INTERMITTENT PERITONEAL DIALYSIS Between 1 and 2 liters of fluid are introduced into the abdominal cavity during intermittent peritoneal dialysis. The fluid is allowed to remain in the abdomen for about 30 minutes and then drained from the body by gravity. One complete exchange takes about an hour. This process is repeated until the blood urea nitrogen level drops.

CONTINUOUS AMBULATORY PERITONEAL DIALYSIS Continuous ambulatory peritoneal dialysis (CAPD) is the dialysis method chosen by many patients. This is a form of self-dialysis. About 1 liter of dialysate is introduced into the abdominal cavity. The fluid remains in the cavity for 4 to 6 hours while the waste products diffuse into the dialysate. The dialysate is then replaced with a new solution. Patients can move about and pursue their activities of daily living during CAPD. The term "continuous" means that the patient is dialyzing constantly. The advantage of CAPD is that the patient's blood levels of sodium, potassium, creatinine, and nitrogen are kept within a much more stable range. Large shifts in fluid balance are also avoided.

Continuous ambulatory peritoneal dialysis (CAPD)—Method of self-dialysis chosen by many patients. The lining of the peritoneal cavity is used as the dialysis membrane.

Kidney Transplant

A kidney transplant can restore full renal function. Immunosuppressants to prevent rejection of the transplanted kidney are necessary. Some commonly used immunosuppressants are azathioprine, corticosteroids, and/or cyclosporine. These medications have many side effects, including diarrhea, nausea, and vomiting, which influence nutrient intake and absorption.

NUTRITIONAL CARE OF THE RENAL PATIENT

The nutritional needs of patients with renal diseases are changing constantly. The reason for the change is that the disease state and treatment approach are not static. Patients with kidney disease require constant assessment, monitoring, and counseling. In addition, it is an ongoing challenge to provide quality nutritional care to these patients, who frequently must be coaxed to eat. Anorexia, nausea, and vomiting are frequent complaints. It is common for the dietitian to see these patients more than once per day for nutritional problems during hospitalization.

Goals of Nutrition Therapy

Well-planned nutritional management is a fundamental part of any treatment for renal disease. Every patient with renal disease requires an individualized diet based on the following goals:

1. Attain and maintain optimal nutritional status.
2. Prevent net protein catabolism.
3. Minimize uremic toxicity.
4. Maintain adequate hydration status.
5. Maintain normal serum potassium levels.
6. Control the progression of renal osteodystrophy (see below).
7. Modify diet to meet other nutrition-related concerns such as diabetes, heart disease, gastrointestinal tract ulcers, and/or constipation.
8. Retard the progression of renal failure and postpone the initiation of dialysis.

No single diet is appropriate for all renal patients. Every patient requires an individual assessment.

Dietary Components

Several basic components need to be monitored and, if possible, controlled in renal diets. These components are:

- Kilocalories
- Protein
- Sodium
- Potassium
- Phosphorus and calcium
- Fluid
- Saturated fat and cholesterol
- Iron, vitamins, and minerals

The need to restrict or encourage the consumption of any of the above nutrients changes according to the patient's medical status and treatment approach. For example, it may not be necessary for a patient to control his or her phosphorus intake at one time but vital at another time.

Kilocalories

Intake of kilocalories is often increased for patients with renal disease. Patients on high-kilocalorie diets are usually given all the simple carbohydrates and monounsaturated and polyunsaturated fats they will eat. The end products of fat and carbohydrate catabolism are carbon dioxide and water. Neither of these dietary constituents imposes a burden on the patient's compromised excretory ability. Inadequate nonprotein kilocalories will, however, encourage tissue breakdown and aggravate the uremia. An adequate intake of kilocalories is crucial to the success of the dietary treatment.

Some individuals with diabetes mellitus and renal diseases still need to have their blood sugar levels controlled. For these patients, it may or may not be advisable to increase simple carbohydrates. The need to control the blood sugar is sometimes a secondary concern. In some situations, the primary nutritional goal is to decrease the uremia. Uremic diabetic patients may have relatively high amounts of sugar planned into their diets.

Some renal patients require an alternate feeding route to attain and maintain optimal nutritional status. Accordingly, some physicians order a peripheral intravenous infusion of lipids to supplement oral feedings. Total parenteral nutrition solutions for renal patients are commercially available.

Protein

A primary goal of nutritional therapy in renal patients is control of nitrogen intake. Control may mean an increase or decrease of dietary protein as the patient's medical condition and treatment approach change. In addition, the kind of protein fed to the patient may be important. High-biological-value protein is indicated for patients with an extremely high blood urea nitrogen (BUN) level. Eggs, meat, and dairy products are examples of foods that contain protein of high biological value. Protein restrictions are only effective if the patient also consumes adequate kilocalories. Beginning renal insufficiency is usually referred to as a predialysis situation and requires a restriction of protein intake.

The treatment approach selected by the patient and the physician influences protein requirements. Hemodialysis patients sometimes need increased protein because hemodialysis results in a loss of 1 to 2 grams of amino acids per hour of dialysis. A patient on CAPD has an even higher protein need because he or she dialyzes continuously. During dialysis, protein passes out of the blood with the waste products and into the dialysate fluid. When the dialysate fluid is discarded, a significant amount of protein is lost from the body. A high-protein diet is necessary to replenish these losses.

Sodium

The desirable sodium intake of renal patients depends on individual circumstances and is usually determined by repeated measurements of sodium in the serum and in the urine (if any). The sodium intake of many patients with renal failure must be restricted to prevent sodium retention in the body with consequent generalized edema (Burton and Hirschman, 1983).

The disease that precipitated the renal failure plays a role in determining the need for a sodium restriction. Because glomerulonephritis, for example, is more likely to produce hypertension and fluid retention, a sodium restriction is often necessary. Other renal diseases, such as pyelonephritis, are often characterized by low levels of sodium, absence of edema, and normal or low blood pressure. Pyelonephritis is an inflammation of the central portion of the kidney. In this situation, sodium intake should be higher than in the other groups of diseases but individualized to the patient's needs.

Potassium

Dietary potassium, like sodium, needs to be evaluated on an individual basis. Hypokalemia (low blood potassium level) needs to be avoided because it introduces the danger of cardiac arrhythmias and eventually cardiac arrest.

Table 18–1 lists foods high and low in potassium. Salt substitutes are very high in potassium and should be *avoided* by most renal patients. Generally the need to restrict potassium increases with decreased urinary output.

The potassium content of fruits and vegetables varies according to the form eaten and the method of food preparation. For example, ½ cup of canned pears in heavy syrup has a potassium content of about 80 milligrams, while one fresh pear has a potassium content of about 200 milligrams. Potassium is water soluble. For this reason, some renal patients on very potassium-restricted diets are taught to use large amounts of water when preparing vegetables and to discard the water after cooking. This decreases the potassium content of the vegetables. Unfortunately, it also decreases the water-soluble vitamins in the food. This is one reason why most renal patients need vitamin supplements. Patients should be taught to eat the fruits or vegetables in the form given on the list.

Phosphorus, Vitamin D, and Calcium

Phosphorus, vitamin D, and calcium are all normally balanced in the body. In patients with kidney disease, vitamin D cannot be activated. This leads to a low serum calcium level. At the same time, the kidneys cannot excrete phosphorus. This leads to an elevated serum phosphorus level. When the serum calcium level drops, calcium is released from the bones because of the increased secretion of parathyroid hormone (PTH). PTH is secreted in an effort to correct the calcium imbalance. This chain of events may lead to **renal osteodystrophy,** which is a complication of chronic renal disease. Renal osteodystrophy leads to faulty bone formation.

Renal osteodystrophy—Pathological changes in bone which often accompany renal failure in which calcium is lost from the bones.

Control of the blood levels of calcium and phosphorus involve four treatment approaches. First, patients with hypocalcemia and hyperphosphatemia are currently given calcitriol, the activated form of vitamin D. Second, phosphate binders are frequently used if the phosphorus level of the blood is elevated. Phosphate binders work in the intestinal tract by binding dietary phosphorus and preventing its absorption into the blood. Phosphate binders are high in aluminum, which has been found to be elevated in the brains of patients receiving aluminum hydroxide or aluminum carbonate binders. Some researchers link the high levels of aluminum in the tissues of dialyzed patients to dialysis dementia. Dialysis dementia is a progressive loss of mental function seen in patients who have been on dialysis for a number of years. The third treatment approach is a dietary phosphorus restriction. Dietary phosphorus restriction is currently recommended over the use of phosphate binders; the intent is to minimize the problem of dialysis dementia. Fourth, calcium supplements and/or a high-calcium diet is frequently prescribed if the serum phosphorus is under control.

Phosphorus is found mainly in meat and dairy products. Patients on protein-restricted diets generally do not eat enough phosphorus to cause hyperphosphatemia. Patients on chronic renal dialysis with a more liberal protein intake may need to limit the intake of dairy products that are high in phosphorus.

Fluid

Predialysis (renal-insufficiency) and dialysis patients generally must restrict fluid intake because their kidneys can no longer excrete excess fluid. Fluids

TABLE 18–1 *Foods High and Low in Potassium*

HIGH-POTASSIUM FOODS TO AVOID

Dairy products	(In excess)
Meats	(In excess)
Starches	Bran cereals and bran products
Fruits	Avocado
	Bananas
	Orange, fresh
	Mango, fresh
	Nectarines
	Papayas
	Dried prunes
	(All others if eaten in excess of allowance)
Vegetables	Bamboo shoots
	Beet greens
	Baked potato, with skin
	Sweet potato, fresh
	Spinach, cooked
	(All others if eaten in excess of allowance)
Others	Chocolate, cocoa
	Molasses
	Salt substitute
	Low-sodium broth
	Low-sodium baking powder
	Low-sodium baking soda
	Nuts

LOW-POTASSIUM FOODS*

Gum drops
Hard clear candy
Nondairy topping
Honey
Jams and jellies
Jelly beans
Lollipops
Marshmallows
Suckers
Sugar
Lifesavers
Chewing gum
"Poly-Rich"
Cornstarch
Low-Potassium Beverages
   Carbonated beverages
   Lemonade
   Limeade
   Cranberry juice
   Popsicles (1 stick = 60 milliliters of fluid)
   Hawaiian punch
   Kool-Aid
Low-Potassium Unsweetened Beverages
   Diet carbonated beverages
   Diet lemonade
   Diet Kool-Aid

*Note: Foods with sugar should not be eaten freely by diabetics.

need to be allocated between meals and medications. Table 18–2 lists guidelines to follow for distributing fluids between meals and medications. Patients on hemodialysis are restricted to "500 to 1000 milliliters plus 24-hour urinary output." This allows for some fluid gain between dialysis treatments. For predialysis patients, fluid restrictions are usually "500 milliliters plus output." For patients on CAPD, fluid restriction is "as tolerated" according to their daily weight fluctuations and blood pressure.

Saturated Fat and Cholesterol

Patients with renal disease frequently have hyperlipoproteinemia. High serum lipid levels are thought to aid in the progression of renal disease which contributes to an increased risk of cardiovascular disease. Total cholesterol levels may be increased tenfold (American Dietetic Association, 1992).This is believed to be especially a problem in patients with nephrotic syndrome, diabetes, and for an LCAT deficiency. LCAT is an enzyme that transports cholesterol from tissues to the liver for removal from the body. Most patients with an LCAT deficiency develop progressive glomerular injury.

Significant hypertriglyceridemia is often present in patients with a history of renal disease. The nutritional care of patients with elevated triglycerides (type 4 hyperlipoproteinemia) includes a modified fat diet and a modification of carbohydrate intake. Patients are usually counseled to avoid saturated fat and to increase their intake of polyunsaturated and monounsaturated fat. Thirty to 35 percent of the total kilocalories are provided as fat because excessive carbohydrate could worsen the hypertriglyceridemia (Moore, 1993). Simple sugars and alcohol are usually limited for the same reason.

TABLE 18–2 *Guidelines for Fluid-Restricted Patients*

If the Fluid Restriction Is:	Use This Amount of Fluids with Meals:	Use This Amount of Fluids with Medication:
1000 milliliters (4 cups)*	600 milliliters (2½ cups)	400 milliliters (1½ cups)
1200 milliliters (5 cups)	700 milliliters (3 cups)	500 milliliters (2 cups)
1500 milliliters (6 cups)	1000 milliliters (4 cups)	500 milliliters (2 cups)
2000 milliliters (8 cups)	1000 milliliters (4 cups)	1000 milliliters (4 cups)

All foods contain some fluids, but it is especially important to count the following as part of the fluid allowance:

Milliliters of Fluid per ½ Cup

Water	120		All juices	120		Watermelon	100
Coffee	120		pop	120		Sherbet	65
Tea	120		Ice	60		Ice cream	40
Sanka	120		Gelatin	100		Ice milk	40
Milk	120		Soup	120		Popsicle	80

*Approximate

Iron

The anemias seen in patients with renal disease may be due to a lack of ery-thropoietin; a decreased oral iron intake, which often occurs as a result of dietary restriction; or blood loss. Epoetin alfa, a pharmaceutical form of ery-thropoietin, may be used to increase red blood cell production and thereby correct the anemia. The treatment for iron-deficiency anemia is oral or par-enteral iron products and an increase in dietary sources of iron. A diagnosis of iron-deficiency anemia can be made by a laboratory measure of <u>ferritin.</u> Fer-ritin is the storage form of iron found primarily in the liver. A small amount of ferritin circulates in the blood and reflects the amount of iron in body stores. A laboratory value of less than 12 micrograms per liter suggests iron deficiency.

Nutritional therapy with iron supplements consists of 200 milligrams of ferrous iron salts per day divided among three to four doses. Absorption is enhanced when iron supplements are taken on an empty stomach or with vitamin C.

Vitamin and Mineral Supplementation

Patients with renal disease may require vitamin-mineral supplementation. Poor food intake may occur due to anorexia or as a result of dietary restric-tions. Vitamin C, B_6, zinc, and folic acid may be lost during dialysis. A potas-sium restriction may impede adequate intake of both vitamin C and folic acid. A low zinc intake may be caused by a low protein intake. In addition, blood loss and infections may increase the individual's requirements.

National Renal Diet

The American Dietetic Association and the National Kidney Foundation introduced the "National Renal Diet" in the fall of 1993. Because the dietary management of renal disease is tailored to the stage of disease and treatment approach, six meal-planning systems were developed. They are: renal insufficiency without diabetes; renal insufficiency with diabetes; hemodialysis without diabetes; hemodialysis with diabetes; peritoneal dialy-sis without diabetes; and peritoneal dialysis with diabetes. These national meal-planning systems offer standardized guidelines for nutrition interven-tion and patient education.

Each system provides food lists and calculation figures (derived from the average nutrient content of foods included in each list). Although the food lists developed for the patient booklets were patterned after the *ADA Exchange Lists*, the varied nutritional requirements of patients with renal dis-ease at different stages of treatment necessitated creation of specific food lists for each treatment modality. Box 18–1 shows the General Dietary Rec-ommendations for Renal Patients by treatment approach. In addition, sepa-rate calculation figures and food lists were devised for patients with diabetes receiving each treatment modality, because foods high in sugars were excluded from the food lists for patients with diabetes.

Box 18–2 is an example of the calculation of a diet for a patient receiv-ing hemodialysis without diabetes (one of the six meal-planning systems). A case study and sample meal plan are shown. Box 18–3 is a condensed food list for the patient with chronic renal failure who is receiving hemodialysis treatments. A sample menu derived from the condensed renal food list and the sample daily meal plan follow.

BOX 18–1

General Dietary Recommendations for Renal Patients

Dietary Component	Renal Insufficiency	Hemodialysis	Peritoneal Dialysis
Protein (grams per kilogram HBW)*	0.6–0.8†	1.1–1.4	1.2–1.5
Energy (kilo-calories per kilogram HBW)	35–40	30–35	25–35
Phosphorus (milligrams per kilogram HBW)	8–12‡	≤17§	≤17
Sodium (milligrams per day)	1000–3000	2000–3000	2000–4000
Potassium (milligrams per kilogram HBW)	Typically not restricted	40	Typically not restricted
Fluid (milliliters per day)	Typically not restricted	500–750 plus daily urine output or 1000 if anuric	≥2000
Calcium (milligrams per day)	1200–1600	Depends on serum level	Depends on serum level

*HBW = healthy body weight.

†The upper end of this range is preferred for patients with diabetes or malnutrition. Suggested protein intake for persons with nephrotic syndrome is 0.8 to 1.0 grams per kilogram HBW.

‡Intake of 5 to 10 milligrams phosphorus per kilogram HBW is frequently quoted in the scientific literature, but 5 milligrams per kilogram HBW is practical only when used in conjunction with a very low-protein diet supplemented with specially formulated commercial feedings.

§It may not be possible to meet the optimum phosphorus prescription on a higher protein diet.

Source: Monsen, ER: Meeting the challenge of the renal diet. Copyright The American Dietetic Association. Reprinted by permission from Journal of the American Dietetic Association, vol. 93;6, p 638, 1993.

BOX 18–2

Calculating the Renal Diet: Hemodialysis Case Study

▼Average Calculation Figures for Renal Diets (No Diabetes)*

Food Choices	Energy kcal	PRO g	CHO g	FAT g	Na mg	K mg	P mg
Milk	120	4	8	5	80	185	110
Nondairy milk-substitute	140	0.5	12	10	40	80	30
Meat	65	7	...	4	25	100	65
Starch	90	2	18	1	80	35	35
Vegetable							
Low potassium	25	1	5	tr	15	70	20
Medium potassium	25	1	5	tr	15	150	20
High potassium	25	1	5	tr	15	270	20
Fruit							
Low potassium	70	0.5	17	...	tr	70	15
Medium potassium	70	0.5	17	...	tr	150	15
High potassium	70	0.5	17	...	tr	270	15
Fat	45	...	...	5	55	10	5
High-calorie	100	tr	25	...	15	20	5
Salt	...	...	...	...	250	...	...

▼Case Example

The patient is a 55-year-old man who works full-time and has a sedentary lifestyle. He is 5 feet 10 inches tall, has a medium frame, and weighs 68 kilograms. His ideal and usual weight is 76 kilograms. During the past 6–9 months, he has been anorectic and has had intermittent nausea and episodes of vomiting. He receives 4 hours of hemodialysis 3 times per week. His predialysis blood chemistry values were blood urea nitrogen, 22.50 millimoles per liter (63 milligrams per deciliter); sodium, 135 millimoles per liter (135 milliequivalents per liter); potassium, 4.0 millimoles per liter (4.0 milliequivalents per liter); phosphorus, 2.0 millimoles per liter (6.2 milligrams per deciliter); calcium, 2.25 millimoles per liter (9.0 milligrams per deciliter); and albumin, 33 grams per liter (3.3 grams per deciliter). His urine output ranges between 800 and 1000 milliliters per day.

Box continued on next page.

BOX 18–2 *(Continued)*

Calculating the Renal Diet: Hemodialysis Case Study

▼Daily Renal Diet Plan Goals

Nutrient	Level	Rationale
Energy (kcal)	3000	40 kcal per kg HBW
Protein (g)	91	1.2 g per kg HBW
Sodium (mg)	2000	Control fluid weight gain
Potassium (mg)	3000(75 mEq)	−40 mg per kg HBW
Phosphorus (mg)	1300	≤17 mg per kg HBW
Fluid (mL)	1500–1750	750 mL plus urine output

▼Sample Calculation of Renal Diet Plan For Hemodialysis

Food Choices	Choices no.	Energy kcal	PRO g	Na mg	K mg	P mg
Milk	1	120	4	80	185	110
Nondairy milk-substitute	1	140	0.5	40	80	30
Meat	9	585	63	225	900	585
Starch	10	900	20	800	350	350
Vegetable	2	50	2	30	...	40
Low potassium		...	...	...	...	...
Medium potassium	(1)	...	...	...	150	...
High potassium	(1)	...	...	...	270	...
Fruit	3	210	1.5	...	...	45
Low potassium		...	...	...	...	...
Medium potassium	(1)	...	...	...	150	...
High potassium	(2)	...	...	...	540	...
Fat	10	450	...	550	100	50
High-calorie	5	500	...	75	100	25
Salt	1	...	...	250	...	...
Totals		2955	91	2050	2825	1235

*Because control of fat and carbohydrate intake is not a priority for all patients, practitioners may include their calculation in the meal plan on a case-by-case basis. Table abbreviations: PRO = protein, CHO = carbohydrate, Na = sodium, K = potassium, P = phosphorus, tr = trace, HBW = healthy body weight.

Source: Monsen, ER: Meeting the challenge of the renal diet. Copyright The American Dietetic Association. Reprinted by permission from Journal of theDietetic Association, Vol. 93: 6, p. 638, 1993.

BOX 18–3

Condensed Renal Food Lists for Chronic Renal Failure, Hemodialysis

Milk List

Approximate Nutrient Content: 4 grams protein, 120 kilocalories, 80 milligrams sodium (Na), 185 milligrams potassium (K), 110 milligrams phosphorus (P)

Item	Amount
Milk	½ cup
Alterna	1 cup
Cream cheese	3 tablespoonfuls

Nondairy Milk Substitutes

Approximate Nutrient Content: 0.5 grams protein, 140 kilocalories, 40 milligrams Na, 80 milligrams K, 30 milligrams P

Liquid nondairy creamer, polyunsaturated	½ cup
Dessert topping, nondairy, frozen	½ cup

Meat List

Approximate Nutrient Content: 7 grams protein, 65 kilocalories, 25 milligrams Na, 100 milligrams K, 65 milligrams P

Low-cholesterol egg substitute	¼ cup
Lean beef, pork, poultry	1 ounce
Unsalted canned tuna	¼ cup

Starch List

Approximate Nutrient Content: 2 grams protein, 90 kilocalories, 80 milligrams Na, 35 milligrams K, 35 milligrams P

Bread (white, light rye, sourdough)	1 slice
Saltines, unsalted	4
Puffed wheat	1 cup
Rice, cooked	½ cup
Angel Food Cake	1 ounce

Box continued on next page.

BOX 18–3 *(Continued)*

Vegetable List

Approximate Nutrient Content: 1 gram protein, 25 kilocalories, 15 milligrams Na, 20 milligrams P; serving size is ½ cup unless otherwise noted; prepared or canned without salt

Low Potassium
(0 to 100 milligrams K)

Lettuce, all varieties	1 cup
cucumber, peeled	

Medium Potassium
(101 to 200 milligrams K)

Carrots	1 small, raw
Corn	½ ear
Broccoli	½ cup

High Potassium
(201 to 350 milligrams K)

Tomato	1 medium
Potato, baked	½ medium
Spinach, cooked	

Fruit List

Approximate Nutrient Content: 0.5 grams protein, 70 kilocalories, 15 milligrams P; serving size is ½ cup, unless otherwise noted

Low Potassium
(0 to 100 milligrams K)

Applesauce

Pears, canned

Medium Potassium
(101 to 200 milligrams K)

Apple, fresh	1 small
Watermelon	1 cup

High Potassium
(201 to 350 milligrams K)

Orange juice	
Pear, fresh	1 medium

Box continued on next page.

BOX 18–3 *(Continued)*

Fat List

Approximate Nutrient Content: trace protein, 45 kilocalories, 55 milligrams Na, 10 milligrams K, 5 milligrams P

Unsaturated Fats

Margarine	1 teaspoonful
Mayonnaise	1 teaspoonful

Saturated Fats

Coconut	2 tablespoonfuls
Powdered coffee whitener	1 tablespoonful

High-Kilocalorie Choices

Approximate Nutrient Content: 100 kilocalories, 15 milligrams Na, 20 milligrams K, 5 milligrams P

Carbonated beverages, fruit flavors, root beer	1 cup
Kool-Aid	1 cup
Lemonade	1 cup
Tang	1 cup
Gum drops	15

Chronic Renal Failure, Hemodialysis Meal Plan and Sample Menu

Meal Plan	Sample Menu
Breakfast	
1 nondairy milk substitute	½ cup liquid nondairy creamer, polyunsaturated
1 high-potassium fruit	½ cup orange juice
2 starches	1 cup puffed wheat and 1 slice light rye toast
1 meat	¼ cup low-cholesterol egg substitute
2 fats	2 teaspoonfuls margarine
Morning Snack	
1 high-kilocalorie	1 cup Tang

Box continued on next page.

BOX 18–3 *(Continued)*

Chronic Renal Failure, Hemodialysis Meal Plan and Sample Menu

Meal Plan	Sample Menu
Breakfast	
1 nondairy milk substitute	½ cup liquid nondairy creamer, polyunsaturated
1 high-potassium fruit	½ cup orange juice
2 starches	1 cup puffed wheat and 1 slice light rye toast
1 meat	¼ cup low-cholesterol egg substitute
2 fats	2 teaspoonfuls margarine
Morning Snack	
1 high-kilocalorie	1 cup Tang
Lunch	
1 medium-potassium vegetable	1 small raw carrot
1 medium-potassium fruit	1 small apple
2 starches	2 slices of sourdough white bread
4 meats	4 ounces unsalted lean beef
2 fats	2 teaspoonfuls mayonnaise
1 high-kilocalorie	1 cup lemonade
Afternoon Snack	
1 high-kilocalorie	1 cup Kool-Aid
Supper	
1 high-potassium vegetable	½ cup cooked drained spinach
1 high-potassium fruit	1 fresh pear
2 starches	½ cup rice and 1 ounce angel-foodcake
4 meat	4 ounce broiled chicken breast
2 fats	2 teaspoonfuls margarine (used on chicken)
1 high-kilocalorie	1 cup root beer
Bedtime Snack	
1 milk	½ cup low-fat milk
2 starches	8 unsalted saltine crackers
1 meat	¼ cup unsalted canned tuna
2 fats	2 teaspoonfuls mayonnaise (for tuna salad)
1 high-kilocalorie	1 cup limeade

Nutrient Guidelines for Adults with Renal Disease

As you can see, the nutritional care of renal patients is complex. Table 18–3 is a summary that lists clinical situations, dietary interventions, and the rationale for nutrient control.

Renal Disease in Children

Growth failure is commonly seen in children with chronic renal failure treated with dialysis, but it is not an inevitable complication. Inadequate kilocaloric consumption and/or metabolic acidosis are reasons for the poor growth. These children often need to have their sodium, potassium, and protein intake rigidly controlled, and this may contribute to poor food intake. Anorexia and emotional disturbances are also contributing factors. Suggestions for improving children's intake might include involving the children in selecting and preparing foods (insofar as possible); serving meals in an

TABLE 18–3 *Clinical Situation, Dietary Intervention, and Rationale for Nutrient Control*

Clinical Situation	Rationale	Intervention
Proteinuria	Protein lost in urine	Increase dietary protein
CAPD	Protein lost in dialysate	Increase dietary protein
Elevated BUN and creatinine	Body unable to excrete waste generated from protein	Decrease dietary protein Increase nonprotein kilocalories
Uremia	metabolism in the amounts eaten and/or catabolized	Emphasis on proteins with high biological value
Edema	Body unable to reabsorb and	Fluid restrictions
Anuria	excrete sodium and fluid in the amounts consumed	Sodium restriction
Hyperkalemia	Body unable to excrete potassium	Potassium restriction
Hyperphosphatemia	May be related to an inability to activate vitamin D Body unable to excrete the amounts of phosphorus consumed and absorbed	Phosphorus restriction Phosphate binders
Low ferritin levels	Iron deficiency; may be caused by blood loss and/or poor food intake	Increase kilocalories Increase nutrient density Iron supplements Vitamin C enhances iron absorption and should be consumed with meals
Poor growth, especially in children	Insufficient energy	Increase kilocalories to spare protein
Low number of red blood cells with normal ferritin level	Inability to manufacture erythropoietin	Epoetin alfa supplement
Elevated triglyceride levels	Common in renal patients	Type 4 hyperlipoproteinemia diet with modifications in fat and carbohydrate intake

appealing, attractive manner (e.g., serving contrasting colors and textures of foods, using decorative tableware and dishes; serving small, frequent meals; ensuring that the child has someone with him or her at mealtime; and planning special mealtime events such as picnics (even if they have to be held in the hospital playroom).

KIDNEY STONES

Kidney stones may be found in the bladder, kidney, ureter, or urethra. During urine formation, the urine moves from the collecting tubules and into the renal pelvis. From the renal pelvis, the urine moves down the ureter and into the urinary bladder. Finally, urine passes from the bladder, down the urethra, and exits the body. A stone, also called a **urinary calculus,** is a deposit of mineral salts held together by a thick, syrupy substance. A urinary calculus can block the movement of urine out of the body. Symptoms of a blockage include sudden severe pain with chills, fever, hematuria (blood in the urine), and an increased desire to urinate. A kidney stone can also pass out of the body via the urine.

Urinary calculus—Calculus (stone) in any part of the renal system, which can block the movement of urine out of the body.

Causes

The cause of most kidney stones is unknown. Some possible causes include an abnormal function of the parathyroid gland, disordered uric acid metabolism (as in gout), an excessive intake of animal protein, and immobility. At higher risk for kidney stones are men, people with a sedentary lifestyle, and people of the Oriental or white race. Typically, kidney stones occur in patients who are between ages 30 and 50. A determination of the stones's composition may lead to a restriction of dietary substrates (the substance acted on). Frequent dietary substrates of kidney stones are oxalic acid and purines.

Treatment

All patients with kidney stones should be advised to drink sufficient water to keep the urine volume above 2 liters per day. About 3000 milliliters or 13 cups of water per day are necessary to produce this amount of urine. The primary reason for increasing fluid intake is to prevent formation of concentrated urine, in which crystals are more likely to combine and precipitate.

Oxalates

A diet low in oxalates (see Table 12–2) is frequently prescribed for patients with kidney stones if laboratory analysis of a surgically removed or passed stone is found to be high in oxalates.

Calcium

Historically, if laboratory analysis of a surgically removed or passed stone was found to be high in calcium, a low-calcium diet was prescribed (600 milligrams per day). Recent research has shown, however, that there is no benefit to the time-honored advice to eat a diet low in calcium (Lemann, 1993). In fact, calcium restriction increases the absorption of oxalate in the gastrointestinal tract and leads to an increase in urinary oxalate excretion. Urinary oxalate may be more important than urinary calcium for stone formation, because calcium oxalate saturation of urine increases rapidly with small increases in the oxalate concentration (Curhan, et al, 1993).

Uric Acid Stones

Stones composed of uric acid are sometimes a complication of **gout**. Gout is a hereditary metabolic disease that is a form of arthritis. One symptom of gout is inflammation of the joints. The metabolism of uric acid is related to dietary purines. **Purines** are an end product of protein digestion. Thus, a purine-restricted diet is often prescribed for gout. Table 18–4 shows foods that are high, moderate, and low in purines.

Gout—Hereditary metabolic disease that is a form of acute arthritis. Marked by inflammation in the joints.

Purines—End product of nucleoprotein digestion. Purines may be synthesized in the body. A purine-restricted diet is often prescribed for gout.

TABLE 18–4 *Purines in Food*

GROUP A: HIGH CONCENTRATION (150 to 1000 milligrams per 100 grams)	
Liver	Sardines (in oil)
Kidney	Meat extracts
Sweetbreads	Consommé
Brains	Gravies
Heart	Fish roes
Anchovies	Herring

GROUP B: MODERATE AMOUNTS (50 to 150 milligrams per 100 grams)	
Meat, game, and fish other than those mentioned in Group A	
Fowl	Asparagus
Lentils	Cauliflower
Whole-grain cereals	Mushrooms
Beans	Spinach
Peas	

GROUP C: VERY SMALL AMOUNTS. NEED NOT BE RESTRICTED IN DIET OF PERSONS WITH GOUT.	
Vegetables other than those mentioned above	
Fruits of all kinds	Coffee
Milk	Tea
Cheese	Chocolate
Eggs	Carbonated beverages
Refined cereals, spaghetti, macaroni	Tapioca
Butter, fats, nuts, peanut butter*	Yeast
Sugars and sweets	
Vegetable soups	

*Fats interfere with the urinary excretion of urates and thus should be limited when attempting to promote excretion of uric acid.

Source: From Thomas, CL (ed): Taber's Cyclopedic Medical Dictionary, ed 16. FA Davis, Philadelphia, 1985, p 1528, with permission.

Surgery

Surgery is sometimes necessary to remove large kidney stones. Surgical removal of the stones prevents infection, reduces pain, and prevents a loss of kidney function.

URINARY TRACT INFECTIONS

Urinary tract infection—Infection of the urinary tract with microorganisms.

One form of **urinary tract infection** (UTI) is <u>cystitis,</u> or an inflammation of the bladder. This condition is prevalent in young women. Recurrent UTI means that the woman has three or more bouts of infection per year. A general nutrition measure includes acidifying the urine by taking large doses of vitamin C. The common practice of drinking cranberry juice to acidify the urine has not been demonstrated to be more effective than other fluid intake. Patients with UTIs should be encouraged to drink extra fluids.

Summary

The basic functional unit of the kidney is the nephron. Millions of nephrons work together to form urine and remove unnecessary substances from the blood. Glomerular filtration rate (GFR) is a measure of kidney function. The kidneys also are the site where vitamin D_3 (calcitriol) and erythropoietin are activated. No other body organ can replace the kidneys. Kidney disease is a feared complication of many disease states such as atherosclerosis, diabetes, hypertension, and septic shock. Kidney failure can be acute or chronic. Chronic renal disease is progressive. Much research is aimed at finding a way to stop the downward spiral in GFR in patients diagnosed with chronic renal failure. Current research is focused on the relationship of dietary protein and phosphorus on the progression of kidney failure. Treatment for kidney failure is dialysis or a kidney transplant.

Nutritional management of patients with renal disease is a fundamental part of treatment. Patients with kidney disease require constant assessment, monitoring, and counseling. The dietary components that may need modification are kilocalories, protein, sodium, potassium, phosphorus, fluid, cholesterol, and saturated fat. Vitamin and mineral supplements are often prescribed. Frequently, the diet these patients follow must be further modified as their medical condition and treatment approach changes. Recently, a National Renal Diet was developed for use by these patients.

Some nutritional intervention is necessary for patients with kidney stones and UTIs. The fluid intake of these patients should be high. Usually, patients with kidney stones need to avoid foods that contain substances likely to form stones.

A case study and a sample plan of care appear below. Both are designed to show you how the information you have studied in this chapter can be used in nursing practice.

CASE STUDY 18–1

Mr. U., a 25-year-old man, was admitted to the hospital from his doctor's office for a shunt implantation with subsequent hemodialysis planned. A college graduate, he is employed as an engineer. His medical record indicates that he had an episode of acute glomerulonephritis about 10 years ago. He contracted the disease after a streptococcal throat infection. At that time his symptoms were hematuria, oliguria, proteinuria, hypertension, and edema. He was discharged on a 4-gram sodium diet.

Mr U. now complains of swollen ankles, headaches, and fatigue. He reports to have had a 10-pound weight gain over the past 6 weeks. His usual body weight is 170 pounds; he is 5 feet 10 inches tall and has a large frame. He now weighs 181 pounds. His blood pressure is 155/99. Laboratory test results follow:

Test	Results	Normal Range
BUN	75 milligrams per deciliter	9–25 milligrams per deciliter
Creatinine	2 milligrams per deciliter	0.6–1.5 milligrams per deciliter
Serum phosphorus	4.4 milligrams per deciliter	3.0–4.5 milligrams per deciliter
Serum calcium	3.5 milligrams per deciliter	3.5–5.0 milligrams per deciliter
Hemoglobin	6 milligrams per deciliter	14–18 grams per deciliter
Hematocrit	19 percent	42–52 percent
Potassium	4.0 milliequivalents per liter	3.5–5.0 milliequivalents per liter
Albumin	3.5 grams per deciliter	3.5–5.5 grams per deciliter
Urine volume	900 milliliters per day	1000–1500 milliliters
Proteinuria	1+	None
GFR	10 milliliters per minute	125 milliliters per minute
Cholesterol	280 milligrams per deciliter	< 200 milligrams per deciliter
Triglycerides	140 milligrams per deciliter	40–150 milligrams per deciliter

The doctor has prescribed a 60-gram protein, 2000-kilocalorie, 2-gram sodium, low-saturated-fat, low-cholesterol diet and a fluid restriction of output plus 500 milliliters. Hemodialysis is ordered for three times a week. His medications include docusate sodium, furosemide, a multivitamin, vitamin B_6, and folic acid. Mr U. stated that the protein, fluid, saturated fat, and cholesterol restrictions are new to him.

NURSING CARE PLAN FOR MR U.

Assessment

Subjective: Patient complains of headaches, swollen ankles, and fatigue.
Objective: Patient has an elevated BUN, phosphorus, blood pressure, and creatinine. The patient also has edema; a decreased GFR, hemoglobin, and hematocrit; and a decreased urinary output.

Nursing Diagnosis

Fluid volume excess: related to renal insufficiency as evidenced by patient complaints of headaches, swollen ankles, fatigue and decreased urinary output, edema formation, and hypertension.

Desired Outcome/Evaluation Criteria

1. The patient will demonstrate a stabilized fluid volume, with balanced intake and output, and a decrease in BUN/creatinine. Vital signs will decrease from admission values within 24 hours.
2. The patient will verbalize knowledge of condition and therapy regimen.
3. The patient will demonstrate behaviors consistent with dietary program.

Nursing Actions/Interventions with Rationales in Italics

Assist patient in the restoration of homeostasis.

1. a. Measure urinary output q shift (q = every). *Patient's urinary output may vary, and fluid intake must be adjusted accordingly.*
   b. Plan fluid intake with patient; monitor fluid intake and body weight. *Fluid intake must be controlled to prevent excessive edema and control blood pressure. Daily weight is best measure of fluid balance.*
   c. Monitor BUN/creatinine results, as needed. *The patient is currently unable to excrete waste generated from protein metabolism in amounts eaten and/or catabolized. As the patient begins dialysis treatments, the BUN/creatinine levels should decrease, and the protein content of the diet will need to be adjusted accordingly.*
   d. Assess mentation using standard tool q shift. Provide for dietary restrictions as prescribed, while providing adequate kilocalories to meet the body's needs. *The patient's mental status may be altered by increased BUN/creatinine levels which in turn are increased by a kilocalorie deficit.*
   e. Monitor blood pressure, pulses, lung sounds q 4 hours. *The patient's fluid volume excess and decreased GFR may increase secretion of renin and raise blood pressure.*
   f. Encourage adequate kilocaloric intake. *The diet will not be effective in controlling BUN/creatinine levels unless adequate kilocalories are consumed.*
2. Discuss necessary changes in lifestyle and assist patient to incorporate disease management into activities of daily living.
   a. Teach patient to measure urinary output. *The patient will need to learn to measure his own urinary output.*
   b. Teach patient to measure fluid intake daily; fluid intake should be 500 milliliters plus urinary output in milliliters. *The patient will need to learn how to calculate his daily fluid intake based on his urinary output and insensible losses of fluid.*
   c. Discuss with patient the relationships of his symptoms (headaches, swollen ankles, fatigue) and signs (edema; decreased GFR, hemoglobin, hematocrit, urinary output; and elevated BUN/creatinine to treatment approaches (hemodialysis and dietary restrictions). *Because the patient has a chronic disease, long-term compliance with the treatment approach will be necessary. Relating signs and symptoms to the patient's treatment approach will assist him in understanding his treatment regimen.*
   d. Refer patient to the dietitian for dietary teaching. *The patient's needs will best be met if referral to the dietitian is made as soon as possible. A diet as complicated as this patient's will require several hours of instruction. Information is usually better retained if small amounts of information are given at frequent intervals.*
   e. Discuss with the patient the importance of regular hemodialysis treatments. *Failure to received regular hemodialysis treatments will result in an excessive fluid gain and abnormal laboratory values between treatments. Subsequent efforts to remove this excess fluid may result in a dangerous drop in blood pressure during the dialysis treatment.*
3. Monitor patient's food intake. *The best method to evaluate whether the patient has learned his dietary restrictions is to monitor food intake.*

STUDY AIDS

Chapter Review Questions

1. Which of the following is not always a nutritional goal for a child with renal disease?
   a. Promote normal growth and development.
   b. Maintain current hydration status.
   c. Minimize uremic toxicity.
   d. Stimulate patient well-being.

2. Kidney disease *cannot* be caused by:
   a. Consumption of toxic metals.
   b. Habitual consumption of water
   c. Consumption of a diet habitually high in protein
   d. Trauma

3. Kilocalories usually need to be increased in protein-restricted diets because an adequate kilocalorie intake _____.
   a. Assists in the control of serum potassium
   b. Is necessary to prevent the renal anemia
   c. Controls and prevents osteodystrophy
   d. Spares protein

4. A normal glomerular filtration rate is approximately:
   a. 125 milliliters per minute
   b. 90 milliliters per minute
   c. 25 milliliters per minute
   d. 10 milliliters per minute

5. Compared with renal failure patients who are not on dialysis, patients on continuous ambulatory peritoneal dialysis require:
   a. The same amount of dietary protein
   b. Less dietary protein
   c. More dietary protein
   d. A different kind of protein

6. Which of the following would be a good snack for a patient with acute renal failure who is not on dialysis?
   a. Hard candy
   b. Cheese
   c. Milk
   d. Oranges

7. Some renal patients need to avoid salt substitutes because these often contain:
   a. Phosphorus
   b. Potassium
   c. Protein
   d. Calcium

8. The _____ intake from food is not monitored in renal patients.
   a. Vitamin D
   b. Fluid
   c. Protein
   d. Sodium

9. Which of the following are high in potassium?
   a. Grapes

    b. Cranberry juice

    c. Baked potatoes

    d. Canned pears

10. The most important nutritional consideration in treating patients with kidney stones is to:
    a. Limit calcium intake.
    b. Restrict all end products of protein metabolism.
    c. Restrict all food sources of calcium, oxalic acid, and purines.
    d. Increase fluid intake.

NCLEX-Style Quiz

Situation One

Bill, age 10, has acute glomerulonephritis. His mother explains that Bill had a streptococcal infection 1 week prior to the illness.

1. When planning Bill's care, the nurse recognizes that he needs help in understanding his diet. Bill's restrictions will include:
    a. A low-fat diet
    b. A potassium restriction
    c. Measuring urine output (if any) daily and planning his fluid intake
    d. A high-protein diet

Situation Two

2. Marie has had four urinary tract infections during the past year. The nurse should instruct Marie to:
    a. Abstain from sexual intercourse.
    b. Drink at least 13 cups of fluid daily.
    c. Avoid milk, meat in excess, and meat extracts.
    d. Drink cranberry juice daily.

Situation Three

3. Mr. Jones, a 49-year-old mechanic, has been admitted to the hospital with diagnosis of renal failure. Mr. Jones has been following a 40-gram protein, 2-gram sodium, 2-gram potassium, 1000-milliliter fluid restriction for the past 5 years. Mr. Jones is scheduled for surgery tomorrow to have a permanent shunt implanted for hemodialysis. Mr. Jones's nutritional needs will most likely change after he is maintained on hemodialysis so as to:
    a. Include more oranges, bananas, and baked potatoes.
    b. Include more lean meat, eggs, low-fat milk, and low-fat cheeses.
    c. Include less starches, breads, and cereals.
    d. Include less margarine, oil, and salad dressings.

4. Mr. Jones is found to have an elevated serum phosphorus level after 6 months on hemodialysis. He should:
    a. Restrict his intake of dairy products.
    b. Restrict his intake of red meats.
    c. Increase his intake of sugar, honey, jam, jelly, and other simple sugars.
    d. Discontinue his phosphate binders.

5. The nurse is helping Mr. Jones fill out his menu. Which lunch would best meet his needs?
    a. Roast beef, noodles, a sliced fresh orange, and milk

b. Baked chicken, rice, fresh grapes, and cranberry juice
c. Macaroni and cheese, a bran muffin, cooked spinach, apricot halves, and lemonade
d. Hamburger on a whole-grain bun, potato chips, a dill pickle, and a cola beverage

BIBLIOGRAPHY

Ahmed, FE: Effect of Diet on Progression of Chronic Renal Disease. J Am Diet Assoc 10, 1266, 1991.

American Dietetic Association: Manual of Clinical Dietetics, ed 4. American Dietetic Association, Chicago, 1992.

Burton, BT and Hirschman, GH: Current concepts of nutritional therapy in chronic renal disease: An update. J Am Diet Assoc 82:4, 1983.

Curhan GC, et al: A prospective study of dietary calcium and other nutrients and the risk of symptomatic kidney stones. N Engl J Med 328:12, 1993.

Doenges, M and Moorhouse, M: Nursing Diagnoses with Interventions, ed 2. FA Davis, Philadelphia, 1985.

Feldman EB: Essentials of Clinical Nutrition. FA Davis, Philadelphia, 1988.

Guyton, AC: Textbook of Medical Physiology, ed 7. WB Saunders, Philadelphia, 1986.

LeMann, J: Composition of diet and calcium kidney stones. N Engl J Med 328:12, 1993.

Monsen, ER: Meeting the challenge of the renal diet. J Am Diet Assoc 93:6, 1993.

Moore MC: Pocket Guide to Nutrition and Diet Therapy, ed 2. Mosby Year Book, St Louis, 1993.

National Live Stock and Meat Board: Iron in Human Nutrition. National Live Stock and Meat Board, Chicago, 1990.

Robinson, CH and Weigley, ES: Basic Nutrition and Diet Therapy, ed 6. Macmillan, New York, 1989.

Ross Laboratories: Specialized Nutrition for Patients with Renal Disease. Ross Laboratories, Columbus, OH, 1990.

Wesley, JR, et al: Parenteral and Enteral Nutrition Manual, ed 4. University of Michigan Medical Center, 1986.

Williams, SR: Essentials of Nutrition and Diet Therapy, ed 5. Times Mirror/Mosby St Louis, 1990.

Zeller, K, et al: Effect of restricting dietary protein on the progression of renal failure in patients with insulin-dependent diabetes mellitus. N Engl J Med 324:78, 1991.

Chapter Outline

Key Terms

As a study aid, each key term is followed by the page number where the term is defined in the chapter. Terms that appear in **boldface** or <u>underscored</u> in the chapter text are located in the glossary.

Diet in Surgery and in Gastrointestinal Disease

After completing this chapter, the student should be able to:

1. Distinguish the dietary preparation for gastrointestinal surgery from dietary preparation for surgery on other body systems.
2. Identify nutritional deficiencies that may accompany diseases of or resection of regions of the gastrointestinal tract.
3. Describe nutritional deficiencies associated with steatorrhea.
4. List several nutritional consequences of cirrhosis of the liver.
5. Discuss dietary modifications for common gastrointestinal diseases treated medically and surgically.

*M*any disorders that affect the gastrointestinal tract and its accessory organs influence the nutritional status of patients. Most surgical procedures have an impact on gastrointestinal tract function and require special dietary measures, both preoperatively and postoperatively. Disorders of the accessory organs of the gastrointestinal tract (liver, gallbladder, and pancreas) influence gastrointestinal tract function and have dietary implications. This chapter discusses diet modifications for surgical patients and for patients with common gastrointestinal diseases.

DIETARY CONSIDERATIONS WITH SURGICAL PATIENTS

As many as 50 percent of surgical patients are malnourished before they enter the operating room. Postoperatively, the healing process requires increased protein, vitamins C and K, and zinc, along with adequate amounts of other nutrients. Vitamin C is necessary for collagen formation; vitamin K for blood clotting; and zinc for tissue growth, bone formation, skin integrity, cell-mediated immunity and generalized host defense.

Protein depletion causes increased risk of infection and shock. Protein is essential for the manufacture of antibodies and white blood cells, which help the body fight infection. Hypoalbuminemia (low serum albumin) impedes the return of interstitial fluid from the tissue to the venous system, decreasing intravascular fluid. This results in an increased risk of shock due to low intravascular volume. Local edema, which accompanies any trauma, including surgery, hampers circulation and healing. A low serum albumin level will increase the time needed to reduce the edema. The serum albumin level, then, becomes a useful and readily available measure of protein status. Clinical Application 19–1 elaborates the possible consequence of malnutrition in surgical patients.

CLINICAL APPLICATION 19–1
Surgical Patients with Rampant Dental Caries

Within a period of weeks, three patients on a particular gynecological surgical unit suffered postoperative wound disruptions. Each disruption was a dehiscence, a separation of the wound edges. Dehiscence occurs most frequently between the fifth and twelfth postoperative days. Risk factors for dehiscence include obesity, malnutrition, dehydration, abdominal distention, increased abdominal pressure from improper deep breathing and coughing, and infection.

All three patients had at least one of the risk factors. One patient ran a postoperative fever, which could have been caused by infection or dehydration. The other two patients had such severely carious teeth it would have been difficult for them to chew much meat in the months before surgery. They probably were malnourished.

Nurses, then, would be wise to refer preoperative patients with marked dental caries to the dietitian for nutritional assessment. Carious teeth can both cause and be caused by poor eating habits.

Persons with gastrointestinal disease are at special risk when facing surgery because their diseases interfere with nutrition. In cases involving gastrointestinal surgery the gastrointestinal tract is incised and sutured, so postoperative feeding is postponed to allow healing. This delay also contributes to nutritional risk.

Special notice should be given to the surgical patient with liver disease. The liver has many functions, which are reviewed in Table 19–1. Because of the liver's role in metabolizing and detoxifying drugs, the patient with liver disease must be carefully managed when surgery is necessary. Drugs may accumulate in the bloodstream because the liver cannot degrade them. Some anesthetics, analgesics, and anti-infectives are toxic to the liver.

TABLE 19–1 *Liver Functions*

Related to	Produces	Stores	Breaks Down
Carbohydrate	Glucose from galactose and fructose	Glycogen	
	Glucose from glycogen		
	Glucose from glycerol and protein		
Fat	Fat from glucose	Fat	
	Cholesterol		
	Fatty acids and glycerol from cholesterol, phospholipids, and lipoproteins		
	Lipoproteins		
	Water-soluble bilirubin (from fat-soluble)		
	Bile		
Protein	Albumin		
	Some globulins		
	Prothrombin		
	Fibrinogen		
	Transferrin		
	Enzymes to convert ammonia to urea		
Vitamins	Retinol-binding protein	A, D, E, K	
	Other transport proteins	Thiamin	
	Activate thiamin	Riboflavin	
	Activate pyridoxine	Pyridoxine	
		Folic acid	
		B_{12}	
		Biotin	
Minerals		Iron	Worn-out red blood cells
Other			Bacteria
			Aldosterone
			Glucocorticoids
			Estrogen
			Progesterone
			Alcohol
			Morphine
			Barbiturates
			Some anesthetics
			Acetaminophen

TABLE 19–2 *Low-Residue Diet*

Food Group	Allowed	Foods to Avoid
Beverages	Coffee, tea, decaffeinated coffee, juices, soda, milk beverages limited to 2 cups per day	Alcohol, prune juice, milk in excess of 2 cups
Breads	All breaded products made from finely milled grain (white bread), crackers made without whole grains or seeds	Whole-grain breads; breads with seeds or nuts; bread made with bran
Cereals	Cooked cereals without whole grains such as Cream of Wheat; dry cereals made from finely milled grains, such as Rice Krispies and puffed wheat	Whole-grain cereals
Desserts	All without dried fruit, seeds, skins, nuts, coconut, or fruits with seeds; gelatin; desserts made from milk (e.g., custard) only if deducted from the milk allowance	Any desserts containing seeds, nuts, coconut or dried fruits
Fats	Butter, margarine, oils, cream, if deducted from the milk allowance	Nuts and olives
Fruits	All fruit juices and strained fruits; banana, cooked and canned apples, apricots, Royal Anne cherries, peaches, pears	Fruits not on the "allowed list"
Meat and substitutes	Tender or ground beef, pork, lamb, poultry, fish, and veal that has been roasted, baked, or broiled; smooth peanut butter	Tough, fried, or spiced meats
Nuts	None	All
Potatoes and substitutes	White and sweet potatoes without skins; rice, noodles, macaroni, spaghetti	Potato skins, potato chips, fried potatoes, whole-grain rice or pasta
Soups	Broth-based soups made with allowed ingredients, cream soups made with allowed ingredients (deduct from milk allowance any amount of milk used)	Soups made with "foods to avoid"; cream soups in excess of milk allowance
Sweets	Sugar, honey, jelly, gumdrops, hard candy, plain chocolates	Sweets made with seeds, nuts, coconut, skins, and dried fruit; jam; marmalade
Vegetables	All vegetable juices and strained vegetables; cooked or canned asparagus, green and wax beans, beets, carrots, peas, pumpkin, spinach, and winter squash	Vegetables not on the "allowed list"
Miscellaneous	Salt, pepper, ground seasonings, plain gravy, milk sauces only if deducted from the milk allowance	Chili sauce, rich gravies, horseradish, pepper, popcorn, seeds of any kind, whole spices, whole-grain snack foods, radishes, vinegar

Preoperative Nutrition

Before elective surgery is undertaken nutritional deficiencies should be corrected. Many obese patients are instructed to lose weight to reduce the risk of surgery. If the patient is anemic, an iron preparation can be prescribed. Other nutrients can be provided as needed. At least 2 to 3 weeks are required for objective evidence of the effectiveness of nutritional therapy. All surgical patients should be instructed to have adequate nutritional intake in the weeks before surgery.

If general anesthesia is employed, the stomach should be empty to prevent aspiration of gastric contents into the lungs. The usual procedure is to have the patient take nothing by mouth (NPO) during the 8 hours prior to surgery. Surgery of the gastrointestinal tract demands additional bowel preparation. Anti-infectives such as neomycin sulfate, which remain predominantly in the bowel, may be given to kill intestinal bacteria. A low-residue diet for 2 to 3 days will minimize the feces left in the bowel.

A low-residue diet reduces the fecal bulk by reducing food residue. Residue refers to the total solid material in the large intestine after digestion; it includes not only undigestible or unabsorbable components of the diet such as fiber but also foods that result in an increased stool volume, such as milk. A low-residue diet usually consists of foods that are easily digested and absorbed. Table 19–2 shows foods allowable and foods to be avoided on a low-residue diet. Meats should be tender or ground and free of tough connective tissue and must be baked, boiled, or broiled. Cooked vegetables should be mild in flavor and without coarse fibers. Milk and milk products are high in residue and are limited to a total of 2 cups per day. In addition to preoperative bowel preparation, a low-residue diet is indicated for severe diarrhea, partial intestinal obstruction, preoperative and postoperative colonic surgery, and acute phases of inflammatory bowel diseases.

Postoperative Nutrition

Intravenous fluids are continued after surgery. The usual minimum replacement is 2 liters of 5 percent glucose in water in 24 hours. This amount contains 100 grams of glucose and delivers 340 kilocalories. Although this will not meet a person's resting energy expenditure, it will prevent ketosis. Most adults have nutrient reserves for 3 to 4 days of semistarvation. To prevent excessive muscle protein from being used for energy, adequate nourishment must be delivered in some form to the patient within 3 days.

To avoid abdominal distention, oral feedings are delayed until peristalsis returns and is detected by listening through a stethoscope. Another sign of peristalsis is the passage via the rectum of flatus (gas). Ambulation as permitted will help the patient pass the flatus and avoid uncomfortable distention of the bowel and abdomen due to gas.

Flatus—gas in the digestive tract, averaging 400 to 1200 ml/day.

Patients are usually progressed from clear liquids to a regular diet as soon as possible. If "diet as tolerated" is ordered, ask the patient what foods sound good. Sometimes, presenting a full dinner tray when the patient does not feel well "turns off" the appetite. After gastrointestinal surgery, oral food and fluids are deferred longer than with other surgeries, to allow healing. One particular precaution is often taken. After surgery on the mouth and throat, tonsillectomy, for example, no red liquids are given to prevent vomitus being mistaken for blood or vice versa.

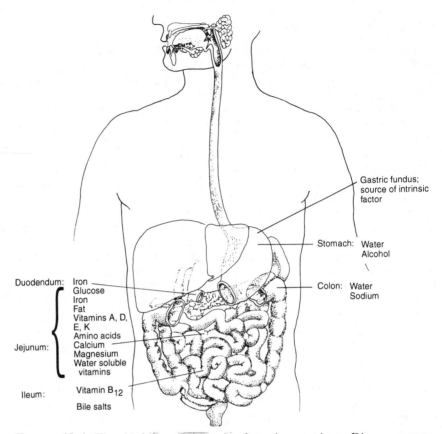

FIGURE 19–1. The chief sites of absorption for various nutrients. Disease or resection of an area will increase the risk of deficiency of specific nutrients. (Adapted from Scanlon, VC and Sanders, T: Student Workbook for Essentials of Anatomy and Physiology, FA Davis Company, Philadelphia, 1991, p 299, with permission.)

Surgical removal of a specific part of the gastrointestinal tract, such as the stomach, duodenum, jejunum, or ileum, may result in malabsorption of specific nutrients, as illustrated in Figure 19–1. For example, intrinsic factor, which is secreted by the stomach, is necessary for the utilization of vitamin B_{12}. Iron absorbed from the duodenum and the jejunum is necessary for hemoglobin synthesis. Glucose, amino acids, fat- and water-soluble vitamins, calcium, and magnesium, all absorbed in the jejunum, are necessary for metabolism. Vitamin B_{12} and bile salts are absorbed in the ileum. Although the loss of bile salts in the feces may seem harmless, the body ordinarily recycles these salts over and over in the management of fats. Prolonged impaired absorption of bile salts can result in failure to absorb fat and fat-soluble vitamins.

DISORDERS OF THE MOUTH AND THROAT

Varied conditions such as dental caries, oral surgery, surgery of the head and neck, fractured jaw, and cancer chemotherapy or radiation therapy can cause difficulty with chewing and swallowing. Often the patient will require a feeding tube. The different types of tube feedings were discussed in Chapter 13.

When patients can begin to take oral nourishment, they often can swallow thick liquids better than thin liquids. Baby cereals or special dietary preparations can be used to achieve the correct consistency. Tasteless or slippery foods do not present enough stimulus to coordinate movements and may also be difficult to swallow. If patients lean forward and hold their breath while trying to swallow, it may make the task easier.

DISORDERS OF THE ESOPHAGUS

Three esophageal disorders, achalasia, esophageal reflux, and hiatal hernia are discussed in this section.

Achalasia

Failure of the gastrointestinal muscle fibers to relax where one part joins another is called **achalasia.** Often the term is applied to the cardiac sphincter, which separates the stomach from the esophagus. Sometimes the condition is termed cardiospasm. The cause of achalasia is unknown. Very hot or cold foods may trigger esophageal spasm, and anxiety seems to aggravate the condition. Symptoms are described as "something sticking in my throat" and a feeling of fullness behind the breastbone (sternum). Vomiting is associated with achalasia, and aspiration of vomitus can cause pneumonia.

Achalasia–failure of the gastrointestinal muscle fibers to relax where one part joins another.

In mild cases, avoiding spicy foods and dietary bulk may be effective. Diets for these patients require much individual attention. Rarely does one achalasia patient display an intolerance for the same foods as another patient. Plenty of liquids with small, frequent meals may help. Treatment of more severe cases involves stretching the cardiac sphincter or surgically slitting it.

Cardiac sphincter—The circular muscle between the esophagus and the stomach.

Esophageal Reflux

Esophageal reflux refers to the regurgitation of the stomach contents into the esophagus. Esophageal reflux can usually be managed without surgery. This regurgitation is common in infancy and disappears with age. In infants, usually no treatment is undertaken unless there is evidence of aspiration of food into the respiratory tract or of failure to thrive. In adults, the most common underlying cause of esophageal reflux is hiatal hernia, which is discussed in the next section. Some experts believe that esophageal reflux may be caused by failure of the lower esophageal sphincter to operate properly. The stomach is normally protected from hydrochloric acid by a thick layer of mucus. Because the esophagus is not so protected, esophageal reflux can lead to ulcer formation. The prominent symptom is heartburn. Pain occurs behind the sternum or breastbone. Sometimes the pain radiates to the neck and the back of the throat. Lying down or bending over may increase reflux and aggravate the pain.

Esophageal reflux—Regurgitation of the stomach contents into the esophagus.

Treatment involves a number of conservative measures. Small, frequent meals are often recommended. No specific foods are associated with tightening of the cardiac sphincter. Foods often avoided because they relax the sphincter are fat, alcohol, caffeine, peppermint, spearmint, and chocolate. Smoking also relaxes the sphincter. Decaffeinated coffee and pepper are frequently avoided because they stimulate gastric secretion. Acidic juices, such as citrus juices and tomato juice, may also be irritating.

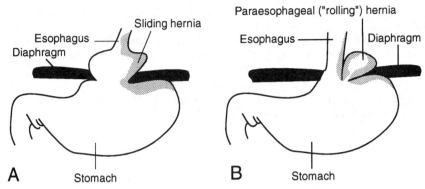

FIGURE 19–2. In hiatal hernia the upper part of the stomach squeezes into the chest cavity through the esophageal opening in the diaphragm. (A) Sliding Hernia (B) Paraesophageal hernia (From Long and Phipps, p 885, with permission.)

Eating behaviors may assist in the control of esophageal reflux. Chewing the food thoroughly, not eating within 3 hours of bedtime, and sitting upright for 2 hours after meals may increase food tolerance. Raising the head of the bed 6 to 8 inches enables gravity to help keep stomach contents contained. Overweight patients with esophageal reflux may experience some relief from symptoms with a loss of weight.

Hiatal Hernia

Hiatal hernia—protrusion of part of stomach into chest cavity.

The esophageal hiatus is the opening in the diaphragm through which the esophagus is attached to the stomach. A **hiatal hernia** is a protrusion of the stomach through the esophageal hiatus into the chest cavity (Fig. 19–2). The symptoms of hiatal hernia are similar to those of esophageal reflux and its medical treatment is the same. Persistent symptoms despite conservative treatment might lead the patient to elect surgical repair of the hernia.

DISORDERS OF THE STOMACH

Disorders of the stomach often require diet modification and in some cases, surgery. In this section we will discuss gastritis and peptic ulcers.

Gastritis

Gastritis—inflammation of the stomach.

Epigastric region—central region of the abdomen above the umbilicus.

Inflammation of the stomach is **gastritis.** Common causes of gastritis are the chronic use of aspirin and alcohol abuse. Other conditions that result in gastritis are food allergies, food poisoning, infections, radiation exposure, and stress. Symptoms of gastritis are anorexia, nausea, a feeling of fullness, and epigastric pain. Look at Figure 19–3 to locate the epigastric region. Abdominal findings are often described according to their location within the four quadrants (top view) or nine regions (bottom view) shown in the figure. As you compare the two views, you can see that the epigastric region is located neither to the left nor to the right, but centrally. Signs of gastritis are vomiting and eructating (belching).

The dietary treatment plan for gastritis includes having the patient:

1. Eat at regular intervals.
2. Chew food, especially fibrous food, slowly and thoroughly.

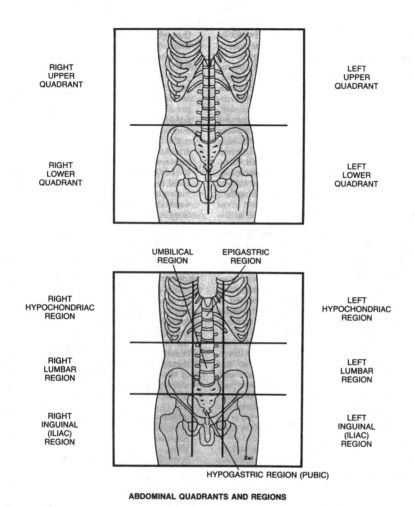

UMBILICAL REGION   EPIGASTRIC REGION

HYPOGASTRIC REGION (PUBIC)

ABDOMINAL QUADRANTS AND REGIONS

FIGURE 19–3. Quadrants and regions of the abdomen which are used to describe locations of signs and symptoms. (From Thomas, p 4, with permission.)

3. Avoid foods that cause pain.
4. Avoid foods that cause gas, especially vegetables in the cabbage family, including broccoli, cauliflower, and brussels sprouts.
5. Avoid gastric irritants such as caffeine (found in coffee, tea, cola beverages, and chocolate); alcohol; nonsteroidal anti-inflammatory drugs (NSAIDs) such as aspirin; and strong spices, including nutmeg, pepper, garlic, and chili powder.
6. Eat in a relaxed manner.

More often than not, discovering which foods are responsible for the pain and discomfort of gastritis is a trial-and-error process. Individual tolerances will vary from person to person and should be respected.

Peptic Ulcers

Here we will discuss both gastric (stomach) and duodenal ulcers. Both are known as peptic ulcers.

Occurrence

Peptic ulcers affect 10 percent of the population worldwide. Men are two to three times more likely than women to have peptic ulcers. Positive family history increases a person's risk of peptic ulcer threefold. Patients can be of any age, but the highest incidence occurs between the ages of 45 and 55. Half of the patients hospitalized for bleeding ulcers are over age 65.

Pathophysiology

An ulcer patient's mucosa is not sufficiently resistant to the acids secreted by the stomach. If just the superficial cells are involved, the lesion is called an erosion. Once the muscular layer of the stomach or duodenum is involved, the person has an **ulcer.**

Gastric ulcers are most common on the lesser curvature or right side of the stomach, rather than on the greater curvature. Duodenal ulcers account for 80 percent of all ulcers. Of the two, duodenal ulcers are associated with increased acidity of the stomach, but gastric ulcers are more likely to require surgery.

The exact cause of peptic ulcers is unknown. Factors predisposing a person to ulcer formation, besides ancestry, are smoking, caffeine, and alcohol. Stress and lack of rest contribute to ulcer development. Although the stereotypical ulcer patient is a hard-driving executive, ulcers are actually more common in the lower socioeconomic class. Low socioeconomic status is seen as a risk factor and may be linked with two other risk factors, poor nutrition and stress. The latter two factors may be related to irregular consumption of meals, which may contribute to ulcer formation in susceptible patients. Long-term use of certain medications is associated with ulcer formation. Among these are aspirin, potassium chloride, and corticosteroids.

Signs and Symptoms

A gnawing, burning epigastric pain when the stomach is empty is characteristic of peptic ulcer. This occurs 1 to 3 hours after eating or at night. One quarter of ulcer patients experience bleeding, more often with duodenal than with gastric ulcers. If the blood is vomited immediately, it is bright red. If it stays in contact with digestive juices for a while, the vomitus will resemble coffee grounds. The medical term for this is "coffee-ground emesis." Other symptoms of peptic ulcer are nausea, anorexia, and sometimes, weight loss.

Complications of Peptic Ulcers

Hemorrhage is a common complication of peptic ulcers. Scar tissue from a healed ulcer can restrict the gastric outlet, causing pyloric obstruction. If the ulcer continues to erode through the entire stomach or intestinal wall, the result is a **perforated ulcer.** Spilling gastrointestinal contents into the sterile abdominal cavity causes peritonitis, an inflammation of the peritoneum, the lining of the abdominal cavity.

Treatment of Peptic Ulcers

Usually a course of medical treatment is prescribed at first. Only if such treatment should prove ineffective is surgery recommended.

MEDICAL TREATMENT   Before the advent of antiulcer medications, patients with peptic ulcers were usually advised to take antacids every 2

Erosion—destruction of the surface of a tissue either on the surface of or inside the body.

Ulcer—open sore or lesion of skin or mucous membrane.

Perforated ulcer—condition in which an ulcer penetrates completely through the stomach or intestinal wall, spilling the organ's contents into the peritoneal cavity.

Peritonitis—inflammation of the peritoneal cavity.

hours, alternating with milk and cream. New medications have revolutionized the treatment. They are almost always effective without a drastic change in diet. Two often-prescribed medications are cimetidine and ranitidine, which block histamine-stimulated gastric acid secretion.

Diet does require some modification, however. Some experts recommend only three regular meals with no snacking. This is because food, including milk, stimulates gastric secretion. Other authorities allow midmorning and midafternoon snacks. In both regimens, substances that cause gastric irritation are avoided. These include the same gastric irritants discussed in the section on gastritis. Patients should be encouraged to avoid or limit spices or foods that are not well tolerated.

Definite changes in the ulcer patient's lifestyle will improve chances of successful treatment. Patients need counseling for stress reduction. They should obtain enough sleep. Since smoking stimulates secretion of gastric acid, ulcer patients should not smoke.

SURGICAL TREATMENT   When surgery is necessary, the ulcer is removed and the remaining gastrointestinal tract is sutured together. Surgical procedures designed to eliminate the diseased area include the gastroduodenostomy (stomach and duodenum anastomosed), the gastrojejunostomy (stomach and jejunum anastomosed) and the total gastrectomy (esophagus and duodenum anastomosed). **Anastomosis** is the surgical connection between tubular structures. Figure 19–4 illustrates these three procedures.

Anastomosis—A surgical connection between tubular structures.

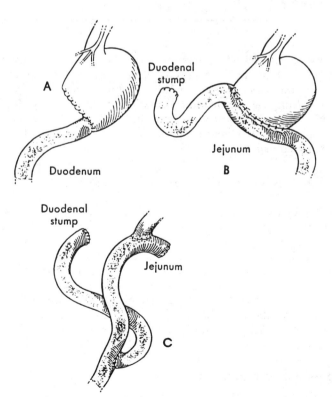

FIGURE 19–4. Common gastric resection procedures. (A) Gastroduodenostomy, Bilroth I (B) Gastrojejunostomy Bilroth II (C) Total gastrectomy. (From Long and Phipps, p 914, with permission.)

CLINICAL APPLICATION 19–2
The Dumping Syndrome

When a concentrated liquid suddenly enters the intestine, water is pulled from the bowel just as in osmotic diarrhea. Local effects are hyperperistalsis, diarrhea, abdominal pain, and vomiting 30 to 60 minutes after a meal. Systemic effects are those of fluid balance deficit: weakness, dizziness, sweating, decreased blood pressure, tachycardia, and palpitations. The dumping syndrome is most often associated with total gastrectomy or resection of two thirds of the stomach. The same signs and symptoms can occur in a patient receiving a tube feeding if the nasogastric tube is carried down into the duodenum accidentally.

Dietary treatment of the dumping syndrome attempts to delay gastric emptying and to spread out the increased osmolality in the bowel. This can be achieved by limiting the intake of simple sugars, consuming frequent meals, and limiting fluids with meals. Simple sugars increase the osmolality of the gastric contents and enhance the movement of food out of the stomach. Small, frequent meals will reduce the load on the intestine. Liquids should be taken between, rather than with, meals. Beverages should be low in simple carbohydrate. Very hot or cold foods will stimulate peristalsis and should be avoided. A nondietary intervention also helps to control the symptoms of the dumping syndrome. Lying down for 30 to 60 minutes after eating retains the meal in the stomach longer.

Dumping syndrome—condition in which the stomach contents move into the duodenum too rapidly; often associated with gastric resections.

Following gastric surgery, parenteral and tube feeding are used singly or in combination. If a tube feeding is used, the tube must be inserted beyond the area resected. Once a patient is advanced to an oral diet, he or she may experience **dumping syndrome.** Dumping syndrome may develop as a complication of any surgical procedure that removes, disrupts, or bypasses the pyloric sphincter. Clinical Application 19–2 describes dumping syndrome in more detail.

DISORDERS OF THE INTESTINES

Much preparation of the patient precedes diagnostic x-ray study of the gastrointestinal system. Often it is imperative to empty the bowel for clear visualization. This is accomplished by laxatives and enemas. Often the patient is advised to follow a low-residue diet for several days prior to diagnostic x-rays studies of the GI tract. Explaining the procedures and the necessity for them is helpful in gaining the patient's cooperation. Follow the instructions from the radiography department or the institution's diet manual for specifics. Above all, be creative and persistent in ensuring that the patient receives maximum nourishment when tests are completed for the day. Frequently, another series of tests is scheduled for the next day.

Problems with Elimination

Several problems with frequency and consistency of bowel movements are common. These include irritable bowel syndrome, diarrhea, and constipation.

Irritable Bowel Syndrome

Signs and symptoms of <u>irritable bowel syndrome</u> are diarrhea, constipation, or alternating diarrhea and constipation; abdominal pain; and flatulence. Investigation often reveals no organic cause for the symptoms. Irritable bowel syndrome is often related to stress and emotional tension triggering overactivity of the nervous system.

> **Irritable bowel syndrome**—diarrhea, or alternating constipation-diarrhea with no discernable organic cause.

    Treatment is symptomatic. Offending foods should be identified and avoided. Stress management techniques and bowel hygiene principles should be part of the teaching plan. A high-fiber diet helps to avoid both constipation and an increase in pressure on the walls of the intestine. This often provides symptomatic relief. You will learn more about this process later in the chapter.

Diarrhea

Diarrhea was discussed in previous chapters. Of special note here are the foods that are risky for travelers. Especially in primitive areas, travelers are well advised to avoid raw vegetables, raw meat, raw seafood, tap water, ice, and unpasteurized dairy products. If a person is in little jeopardy from electrolyte imbalance, self-treatment for diarrhea by following the regimen listed in Table 19–3 is appropriate. If a patient has medical conditions for which dehydration is a hazard, a physician should be consulted.

Constipation

A person is constipated when bowel movements are so infrequent that defecation is difficult. Over time each person develops a usual bowel pattern. A bowel movement every second or third day may be perfectly normal for a

TABLE 19–3 *Self-Treatment for Diarrhea**

Time	Oral Intake	Comments
1st 12 hours	Nothing by mouth	Anything additional in the GI tract will stimulate peristalsis.
2nd 12 hours	Clear liquids	If up to 5 percent body weight lost; if more than 5 percent lost, seek medical attention.
3rd 12 hours	Full liquids	Experiment with milk in case lactose intolerance has developed.
4th 12 hours	Soft diet	Include applesauce or banana for pectin; rice, pasta, and bread without fat (digested by enzymes usually unaffected by gastroenteritis).
By 48th hour	Regular diet	If diarrhea has not resolved and regular diet is not tolerated, seek medical treatment.

*Appropriate for healthy adults.

given individual. Objective evidence of constipation is stool that is hard and dry, with small round pieces like marbles. It is essential that changes in bowel habits be investigated thoroughly to discover possible bowel cancers. Aside from disease conditions, the causes of constipation are lack of water and fiber in the diet, lack of exercise, and voluntary retention.

Treatment for constipation involves dietary and lifestyle changes, not laxatives. Unfortunately, the message has not yet been widely heard, especially by the elderly. Up to 50 percent of adults over age 70 regularly use laxatives. Overall, Americans spend $250 million on laxatives each year. Increasing the fiber in the diet, drinking adequate amounts of water, and exercising regularly are the keys to overcoming constipation. Even laxative habits established for years can be overcome this way.

Problems with Absorption

Two conditions are discussed in this section, fat malabsorption and celiac disease. Fat malabsorption may follow many diseases that damage the intestine. Celiac disease, or nontropical sprue, is a specific response to gluten-containing foods.

Fat Malabsorption

Several conditions hinder fat absorption. Many of the resulting symptoms are similar despite the differences in the underlying pathology.

When fat is not well absorbed, the fat-soluble vitamins also are poorly absorbed. Fat content of the feces is increased. These extra fatty acids bind with calcium and magnesium to form soaps in the bowel. (A chemical soap results from the union of fatty acid and alkali.) The calcium bound in the soap is thus unavailable to bind with oxalate. An increased amount of oxalate is excreted through the kidney. This is not a harmless rerouting, however, because oxalate kidney stones can form as a result.

Treatment centers upon careful selection of fats in the diet and appropriate supplementation of unavailable nutrients. Low-fat diets will be discussed later in the chapter. Medium-chain triglycerides (MCTs) are often given to increase kilocalories. They do not need pancreatic lipase or bile for digestion and absorption. MCTs are absorbed into the portal vein, as are amino acids and monosaccharides, rather than into the lymphatic system as are other lipids. Usually, MCTs are added to salad dressings, skimmed milk, or desserts. Because linoleic acid, an essential fatty acid, is missing from MCT, some regular fat is still needed in the diet. Supplements of the fat-soluble vitamins should be given in water-soluble form. To overcome malabsorption, the commonly used dose of supplements is twice the RDA.

Celiac Disease

Celiac disease (Gluten enteropathy)— intolerance to dietary gluten which damages the intestine and produces diarrhea and malabsorption.

Celiac disease is also called gluten enteropathy or nontropical sprue. The cause is unknown. The affected person is sensitive to gluten, a protein in wheat, oats, rye, and barley. As little as 3 grams per day may cause symptoms. Ingestion of gluten by these sensitive people causes atrophy of the intestinal villi in the jejunum. What follows is malabsorption of all the classes of nutrients except water. Celiac disease affects the absorption of fat, protein, carbohydrate, fat-soluble vitamins, and folic acid, and the minerals iron, calcium, magnesium, and zinc.

The outstanding sign of celiac disease is <u>steatorrhea,</u> or excessive fat in the stools. The result is foul-smelling, frothy, bulky stools. Patients complain of bloating, diarrhea, and cramping abdominal pain. Some of this may be temporary, the result of lactase insufficiency. Untreated, the patient's anorexia leads to weight loss and malnutrition marked by anemia, muscle wasting, edema from hypoalbuminemia, bleeding due to vitamin-K deficiency, and bone pain and tetany from hypocalcemia.

The treatment is simply to remove gluten permanently from the diet. The disease is not outgrown, and damage to the villi continues even without symptoms. Removing gluten from the diet is easier said than done, however. It involves analyzing the label of every food the patient takes. Table 5–5 contains a list of gluten-free foods. Fortunately, this treatment reverses the pathology almost completely, but it might take 3 to 6 months. Sometimes, a secondary lactose intolerance results from mucosal damage and requires long-term management.

Inflammatory Bowel Diseases

Inflammatory bowel diseases are a group of syndromes that share similar characteristics but have some major differences. The two most common inflammatory bowel diseases are **Crohn's disease,** also known as ileitis or regional enteritis, and **ulcerative colitis.** Although the cause of both of these conditions is unknown, autoimmunity and genetic susceptibility may be partially responsible. The signs and symptoms of both Crohn's disease and ulcerative colitis include anorexia, weight loss, fever, and diarrhea. Differences between the two diseases include their location in the gastrointestinal tract, the type of lesions involved, and complications (Table 19–4). The nutritional care of patients with inflammatory bowel disease is variable and dependent on the nutritional status of the individual, the location and extent of the disease, and the nature of the surgical and medical management

Crohn's Disease—inflammatory disease appearing in any area of the bowel, with diseased areas alternating with healthy tissue.

Ulcerative colitis—Inflammatory disease of the large intestine which usually begins in the rectum and spreads upward in a continuous pattern.

Nutritional Therapy in Crohn's Disease

Crohn's disease may involve either the small or large intestine or both, as well as the stomach and esophagus, in some cases. The emphasis of treatment is (1) to support the healing of tissue, (2) to avoid and/or prevent nutritional deficiencies, and (3) to prevent local trauma to inflamed areas. Par-

TABLE 19–4 *Differences between Crohn's Disease and Ulcerative Colitis*

	Crohn's Disease	Ulcerative Colitis
Location	Anywhere in bowel Diseased areas alternate with healthy tissue	Large intestine Usually starts in rectum and spreads upward in continuous pattern
Lesions	Involves all layers of intestinal wall	Confined to mucosal and submucosal layers
Complications	Fistula, obstruction, stricture	Toxic megacolon, fistula Increased risk of colon cancer.

enteral and tube feedings may be used together or separately to meet nutritional goals. The diet modifications are usually based on high-kilocalorie, high-protein, low-fat, and low-fiber or low-residue intake. Small, frequent feedings may assist in promoting comfort and adequate nutrition. Seasonings and chilled foods often aggravate symptoms. Because of damage to the intestinal wall, lactose intolerance may develop.

Nutritional Therapy in Ulcerative Colitis

During an acute exacerbation of ulcerative colitis, tube feedings or TPN are often given. A 4- to 6-week course of TPN achieves complete bowel rest. This choice is necessary when the patient has a fistula, obstruction, or abscess. As many as 60 to 80 percent of patients undergo remission with these therapies. Convalescent patients with ulcerative colitis must avoid irritating foods. Dietary modification is usually based on patient tolerance. To maintain nutritional status, foods should not be eliminated from the diet without a fair trial. Restrictions should be limited to foods that produce gas or loose stools. Suspected foods should be tried in small amounts to determine tolerance levels. Parenteral supplements of iron and vitamin B_{12} may also be prescribed for these patients.

Surgical Treatment in Inflammatory Bowel Disease

Colectomy—Surgical removal of all or part of the colon.

Surgery may be recommended when inflammatory bowel disease becomes medically unmanageable. The portion of the bowel that is inflamed can be surgically removed (resected). This results in a shorter gut. Resection of the small intestine may create additional nutritional hazards for the patient (Clinical Application 19–3). A colectomy is the surgical removal of part or all of the colon. Other surgical procedures include ileostomy and colostomy. Both procedures may be either permanent or temporary.

CLINICAL APPLICATION 19–3
Short-Gut Syndrome

Because the small intestine is 16 to 20 feet long in the adult, up to 50 percent can be removed, if necessary. Depending on the site of resection, the remaining bowel adjusts by becoming longer, thicker, and wider to increase its absorptive capacity. However, this process may take up to 6 months and will occur only if the patient receives food or tube feedings. In cases in which the ileocecal valve and/or 80 percent of the small bowel is removed, the body cannot completely compensate for the loss.

Certain nutrients are absorbed at specific locations in the small bowel. Thus, removing a section of the bowel eliminates the absorption of those nutrients usually absorbed in that particular portion, until the body can adapt to the change. When the duodenum is resected, iron absorption is deficient. When more than 8 feet of the proximal jejunum is resected, absorption of glucose, protein, fat, fat-soluble vitamins, calcium and magnesium is impaired. When the ileum is resected, vitamin B_{12} is not absorbed. This function is not assumed by other segments of

Box continued on next page.

CLINICAL APPLICATION 19–3 *(continued)*
Short-Gut Syndrome

the bowel, so the patient must receive vitamin B_{12} injections. Bile salt-salso are reabsorbed into the bloodstream in the ileum. When the ileum is resected and bile salts are inappropriately excreted in the feces, a smaller quantity is available for fat metabolism. The excess bile salts in the feces also can cause osmotic diarrhea, dehydration, and anal excoriation.

If, in addition, the ileocecal valve, which separates the small and large intestines, must be removed, nutrients move through the gastrointestinal tract very quickly. This anatomical change worsens the prognosis and greatly increases the chance of malabsorption.

Signs and symptoms of short-gut syndrome are diarrhea, weight loss, and muscle wasting. These are related to protein and fat malabsorption. Poor iron, calcium, and magnesium absorption lead to anemia, hypocalcemia, and hypomagnesemia.

Treatment of short-gut syndrome can become intensive. The patient needs up to 175 grams of protein and 5000 kilocalories per day. Early nourishment is provided by total parenteral nutrition. When enteral feedings begin, elemental predigested formulas are used because they are completely absorbed in the proximal small intestine. When food is taken, it should be eaten as small low-fat meals, with medium-chain triglycerides replacing regular fats.

In an <u>ileostomy,</u> the end of the remaining portion of the small intestine (the ileum) is attached to a surgically established opening in the abdominal wall called a <u>stoma,</u> from which the intestinal contents are discharged. In a <u>colostomy,</u> a part of the large intestine is resected and a stoma is created on the abdomen. Patients who have surgery to divert intestinal contents onto the abdominal wall may suffer both physical and psychological trauma.

ILEOSTOMY   An ileostomy produces liquid drainage. This drainage is irritating to the skin because of the active enzymes it contains. In addition, nutrient losses are great. A loss of as much as 2 liters of fluid per day immediately following surgery is possible. Read Clinical Application 19–4 for more information on innovations for controlling ileostomy drainage. Over

Ileostomy—surgical procedure in which an opening to the small intestine (ileum) is constructed on the abdomen.

Stoma—A surgically created opening in the abdominal wall.

Colostomy—surgical procedure in which an opening to the large intestine is constructed on the abdomen.

CLINICAL APPLICATION 19–4
Continent Ileostomies

Ordinarily if an ileostomy is performed, the patient must wear an appliance to contain the loose drainage. Other procedures afford a measure of control of the drainage. Continent ileostomies sometimes can be constructed from the remaining intestine, creating an intestinal reservoir just inside the abdominal wall. The reservoir is emptied by inserting a catheter into the stoma several times a day. Sometimes an ileoanal anastomosis is done so that the anal sphincter can be used to control elimination. Even after the bowel adapts to its shorter length, the patient has 7 to 10 bowel movements per day.

time the bowel adapts to some extent, and drainage decreases to 300 to 500 milliliters. This amount, however, is more than the 100 to 200 milliliters in the normal stool. Additional nutrient losses in ileostomy patients are those of sodium, potassium, and vitamin B_{12}.

COLOSTOMY   In contrast to an ileostomy, a colostomy, after the convalescent period, may be so continent that a dry dressing is all that is necessary to cover the stoma. The patient may do daily irrigations or not, as the surgeon suggests. Sometimes the patient knows best, after the initial learning process.

DIETARY GUIDELINES FOR OSTOMY PATIENTS   A soft or general diet is usually served to ostomy patients after recovery from surgery. Stringy, high-fiber foods are initially avoided until a definite tolerance has been demonstrated. Stringy, high-fiber foods include celery, coconut, coleslaw, membranes on citrus fruits, peas, popcorn, spinach, dried fruit, pineapple, seeds, and fruit and vegetable skins. Some patients complain that fish, eggs, beer, and carbonated beverages produce excessive odor.

Patients with ostomies should be encouraged to (1) eat at regular intervals; (2) chew food well to avoid blockage at the stoma site; (3) drink adequate amounts of fluid; (4) avoid foods that produce excessive gas, loose stools, offensive odors and/or undesirable bulk; and (5) avoid excessive weight gain. Dietary restrictions are usually based on individual tolerance.

Diverticular Disease

Diverticulum—A sac or pouch in the walls of an organ of the alimentary canal.

A **diverticulum** (plural—diverticula) is an outpouching of intestinal membrane through a weakness in the intestine's muscular layer. Diverticula are present in 10 percent of the United States population. About one third to one half of the elderly have diverticula, 60 percent among people older than 80. A low-fiber diet is believed to increase the risk for diverticula. A low-fiber diet contains less than 15 grams of fiber per day.

Diverticulosis

Diverticulosis—presence of one or more diverticula (outpouching of the inner mucosa through a weakness in the gastrointestinal muscle).

The presence of diverticula is called **diverticulosis.** The usual site is the sigmoid colon (Fig. 19–5). Diverticula often occur at the points at which blood vessels enter the intestinal muscle. A proposed cause for diverticulosis is the increased force needed to propel insufficient intestinal contents through the lumen. Often the person with diverticulosis has no signs or symptoms. Once an individual knows the diverticula are present, a high-fiber diet of 30 grams per day is advised. This should be accompanied by an adequate fluid intake.

Diverticulitis

Diverticulitis—inflammation of a diverticulum.

When diverticula become inflamed, the condition is termed **diverticulitis.** This happens in 15 to 30 percent of diverticulosis cases. Inflammation occurs in the elderly at about the same rate as in younger people with diverticulosis, 25 percent. Following the prescribed diet improves the condition of 85 percent of the patients.

Signs and symptoms of diverticulitis, with the exception of fever, are focused in the abdomen. The patient complains of cramps, pain in the lower left quadrant, dyspepsia, nausea and vomiting, distention and flatus, and

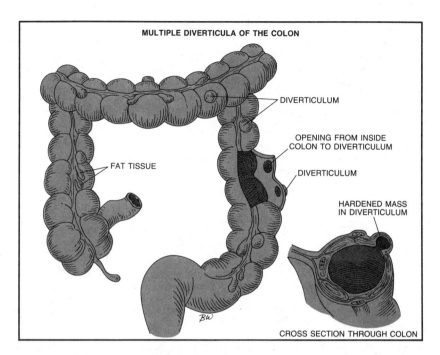

FIGURE 19-5. Diverticula of the transverse and descending colon (From Thomas, p 523, with permission)

alternating constipation and diarrhea. Some serious complications can follow diverticulitis. The inflammatory process can lead to adhesions or fistulas. A thickened intestinal wall from the scar tissue can cause an obstruction. Rupture of a diverticulum can initiate peritonitis.

Dietary treatment of diverticulitis has changed radically over the years. Whereas once a low-fiber diet was the rule, now it is only a temporary measure. While the inflammation is severe, elemental or predigested formulas or a low-fiber diet is given. After that, a high-fiber diet as for diverticulosis is prescribed. Although not proven to be helpful, avoiding foods with small seeds that could get caught in the diverticulum may be recommended.

DISEASES AND CONDITIONS OF THE LIVER AND GALLBLADDER

Anatomically, the liver and gallbladder are closely aligned. Of the two, the liver is more essential for life.

Diseases and Conditions of the Liver

The liver is a workhorse for the body. Disease in the liver probably produces more diverse symptoms than disease of any other organ.

Functions of the Liver

If you refer again to Table 19–1, you can see that the liver is involved with the metabolism of all the nutrients. All digested substances go to the liver for the next step in processing. The liver is also the major organ of drug detoxification.

The liver is the sole site of albumin production. Serum albumin maintains intravascular volume by exerting osmotic pressure on interstitial fluid. It also binds with certain drugs. The half-life of albumin is 14 days. Clotting proteins, however, have a relatively short half-life of 24 to 36 hours. Thus, blood levels of albumin and prothrombin are helpful in diagnosing liver disease. In acute toxicity or injury, prothrombin level falls before albumin level because the clotting proteins have a shorter half-life and are rapidly expended. By contrast, in chronic liver disease, blood albumin level falls before that of prothrombin.

Fatty Liver

Fatty liver—accumulation of triglycerides in the liver cells; usually reversible if the cause, of which there are many, is removed.

The infiltration of liver cells by fat is called <u>fatty liver.</u> Many situations can cause fatty liver, including a low-protein or starvation diet (because of the breakdown of adipose tissue for energy) and alcoholism. Usually no harm is done by fatty liver unless it progresses. Treatment is to correct the cause. If it is alcohol consumption, abstinence reverses the pathology.

Hepatitis

Hepatitis—inflammation of the liver, caused by viruses, drugs, alcohol, or toxic substances.

Inflammation of the liver, or **hepatitis,** It can result from viral infections, alcohol, drugs, and toxins. The two well-known viral infections are hepatitis A and hepatitis B. Hepatitis A is spread by both the fecal-oral route and, rarely, by blood transfusion. It was discussed in Chapter 12. Hepatitis B is spread by body fluids such as blood, saliva, semen, and vaginal secretions.

SIGNS AND SYMPTOMS OF HEPATITIS Regardless of cause, the body responds to liver inflammation according to the following pattern. Symptoms are anorexia, nausea, epigastric discomfort, and weakness. Signs of hepatitis are vomiting, diarrhea, and jaundice due to inability of the liver to convert fat-soluble bilirubin to a water-soluble (conjugated) form. The degree of jaundice gives a rough estimate of the severity of the disease. Physical examination will show an enlarged and tender liver and an enlarged spleen.

TREATMENT OF HEPATITIS Currently, no specific medications can be given to cure hepatitis. Bed rest, abstinence from alcohol, and optimum nutrition are the keys to treatment. Convalescence may take from 3 weeks to 3 months. Patients on bed rest, especially debilitated patients, are more susceptible to pressure ulcers than the average patient. The reason for this is the decreased protein synthesis of albumin and the globulins. If the patient abstains from alcohol, the hepatitis is often reversible.

A high-kilocalorie, high-protein, and moderate-fat diet is frequently prescribed for the hepatitis patient. Energy intake should come from as much as 400 grams of carbohydrate daily. Protein in amounts up to 100 grams will help heal the liver. Emulsified fats in dairy products and eggs may be accepted better by the patient than other fats. Up to 35 percent of kilocalories in fat will provide high energy in a lower volume of food. Fluid intake should be 3 to 3.5 liters per day.

Coaxing a person with hepatitis to accept such a substantial meal pattern is an enormous task, in view of the anorexia and nausea that accompany the disease. Since the nausea is often less in the morning than later in the day, the hepatitis patient should be encouraged to eat a big breakfast. Polymeric oral feedings which are high in kilocalories and protein are widely used for between meal feedings.

Cirrhosis of the Liver

The word cirrhosis comes from a French word for orange. In **cirrhosis** the liver becomes fibrous and contains orange-colored nodules.

    In the United States, chronic alcohol abuse is the most common cause of cirrhosis. About half of the 10 million alcoholics in this country will develop cirrhosis. As a cause of death, chronic liver disease and cirrhosis rank ninth. Cirrhosis is not the only consequence of alcohol consumption producing suffering and death. Accidents are the fourth leading cause of death. Though not all accidents involve motor vehicles, alcohol is involved in half of the fatal motor vehicle accidents.

    Alcohol is toxic to all body tissues, including the liver. For a summary of the nutritional effects of alcoholism on the liver and other body organs and systems, see Clinical Application 19–5.

Cirrhosis— chronic disease of the liver in which functioning cells degenerate and are replaced by fibrosed connective tissue.

🌾 CLINICAL APPLICATION 19–5 🌾
Nutritional Effects of Alcohol

    Alcoholism is a disease of alcohol consumption that produces tolerance, physical dependence, and characteristic organ pathology in the body. Ingestion of prodigious amounts of alcohol is not necessary for someone to become an alcoholic. The disease may be produced in some persons by 3 to 5 ounces of whiskey per day. The first notion to dispel is the cliché of the skid-row alcoholic. There still are alcoholics on skid row, of course, but the disease is far more pervasive than that. In an affluent society alcoholics may be obese, usually early in the disease, rather than later.

    In the United States, alcoholism is the single most important factor in nutrient deficiencies. Associating the numerous functions of the liver with the fact that alcohol is toxic to all body cells, the nutritional havoc accompanying alcoholism becomes obvious. Widespread vitamin deficiencies occur. Even without liver damage, alcohol injures the intestine, thereby reducing absorption of vitamins A, D, K, thiamin, pyridoxine, folic acid, and B_{12}.

    Folic acid deficiency is the most common vitamin deficiency in the world. It also is the most common vitamin deficiency in alcoholics, affecting 50 to 80 percent of them.

    The vitamin deficiency that is almost synonymous with alcoholism is that of thiamin. In the United States, thiamin deficiency is seen almost exclusively in alcoholics, affecting from 30 to 80 percent of them. The neurological symptoms of thiamin deficiency present a disheartening picture. Patients have atrophy of many nerves, weakness in the ankles and toes, and numbness and tingling in the feet.

    The behavior of an intoxicated person indicates that alcohol penetrates the blood–brain barrier. In fact, brain damage may occur before severe liver damage. The Wernicke-Korsakoff syndrome is a disorder of

Box continued on next page.

the central nervous system caused by thiamin deficiency in alcoholics. The patients display disorientation, memory dysfunction, and ataxia. Weakness of the muscles controlling the eyes produces double vision (diplopia) and abnormal movements of the eyeball (nystagmus). Thiamin helps to oxidize glucose and to metabolize alcohol to energy. This is a critical piece of information for healthcare workers taking care of alcoholics. These patients are deficient in thiamin when treatment is begun. Administering a simple solution of glucose intravenously can precipitate symptoms of Wernicke-Korsakoff syndrome. For this reason you will find that thiamin is routinely administered parenterally to alcoholics.

Other vitamin deficiencies in alcoholics, in order of frequency after folic acid and thiamin, are pyridoxine, niacin, vitamin C, and vitamin A. Niacin deficiency occurs in one third of alcoholics. Scurvy in the United States is almost exclusively found in alcoholics. Vitamin C, besides being necessary for tissue repair, plays a role in folic acid metabolism and in iron absorption. Storage of vitamin A in the liver is impaired. A prominent result of hypovitaminosis A is night blindness. Night blindness and intoxication in an automobile driver are a deadly duo.

Other nutritional effects possible in alcoholics are bone loss and bleeding tendencies. One half of alcoholics show bone loss. Albumin carries calcium in the bloodstream. Hypoalbuminemia, reduced stores and faulty metabolism of vitamin D, low calcium intake, and steatorrhea causing binding of calcium in the intestine may all combine to produce bone loss.

Prothrombin, normally manufactured by the liver using vitamin K, is necessary for blood clotting. Vitamin-E deficiency produces neurological changes, cerebellar degeneration, and peripheral neuropathy.

Potassium, phosphorus, and magnesium are the most common major mineral deficiencies in alcoholics. Because some of the symptoms of delirium tremens are the same as symptoms of magnesium deficiency, it was postulated that magnesium deficiency causes delirium tremens. At present, there is no consensus on this issue.

Iron and zinc are the trace minerals most often deficient in alcoholics. Low iron stores are related to gastrointestinal bleeding, rather than poor absorption. Alcohol damages the intestinal mucosa and thereby permits increased absorption of iron. With low folic acid levels, however, red blood cell production cannot proceed normally. Anemia or bone marrow abnormalities have been found in 75 percent of patients hospitalized with alcoholism.

Up to 50 percent of alcoholic patients are deficient in zinc. Zinc is needed for many enzymes that serve a function in DNA and RNA metabolism. It plays a vital role in the growth and repair of essential organs, such as the liver. Zinc is also necessary to convert vitamin A to a functional form in the retina. Sometimes a patient with night blindness is deficient in zinc, not vitamin A.

Lastly, alcoholics suffer from protein-energy malnutrition. Even in early alcoholism, albumin levels are low-normal. The typical alcoholic consumes only 75 percent of required energy. The result of low-protein, low-energy intake is muscle wasting. Fat is not an adequate source of energy for alcoholics, owing to malabsorption. Steatorrhea is seen in half the patients.

This summary of the extensive effects of alcohol on nutrition is intended to provide a basis for understanding the many diverse signs and symptoms alcoholic patients display. Intensive nutritional support is needed by patients with advanced alcoholism and cirrhosis.

Alcoholic patients may not be truthful when asked about their intake of alcohol. Nevertheless, that does not excuse the healthcare worker from trying to discover if a problem exists. Asking the right questions is more likely to yield honest answers. Clinical Application 19–6 offers suggestions on the assessment of drinking habits.

A diagnosis of cirrhosis cannot always be linked to alcoholism. Cirrhosis may occur in nonalcoholics. Such insults to the liver as infection, biliary obstruction, and toxic chemicals, including medications, may precede cirrhosis.

CLINICAL APPLICATION 19–6
Assessment of Drinking Habits

It sometimes is more fruitful to approach the subject of alcohol consumption through the family history. Patients may feel less defensive and less likely to "cover up" a relative's excessive drinking than their own.

Asking every question is not necessary; the following items are intended to stimulate your thinking. Use of a "laundry list" in a sensitive area is likely to be unproductive.

FAMILY HISTORY

How often is alcohol served in your house?
Who partakes?
What is served most often?
How much does the heaviest drinker consume? The least heavy drinker?
Who is most likely to drink alcohol away from home?
Where is that likely to be?
Who are the drinking companions?
How often is alcohol consumed outside the home?
How much alcohol is usually consumed?

While the healthcare worker is focusing on the family, the patient is focusing on the healthcare worker. If the attitude is nonjudgmental, chances are increased that more personal inquiries will be answered frankly.

INDIVIDUAL CONSUMPTION

How much alcohol do you drink? (Try to get specific answers: ounces, a pint, a fifth. To an alcoholic, a "drink" might be a quart of beer rather than 12 ounces, or a fifth of wine rather than 4 ounces.)
What do you drink? (If mixed drinks, inquire about the proportions of whiskey to mixer.)
When do you drink?
Who are your drinking companions?
How much do you drink in 24 hours?

Box continued on next page.

CLINICAL APPLICATION 19–6 *(continued)*
Assessment of Drinking Habits

What is the most you have drunk in a 24-hour period?
Have you ever had blackouts?
How often do you gulp drinks?
Have you ever tried to quit drinking?
When did you have your last drink?
What was it?
How much did you drink?

It might be helpful to ask the patient to define an alcoholic. Some of us have narrow definitions to satisfy our personal needs. For instance, we might define an alcoholic as someone who drinks alone, drinks in the morning, or goes on binges.

These are defense mechanisms. As long as our own drinking does not fit "alcoholism" as personally defined, the denial is maintained.

There is no score for this questionnaire. There is no one answer that is diagnostic of alcoholism. The healthcare workers look for a pattern of dependence on alcohol. It will take some experience to become adept at interviewing suspected alcoholics. The right questions must be asked to avoid participating in the patient's denial.

PATHOPHYSIOLOGY Alcohol needs no digestion. It is absorbed rapidly, 20 percent from the stomach and 80 percent from the small intestine. Immediately after absorption, the alcohol is carried to the liver. The rate of breakdown by the liver is 0.5 ounce of alcohol per hour. This refers to the alcohol content, not the whole beverage. This step cannot be rushed. So giving coffee or other stimulants to an intoxicated person will not induce sobriety, merely a "wide-awake drunk."

If the cause of the illness is not corrected, dying liver cells, are replaced by scar tissue. Figure 19–6 traces the path from cell death to several cardinal signs of cirrhosis. Because of the multiple functions of the liver, one pathological change reinforces another. The ascites is worsened by hypoalbuminemia and is partly caused and also worsened by sodium retention. Depressed plasma protein production, as evidenced by decreasing albumin levels, indicates a poor patient outcome.

SIGNS AND SYMPTOMS OF CIRRHOSIS Cirrhosis causes anorexia, epigastric pain, and nausea that worsens as the days go on. Signs of the disease are abdominal distention, vomiting, steatorrhea, jaundice, ascites, edema, and gastrointestinal bleeding. Of patients with advanced cirrhosis, 70 percent develop esophageal varices, varicose veins of the esophagus. Muscle tremors result from hypomagnesemia. Laboratory tests will show hypoglycemia and elevated serum triglyceride levels. The lack of enzymes for converting noncarbohydrate sources to energy causes hypoglycemia. Insufficient lipoprotein synthesis causes the elevated triglycerides and fatty liver. The end result of cirrhosis is liver failure, which leads to hepatic coma (Clinical Application 19–7).

TREATMENT OF CIRRHOSIS Absolutely no alcohol is permitted. Treatment is ineffective if the patient continues to drink. Even so, once por-

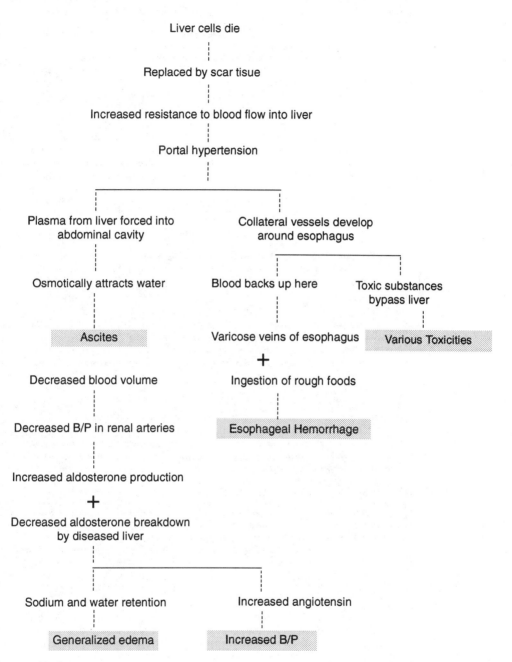

FIGURE 19–6. The progression of pathology leading to the classic symptoms of cirrhosis of the liver. The signs and symptoms are shaded.

Hepatic Encephalopathy

Hepatic encephalopathy, or hepatic coma, is the result of liver failure. The precise mechanism involved in the pathology is uncertain. Because hepatic encephalopathy is associated with increased serum levels of ammonia and aromatic amino acids, treatments to control one or both of these factors have been suggested.

Ammonia is produced by intestinal bacteria, and by digestive enzymes breaking down protein. Even if the person consumes no protein foods, the bacteria work on the cast-off cells of the gastrointestinal tract and on the blood from gastrointestinal bleeding, which is so common in alcoholic cirrhosis. Ordinarily, the liver degrades ammonia to urea, which is then excreted by the kidneys in urine. In liver failure, blood ammonia levels rise. Ammonia is toxic to all cells, including those of the liver and the brain. The laboratory values are not clearly correlated with the degree of encephalopathy, so a series of tests is necessary to monitor each patient.

The liver normally breaks down amino acids. The patient with liver failure exhibits a change in the ratio of aromatic amino acids (phenylalanine, tryptophan, and tyrosine) to branched-chain amino acids (leucine, isoleucine, and valine). In the healthy patient this ratio is approximately 1:1; in hepatic coma it is 3:1 or higher. The elevated levels of aromatic amino acids interfere with the formation of the neurotransmitters dopamine and norepinephrine, and may contribute to hepatic coma.

Some signs of hepatic encephalopathy can be observed prior to the onset of coma. These are personality changes, irritability, weakness, apathy, confusion, and sleepiness. More specific signs are asterixis and fetor hepaticus. Asterixis, or liver flap, refers to involuntary jerking movements or a flapping of the hand when the arm is outstretched. Fetor hepaticus is a fecal odor to the breath. Lastly, there is coma.

Treatment consists of medications and dietary modifications, along with symptomatic care. Oral neomycin kills the bacteria in the intestine, thereby decreasing ammonia production. Lactulose acidifies the large intestine, causing ammonia to be converted to ammonium ions, which are not absorbed. Diet must be carefully planned. Some foods produce higher ammonia levels than most others. These include chicken, salami, ground beef, ham, bacon, gelatin, peanut butter, potatoes, onions, lima beans, egg yolk, buttermilk, and blue and cheddar cheese.

When coma is approaching, protein is limited to 40 to 60 grams of high-quality protein per day. Because they contain fewer aromatic amino acids, vegetable proteins may be tolerated better than animal protein. If enteral feeding is necessary, special preparations low in aromatic amino acids are available. Two of them are Hepatic-Aid II and Travasorb-Hepatic. According to theory, these should be beneficial, but more data are being collected. Although weight reduction is probably not a focus of concern on the part of patients as sick as these, note should be made that aspartame (NutraSweet) contains phenylalanine, an aromatic amino acid. If the theory holds, it too should be avoided.

If the patient's condition continues to deteriorate, even greater restrictions are placed on diet. Adequate kilocaloric intake, 1500 to 2000 kilocalories, must be maintained to prevent tissue protein from being used for energy. Dietary protein is decreased to 10-20 grams per day. As the patient recovers, dietary protein is added in increments of 10 grams every 2 days. If signs of encephalopathy occur, protein is reduced to the previous restriction (American Dietetic Association, 1992).

tal hypertension has set in, abstinence does not halt the progression of cirrhosis.

A protein-restricted diet is prescribed if the liver is unable to process the end products of protein metabolism. Anywhere from 20 to 40 grams of protein per day may be prescribed. After extremely low intake of foods, the cirrhosis patient may not be able to tolerate anything resembling a normal diet. If the patient has esophageal varices, the diet also must be soft.

As the patient improves, the protein content of the diet can sometimes be increased. It is necessary to monitor the patient carefully for signs of excessive protein intake. If residual liver function is sufficient, the diet should contain 1 to 1.5 grams of protein per kilogram of body weight to aid in regeneration of liver cells. This is enough for tissue renewal but not enough to build up ammonia in the bloodstream. Enough fat is offered for palatability. Fats that are already emulsified, such as those in homogenized milk and eggs, need less bile for digestion.

Fluid and electrolyte balance demands careful attention. If the patient has ascites, sodium will likely be restricted. An amount of 0.25 to 1 gram (250 to 1000 milligrams) is frequently used. Fluid is restricted also. A commonly prescribed amount is 1.5 to 2 liters in 24 hours. If the serum sodium level is low, fluid may be limited to 1 to 1.5 liters. Monitoring the signs of ascites reduction includes measuring abdominal girth and weighing daily. If the patient has ascites without peripheral edema, a reasonable goal for weight loss is 0.5 kilogram (1.1 pounds) per day. If both ascites and peripheral edema are displayed, the goal for weight loss is 1 kilogram per day.

The effects of alcohol on vitamin metabolism are extensive and serious. For this reason, cirrhosis patients are given supplemental vitamins daily. Up to five times the RDA of water-soluble vitamins may be necessary.

Protein-Controlled Diets

The need to control protein intake changes with liver function. Protein is severely restricted in liver failure but encouraged in mild liver disease. The goal of a severely protein-restricted diet is to decrease blood ammonia levels, reduce the clinical manifestations of liver failure, and minimize the risks of severe malnutrition. The goal of a high-protein diet is to support liver regeneration. Table 19–5 displays various protein-controlled diets that contain from 20 to 80 grams of protein.

Sufficient kilocalories must be provided to prevent protein from being catabolized for energy. The goal is to promote positive nitrogen balance while preventing further exacerbation of liver disease. For this reason, the protein restriction should be used for only a short period. Adequate kilocalories are crucial to spare protein and promote liver regenation. Intake of simple carbohydrates should be encouraged. Fats may be given according to patient tolerance. The sample menu in the table assumes that the patient can tolerate fats.

For severely protein-restricted diets, the protein content of fruits and vegetables is usually calculated as 0.5 gram per fruit exchange and selected vegetable exchanges as 1 gram per exchange. Other vegetables are considered 2 grams per exchange. Starches are calculated as 2 grams of protein per exchange. In addition to a protein restriction, sodium, potassium, and fluids may need to be restricted in some patients.

TABLE 19–5 *Meal Plan for Various Levels of Protein Restriction*

Meal Plan	Sample Menu

20-GRAM PROTEIN DIET

Breakfast
½ cup milk — ½ cup whole milk
1 fruit — ½ cup orange juice with 2 tablespoons modular carbohydrate supplement*
2 starches — ½ cup Cream of Wheat with 1 tablespoon modular carbohydrate supplement and 1 slice of toast with 1 tablespoon margarine and jelly
Fat (as tolerated) — 2 tablespoons cream
Beverage — As tolerated and per fluid restriction
Lunch
2 starches — 1 cup rice with ¼ cup unsalted tomato sauce and 1 tablespoon olive oil
Vegetable — ½ cup green beans with 1 teaspoon margarine
Fruit — ½ cup canned peaches with 1 tablespoon modular carbohydrate supplement
Beverage — As tolerated and per fluid restriction
Dinner
2 starches — 1 baked potato with 2 tablespoons sour cream and 1 slice of bread with 1 teaspoon margarine and jelly
Vegetable — ½ cup mushrooms (for potato topping)
Fruit — ½ cup strawberries with 1 tablespoon modular carbohydrate supplement
Beverage — As tolerated and per fluid restriction

40-GRAM PROTEIN DIET

Add to the Above:
½ cup milk
2 meat exchanges
1 starch exchange

60-GRAM PROTEIN DIET

Add to the 20-Gram Protein Diet Meal Plan:
2 cups milk
1 starch exchange
1 vegetable exchange
3 meat exchanges

80-GRAM PROTEIN DEIT

Add to the 20-Gram Diet Meal Plan:
2 cups milk
5 meat exchanges
1 vegetable exchange
4 starch exchanges

*Polycose, Sumacal, and Moducal are all modular carbohydrate supplements.

Gallbladder Disease

On the underside of the liver is a small pouch-like organ called the gallbladder. Its function is to concentrate and store bile until it is needed for digestion. The liver secretes 600 to 800 milliliters of bile per day. The gallbladder reduces this to 60 to 160 milliliters.

Gallbladder disease is usually related to gallstones. The presence of gallstones is called **cholelithiasis.** One third of adults over 70 years of age have gallstones. Gallstones form when the bile is too scant or too concentrated. When the gallbladder becomes inflamed from the stones' irritation, the condition is labeled **cholecystitis.**

Cholelithiasis— the presence of gallstones.

Cholecystitis— inflammation of the gallbladder.

Causative Factors

Women are three times more likely than men to have gallbladder disease. Heredity and hypercholesterolemia are associated with gallstones. Obesity is the only nutritional factor definitely linked to gallbladder disease in humans. Other conditions associated with gallbladder disease include cardiovascular disease, diabetes mellitus, ileal disease or resection, long-term total parenteral nutrition, multiple pregnancies, and oral contraceptive use. Some of these, once present, are unchangeable risk factors. Gallstone disease is also associated with a habitual long overnight fast, with dieting, and with a low fiber intake. A long fast between the evening meal and the first meal of next day could be modified by a light bedtime snack and/or drinking 2 glasses of water on arising if breakfast will be delayed. Either practice will stimulate the gallbladder to empty, thus decreasing the likelihood of very concentrated bile.

Symptoms of gallbladder disease

The cardinal symptom of gallbladder disease is pain after ingestion of fat. The pain is located in the right upper quadrant and often radiates to the right shoulder.

Treatment of gallbladder disease

Dietary modification and medical and surgical interventions are used to treat gallbladder disease. Usually, conservative medical management is tried for a time before surgery.

DIETARY MODIFICATIONS   Conservative treatment of gallbladder disease is dietary modification. Some patients obtain relief with the restriction of dietary fat; others do not. Meals should be well balanced. A 50-gram fat diet is often prescribed. Patients usually can identify foods that cause pain. Fried foods are the worst offenders. During an acute attack, a full liquid diet with minimal fat is recommended. For chronic gallbladder disease, the patient should limit fat and correct obesity. Table 19–6 identifies some foods that are low in fat and some that are high. The high-fat list contains four times as much fat as the possible substitutions on the low-fat list.

MEDICAL INTERVENTIONS   New procedures have been devised to treat gallstones without surgery. One technique involves injecting solvents into the gallbladder. Another method is to break up the stones using shock

TABLE 19–6 *Comparison of Fat Content of Selected Foods*

Low-Fat Foods	Fat (Grams)	High-Fat Foods	Fat (Grams)
	STARCH/BREADS		
Angel food cake, 1/12	<1	Pecan pie, 1/6 of pie	24
Italian bread, 1 slice	<1	Bread stuffing, 1/2 cup	13
English muffin, 1	1	Danish pastry	12
Raisin toast, 1 slice	1	Croissant, 1	12
Pancake, 4-inch, 1	2	Glazed raised donut, 1	13
	MEATS, FISH, AND POULTRY		
Beef round, 3 ounces lean roasted	9	Beef prime rib, 3 ounces, lean only	24
Chicken breast, 3 ounces roasted, without skin	9	Chicken, deep-fried thigh, 1	14
Boiled ham, 3 ounces	9	Spare ribs, 3 ounces	24
Tuna, 1/2 cup water-packed	6	Tuna, 1/2 cup oil-packed, drained	24
	FRUITS AND VEGETABLES		
Banana, 8¾ inches long, 1	1	Avocado, 1	30
Raisins, 1 cup	1	Coconut, dried, 1 cup	50
Potato, baked, 1	<1	French fried potato, 2 × 3½ inches, 15 pieces	12
Onion, raw, sliced, 1 cup	<1	French fried onion rings, 4	10
	MILK PRODUCTS		
Cottage cheese, 1 percent, 1/2 cup	1	Cottage cheese, 4 percent, 1/2 cup	5
Mozzarella, part skimmed, 1 ounce	5	Cheddar, 1 ounce	9
Skimmed milk, with added milk solids, 1 cup	1	Whole milk, 1 cup	8
Frozen yogurt, low-fat, 1 cup	4	Ice cream, regular, hard, vanilla, 1 cup	14
	FAST FOODS		
Arby's			
Regular roast beef sandwich	15	Chicken breast sandwich	26
Burger King			
Whopper Junior	17	Whopper with cheese	48
McDonald's			
Chicken McNuggets, 6	16	Quarter pounder with cheese	29
Wendy's			
Chili, 1 cup	9	Bacon cheeseburger	28

waves. Patients and physicians still may opt for removal of the gallbladder, cholecystectomy, through a laparoscope or the traditional abdominal incision.

Postoperative diet routines are similar to those for other gastrointestinal surgery. When the patient begins to take oral nourishment, clear liquids are given for 24 hours. The diet is progressed as tolerated. Because bile enters the duodenum continuously, balanced meals should be well tolerated. Many patients can eat a regular diet without difficulty 1 month after surgery. Patients who became nauseated after eating certain foods preoperatively, however, may avoid them postoperatively because of the association.

DISEASES AND DISORDERS OF THE PANCREAS

The pancreas is located in the left upper quadrant of the abdomen. It produces the endocrine secretions insulin and glucagon, along with digestive enzymes (pancreatic juice). Disorders of the pancreas include pancreatitis and cystic fibrosis.

Pancreatitis

When the blood vessels of the pancreas become abnormally permeable, plasma and plasma protein leak into the interstitial spaces. The resulting edema damages the pancreatic cells. Normally, the pancreatic enzymes necessary for digestion are inactive in the pancreas and become activated only upon entering the duodenum. Otherwise, the active enzymes would digest the pancreas itself. In **pancreatitis,** the retained pancreatic enzymes, especially trypsin, become do activated and digest the pancreatic tissue.

Pancreatitis— inflammation of the pancreas.

Alcoholism is the most common cause of pancreatitis, inciting up to 75 percent of the cases. Other conditions that can lead to pancreatitis are biliary tract disease or surgery; stomach surgery; and the administration of cancer chemotherapy, steroids, thiazides, or estrogens. In some cases, viral infection, pregnancy, or trauma have preceded pancreatitis. The characteristic symptom of pancreatitis is excruciating pain in the left upper quadrant. Nausea and vomiting accompany an attack. Laboratory tests reveal elevated levels of serum amylase and lipase.

In the treatment of pancreatitis, the patient is advised to avoid alcohol. The acutely ill patient is usually allowed nothing by mouth for 24 to 48 hours to reduce secretions. A nasogastric tube is used to suction stomach contents. Ice chips may be prescribed to lessen dryness of the mouth. Because plain water stimulates gastric secretions, the ice chips may be made by freezing electrolyte solutions instead. Increased secretions when administering gastric suction would only escalate electrolyte losses. If necessary, the patient is maintained on intravenous or TPN feedings until the acute phase subsides.

When the pain subsides and bowel sounds return, oral intake is started. Clear liquids, progressing to a low-fat, high-carbohydrate diet, are given. The use of elemental formulas may be necessary. Medium-chain triglycerides may be a better tolerated source of fats than normal dietary fats. Six small meals per day is the usual pattern. The patient's comfort level is monitored, and serum amylase concentrations are periodically checked. If the patient's condition worsens, the acute care regimen is reinstituted.

Acute pancreatitis may or may not progress to chronic pancreatitis. For chronic pancreatitis patients, no alcohol is permitted. A 50- to 70-gram fat diet is prescribed. Pancreatic enzymes can be given orally before or with meals to aid digestion. Because vitamin B_{12} is not absorbed adequately by pancreatitis patients, it is given parenterally.

Cystic Fibrosis

Cystic fibrosis— hereditary disease often affecting the lungs and pancreas in which glandular secretions are abnormally thick.

The most common cause of pancreatic insufficiency in children and young adults is **cystic fibrosis.** It occurs once in 2500 live births. One in 20 white people carries the recessive gene for this disorder.

Pathophysiology

The underlying pathology of cystic fibrosis is thick glandular mucus production. This dense mucus affects the pancreas, lungs, liver, heart, gallbladder, and small intestine. The mucus plugs the ducts through which it is supposed to flow. The stagnant secretions then become a hospitable environment for bacteria. Fifty percent of children with cystic fibrosis show lung symptoms. Lung infection is the most common cause of death.

The pancreas is affected in 80 percent of the cases. Here the thick mucus interferes with digestive secretions, leading to malabsorption of many nutrients and stunted growth. The sign of cystic fibrosis related to the gastrointestinal tract is the passage of bulky, fatty, foul-smelling feces. This is caused by the impairment of fat digestion. With increased life expectancy a greater number of cystic fibrosis patients display hyperglycemia or diabetes mellitus.

The sweat of cystic fibrosis patient has more sodium chloride than normal. A sweat chloride level greater than 60 milliequivalents per liter is diagnostic of cystic fibrosis. The high electrolyte content of the sweat also puts the patient at increased risk of imbalance during hot weather, fever, or bouts of diarrhea.

Treatment of Cystic Fibrosis

Supportive care is the foundation of cystic fibrosis treatment. Pulmonary congestion and infections are treated as required. The patient's energy needs may be double those of others the same age. When the lungs are involved, much of the patient's energy is expended in respiratory effort. Because starches require amylase for digestion, carbohydrates in the form of simple sugars are a better source of energy. If the patient also has diabetes mellitus, the diet may still include more simple sugars than the usual diet for diabetes mellitus. Intensive therapy of the diabetes mellitus can be maintained with self-monitoring of blood glucose and multiple doses of insulin (Hayes, 1994).

For the cystic fibrosis patient, protein needs are double the RDA. Fat content should be as high as possible because it is a concentrated energy source. If necessary, medium-chain triglycerides can be used to increase fat intake without overtaxing the weak digestive system.

Pancreatic enzymes are administered orally. These help, but they do not completely substitute for a normally functioning pancreas. Fat-soluble vitamins are supplemented in water-miscible form. Some nutrients merit special mention. Riboflavin needs are increased because of the patient's high energy expenditure. Vitamin A should be readily available, to help maintain the integrity of the respiratory and gastrointestinal mucosa. Vitamin K is required because frequent courses of antibiotics kill the intestinal flora. Mineral intake is watched carefully if the weather is hot or the patient is feverish. Extra salt is given if sweat losses are increased. Zinc levels often are low as a result of loss in the feces. Deficiency of zinc contributes to failure of bone growth and to increased susceptibility to infection.

Summary

Diseases of other body systems may be more immediately life-threatening, but over the long term, gastrointestinal diseases can profoundly affect quality of life and life expectancy. Healthcare workers should make nutrition a priority for patients undergoing diagnostic tests or surgery.

Almost everyone with a gastrointestinal disorder benefits from small, frequent meals. Hiatal hernia patients should take liquids with meals and remain upright afterwards. In contrast, postgastrectomy patients with dumping syndrome are treated with frequent dry meals, low in simple sugar, and should maintain a horizontal position following meals.

Celiac disease and cystic fibrosis are gastrointestinal diseases found in children as well as in adults. In celiac disease, gluten destroys the intestinal villi, causing major malabsorption problems. In cystic fibrosis, thick glandular secretions plug the pancreatic ducts, causing malabsorption. The excessive mucus produced in the lungs by cystic fibrosis is even more life-threatening, however.

Nourishing patients with Crohn's disease and ulcerative colitis poses significant challenges. Use of elemental formulas or total parenteral nutrition is often necessary to permit healing. In intractable cases, colon resection and ileostomy may be performed. This drastic surgery presents a new set of management problems, including fluid balance, odor control, and skin integrity.

In cirrhosis, the liver becomes scarred and hard. The result is portal hypertension, absorption of toxins through collateral channels, esophageal varices, ascites, bleeding problems, and possible hepatic coma. Alcohol abuse underlies most cases of cirrhosis and pancreatitis. Treatment is abstinence and supportive therapy. Diet is modified according to the patient's current clinical status.

A case study and a sample plan of care appear below. Both are designed to show you how the information you have studied in this chapter can be used in nursing practice.

CASE STUDY 19–1

An outpatient, Ms. C., a 40-year-old white woman, has just been evaluated for right upper quadrant pain. The pain occurs after meals and radiates to the right shoulder. Ms. C. has noticed her stools have become pale gray in the past 2 months. Ms. C. is 5 feet 4 inches tall, has a medium frame, and weighs 151 pounds.

Ultrasound examination of the gallbladder showed the presence of numerous stones. None is obstructing the duct system yet.

Ms. C. is a single parent of four children, aged 4 to 17, and is employed as a secretary. If surgery does become necessary, she would like to delay it until the youngest child is in school. For that reason, she is electing conservative treatment.

The nurse taking a dietary history discovers that Ms. C. seldom eats breakfast, substituting a doughnut and coffee during her morning coffee break. Lunch is generally a bologna sandwich with chips. Dinner at home often consists of hamburgers or pizza or macaroni and cheese. Ms. C told the nurse she does not know much about nutrition, that she shops as her mother did, and cooks food her children will eat.

NURSING CARE PLAN FOR MS. C.

Assessment

Subjective

Pain in right upper quadrant immediately after eating
Pale stools for 2 months by history
High-fat, low-fiber diet by history
Admitted lack of knowledge about nutrition

Objective:

Gallstones per ultrasound
115 percent of healthy body weight

Nursing Diagnosis

Knowledge deficit, related to prescribed low-fat diet for cholecystitis as evidenced by admitted lack of knowledge about nutrition

Desired Outcome/Evaluation Criteria

Patient will verbalize foods to avoid to maintain low-fat diet by end of teaching session.
Patient will state means of modifying meals to accommodate prescribed diet by end of teaching session.
Patient will return to follow-up session in 1 week with report of the week's meals and any questions she may have.

Nursing Actions/Interventions with Rationales in Italics

1. Explain 50-gram fat diet. Provide written instructions for patient to take home. *Having written instructions available as a teaching tool structures the session and may stimulate questions the patient would not think of otherwise. Her taking the material home will reinforce the instruction.*
2. Explore Ms. C.'s preferences for adding fiber to her diet. *Soluble fiber will combine with cholesterol, which comprises most gallstones, and carry it out of the body. Building on the patient's choices increases chances of compliance.*
3. Obtain patient's reaction to diet and offer alternatives to her present meal pattern. *Considering the patient's wishes affirms her status as an individual. Personalizing the diet for her circumstances will increase the chances of success.*
4. Suggest Ms. C. either eat breakfast or drink 2 glasses of water first thing in the morning. *Either of these actions will stimulate the gallbladder to empty and rid itself of the concentrated bile that has accumulated overnight.*
5. Try to obtain a commitment to return for follow-up in 1 week. *This is quite a radical change from Ms. C.'s usual eating habits. Follow-up in 1 week will give the nurse an opportunity to reinforce the teaching, answer questions, and counsel the patient to remain committed to the therapeutic regimen.*

STUDY AIDS

Chapter Review Questions

1. Which of the following would tend to relax the cardiac sphincter in esophagitis patients?
   a. Whole wheat bread
   b. Orange juice
   c. Milk
   d. Peppermint tea

2. Which of the following foods would be allowed for a patient on a low-residue diet?
   a. 8 ounces of milk with each of the three main meals
   b. Minestrone soup containing peas and lentils
   c. Ground beef on a white bun
   d. A fresh fruit salad

3. A new method of treating peptic ulcers is three meals a day rather than many feedings. This change was introduced because:
   a. Any food increases gastric secretions.
   b. Patients fed every 2 hours gained too much weight.
   c. Feedings of half-and-half every 2 hours caused too much cardiovascular disease.
   d. Larger, less frequent meals dilute the irritating substances contained in them.

4. A patient has been receiving a gravity (bolus) feeding of a complete liquid diet by nasogastric tube for several days without ill effects. Today after starting the feeding, the patient complained of abdominal pain. The nurse noticed the patient was sweating and again checked the patient's vital signs. The pulse was more rapid and the blood pressure lower than at the beginning of the shift. The nurse would notify the physician because:
   a. The patient may be developing an intolerance to the milk-based feeding.
   b. The patient will need an intravenous for replacement of fluid lost from the sweating.
   c. A pump is needed to better control the rate of administration of the tube feeding.
   d. The nasogastric tube may have inched its way into the small intestine.

5. Increased fat in the bowel due to absorption problems may lead to kidney stones because:
   a. Fatty acids form the core of kidney stones.
   b. Less calcium is available to bind with oxalate to promote its excretion.
   c. The bile supply cannot meet demand, so fats are absorbed without emulsification.
   d. Waste material moves through the intestine so fast that insufficient water is absorbed to keep the urine dilute.

6. The advantage of medium-chain triglycerides (MCT) in treating fat absorption problems is that MCT:
   a. Needs no pancreatic lipase or bile for absorption
   b. Is a complete fat supplement in a concentrated form
   c. Adds palatability to the diet
   d. Will deodorize and solidify the foul, bulky stools of these patients

7. Patients who have had resection of the ileum must be protected from:
   a. Iron-deficiency anemia
   b. Fat-soluble vitamin deficiency

c. Calcium and phosphorus deficiency

d. Vitamin B$_{12}$ deficiency

8. Which of the following are least likely to cause the ostomy patient problems?

a. Wine, green pepper, and corn

b. Cheese, buttermilk, and yogurt

c. Beans, onions, and diet soda pop

d. Broccoli, cauliflower, and peanuts

9. A patient with cirrhosis of the liver should be asked if _____ has been experienced before ordering a diet.

a. Headache

b. Vomiting of blood

c. Vomiting followed by pneumonia

d. Delirium tremens

10. The disease in which the underlying pathology is secretion of abnormally thick glandular mucus is:

a. Celiac disease

b. Cholecystitis

c. Crohn's disease

d. Cystic fibrosis

NCLEX-Style Quiz

Mr. W. is a 55-year-old white man admitted to the acute care unit with jaundice and ascites secondary to cirrhosis of the liver. He has gained 15 pounds in the last 3 weeks. He is a known alcoholic who went through detoxification several times in the past 5 years. The dietitian has instructed Mr. W. on a 1000-milligram sodium diet with a fluid restriction of 1000 milliliters per day.

1. When the nurse does the beginning of shift assessment, Mr. W. says he has tried "cutting down on salt" when he started gaining weight, but it didn't work. Which of the following statements best reflects the nurse's understanding of Mr. W.'s pathology and treatment?

a. Just cutting out added salt is not enough, because many foods are naturally high in sodium.

b. Fluids are always restricted with a low-sodium diet.

c. The ascites is caused by the inability of the liver to produce water-soluble bilirubin.

d. Besides retaining sodium, Mr. W. has ascites due to decreased blood pressure in the liver and lack of blood proteins.

2. Mr. W. vomits immediately after his next meal. The physician then orders a hydrating solution of 5 percent dextrose in water intravenously. If thiamin is not included in that order, the nurse should inquire about it because:

a. Thiamin is necessary to predigest the dextrose for immediate absorption.

b. Intravenous glucose without thiamin in the cirrhosis patient can precipitate the Wernicke-Korsakoff syndrome.

c. Thiamin prevents folic acid stores from being diluted by the hydrating solution.

d. Deficiency of thiamin causes delirium tremens.

3. Mr. W.'s serum ammonia level is 150 micrograms per deciliter (normal 40 to 120 micrograms). On his nursing care plan the nurse writes "Observe for signs and symptoms of hepatic encephalopathy." Besides looking for irritability and decreased mentation, the nurses would check for

a. Bloody diarrhea and decreased blood pressure

b. Projectile vomiting

c. Involuntary jerking movements of the hands

d. "Uremic frost" on the skin of the face

4. Mr. W.'s condition worsens. He is placed on a 30-gram protein diet. Mrs. W. has been told the purpose of the protein restriction. The next day, Mrs. W asks the nurse, "If protein breakdown is causing the problem, why is he getting any at all?" Which of the following responses from the nurse would be most accurate?

a. Some protein is necessary to spare glucose for basic energy needs.

b. If the body receives no protein, it will break down muscle tissue to obtain it.

c. The proteins in this diet are predigested and more easily absorbed.

d. Laboratory tests show the doctor how much and what kinds of protein can be tolerated.

5. Mr. W. slowly recovers. His diet is increased to 50 grams of protein per day. He still is bothered with anorexia and nausea. If his symptoms parallel those of other cirrhosis patients, the healthcare worker should encourage his biggest meal to be:

a. Breakfast

b. Lunch

c. Dinner

d. Bedtime snack

CHARTING TIPS 19–1: ALERTING ADMINISTRATION TO HAZARDS

Charting on the patient's medical record is only part of our responsibility as nurses.

✓ If you notice hazards in your institution, you are obliged to report them. An oral report is inadequate.

✓ You should send a written memo to your supervisor with specific details, and keep a copy for yourself. Administration should be apprised of the possibility and is responsible for investigating. Keeping a copy of your documentation memo will prove that you fulfilled your obligation.

✓ In the cases of dehiscence described in Clinical Application 19–1, several similar, unexplained occurrences within a short time might point to an environmental hazard such as contamination in the operating room.

BIBLIOGRAPHY

American Dietetic Association: Manual of Clinical Dietetics, ed 4. The American Dietetic Association, Chicago, 1992.

Bates, B: A Guide to Physical Examination and History Taking, ed 4. JB Lippincott, Philadelphia, 1987.

Blackburn, GL, et al: Surgical nutrition. In Halpern, SL (ed): Quick Reference to Clinical Nutrition. JB Lippincott, Philadelphia, 1987.

Bullock, BL and Rosendahl, PP: Pathophysiology, ed 3. JB Lippincott, Philadelphia, 1992.

Burtis, G, Davis, J, and Martin, S: Applied Nutrition and Diet Therapy. WB Saunders, Philadelphia, 1988.

Cella, JH and Watson, J: Nurse's Manual of Laboratory Tests. FA Davis, Philadelphia, 1989.

Cerrato, PL. Surgery, stress, and metabolism. RN 54(8):63, 1991.

Committee on Diet and Health. Food and Nutrition Board. Commission on Life Sciences. National Research Council: Diet and Health: Implications for Reducing Chronic Disease Risk. National Academy Press, Washington, DC, 1989.

Deglin, JH and Vallerand, AH: Davis's Drug Guide For Nurses, ed 3. FA Davis, Philadelphia, 1993.

Feldman, EB: Essentials of Clinical Nutrition. FA Davis, Philadelphia, 1988.

Ferry, GD and Price-Jones, BA: Nutrition and disorders of the colon. In Halpern, SL (ed): Quick Reference to Clinical Nutrition. JB Lippincott, Philadelphia, 1987.

Gylys, BA and Wedding, ME: Medical Terminology, ed 2. FA Davis, Philadelphia, 1988.

Hamilton, EMN, Whitney, EN, and Sizer, FS: Nutrition Concepts and Controversies, ed 2. West, St Paul, 1991.

Hayes, DR et al: Management dilemmas in the individual with cystic fibrosis and diabetes. JAm Dietc Assoc 94(1): 78, 1994.

Horne, MM, Heitz, UE, and Swearingen, PL: Fluid, Electrolyte, and Acid-Base Balance. Mosby Year Book, St Louis, 1991.

Hotter, AN. Wound healing and immunocompromise. Nurs Clin North Am 25(1):193, 1990.

Kasprisin, CA and Kasprisin, DO: Clinical Human Genetics. Medical Examination Publishing, New Hyde Park, NY, 1982.

Klish, WJ and Montandon, CM: Nutrition and upper gastrointestinal disorders. In Halpern, SL (ed): Quick Reference to Clinical Nutrition. JB Lippincott, Philadelphia, 1987.

Kuhn, MM: Pharmacotherapeutics: A Nursing Process Approach, ed 2. FA Davis, 1991.

Lee, KA and Stotts, NA. Support of the growth hormone–somatomedin system to facilitate healing. Heart Lung 19(2):157, 1990.

Lewis, SM and Collier, IC: Medical-Surgical Nursing, ed 2. McGraw-Hill, New York, 1987.

Long, BC and Phipps, WJ: Medical-Surgical Nursing, A Nursing Process Approach, ed 2. CV Mosby, St Louis, 1989.

O'Brien, S: Panel recommends blood cholesterol health screening and education guidelines for children and adolescents. American Association of Occupational Health Nurses Journal 39(6):296, 1991.

Pemberton, CM, et al: Mayo Clinic Diet Manual, ed 6. BC Decker, Philadelphia, 1987.

Reisner, EH: Nutrition and the anemias. In Halpern, SL (ed): Quick Reference to Clinical Nutrition. JB Lippincott, Philadelphia, 1987.

Rosenberg, CS. Wound healing in the patient with diabetes mellitus. Nurs Clin North Am 25(1):247, 1990.

Rudman, D et al. Ammonia content of food. Am J Clin Nutr 26(5):487, 1973.

Scanlon, VT and Sanders, T: Essentials of Anatomy and Physiology. FA Davis, Philadelphia, 1991.

Scanlon, VC and Sanders, T: Student Workbook for Essentials of Anatomy and Physiology. FA Davis, Philadelphia, 1991.

Shaw, EW and Maddrey, WC: Nutritional therapy in patients with liver disease. In Halpern, SL (ed): Quick Reference to Clinical Nutrition. JB Lippincott, Philadelphia, 1987.

Shlafer, M and Marieb, E: The Nurse, Pharmacology, and Drug Therapy. Addison-Wesley, Redwood City, CA, 1989.

Sichieri, R, Everhart, JE, and Roth, H. A prospective study of hospitalization with gallstone disease among women: Role of dietary factors, fasting period, and dieting. Am J Public Health 81(7):880, 1991.

Smeltzer, SC and Bare, BG: Brunner and Suddarth's Textbook of Medical-Surgical Nursing, ed 7. JB Lippincott, Philadelphia, 1992.

Stotts, NA and Whitney, JD. Nutritional intake and status of clients in the home with open surgical wounds. Journal of Community Health Nursing 7(2):77, 1990.

Tamburro, CH: Nutritional management of alcoholism, drug addiction, and acute toxicity syndromes. In Halpern, SL (ed): Quick Reference to Clinical Nutrition. JB Lippincott, Philadelphia, 1987.

Thomas, CL, ed: Taber's Cyclopedic Medical Dictionary, ed 17. FA Davis, Philadelphia, 1993.

United States Bureau of the Census: Statistical Abstract of the United States, ed 110. US Department of Commerce, Washington, DC, 1990.

Whitney, EB, Cataldo, CB, and Rolfes, SR: Understanding Normal and Clinical Nutrition, ed 3. West, St Paul, 1991.

Williams, SR: Nutrition and Diet Therapy, ed 6. Times Mirror/Mosby College, St Louis, 1989.

Chapter Outline

Key Terms

As a study aid, each key term is followed by the page number where the term is defined in the chapter. Terms that appear in **boldface** or <u>underscored</u> in the chapter text are located in the glossary.

Cachexia (623)
Carcinogenic (618)
Carcinoma (616)
Initiation (616)
Metastasis (616)
Neoplasm (616)
Oncogenes (616)
Promotion (616)
Sarcoma (616)
T-lymphocytes (625)
Thymus gland (625)

Chapter Twenty
Diet in Cancer

Learning Objectives

After completing this chapter, the student should be able to:

1. Describe the ways in which foods are implicated in the development of cancer.
2. List several correlations between dietary intake and cancers of specific sites.
3. Interpret dietary guidelines on the prevention of cancer.
4. Name several factors thought to contribute loss of appetite in cancer patients.
5. Discuss measures to increase oral intake for patients with cancer.

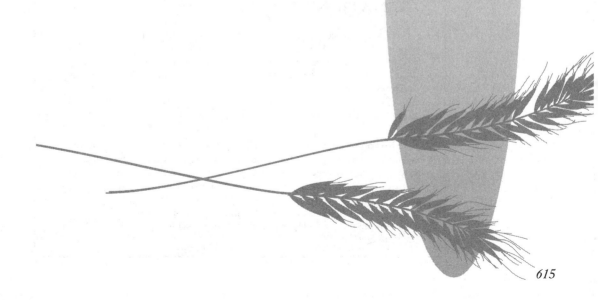

Neoplasm—A new and abnormal formation of tissue (tumor) that grows at the expense of the healthy organism.

Carcinoma—A malignant neoplasm that occurs in epithelial tissue.

Metastasis—the "seeding" of cancer cells to distant sites of the body by blood and lymph vessels or by spilling into a body cavity.

Cancer has been known since 3400 B.C. Its name means crab, for the creeping way in which it spreads. Cancer encompasses more than 100 types of malignant neoplastic disease. Cancer is a *neoplasm*, a new and abnormal formation of tissue (tumor} that grows at the expense of the healthy organism. Two of the main types of cancer are sarcomas and carcinomas. *Sarcomas* arise from connective tissue, such as muscle or bone. *Carcinomas* occur in epithelial tissue, such as skin and mucous membranes. The characteristics common to all types of cancer are uncontrolled growth and the ability to spread to distant sites (to *metastasize*). Clinical Application 20–1 discusses the transformation of normal cells into cancer cells.

Cancer is the second most common cause of death in the United States. One in three persons now alive will contract cancer (American Cancer Society, 1991). Patients who are alive and without recurrence of cancer 5 years after diagnosis are considered cured. This is termed the 5-year survival rate. It is now 40 percent. There are major differences in survival rates, depending on the site in which the cancer occurs.

Oncogene—a gene found in tumor cells making the host cells susceptible to initiation and promotion by carcinogens.

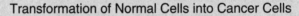

CLINICAL APPLICATION 20–1

Transformation of Normal Cells into Cancer Cells

When the reproductive processes of the cell malfunction, why does it happen to some persons and not others? Within all cells are genes that make up the DNA molecule. Genes carry the traits that the individual inherited from his or her parents. Within tumor cells, *oncogenes* have been located which transform normal cells into cancer cells. Forty different oncogenes have been identified. Just having an oncogene is not enough to produce a cancer. The transformation of normal cells to cancer cells is a two-step process. The first step is *initiation*. The second step is promotion.

INITIATION

Physical forces, chemicals, or biological agents can cause an alteration in the cell's DNA, resulting in a permanently altered gene. This altered gene is not significant until the second step of *promotion* takes place. In fact, 10 to 30 years may elapse between initiation and the diagnosis of cancer.

PROMOTION

For promoters to enhance the expression of the altered gene, they must be present in high levels for a prolonged period. Repeated exposure to promoting agents causes expression of the altered gene. Promoters are tissue-specific; for instance, bile acids for colon cancer and saccharin for cancer of the urinary bladder. In contrast to initiation, which results in permanent change, the process of promotion is reversible. Reducing exposure to high levels of promoters allows the body to repair the damaged cells.

EVIDENCE LINKING CANCER TO DIET

The causes of cancer are complex and often poorly understood. Some convincing evidence, however, connects dietary practices to the incidence of cancer. Certain cancers appear in great numbers in particular countries. Clinical Application 20–2 summarizes some of these findings.

Dietary Components Associated with Cancer

It is difficult to assess the role of dietary components without also considering the other factors that might contribute to the development of cancer. Diet is, after all, part of total lifestyle. Nevertheless, some experts claim that 50 percent of cancers may be related to diet, including 60 percent of cancers in women, and 40 percent of those in men.

 CLINICAL APPLICATION 20–2

Diet-Cancer Links in Various Populations

Certain cancers occur with greater frequency in some countries than others. When this was noted, the search began for dissimilarities in environment that could explain the differences in cancer occurrence. Because hereditary factors could confound the results, the study of immigrants is particularly enlightening.

In Japan there is more stomach cancer and less colon cancer than in the United States. In second-generation Japanese immigrants to the United States, however, the distribution of cancers becomes similar to that of other Americans.

Stomach and esophageal cancers are common where nitrates and nitrites are prevalent in food and water, or where cured and pickled foods are popular. Some of these areas are China, Japan, and Iceland.

A low rate of colon cancer is seen in Africa. The diet there is high in fiber, and the Africans pass bulky stools. The theory is that the fiber both dilutes the carcinogens in the feces and pushes them out of the body faster than a low-fiber diet would.

In the United States, breast and colon cancer occur five to eight times more frequently than in other countries. Studies have correlated these cancers with fat intake. American women eat three times as much fat as Japanese women and have three times the incidence of breast cancer. New studies of American women have not connected fat or fiber intake with the incidence of breast cancer, but these women consumed the American, not Japanese, proportions of dietary fat. It may be that 20 percent of kilocalories is a healthier maximum than 30 percent (Weisburger, 1991). The link between fat intake and colon cancer has not been challenged.

The Finnish people consume a diet high in saturated fat, but their colon cancer rate resembles that of Japan and their breast cancer rate is less than that of Denmark. One plausible explanation is related to the large amount of cereal bran consumed by the Finnish people.

Excesses of Certain Substances

Some substances are associated with cancer when they are consumed in large quantities. This is the case with fat, alcohol, and pickled and smoked foods. The cooking method also may influence the development of cancer.

FAT   Of all dietary components, fat is the most definitely linked to cancer. A high-fat diet contains more than 40 percent of kilocalories as fat. It is thought that the end products of fat metabolism are *carcinogenic*. That, plus the slow intestinal transit time, which increases the duration of exposure to the carcinogen, may contribute to the development of bowel cancer. Intake of either saturated or unsaturated fat is associated with breast, prostate, and colon cancers. In the breast and prostatic cancers, fat is thought to act on the endocrine system and affect hormonal activity.

Linoleic acid, an essential fatty acid, is classified as a promoter of cancer rather than an initiator. Although some polyunsaturated fats are recommended for protection against heart disease, excessive intakes of polyunsaturated fats have been connected to cancer. In animal studies, the omega-3 fatty acids have been protective against cancer development, and monounsaturated fatty acids have been neutral, neither promoting nor protecting.

Closely linked to fat intake is kilocaloric intake. In both animals and humans, restricted kilocaloric intake was associated with lower rates of tumor incidence. With animals particularly, the experimenter can vary the components of the diet. Even when fed high-fat diets, animals on kilocaloric restrictions had fewer tumors than those given an equal amount of fat but more kilocalories.

ALCOHOL   Alcohol-induced cirrhosis, with resulting increased liver cell turnover, is associated with liver cancer. Heavy beer drinking is identified with colorectal cancer. Risk of esophageal cancer increases two to four times if 41 to 80 grams of alcohol is ingested per day, and 18 times if more than 80 grams per day is drunk. When combined with cigarettes or chewing tobacco, alcohol increases the risk of mouth, larynx, and throat cancers.

PICKLED AND SMOKED FOODS   Cancers of the esophagus and stomach are correlated with large intakes of pickled and smoked foods. It is postulated that the process of smoking foods may result in their absorbing tar similar to that in tobacco smoke. Charcoal broiling presents the same type of danger, in that carcinogens may be deposited on the surface of the food.

CARCINOGENS RELATED TO COOKING   Recent data have shown that high-temperature cooking of meat—frying, broiling, and grilling—produces substances known to produce cancer in animals. Low-temperature, high-moisture cooking, such as stewing and pot roasting, does not produce the same level of carcinogens.

Protective Nutrients

Excessive amounts of a cancer-promoting food seems to be neutralized by other foods. Of particular note are fiber, vitamin A and carotene, and vitamin C.

FIBER   Low-fiber diets are associated with colon cancer. It has been suggested, however, that all fiber is not of equal value, and that perhaps a particular subset of fiber, as yet unspecified, confers all the protection.

VITAMIN A AND CAROTENE   High intakes of vitamin A and carotene may reduce the risk of lung, larynx, esophagus, bladder, upper gastrointestinal tract, and breast cancers. Vitamin A may control cell differentiation or influence host immune defenses; carotene may protect against oxidation. Studies have shown that individuals with the overall highest cancer rates have lower serum retinol levels than other people. A current trial is testing the influence of beta carotene versus a placebo on cancer rates.

VITAMIN C   Diets high in fruits and vegetables are associated with a decreased incidence of cancers of the stomach and esophagus. Clinical Application 6–7 showed that vitamin C may inhibit the formation of nitrosamines in stomach.

VITAMIN E AND SELENIUM   Vitamin E and selenium are both antioxidants that protect cells against breakdown. These two nutrients have a reciprocal sparing relationship, so relating one or the other to cancer is a complicated process. Although little is known about the role of vitamin E in cancer prevention, the subject is currently being investigated by researchers.

People with the highest intakes of selenium had half the cancer risk of people with the lowest intakes (Feldman, 1988). Selenium, along with other antioxidants, namely vitamins A, E, and C, is found in cruciferous vegetables. Conversely, selenium in drinking water was positively correlated with colorectal cancer. Because of the small database and selenium's narrow margin of safety, selenium supplementation is not recommended. Clinical Application 20–3 gives a synopsis of the role of vegetable intake in cancer prevention.

 CLINICAL APPLICATION 20–3
The Role of Vegetables in Cancer Prevention

Low intakes of vegetables have been associated with stomach and colon cancers. In Japan, smokers who ingested yellow or green vegetables every day had 20 to 30 percent lower lung cancer rates than smokers who did not consume those vegetables every day.

Vegetables contain several substances that may contribute to cancer prevention. Some of these substances are carotene, indoles, and antioxidants.

Carotene, the precursor of vitamin A, is present in many green and deep-yellow vegetables. Vitamin A plays a role in cellular differentiation, the process that is faulty in cancer. Thus, a high intake of carotene may be instrumental in preventing cancer.

Cruciferous vegetables, those of the cabbage family, are specifically recommended for cancer prevention. These vegetables contain compounds called *indoles*, which activate enzymes to destroy carcinogens. Members of the cruciferous family include brussels sprouts, broccoli, cabbage, cauliflower, and turnips.

Vitamins A, E, and C and the mineral selenium are all antioxidants. They prevent oxidation of molecules by becoming oxidized themselves. Some molecules become very unstable when oxidized and damage

Indoles—Compounds found in vegetables of the cruciferous family which activate enzymes to destroy carcinogens.

Box continued on next page.

> ## CLINICAL APPLICATION 20–3 *(continued)*
> ### The Role of Vegetables in Cancer Prevention
>
> nearby molecules. This reaction could modify a cell's DNA to set in motion the uncontrolled reproduction of cancer cells. Many vegetables contain vitamins A and C.
>
> It is unclear which of these substances is the best agent for cancer prevention. In fact, it may be determined that another, yet-untested substance in the vegetables is more valuable for cancer prevention than those mentioned here. For these reasons, taking supplements of carotene or vitamin C is not recommended. Eating a variety of vegetables, including those linked to low cancer incidence, is the better method of protecting a person's health.

CALCIUM   In both animals and humans, calcium seems to protect against colon cancer. Experts theorize that calcium reduces cell turnover rates.

Questionable Relationships to Cancer

Studies have produced inconclusive data or conflicting reports on the relationship of certain substances to cancer. Two of these are caffeine and coffee.

Aflatoxins (see Chapter 12) are another factor that is inconclusively linked to cancer. Aflatoxins are contaminants of improperly stored food. Aflatoxin contamination of peanuts and corn is related to primary liver cancer, especially in Africa and Asia. Interpreting this information is complicated, since hepatitis B is endemic to both continents. The cancer may be caused the aflatoxins or by hepatitis B virus, or both. There is no evidence relating aflatoxins to cancer risk in the United States.

Other dietary components have been noticed to be prevalent with certain cancers. Some of these are shown in Table 20–1.

REDUCING THE RISK OF CANCER

There is no single cause of cancer. Nor is there one "magic bullet" that will protect everyone from developing cancer. Based on the evidence, however, certain practices are widely recommended. These practices are identical to those advocated throughout this book.

Food Practices to Avoid

Persons attempting to minimize the risk of cancer should avoid excessive intakes of meat, fat, and alcohol.

Excessive Meat Consumption

Vegetarians have lower cancer rates, even when the effects of smoking and alcohol are eliminated. Population studies link low cancer rates with low

TABLE 20–1 *Diet and Increased Rate of Cancer at Specific Sites*

| Cancer Site | Dietary Constituent | | |
	At Any Level	High Intake	Low Intake
Esophagus	Alcohol	Pickles	Lentils
		Pickled vegetables	Green vegetables
		Moldy food	Fresh fruit
		Very hot beverages	Animal products
		Grains (wheat, corn)	Fat
			Vitamins A
			Vitamin C
			Riboflavin
			Niacin
			Calcium
			Magnesium
			Molybdenum
			Zinc
Stomach	Spiced, pickled, and		Milk
	smoked food		Raw green or yellow
	Nitrates		vegetables
			Vitamin C
Colon/Rectum	Fat		Fiber
	Meat		Cruciferous
	Beer		vegetables
	Cholesterol		
Liver	Alcohol		
	Aflatoxin		
Pancreas	Alcohol		
	Meat		
Gallbladder	Kilocalories		
Lung			Vitamin A
			Carotene
Kidney	Cadmium		
Urinary bladder	Coffee		Vitamin A
	Nonnutritive sweetener		
Breast	Fat		
	Milk products		
	Eggs		
	Meat		
	Kilocalories		
Ovary	Fat		
Uterus, endometrium	Fat		
	Kilocalories		
Prostate	Fat		Vegetables
	Protein		Vitamin A

Source: Adapted from Feldman, 1988, p 53.

meat intake and high intake of vegetables and grains. Seventh Day Adventists and Mormons have a lower incidence of bowel cancer than other Americans, even when caffeine and alcohol differences between the study groups are equalized.

Of particular concern is the consumption of smoked, salted, or nitrate-cured meat. These foods should be consumed infrequently. Matching these preserved foods with a good source of vitamin C to counter the effects of nitrosamines would be wise planning. Likewise, limiting the consumption of meats cooked at high temperature may be desirable.

Excessive Fat Consumption

Cancers of the breast, uterus, colon, and prostate are linked to excessive fat consumption. Limiting fat intake to 30 percent of kilocalories is recommended. Substituting skimmed-milk dairy products for whole-milk products would be a significant change. Selecting lean meats and trimming fat is another step. Limiting fat intake without adding other foods in place of it would also limit kilocalories, which seems to be beneficial.

Alcohol Consumption

Along with tobacco, alcohol is linked to head and neck cancers. Liver cancer risk is increased by alcoholic cirrhosis. Excessive beer consumption is associated with rectal cancer. Some evidence links regular alcohol consumption with breast cancer (Work Study Group, 1991). The recommendation is to drink alcohol moderately, if at all.

Food Practices to Cultivate

Along with food practices to avoid, there are some food practices to cultivate so as to minimize cancer risk. These concern fiber, carotene, and cruciferous vegetables.

Increase Fiber Intake

To reduce the risk of colon cancer, a high-fiber diet is recommended. Fiber promotes bile excretion and speeds up intestinal transit time so that carcinogens are eliminated quicker. The Finnish people have a low cancer rate despite high-fat diets, but their diets are also high in fiber.

Increase Carotene Intake

These precursors of vitamin A have been associated with lower cancer rates. Because of the function of vitamin A in maintaining the integrity of epithelial tissue, carotene intake may help prevent cancers of these tissues. Preformed vitamin A as a supplement is not recommended because of the hazard of toxicity.

Increase Consumption of Cruciferous Vegetables

Cancer patients have been found to eat less cabbage, broccoli, and brussels sprouts than cancer-free persons. The other members of this vegetable family are cauliflower and turnips. Consuming these vegetable regularly may reduce risk of cancer of the gastrointestinal and respiratory tracts.

NUTRITION FOR CANCER PATIENTS

Once a person has cancer, nutrition becomes part of the treatment. Cancer patients have the highest incidence of protein-energy malnutrition (PEM) of any group of sick people. PEM is virtually universal among hospitalized cancer patients (Feldman, 1988).

Cachexia

A state of malnutrition and wasting is called *cachexia*. Often associated with cancer, it is also seen in AIDS, alcoholism, malaria, tuberculosis, and pituitary disease. Cachexia affects one third to two thirds of cancer patients. It occurs despite efforts to nourish the patient, because of the tumor's effects on the patient's metabolism. Figure 20–1 shows a woman with cachexia.

Cachexia—state of malnutrition and wasting seen in chronic conditions such as cancer, AIDS, malaria, tuberculosis, and pituitary disease

Cancer changes the patient's carbohydrate metabolism. Insulin resistance is common. The patient can no longer produce glucose efficiently from carbohydrate but instead uses tissue protein for energy. In traumatized noncancer patients, catabolism of fat for fuel gradually replaces protein breakdown. The cancer patient's body does not make this adaptive change.

Special Needs

Food is therapy for cancer patients. Energy needs are one and a half to two times the resting energy expenditure. Protein needs are 1.5 to 2 grams per kilogram of body weight. Often, increased folate is needed (Theologides,

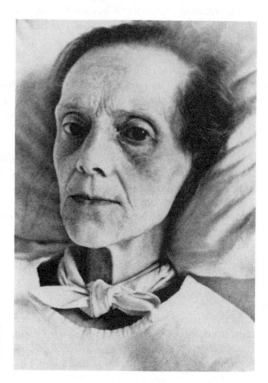

FIGURE 20–1. This woman is cachectic. (From Nutrition Today 16:(3), cover, © by Williams & Wilkins, 1981, with permission.)

1987). Within the cancer patient, the tumor cells are multiplying rapidly and consuming folic acid, which is necessary for DNA formation.

Assessment

Unexplained weight loss is one of the seven danger signals of cancer. Anorexia and changes in the sense of taste often precede the diagnosis of cancer. Because the tumor alters the person's metabolism, it is possible for weight loss to occur without a reduction in food intake. Except for gastric and pancreatic cancers, patients who did not lose weight before beginning chemotherapy had better survival rates than those who lost weight (DeWys, 1980).

Cancer patients develop ascites, as well as accumulation of fluids in other body cavities. Interpreting the weight gain or loss may be more difficult than in patients without third-space sequestering of fluids. Nevertheless, weight is still an important measure of progress.

Serum proteins, particularly albumin, reflect skeletal muscle and visceral protein status. Serum protein levels were lower in patients with pressure ulcers (pressure sores) if they also had cancer than if they did not. Increased breakdown of the body's tissues and catabolism of the albumin will produce low serum albumin levels. Hypoalbuminemia also may be due to nephrotic syndrome or loss of proteins from removal of third-space fluids.

Common Nutritional Problems in Cancer Patients

Some nutritional problems in cancer patients are due to the disease. Some are due to treatment modalities. Common problems affecting meals and nourishments are early satiety and anorexia, taste alterations, local effects in the mouth, nausea, vomiting and diarrhea, and altered immune response.

Early Satiety and Anorexia

Although they may look starved, cancer patients may take a few bites of food and declare that they are full. They may say that they have no appetite at all. The main source of these symptoms is the cancer itself, by a mechanism that is poorly understood (Theologides, 1987). Control of the disease improves the appetite.

Sometimes, though, the physical pressure from the tumor or third-space fluid accumulation may give a feeling of fullness. Relieving those problems may improve food intake.

Some additional factors may interfere with appetite. The psychological stress of dealing with cancer may produce anxiety or depression. The person may be grappling with a body image change and may be going through the grieving process for the loss of a body function or the potential loss of life itself.

Taste Alterations

Cancer patients often have changes in taste perceptions. They have an increased threshold for sweetness and a decreased threshold for bitterness. Accordingly, they will increase the amount of sugar used and often say that beef and pork taste bitter or metallic. These taste changes are due to the cancer and the various modes of therapy.

Local Effects in the Mouth

Patients who are being treated for head and neck cancers often experience mouth ulcers, decreased and thick saliva, and swallowing difficulty. Any of these may interfere with nutritional intake.

Nausea, Vomiting, and Diarrhea

This triad of symptoms often accompany cancer treatment, either radiation or chemotherapy, as well as certain types of tumors. Since the gastrointestinal tract cells are replaced every few days, these rapidly dividing cells are more vulnerable to the cancer treatments than are more slowing reproducing cells. Not all patients suffer these side effects to the same extent. Healthcare workers must be careful not to program patients to be sick.

Altered Immune Response

Sometimes, antineoplastic agents also suppress the patient's immune system. Patients receiving them are at risk of overwhelming infections from organisms that would not affect other persons. Clinical Application 20–4 discusses the role of the immune system in preventing cancer.

Nutritional Interventions

After the disease is controlled, vitamin and mineral deficiencies can be corrected rapidly. Tissue loss responds more slowly to treatment.

For Early Satiety and Anorexia

Many nutrient-dense feedings are offered to the cancer patient. To maximize the nutrition, creative concoctions are in order. For instance, adding $1\frac{1}{3}$

 CLINICAL APPLICATION 20–4

Role of the Immune System in Preventing Cancer

Some experts believe that many cancers begin in a person's lifetime, only to be stopped by the body's defense system. The increased incidence of cancer in organ transplant patients on immunosuppressive drugs offers credence to this theory.

One of the body's defenses is provided by certain white blood cells called *T-lymphocytes*. These cells have the task of recognizing foreign materials, including cancer cells, as "non-self" and acting to destroy the invaders. Some of the T-lymphocytes develop into killer cells, which bind to the foreign cell membrane and release lysosomal enzymes into the cancer cell which destroys it. The T-lymphocytes mature in the *thymus gland* in the chest, hence the name, thymic lymphocytes.

Contributing to the development of cancer in the elderly is the deterioration of the immune system. The thymus gland begins to shrink at sexual maturity. By age 50 only 10 percent of the original gland remains.

T-lymphocytes (T-cells)—white blood cells which recognize and fight foreign cells such as cancer.

Thymus—gland in the chest, above and in front of the heart, which contributes to the immune response, including the maturation of T-lymphocytes.

cup of instant dry skimmed-milk powder to 1 quart of liquid milk increases the nutrient density, with little or no change in palatability.

No appetite-stimulating medication is effective for cancer patients with anorexia (Theologides, 1987). Cancer patients should be encouraged to eat whether they are hungry or not. Food is therapy, too. Appropriate exercise before meals may help to stimulate appetite. Attractively prepared food served in a pleasant environment is enticing. Very small servings, offered frequently, may increase the patient's intake. For inpatients, receiving favorite foods from home or sharing a meal with the family may help overcome the patient's aversion to food. Children sometimes can be coaxed to eat by decorating their food with faces or serving it in the form of designs such as cars or dolls or the child's name. Involving the child in food preparation or in choosing the menu can help to pique the appetite.

To Combat Bitter or Metallic Tastes

Oral hygiene before meals will freshen the mouth. Cooking in the microwave oven or in glass utensils may minimize the metallic taste. As protein sources, eggs, fish, poultry, and dairy products may be better received than beef or pork. Serving meat cold or at room temperature lessens the bitter taste. Sometimes sauces and seasonings added to the meat will improve its palatability for these patients.

For Local Effects about the Mouth

A single canker sore can be remarkably painful. A cancer patient with multiple oral ulcerations may complain of severe pain upon food ingestion. In addition, some patients also have dry mouths and difficulty swallowing. For all of these problems, good oral hygiene, before and after meals, is essential.

MOUTH ULCERATIONS Foods should be soft and mild. Sauces, gravies, and dressings may make foods easier to eat. Cream soups and milk provide much nutrition for the volume ingested. "Dunking" harder textured foods allows more variety in the menu. Cold foods have a somewhat numbing effect and may be better tolerated than hot food. Taking liquids with meals will help to wash down the food. Soda straws may help get the liquids past mouth ulcerations. Substances likely to irritate the mouth ulcerations should be avoided. These may include hot items, salty or spicy foods, and acidic juices.

To maintain oral intake, it may be necessary to resort to an anesthetic mouthwash. If the mouth is anesthetized, patients should be instructed to chew slowly and carefully to avoid biting their lips or tongue or cheeks.

DRY MOUTH Adequate hydration will help keep the mouth moist. Food lubricants can be of value: gravy, butter, margarine, milk, beer, or bouillon may aid in consuming a near-adequate diet when the mouth is dry (Theologides, 1987). Synthetic salivas are available also.

SWALLOWING DIFFICULTY This problem may linger throughout a 6-week course of treatment. To combat it, patients should make swallowing a conscious act. They should inhale, swallow, and exhale. Experiment with head position. Tilting the head backward or forward may help. Foods for these patients should be nonsticky and of even consistency. Lumpy gravy and mixed vegetables are not desirable.

For Nausea, Vomiting, and Diarrhea

Antiemetic medications should be given 6 hours before chemotherapy begins, and continued on a regular schedule. These drugs are most effective if given prophylactically, before the patient becomes nauseated.

Similarly, medications for pain and insomnia must be given liberally. Nausea and vomiting frequently accompany pain in patients without cancer, also. Controlling the pain may alleviate nausea to a great extent.

As with morning sickness, eating dry crackers before arising may help the nausea. Liquids taken between, rather than with, meals will reduce the volume in the stomach. Similarly, a low-fat diet is digested faster, leaving less content in the stomach to cause nausea or be vomited.

Patients should eat slowly and chew thoroughly. Resting after eating helps. Foods the patient especially likes should be saved for times the patient feels good, lest these favorite foods become associated with vomiting.

As with the patient who has gastrointestinal upset, clear liquids should be tried first, after vomiting ceases, and the diet progressed as tolerated. Unconventional mealtimes may be instituted to ensure that the patient receives nourishment when nausea is minimal. If this means that breakfast is eaten at at 2 A.M. and lunch at 6 A.M., so be it. That is truly individualized care.

Diarrhea may be countered by adding pectin-containing foods to the patient's intake. A low-residue diet helps reduce intestinal stimulation. The possibility of lactose intolerance should be considered because of the destruction of the gastrointestinal mucosa. Active cultures of yogurt have been used to repopulate the intestine with bacteria, when the flora normally present have been killed by the therapy or washed out by the diarrheal stools.

For Altered Immune Response

Patients may be placed in protective isolation to minimize their exposure to microorganisms. As for dietary interventions, fresh fruits and vegetables may be restricted since they cannot be disinfected adequately. Other measures are similar to those taken to protect AIDS patients and are discussed in Chapter 22.

Total Parenteral Nutrition or Tube Feedings

The principles of tube feeding and total parenteral nutrition, as presented in Chapter 13, apply to cancer patients as well as patients generally. Patients should be started on appropriate feeding methods before they become severely malnourished. Patients whose weight is 5 kilograms below their healthy body weights and whose serum albumin is less than 3 grams per 100 milliliters should be considered candidates for intensive nutritional support. Charting Tips 20–1 discusses documenting cancer patients' at-home treatment and diet plans.

OTHER NURSING INTERVENTIONS

In your nursing courses, you will learn many techniques to provide comfort and support for patients. We have already mentioned oral hygiene. Two others that are particularly suitable for cancer patients are massage and relaxation. Massage can either stimulate or relax a person, depending on the techniques used. Besides the local effects, the patient receives the benefit of touch from another person. This can be very valuable, since cancer patients sometimes feel, rightly or wrongly, shunned. In one type of relaxation exercise, patients are coached to relax areas of the body in sequence. Another exercise focuses the patient's mind on controlled breathing. These procedures have the added advantage of assisting the patient to achieve some control over an oppressive situation.

Care of the cancer patient can be especially rewarding for nurses. Just as cancers develop and respond to treatment differently, so do patients respond in various ways to nursing interventions. No single technique will work in every situation. Nursing of the cancer patient requires creativity and patience. It also exemplifies one of the magical features of nursing. We often enter patients' lives at critical times. For the most part, they share their hopes and fears with us. As often as not, we can learn as much from them as they can from us. Cancer patients, by confronting a potentially fatal disease, can teach themselves, their families, and their caregivers the truth of the adage that life is a journey, not a destination.

Summary

Cancer is the second leading cause of death in the United States. Many different kinds of cancer exist, but all occur when normal cells reproduce uncontrollably both at the site of origin and in metastatic sites of the body. Substances called initiators and promoters are necessary for cancer to begin.

Dietary guidelines to prevent cancer are similar to those discussed throughout this book. People should avoid excessive consumption of meat fat, kilocalories, and alcohol. Positive dietary steps are to increase intake of fiber, carotene, and cruciferous vegetables, and to consume adequate amounts of vitamin C.

Cancer patients often present difficult nutritional problems. Both the disease and its treatment cause early satiety and anorexia, taste alterations, local effects in the mouth, nausea, vomiting, diarrhea, and altered immune responses. Creative interventions for these problems will make the patient's life significantly more comfortable and can give a sense of accomplishment to the nurse.

A case study and a sample plan of care appear below. Both are designed to show you how the information you have studied in this chapter can be used in nursing practice.

CASE STUDY 20–1

Ms. X. is admitted to the hospital for a third course of chemotherapy. She is divorced, with no children, and lives with her mother, who is very supportive. Hopeful that this therapy will stem the cancer, Ms. X. is determined to complete the prescribed treatments. Nausea and vomiting in the past two courses of chemotherapy caused her to suspend treatment before it was completed.

Ms. X. is 42 years old, 5 feet 5 inches tall, and weighs 123 pounds. Her wrist measurement is 5½ inches. The mucous membranes of her oral cavity are intact. Her favorite foods are ice cream and steak, although for the past 2 months beef has tasted bitter to her.

NURSING CARE PLAN FOR MS. X.

Assessment

Subjective

History of intolerance to chemotherapy due to excessive nausea and vomiting

Taste alteration for beef

Stated determination to complete treatment

Objective

6 percent under healthy body weight of 131 pounds

No breaks in mucous membranes of mouth

Nursing Diagnosis

Nutrition, altered: less than body requirements, related to cancer cachexia as evidenced by 6 percent under healthy body weight for height

Desired Outcomes/Evaluation Criteria

Patient will maintain current weight during chemotherapy treatments.

Nursing Actions/Interventions with Rationales in Italics

1. Give antiemetics on scheduled basis beginning 6 hours before first treatment. *Antiemetics work better as preventive medicine than as curative.*

2. Assess daily the times nausea occurs. Schedule three main meals at other times. Offer dry crackers whenever nausea occurs. *Individualizing meal schedules for patients at high risk of malnutrition takes priority over maintaining hospital routines.*

3. Give gentle oral hygiene every 4 hours. *Keeping the oral cavity clean and in good condition will help maintain intake.*

4. Encourage patient to eat slowly and chew thoroughly. *Eating slowly and chewing thoroughly reduce the incidence and severity of nausea.*

5. Provide a back rub and quiet time after meals. *Rest after eating will lessen pressure on stomach and intestines. Massage induces relaxation.*

6. Teach relaxation exercises and controlled breathing to be used when nausea occurs. *These exercises give the patient some control over her environment. Teaching the exercises before treatments begin will be more effective rather than trying to interrupt the cycle of nausea and vomiting once begun.*

7. Consult with clinical dietitian and physician regarding high-protein, low-fat diet; enteral feeding; or total parenteral nutrition. *Although this patient is not 10 percent below minimum body weight, the loss of an additional 5 pounds will put her there. Aggressive nutritional support should begin before the patient becomes severely malnourished.*

STUDY AIDS

Chapter Review Questions

1. Which of the following practices is suggested to help the cancer patient overcome his aversion to food?
   a. Offering small, frequent feedings, attractively served
   b. Encouraging the patient to consider food as therapy
   c. Collaborating with the physician to control the cancer
   d. All of the above.

2. The structures found in tumor cells which are associated with the transformation of normal cells to cancer cells are:
   a. DNA
   b. Initiators
   c. Oncogenes
   d. Promoters

3. The body's cells responsible for recognizing cancer cells and killing them are the
   a. Antibodies
   b. B-lymphocytes
   c. Platelets
   d. T-lymphocytes

4. Which of the following dietary components is most causally linked to cancer development?
   a. Alcohol
   b. Fat
   c. Sugar
   d. Vitamin A

5. Carotene, ascorbic acid, vitamin E, and selenium all may protect against cancer through their _____ properties.
   a. Antioxidant
   b. Fat-binding
   c. Laxative
   d. Tumor-marking

6. A high-fiber diet is thought to reduce the risk of colon cancer because it:
   a. Absorbs water from the intestinal wall
   b. Promotes the excretion of bile
   c. Stops diarrhea
   d. Is low in kilocalories

7. Vegetables that are specifically thought to protect against cancer are:
   a. Corn, lima beans, and peas
   b. Carrots, green beans, and tomatoes
   c. Brussels sprouts, bean sprouts, and water chestnuts
   d. Broccoli, cauliflower, and cabbage

8. Which of the following foods is likely to be well received by a cancer patient with mouth ulcerations?
   a. Hot chicken noodle soup
   b. Orange juice with orange sherbet
   c. Vanilla milkshake
   d. Soda crackers with cream cheese

9. Which of the following is the best advice to increase oral intake for the chemotherapy patient who suffers from nausea and vomiting?

a. Drink plenty of fluids with the meal
b. Eat high-fat, high-protein meals
c. Take only foods that are well liked
d. Eat slowly and chew thoroughly

10. If visitors brought all of the following to a patient in protective isolation, which should the nurse question?
a. Fruit basket
b. Homemade vegetable soup
c. Apple pie
d. Malted milk and french fries

NCLEX-Style Quiz

Situation One

Ms. P. is a 38-year-old single mother of three who has returned to the clinic for follow-up after a breast biopsy. The tissue removed from her left breast was diagnosed as benign.

Ms. P. is 5 feet 6 inches tall and weighs 180 pounds. Meals at the P. house are often hamburger dishes or ethnic combinations. Italian and Mexican foods are favorites of her children.

Ms. P.'s mother was treated for breast cancer at age 60, but is living and well. When interviewed by the nurse, Ms. P. expressed interest in learning what she could do to lessen her chances of developing a malignancy of the breast.

1. Knowing that too radical a change is likely to be rejected by the patient, the nurse concentrates on one improvement to be made in Ms. P.'s diet. Which of the following is likely to make the biggest difference in Ms. P's health?
a. Substituting vegetable oil margarine for butter
b. Eating bran and lima beans every other day
c. Limiting fats to 30 percent of kilocalories
d. Increasing protein to 20 percent of kilocalories

2. Ms. P. wants to know how cancer starts. The nurse's best reply is:
a. "Nobody knows. It just happens."
b. "Something damages the program that governs cell division."
c. "It's a predisposition that some people are born with."
d. "Most of the time it is caused by exposure to radiation."

3. Ms. P. confides that her mother is a recovering alcoholic. She wonders if heavy alcohol consumption contributed to her mother's breast cancer. Which of the following answers would be best for the nurse to give?
a. "Much evidence has shown alcohol is related to cancers of the gastrointestinal system" but not to breast cancer.
b. "Probably not. Alcohol intake is related to liver cancer only."
c. "Only if she also smoked. Alcohol must be potentiated by cigarettes to produce breast cancer."
d. "It may have played a role in the development of her breast cancer. Alcohol, caffeine, and nicotine all are related to breast cancer occurrence."

4. The measure of successful treatment of cancer is the 5-year survival rate. This is based on the number of patients alive:
a. 5 years after first treatment for cancer
b. 5 years after diagnosis, compared with all cancer patients diagnosed in the same year
c. After 5 years, minus any who died from other causes
d. Without evidence of cancer 5 years after diagnosis

CHARTING TIPS 20–1

When admitting a patient who provides much of his or her own care at home, try to learn all about treatments and dietary preferences and document them. If, later on, the patient becomes less self-sufficient after surgery or after beginning cancer therapy, the staff will not have to ask multiple questions before providing care. Recording this information completely ensures that others besides the nurse who obtained it will be able meet the patient's needs.

BIBLIOGRAPHY

American Cancer Society: Cancer Facts and Figures—1991. American Cancer Society, Atlanta, GA, 1991.

Burtis, G, Davis, J, and Martin, S: Applied Nutrition and Diet Therapy. WB Saunders, Philadelphia, 1988.

Daly, HM and Shinkwin, M: Nutrition and the cancer patient. In Holleb, AI, Fink, DJ, and Murphy, GP (eds): American Cancer Society Textbook of Clinical Oncology. American Cancer Society, Atlanta, GA, 1991.

DeWys, WD: Nutritional care of the cancer patient. JAMA 244:374, 1980.

Feldman, EB: Essentials of Clinical Nutrition. FA Davis, Philadelphia, 1988.

Ferry, GD and Price-Jones, BA: Nutrition and disorders of the colon. In Halpern, SL (ed): Quick Reference to Clinical Nutrition. JB Lippincott, Philadelphia, 1987.

Hamilton, EMN, Whitney, EN, and Sizer, FS: Nutrition Concepts and Controversies, ed 2. West, St Paul, 1991.

Heath, CW, Jr,: Cancer prevention. In Holleb, AI, Fink, DJ, and Murphy, GP (eds): American Cancer Society Textbook of Clinical Oncology. American Cancer Society, Atlanta, GA, 1991.

Ignatavicius, DD and Bayne, MV: Medical-Surgical Nursing. WB Saunders, Philadelphia, 1991.

Kritchevsky, D: Diet and cancer. In Holleb, AI, Fink, DJ, and Murphy, GP (eds): American Cancer Society Textbook of Clinical Oncology. American Cancer Society, Atlanta, GA, 1991.

Patrick, ML, et al: Medical-Surgical Nursing. JB Lippincott, Philadelphia, 1991.

Shils, ME and Young, VR: Modern Nutrition in Health and Disease, ed 7. Lea & Febiger, Philadelphia, 1988.

Smeltzer, SC and Bare, B.G. Brunner and Saddarth's Textbook of Medical-Surgical Nursing, ed 7. JB Lippincott, Philadelphia, 1992.

Smith, TJ, Kelly, KG, and Blackburn, GL: Nutrition and the cancer patient. In Cady, B (ed): Cancer Manual. Massachusetts Division, American Cancer Society, Boston, 1986.

Stewart, GS. Trends in radiation therapy for the treatment of lung cancer. Nurs Clin North Am 27(3):643, 1992.

Theologides, A: Nutrition in cancer. In Halpern, SL (ed): Quick Reference to Clinical Nutrition. JB Lippincott, Philadelphia, 1987.

Waltman, NL, et al: Nutritional status, pressure sores, and mortality in elderly patients with cancer. Oncology Nursing Forum 18(5):867, 1991.

Weisburger, JH and Horn, CL: The causes of cancer. In Holleb, AI, Fink, DJ, and Murphy, GP (eds): American Cancer Society Textbook of Clinical Oncology. American Cancer Society, Atlanta, GA, 1991.

Whitney, EB, Cataldo, CB, and Rolfes, SR: Understanding Normal and Clinical Nutrition, ed 3. West, St Paul, 1991.

Willett, WC, et al: Dietary fat and fiber in relation to risk of breast cancer. JAMA 268:2037–2044, 1992.

Willett, WC et al: Dietary fat and the risk of breast cancer. N Engl J Med 316(1):22, 1987.

Williams, SR: Nutrition and Diet Therapy, ed 6. Times Mirror/Mosby College, St Louis, 1989.

Work Study Group on Diet, Nutrition, and Cancer: American Cancer Society guidelines on diet, nutrition, and cancer. CA 41:334, 1991.

Chapter Outline

Nutrition and Mental Health
Genetics and Mental Health
Not All Stress Is Negative
Chronic Disease
Food Intake
Requirements for Nutrients
The Stress of Starvation
The Stress Response
Ebb Phase
Flow Phase
Recovery or Anabolic Phase
Nutrition and Metabolic Stress from Illness, Trauma, and Infection
Hypermetabolism
Examples of Hypermetabolic Conditions
Nutrition and Respiration
Effects of Impaired Nutritional Status on
   Respiratory Function
Nutritional Therapy
Refeeding Syndrome
Principles of Safe Refeeding of the Mal-
   nourished Patient

Key Terms

As a study aid, each key term is followed by the page number where the term is defined in the chapter. Terms that appear in **boldface** or <u>underscored</u> in the chapter text are located in the glossary.

Atrophy (649)
Chronic obstructive pulmonary disease (COPD) (648)
Dyspnea (654)
Ebb phase (640)
Flow phase (640)
Harris-Benedict equation (643)
Hypermetabolism (642)
Kilocalorie:nitrogen ratios (644)
Paralytic ileus (649)
Pulmonary (648)
Refeeding syndrome (652)
Respiration (648)
Respirator (649)
Sepsis (647)
Stress (636)
Stress factor (643)
Trauma (648)
Uncomplicated starvation (638)
Ventilation (648)

Nutrition during Stress

After completing this chapter, the student should be able to:

1. Explain how people can protect themselves nutritionally from the effects of excessive mental stress.
2. List four hypermetabolic conditions that increase resting energy expenditure and hence, kilocaloric requirements.
3. Discuss the relationship between uncomplicated starvation and resting energy expenditure.
4. Discuss the effects of impaired respiratory function on nutritional status and appropriate nutritional therapy.
5. List six recommendations for the safe refeeding of malnourished patients.

*W*e have all experienced stress. **Stress** is defined as any stimulus or condition that threatens the body's homeostasis. Starvation is one form of stress. The effect of a food deprivation in the absence of disease is discussed in this chapter. Also discussed are the relationships of mental health to nutrtionand that of nutrition to metabolic stress from illness, trauma, and infections. The safe principles of refeeding a nutritionally deprived patient conclude the chapter.

NUTRITION AND MENTAL HEALTH

The effects of mental stress cannot be isolated easily from the effects of physical stress. The physical self is structurally related to the emotional self. For example, in the presence of danger, a series of chemical reactions occurs and is associated with our feeling of fear. The flight-or-flight response discussed in the first chapter is mediated by hormones. In other words, the fear (emotional factor) triggers the hormones (physical factors).

Genetics and Mental Health

Genetics may play a role in our response to stress. For example, one person may perceive a given situation to be more stressful than another person. We all know people who anger easily at events others regard as insignificant. Some individuals may also be more genetically susceptible to the negative effects of stress than others. For example, highly stressful situations have been known to precipitate heart attacks in some people, whereas in others the heart is not affected. In this regard the effect of genetics, although known to have an impact on our response to stress, is poorly understood.

Not All Stress Is Negative

A balanced amount of stress maximizes health. Human beings need some stress for emotional well-being. For example, boredom is stressful to many people. Emotional stress such as ambition, drive, and desire may in fact be perceived as positive. Stress such as strain, tension, and/or anxiety is commonly perceived as negative. The death of a spouse, divorce, unemployment, financial problems, and personal injury are all perceived by most people as negative. Clearly, we cannot control all of the events that affect us. However, we do have some control over how we respond to such events. The relationship between nutritional status and people's response to emotional stress has not been completely researched.

Chronic Disease

Emotional stress does appear to be related to the prevalence of cancer, cardiovascular disease, hypertension, and some forms of gastrointestinal diseases. All of these chronic diseases are related to nutrition. Emotional health is known to be important in reducing the risk of heart disease. People who are ordinarily tense, impatient, and ambitious tend to have a high serum cholesterol level.

Gastrointestinal Complication

Ulcers and some intestinal diseases are aggravated by perceived excessive mental stress. A patient may report that he or she has specific food intolerances when under emotional stress, but that the same food is easily tolerated in the absence of stress. This is partially due to impairment of gastrointestinal function during episodes of stress. Decreased motility often causes development of anorexia, abdominal distention, gas pains, and constipation. These symptoms may contribute to reduced food intake and/or food intolerances. Thus, the effects of emotional stress, including food intolerances, can vary not only from person to person, but also in the same person from time to time.

Food Intake

The volume of food a patient consumes and the desire to prepare food are sometimes related to emotional stress. Some people respond to stress by eating more; others respond by eating less. Mental stress can cause a person to lose interest in food preparation. Thus, mental stress can be related to both overnutrition and undernutrition. An individual's perceived stress should always be taken into consideration when formulating the nutritional component of a care plan.

Requirements for Nutrients

Nutrition experts believe the need for most nutrients is not increased solely as a result of excessive mental activity. The needs for kilocalories, protein, calcium, and vitamins have all received some attention from scientists.

Kilocalories

Mental stress alone does not increase our need for kilocalories. For example, mental effort used in studying demands few if any additional kilocalories (Williams, 1990). Likewise, a single parent coping with financial problems, a job, and child rearing does not require extra kilocalories solely as a result of excessive mental activity. Because mental stress does not require additional kilocalories, our requirement for certain vitamins is not increased solely as a result of mental activity. Thiamin, riboflavin, and niacin requirements are based on kilocalorie requirements; if the need for kilocalories is not increased, neither is the requirement for these vitamins.

A person who responds to mental stress by increased physical movement or muscle activity will require additional kilocalories to maintain his or her body weight. Mental stress may cause a person to sleep less, walk more, tremble, fidget, or otherwise increase the work of the muscles. In this situation, additional kilocalories are needed in underweight patients. Underweight patients who complain of a recent weight loss or an inability to gain weight are likely to need additional kilocalories.

Protein and Calcium Balance

Some research has been done on the effects of emotional stress on both protein and calcium balance. Emotional stress such as fear, anxiety, or anger increases the secretion of epinephrine, which in turn causes a series of changes that result in a loss of nitrogen (Guthrie, 1986). Most Americans consume protein in excess of their recommended dietary allowances. However, large amounts of dietary protein provide no insurance against the effects of a stressful lifestyle, since excessive protein intake is thought to stress kidney function.

Calcium is another nutrient that has been studied in people under stress. In one study, individuals in calcium balance have gone suddenly into negative balance under the stress of student examinations (National Center for Health Statistics, 1967). In another study, a group of emotionally distressed young women was found to require a higher intake of calcium to maintain calcium balance than a comparable group of happy, relaxed women (Guthrie, 1986). Calcium intake varies widely among individuals in the United States (National Research Council, 1989). Many Americans do not routinely consume the recommended dietary allowance (RDA) for calcium. For this reason, the authors do advocate that individuals who find themselves the victims of excessive mental stress pay close attention to their calcium intake.

Vitamins and Minerals

The majority of evidence gathered thus far indicates that vitamins in excess of the RDA do not counterbalance the negative effects of mental stress. An example illustrates this principle. In one study, persons on low thiamin intakes showed pronounced mood changes, vague feelings of uneasiness, fear, disorderly thinking, and other signs of mental depression (Guthrie, 1986). When their diets were supplemented with thiamin, they responded readily. The subjects in this study were not habitually consuming their RDA for thiamin. The results of this study have been erroneously interpreted by some lay consumers to mean that thiamin supplements cure mental ailments. This is not true. The purchase of over-the-counter vitamins and/or minerals for stress has limited scientific basis. A healthy, well-balanced diet with adequate protein, calcium and other minerals, and vitamins is the best insurance against excessive stress. Maintenance of a healthy body weight is an indication that kilocaloric intake is appropriate.

THE STRESS OF STARVATION

Starvation is a form of stress to the human body. In the first chapter we introduced the idea the we have a primitive body. Biologically, our bodies developed to cope with periods of feast or famine. Our response to the stress of starvation evolved slowly over the course of millions of years. The human body's response to a food deprivation differs from the body's response to other forms of stress.

Uncomplicated starvation means that the patient has a food deprivation without an underlying stress state. A stress state may be an underlying disease. During uncomplicated starvation, patients will expend about 70 percent of the kilocalories they normally need to maintain their body weight (American Dietetic Association, 1984). Because of the biochemical adaptation to starvation, these patients require fewer kilocalories than they normally do.

The human body has a well-defined response to starvation. The breakdown or catabolism of nutrient stores to meet energy needs characterizes our response. Every cell within the human body needs a constant supply of energy to function. During starvation, a series of chemical reactions occurs to meet each cell's energy needs. A summary of these chemical reactions follows:

1. Glycogenolysis is the breakdown of glycogen (the liver's carbohydrate stores). This releases glucose into the bloodstream. However, the body's limited glycogen stores will last only a few hours.
2. Gluconeogenesis is the production of glucose from noncarbohy-

drate stores. The primary source of glucose in early starvation is the increased rate of gluconeogenesis (Zeman, 1983).

3. Lipolysis is the breakdown of adipose tissue for energy. This releases free fatty acids into the bloodstream. In prolonged starvation, adaptive mechanisms conserve body protein stores by enabling a greater proportion of energy needs to be met by increased fatty acids, with a decreased requirement for glucose. (See below.)

4. Ketosis is the accumulation in the body of the ketone bodies: acetone, beta-hydroxybutyric acid, and acetoacetic acid. Ketosis results from the incomplete metabolism of fatty acids, generally from carbohydrate deficiency, and is commonly seen in starvation. The body will utilize some ketone bodies for energy during prolonged starvation. This reduces but does not eliminate the need for glucose.

These chemical reactions are summarized in Figure 21–1.

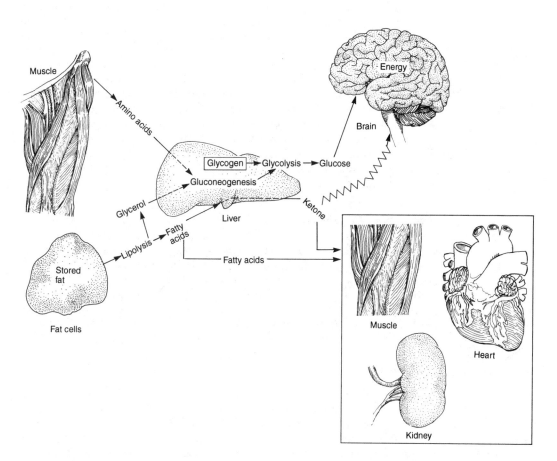

FIGURE 21–1. Origin of fuel and fuel consumption during starvation. The primary source of glucose in early starvation (after the depletion of glycogen stores) is the increased rate of gluconeogenesis. In prolonged starvation, adaptive mechanisms conserve protein by enabling a greater proportion of energy needs to be met by ketone bodies, with a decreased requirement for glucose (after adaptation to starvation).

Each body cell ultimately needs glucose, fatty acids, or the end products of fatty acids and amino acids for energy. Body cells need fuel constantly. Amino acids can be utilized for energy, but only after the liver converts them into glucose and/or fat. Specific organs have a preference for glucose as a fuel source. The brain prefers glucose for energy. Ketone bodies can also be utilized by some cells for energy. The brain will use ketone bodies but prefers glucose. For the most part, the human body can utilize only a very small part of the fat molecule, the glycerol portion, to manufacture glucose. This means that body protein stores must be continually broken down to supply the brain with glucose during starvation after the liver's glycogen stores are depleted.

The heart, kidney, and skeletal muscle tissues prefer fatty acids and/or ketone bodies for their fuel sources. This means that even if a starving person is fed glucose (as in total parenteral nutrition), some dietary fat is still needed to prevent the breakdown of adipose tissue. A balance of the end products of fat and carbohydrate metabolism is necessary for survival.

In prolonged starvation, most body organs will switch to a less preferred fuel source. Even the brain will increasingly begin to utilize more ketone bodies for energy after adaptation to starvation than before. The breakdown of muscle tissue continues in prolonged starvation, but at a much lower rate than previously. The human body also becomes more efficient in reusing amino acids for protein synthesis. Thus, urea nitrogen excretion decreases during prolonged starvation (Zeman, 1984). The rate of tissue breakdown in prolonged starvation also decreases because the metabolic rate and total energy expenditure decrease to conserve energy and prolong life. The catabolic or starved individual will spontaneously decrease physical activity, increase sleep, and run a decreased body temperature. All of these adaptations during prolonged starvation serve one purpose—to prolong life. The human body gets "more miles per gallon" as a result of individual body organs switching to a less preferred fuel source.

THE STRESS RESPONSE

The term *stress response* refers to major changes in metabolism that occur after severe injury, illness, and/or infection. Kilocaloric needs *decrease* during uncomplicated starvation and *increase* (sometimes markedly) as a result of bodily response to stress. The stress response is a dynamic process that has an ebb phase, a flow phase, and an anabolic phase. A patient can progress or regress from one phase to another during his or her clinical course. The need for protein varies according to the patient's stress level.

Ebb Phase

Ebb Phase—The first phase in the stress response; the body reduces blood pressure, cardiac output, body temperature, and oxygen consumption to meet increased demands.

The **ebb phase** begins with an initial stress stimulus and typically lasts for approximately 24 hours. Blood pressure, cardiac output, body temperature, and oxygen consumption are all reduced during the ebb phase (Henningfield, 1991). The body does this so that it has the capacity to meet the increased demands of the environment. These patients require about 1.5 grams of protein per kilogram of body weight per day (Cerra, 1993).

Flow Phase

Flow Phase—The second stage in the stress response; usually lasts from 2 to 10 days and is marked by pronounced by hormonal changes.

Increased cardiac output, increased urinary nitrogen losses, altered glucose metabolism, and accelerated catabolism characterize the flow phase. In addi-

TABLE 21–1 *Hormonal Secretion during Phase Two of the Stress Response and the Metabolic Effect of These Hormones**

Hormonal Secretion	Effect on Metabolism
Increased epinephrine	Rate of lipolysis increased
	Rate of glycolysis increased
	Rate of gluconeogenesis increased
Decreased insulin	Storage of glucose, fatty acids, and amino acids ceases. Glucose delivery to the cells thus decreases. For this reason, hyperglycemia is commonly seen in stressed patients.
Increased glucagon	Rate of gluconeogenesis increases
Increased antidiuretic hormone	Increase in water retention
Increased aldosterone	Increase in sodium retention

*Net effect: decrease in body protein and fat stores.

tion, the flow phase is marked by pronounced hormonal changes. Table 21–1 lists hormones secreted during this stage of the stress response and describes the impact these hormones have on metabolism. These hormonal conditions favor the breakdown of body protein stores to provide glucose. This leads to a rapid loss of nitrogen in the urine as lean body mass is broken down to furnish the cells with glucose. The need for protein is about 2 grams per kilogram of body weight during the flow phase (Cerra, 1993).

Blood flow to the gastrointestinal tract is often diminished during this phase of the stress response. This decreases the supply of both oxygen and nutrients to the GI tract. The secretion of mucus is diminished and the secretion of gastric acid is increased. Cells that line the GI tract waste away and die as a result of these changes. The patient may complain of diarrhea and bloating.

Recovery or Anabolic Phase

The third stage of the stress response, the anabolic phase, is also marked by changes in hormonal secretions. Insulin and growth hormone increase in the bloodstream during the anabolic phases. Secretion of most of the other hormones decreases. The building up of body tissue and nutrient stores (anabolism) characterizes this phase. Protein need during the anabolic phase is between 2 to 3 grams per kilogram of body weight (Cerra, 1993).

Obviously it is desirable for a patient to progress to the third phase of the stress stage as rapidly as possible. Tissue building, or anabolism, is beneficial. The ability of a patient to rebuild tissue after a physical stress depends on several factors. Age is one factor. The patient's prior nutritional status, the severity of the stress, and the duration of the stress particularly influence tissue growth. Patients who have ample nutrient stores to draw on during stress are better able to tolerate the negative effects of the stress. Good nutrition is a form of insurance. The nutrient stores are available to be used if an unexpected stress occurs. Recent research has shown that early supplementation with the amino acid glutamine may enhance the progression to the anabolic phase of the stress response (see Clinical Application 21–1).

Anabolic Phase—The third stage in the stress response in which the body begins to rebuild tissue.

CLINICAL APPLICATION 21–1

Glutamine and Stress

Glutamine is a nonessential amino acid. During stress the body's requirement for glutamine appears to exceed the individual's ability to produce it in sufficient amounts (Lacy and Wilmore, 1991). Current research is exploring the provision of supplemental glutamine to enhance the recovery of the seriously ill patient. Alitraq, manufactured by Ross Laboratories, is a specialized elemental formula for medical use that is high in glutamine.

NUTRITION AND METABOLIC STRESS FROM ILLNESS, TRAUMA, AND INFECTION

Cancer, major surgery, burns, infections, and trauma are the physical stressors that have the greatest impact on metabolism. The needs of patients with cancer were described in the previous chapter. This section of the text focuses on the nutritional needs of patients subjected to surgery, burns, infections and fevers, and trauma. Nutritional support during extreme stress is needed to decrease the length of the stress, prevent complications, and minimize human suffering.

Hypermetabolism

Hypermetabolism—An abnormal increase in the rate at which fuel or kilocalories is burned.

Hypermetabolism is an abnormal increase in the rate at which fuel or kilocalories are burned. Hypermetabolism can be identified by an increased metabolic rate, negative nitrogen balance, hyperglycemia, and increased oxygen consumption. Patients are hypermetabolic during the flow phase of the stress response.

Protein Needs

Protein needs are elevated during hypermetabolism. Injury or illness requires active protein formation. Surgical wounds, tissue repair, replacement of red blood cells and plasma protein lost in hemorrhage, and the immune response to infection all require a constant supply of protein. For these reasons, a patient who is hypermetabolic has an increased need for protein. A hypermetabolic patient may lose as much as 250 grams (about $^1/_2$ pound) of muscle tissue per day (Zemen, 1984).

URINE ASSESSMENT OF PROTEIN STATUS   Total urinary excretion of nitrogen increases with the patient's stress level. Urinary creatinine measurements may be used to estimate muscle protein reserves. One problem common to the use of all urinary measurements is the completion of an accurate 24-hour urine collection. The nurse is typically responsible for collecting a 24-hour urine specimen from the patient. If even one voiding is discarded, measurements will be inaccurate.

Kilocalories and Hypermetabolic Stress

Patients who are hypermetabolic have an increased need for kilocalories. The negative nitrogen balance observed in hypermetabolic patients may be the result of an inadequate kilocalorie intake rather than an insufficient protein intake.

EARLY FEEDING   The use of early nutritional support during the ebb phase of the stress response has been studied (Young, 1988). The use of enteral nutrition shortly after the event that precipitated the stress may be advantageous because it supplies essential nutrients, keeps the GI tract active, and halts the elevation of the catabolic stress hormones (Henningfield, 1991).

KILOCALORIE NEEDS   Energy expenditure means the number of kilocalories that an individual uses to meet the body's demand for fuel. The kilocalorie need of a person is calculated by the following formula:

Resting Energy Expenditure × Activity Factor = Daily Energy Allowance

Clinical Calculations 8–2 and 8–3 demonstrated these calculations. A variation of this formula is used to estimate the kilocalorie needs for the hypermetabolic patient.

The hypermetabolic patient's kilocalorie need has been well researched. Major body stressors increase kilocalorie needs. The kilocalorie need of a hypermetabolic patient is often calculated with the following formula:

Resting Energy Expenditure × Activity Factor × Stress Factor
= Estimated Energy Need

Each part of this formula is discussed in detail below.

RESTING ENERGY EXPENDITURE   The <u>Harris-Benedict equation</u> is widely used to estimate resting energy expenditure (REE) for critically ill patients. The Harris-Benedict equation is presented in Clinical Calculation 21–1 along with an example of these calculations. Please note that different equations are used for male and female patients. These equations are similar to the equations used in Chapter 8 but differ in one important way. The RDA for kilocalories is based on a reference man or woman. The Harris-Benedict equation allows the healthcare provider to calculate kilocalories based on an individual patient's height, age, and weight.

ACTIVITY FACTOR   The Harris-Benedict equation calculates the patient's REE. Physical activity is not included in REE and must be calculated. Table 21–2 shows activity factors for patients confined to bed and for those not confined to bed; kilocalorie needs for physical activity are 0.20, or 20 percent, and 0.30, or 30 percent, respectively.

STRESS FACTOR   Research has shown that different types of stress increase kilocalorie needs differently. A <u>stress factor</u> is a number assigned to

TABLE 21–2 *Activity Factors Commonly Used to Calculate a Patient's Activity Kilocalories*

For a patient confined to bed	0.2, or 20 percent
For a patient out of bed	0.3, or 30 percent

a given pathological state to predict how much a patient's kilocalorie need has increased as a result of the type of stress the patient is experiencing from that state. Table 21–3 lists various types of physical stress and the stress factor used for each disease state.

As you can see in the table, a patient with burns over 50 percent of his or her body has a stress factor of 2.0. This means kilocalorie need is twice (200 percent) his or her resting energy expenditure. By contrast, the stress factor for minor surgery is 1.05. This means a patient who has had minor surgery needs only 5 percent more kilocalories than his or her REE multiplied by the previously determined physical activity factor. Stress factors are convenient to use in estimating kilocalorie needs.

Kilocalorie:Nitrogen Ratios in the Hypermetabolic Patient

Kilocalorie:Nitrogen Ratios—A mathematical relationship expressed as the number of kilocalories to grams of nitrogen provided in a feeding.

Protein requirements cannot be totally separated from energy requirements because protein is used as an energy source in the absence of adequate kilocalories. The current practice is to calculate **kilocalorie:nitrogen ratios** for hypermetabolic patients. As a rule, the average healthy person needs 1 gram of nitrogen per 300 kilocalories (American Dietetic Association, 1984). One gram of nitrogen is equal to 6.25 grams of protein. The hypermetabolic patient needs approximately 1 gram of nitrogen per 100 to 150 kilocalories (American Dietetic Association, 1984). The hypermetabolic patient needs about twice as much protein as the patient not in a state of hypermetabolism.

A variety of commercially produced enteral feedings are available for these patients. Most nutritional supplements have the kilocalorie:nitrogen ratio of the product listed either on the label or in a package insert.

Vitamin Needs

The hypermetabolic patient usually requires an increase in the B vitamins and vitamin C. The hypermetabolic patient who has an increased need for kilocalories also has an increased need for thiamin, riboflavin, and niacin. The B vitamins involved in protein metabolism also need to be increased in

TABLE 21–3 *Stress Factors Commonly Used to Determine a Patient's Need for Kilocalories*

Stressor	Factor
Uncomplicated minor surgery	1.05
Starvation	0.70
For each degree F above 98.6	1.07
Cancer	1.1–1.45
Soft tissue trauma	1.14–1.37
Skeletal trauma (fracture)	1.35
Burns (10–30 percent of body surface area)	1.5
Burns (30–50 percent of body surface area)	1.75
Burns (>50 percent of body surface area)	2.0
Peritonitis	1.2–1.5
Major sepsis	1.4–1.8

the hypermetabolic patient's diet. The B vitamins help release the chemical energy stored in foods. Any time a patient requires increased kilocalories, the need for the B-vitamin complex automatically increases. When anabolism or the building of body tissue is indicated, vitamin C requirements are increased. Hypermetabolic patients usually need to build up depleted tissue stores.

Examples of Hypermetabolic Conditions

The hypermetabolic conditions which influence nutritional needs most profoundly are major surgery, burns, infections and fevers, and trauma. All of these conditions increase resting energy expenditure and hence, kilocalorie requirements. This section of the chapter discusses these conditions.

Surgery

The nutritional needs of the surgical patient were previously discussed in Chapter 19. In this chapter, we will focus on the increased need for kilocalories in the surgical patient. Uncomplicated minor surgery increases the surgical patient's kilocaloric requirement by only 5 percent. Surgery needed to repair a soft tissue trauma requires between a 14 and 37 percent increase in kilocalories. A surgical patient with complications may require a large increase in kilocalories. Please refer again to Table 21–3 for more specific numbers.

Burns

Major burns represent the most extreme state of stress a patient can sustain. They produce a hypermetabolic state that raises kilocaloric needs higher than those of most other stress states. Kilocalorie requirements may be as large as 8000 kilocalories per day. Even a patient who was well nourished before becoming burned may rapidly develop protein-calorie malnutrition. As indicated in Table 21–3, the degree to which the metabolic rate increases is directly related to the body surface area burned. Although it is not reflected in the stress factors listed in the table, the deeper the burn, the higher the patient's kilocalorie need. Burn patients may remain in a hypermetabolic state for many weeks.

Figure 21–2 classifies burns according to the depth of the burn. Determination of the surface area burned is also provided in this figure. Note that a first-degree burn includes minimal depth. Superficial burns, where the damage is limited to the outer layer of the skin, are considered first-degree burns. Second-degree burns include some damage to both layers of the skin; blisters are present. Second-degree burns that become infected, however, may be equivalent to a third-degree burn (Thomas, 1985). Third-degree burns include damage to the tissue beneath the skin. The percentage of body surface area burned is determined by totaling the individual percentages given in the figure.

The increased load of waste products produced in patients with burns is one reason for an increase in fluid requirements. Extra fluids will assist the kidneys in eliminating these waste products. Capillary permeability is increased in the burn patient; hence, plasma proteins, fluids, and electrolytes escape into the burn area and interstitial space, causing edema (Robinson

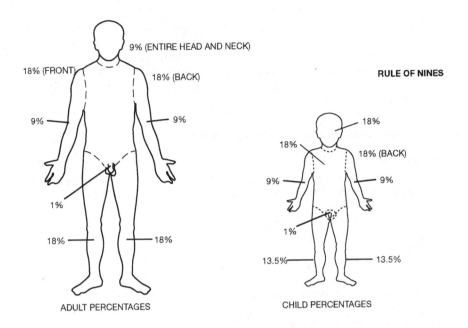

ADULT PERCENTAGES

CHILD PERCENTAGES

RULE OF NINES

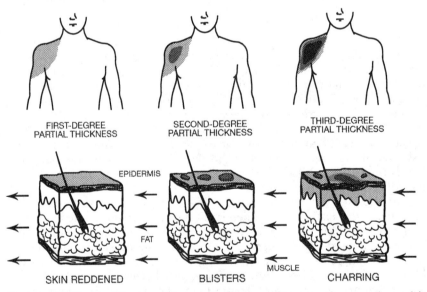

CLASSIFICATION OF BURNS

FIRST-DEGREE
PARTIAL THICKNESS

SECOND-DEGREE
PARTIAL THICKNESS

THIRD-DEGREE
PARTIAL THICKNESS

EPIDERMIS

FAT

MUSCLE

SKIN REDDENED

BLISTERS

CHARRING

FIGURE 21–2. Classification of burns. Percentage of body surface area burned is determined by comparing the body surface area of the patient's burns to percentages given in this chart. For example, if a patient has extensive burns over both legs, the total body surface area burned would be 36% (18% for the first leg plus 18% for the second leg). The depth of the burn determines whether the burn is classified as first, second, or third degree. (From Thomas CL (ed): Taber's Cyclopedic Medical Dictionary, ed 16, FA Davis, Philadelphia, 1993, p 281, with permission.)

and Weigley, 1989). This shift reduces the volume of the plasma, so fluid volume needs to be replaced.

Physicians disagree on the best time to begin feeding the burn patient. Some physicians initiate tube feedings within 4 hours following burn injury. Here, an important consideration is that peristalsis, the wavelike motion that propels food through the gastrointestinal tract, ceases in some burn patients. Until peristalsis returns, the patient's stomach should not be the site of choice for a tube feeding. Instead, the tube should be inserted into the patient's intestines and a very slow continuous drip feeding is used. Rather than beginning the feedings on the day of injury, other physicians resume oral feeding of the patient with the return of normal bowel activity. For most patients this is 2 to 4 days after the initial burn. The burn patient is usually allowed a clear or full liquid diet at this time. Dietary progression begins 4 to 10 days after the injury, as tolerated.

Burn patients are particularly susceptible to **sepsis,** the state in which disease-producing organisms are present in the blood. Major sepsis further increases a patient's metabolic rate. See Table 21–3 for the stress factor to use in determining kilocalorie needs during sepsis.

Stress factors can be multiplied by each other. For example, the formula to use for a patient with greater than 50 percent burns over the body surface area and major sepsis is:

Kilocalorie Need = REE × Activity Factor × Stress Factor No. 1
(2.0 for 50 percent burn) × Stress Factor No. 2 (1.5 for major sepsis)

Sepsis is of course not limited to burn patients; surgical and trauma patients may also suffer from sepsis.

For all burn patients, a nutritional assessment is essential to minimize complications and allow the nutritional therapy to be effectively evaluated. These patients should have their food intake monitored and documented. The kilocalories consumed or taken intravenously should be charted daily.

Most burn patients have a high-protein, high-kilocalorie diet ordered; often the diet is initially offered in six small meals. Complete nutritional oral supplements are commonly used to increase the patient's kilocalorie and protein intake. The protein content of the diet can be increased by providing a between-meal feeding high in protein, a serving of two eggs at breakfast, and a large serving of meat at both lunch and supper. If the patient drinks a full 8 ounces of milk with each meal, this will further increase the protein content of the diet.

Infections and Fever

Malnutrition decreases resistance to infection, and infection aggravates malnutrition by depleting body nutrient stores. Fever characteristically accompanies infection but can also result from a variety of causes, including inflammatory processes within the body, trauma, central nervous system disorders, and dehydration (LaQuatra and Gerlack, 1990). Infection often results in decreased food intake and absorption of nutrients, altered metabolism, and increased urinary losses of nutrients (Suitor and West, 1984). Extra kilocalories are needed by the body during fever because it takes more energy to regulate body temperature. Also, as in any hypermetabolic state, extra kilocalories are needed because the patient's REE increases. Table 21–3 shows a stress fac-

Sepsis—A condition in which disease-producing organisms are present in the blood.

tor of 1 + 0.07 for each degree Fahrenheit the temperature exceeds normal. For example, to determine the kilocalorie need of a patient with a prolonged fever of 104.6°F, the stress factor is 1.49 (1 + 7 degrees × 0.07).

Protein requirements for the patient with an infection are increased. Extra protein is also needed to enable the human body to produce antibodies and white blood cells to fight the infection.

The fluid requirements of a patient with a fever are increased. Perspiration entails a loss of fluids from the body, and patients with fever have increased perspiration. Fluid will also be lost in vomiting and diarrhea. This fluid needs to be replaced.

Trauma

Trauma—A physical injury or wound caused by an external force.

Trauma may be defined as a physical injury or wound caused by an external source or violence. In the United States, trauma is the principal cause of death of persons between the ages of 1 and 38 years (Thomas, 1985). Stab and gunshot wounds, multiple fractures, and motor vehicle accidents that include crushing are some examples of trauma. Victims of these traumas may become hypermetabolic, depending on the severity of the injury. Vitamin supplements may be necessary. These patients are at a nutritional risk and may need extra kilocalories and protein.

NUTRITION AND RESPIRATION

Only recently has the scientific literature addressed the relationship between good nutrition and respiration. Respiration refers to the exchange of gases (oxygen and carbon dioxide) between a living organism and its environment. The air or oxygen inhaled and the carbon dioxide exhaled is the act of ventilation. Ventilation means breathing. Pulmonary means concerning or involving the lungs. **Chronic Obstructive Pulmonary Disease** (COPD) refers to a group of lung diseases with a common characteristic of chronic airflow obstruction. COPD has become the fifth leading cause of death in the United States. The mortality has tripled in the past 30 years (Bullock and Rosendahl, 1992). Malnutrition is commonly seen in patients with respiratory diseases.

Chronic Obstructive Pulmonary Disease (COPD)—A group of chronic diseases with a common chraracteristic of chronic airflow obstruction.

Effects of Impaired Nutritional Status on Respiratory Function

Poor nutrition is related to inadequate pulmonary function in five important ways. First, these patients frequently have an inadequate food intake, which is related to anorexia, shortness of breath, and/or gastrointestinal distress. Shortness of breath during food preparation and consumption of meals may limit kilocalorie intake (Brown and Light, 1983). Inadequate oxygen delivery to the cells causes fatigue. Impaired gastrointestinal tract motility is common in patients with respiratory diseases (see below).

Second, kilocalorie requirements are often increased in patients with pulmonary disease. Recent research has estimated that while the kilocalorie cost of breathing ranges from 36 to 72 kilocalories per day in normal individuals, the kilocaloric cost of breathing increases to 430 to 720 kilocalories per day in patients with COPD (Brown and Light, 1983). Owing to the combined effects of decreased food intake and increased energy requirements, weight loss is commonly seen in these patients. Mortality is significantly greater among patients who have lost weight (Vandenbergh, 1967).

The third important relationship between nutrition and pulmonary function is the effect of catabolism. When kilocalorie intake is decreased, the body begins to break down muscle stores, including those of the respiratory muscles. A loss of the lean mass of any muscle will have an impact on the muscle's function. The lung's structure itself is thus affected as a result of catabolism. Malnutrition may also result in decreased lung-tissue cell replacement or growth.

The gastrointestinal distress common in patients with pulmonary disease may be related to malnutrition. A loss of the structure within the gastrointestinal tract may lead to hemorrhage and **paralytic ileus.** Paralytic ileus is defined as the temporary reduction of peristalsis. This contributes to the feeling of anorexia and decreased food intake. In addition, paralytic ileus may lead to a translocation of bacteria. Decreased peristalsis in the gastrointestinal tract fosters the movement (translocation) of bacteria from the gastrointestinal tract into the bloodstream. This in turn leads to sepsis, or bloodborne infection, a sometimes fatal complication.

Paralytic ileus— A temporary cessation in peristalsis which causes symptoms of intestinal obstruction.

The fourth important relationship between nutrition and pulmonary function is that malnutrition decreases resistance to infection. Lung infection is frequently the cause of death in pulmonary patients (Ross Laboratories, 1984).

In a state of malnutrition, the body decreases the production of antibodies, which are necessary to fight infection. Also, as a result of starvation, the lungs will decrease production of pulmonary phospholipid (a fat-like structure). Phospholipids assist in keeping the lung tissue lubricated and help to protect both lungs from any disease-producing organisms that are inhaled.

The fifth important relationship between nutrition and pulmonary function is that improved nutritional status has been associated with an increased ability to wean patients from respirators or ventilators. A respirator (also called a ventilator) is a machine for prolonged artificial or mechanical respiration. Patients on artificial respirators do not have to use their respiratory muscles to breathe. Active muscle movement stimulates muscle growth via protein stimulus. This is the same principle as physical exercise increasing muscle size. To some extent, all the respiratory muscles atrophy, or waste away, due to inactivity while a patient is artificially breathing.

Patients on ventilators are usually weaned slowly from these machines as their condition improves. Nutritional support improves the likelihood of successful weaning in patients on artificial respiration (Bassili and Dietel, 1981; Larca and Greenbaum, 1982). Some experts have attributed patients' ability to be successfully weaned from respirators to an increase in protein synthesis. Good nutrition stimulates protein synthesis.

Nutritional Therapy

Respiratory disease can affect both food intake and nutrient utilization. Many patients with respiratory diseases also have problems with water balance.

Energy Nutrient Utilization

Many patients with COPD suffer from carbon dioxide retention and oxygen depletion. Such patients are said to be carbon dioxide retainers. The medical goal with these patients is to decrease their blood level of carbon dioxide.

The following formula from Chapter 8 may assist the understanding of this concept:

$$\text{Protein (or Carbohydrate or Fat)} + \text{Oxygen}$$
$$= \text{Heat Energy} + \text{Water} + \text{Carbon Dioxide}$$

Fat kilocalories produce less carbon dioxide than carbohydrate kilocalories. For this reason, a diet high in fat is often used for carbon dioxide retainers. A high-fat diet may also assist the patient with respiratory failure who must be weaned from mechanical ventilation. A high-fat diet may provide as much as 50 percent of the kilocalories in the form of fat. Figure 21–3 illustrates the relationship between nutrition and respiratory status in patients with pul-

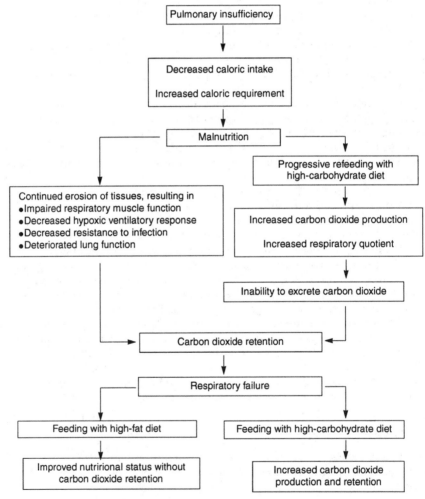

FIGURE 21–3. Interrelationship between nutrition and respiratory status in patients with pulmonary insufficiency. Influence of high-carbohydrate and high-fat diets is shown. (Reprinted with permission of Ross Laboratories, Columbus, OH 43216. From Specialized Nutrition for Pulmonary Patients, December, p 14, 1984, Ross Laboratories.)

monary insufficiency. The influence of high-carbohydrate and high-fat diets is shown.

Some physicians may oppose the use of a high-fat diet for carbon dioxide retainers. This opposition is based on research that has shown that a high fat intake may be immunosuppressive in some patients. (Juskelis, 1991). For this reason, fat in excess of 50 percent of total kilocalories is rarely prescribed.

Care must be taken not to overfeed these patients. Excess intake can raise the demand for oxygen and production of carbon dioxide beyond the capacity of the patient with reduced respiratory function The total number of kilocalories fed to the pulmonary patient should be closely monitored. A nutritional assessment will help predict the patient's kilocalorie need and assist in therapy. Two complete nutritional supplements commonly used to increase kilocaloric consumption for this type of patient are Pulmocare and Isocal HN. These formulas have a greater percentage of kilocalories provided from fat than other complete nutritional supplements.

Vitamins A and C

An adequate intake of vitamins A and C is essential in helping to prevent pulmonary infections and to help decrease the extent of lung tissue damage. (McCauley and Weaver, 1983). Foods high in vitamin A, such as fortified milk, dark green or yellow fruits and vegetables, some breakfast cereals (check the label), cheese, and eggs should be included in the diet. Foods high in vitamin C, such as citrus fruits and juices, strawberries, and fortified breakfast cereals (check the label) should also be included. Sources of vitamins A and C that are used should not produce gas.

Water and Phosphorus

Water balance and serum phosphorus levels need to be closely monitored in these patients. Patients with COPD and acute respiratory failure often need a fluid restriction. A fluid restriction will assist in the control of pulmonary edema or a movement of fluid into interstitial lung tissue. Low serum phosphorus levels or hypophosphatemia are often seen in patients who are respirator-dependent. Phosphorus leaves the intracellular space and moves into the extracellular space during starvation. Serum phosphorus levels are in the normal or near-normal range at this point. With refeeding, phosphate moves back into the intracellular space. At this point, the serum phosphorus level may drop below normal. In the event that this occurs, it is crucial that the patient receive phosphate therapy. Because acute hypophosphatemia has been reported to cause respiratory failure, serum phosphorus levels should be monitored in all patients receiving aggressive nutritional support.

Feeding Techniques

Many of these patients lack the energy to eat. Complaints of fatigue are common. The gastrointestinal distress experienced by these patients contributes to the anorexia. Foods such as onions, peas, melons, and vegetables from the cabbage family may contribute to gastrointestinal distress. (LaQuatra and Gerlach, 1990). Small, frequent feeding of foods with a high nutrient density should be encouraged. Serving food items that require little or no chewing may help with difficulties chewing, breathlessness, and swallowing.

REFEEDING SYNDROME

Many of the types of patients discussed in this chapter will require aggressive nutritional support. Several metabolic and physiological changes occur when refeeding the chronically protein-calorie malnourished patient (Nutrition and the MD, 1991). Improper refeeding of a chronically malnourished patient can result in congestive heart failure and respiratory failure. These complications can occur regardless of the mode of feeding, whether oral, enteral, or parenteral (Nutrition and the MD, 1991).

Refeeding Syndrome has been used to describe a series of metabolic and physiological reactions that occur in some malnourished patients when nutritional rehabilitation is begun. Improper refeeding of a chronically malnourished patient can result in congestive heart failure and respiratory failure. Patients at risk include those with alcoholism, chronic weight loss, hyperglycemia, insulin-dependent diabetes mellitus, or those on chronic antacid or diuretic therapy (Solomon and Kirby, 1990).

Starvation leads to both a loss of the lean body mass in the heart and respiratory muscles and decreased insulin secretion. When carbohydrate intake is low, the pancreas adapts by decreasing insulin secretion. With the reintroduction of carbohydrate into the diet, insulin secretion will increase. The increased insulin secretion is associated with increased sodium and water retention. Other hormones are also activated with carbohydrate feeding. As a result of hormone action, increases in metabolic rate, oxygen consumption, and carbon dioxide production occur (Alfin-Slater, 1991). The net effect of these metabolic changes is an increased workload for the cardiopulmonary system. Refeeding may increase the work of the cardiopulmonary system beyond its diminished capacity (due to the loss of lean body mass) and cause congestive heart failure and respiratory failure.

Starvation also leads to an increase in extracellular fluid and an increased loss of intracellular phosphorus, potassium, and magnesium. The degree of intracellular loss of these minerals reflects the degree of loss of lean body mass (Alfin-Slater, 1991). Before refeeding, serum phosphorus and magnesium levels may remain in the lower range of normal, while the intracellular and total body stores of these minerals are depleted. After refeeding, these minerals are redistributed from the extracellular to the intracellular compartments. Repeated laboratory measurements taken after refeeding is started may show low serum levels of phosphorus, magnesium, and potassium. Failure to correct for these mineral deficiencies may be fatal for the patient.

Principles of Safe Refeeding of the Malnourished Patient

Healthcare workers need to be aware of the dangers of refeeding a malnourished patient. Starved patients can be found in outpatient settings as well as in hospital intensive care units. A high prevalence of malnutrition is common in the outpatient setting (Alfin-Slater, 1991). The following recommenda-

Refeeding Syndrome—a series of metabolic reactions that occur in some malnourished patients when they are refed; characterized by congestive heart failure and respiratory failure.

tions may help the healthcare worker to avoid the refeeding syndrome in malnourished patients:

1. Recognize the "patient at risk." Refeeding syndrome occurs in patients with frank starvation, including war victims undergoing repletion, chronically ill patients who are malnourished, those patients on prolonged intravenous dextrose solutions without other modes of nutritional support, hypermetabolic patients who have not received nutritional support for 1 to 2 weeks, patients who report prolonged fasting, obese patients who report a recent loss of a considerable amount of weight, chronic alcoholics, and patients with anorexia nervosa.

2. Healthcare workers practicing in an outpatient setting and not directly under the supervision of a physician need to develop a referral plan in the event they suspect a patient is a likely candidate for the refeeding syndrome. These patients require the expertise of a physician. Many physicians will accept referrals from any healthcare worker.

3. A physician needs to test for and correct all electrolyte abnormalities before initiating nutritional support, whether by oral, enteral, or parenteral routes. Many physicians depend on other healthcare workers to assist in the monitoring of serum phosphorus, magnesium, and potassium values. For the nurse practicing in the inpatient setting, this means notifying the physician upon receipt of laboratory test results showing low serum levels of these minerals. It is especially important to notify the physician before implementing changes in tube feedings, oral diets, or the rate of hyperalimentation. In larger hospitals, the nutrition support service will perform this service, as described in Chapter 13.

4. The physician needs to restore circulatory volume and to monitor pulse rate and intake and output before initiating nutritional support. Again, many physicians depend on nurses and other healthcare workers to assist in monitoring these parameters.

5. The kilocaloric delivery of previously starved patients should be slow. Tube-fed and parenterally fed patients need to be closely monitored. The rate, the total volume, and the concentration of kilocalories delivered should be carefully monitored and documented. The concentration, volume, or rate of kilocalorie intake should be increased one at a time. Stepwise advancement to a higher kilocalorie intake should not occur unless the patient is metabolically and physiologically stable (Alfin-Slater, 1991).

6. Electrolytes should be monitored before nutritional support is started and at designed intervals thereafter.

Refeeding the malnourished patient requires a team effort. A careful diet history performed by the dietitian can assist in the identification of patients likely to become victims of the refeeding syndrome. Changes in taste, appetite, intake, weight, or consumption of a special diet may indicate significantly altered status (University of Michigan Medical Center, 1986). Correction of electrolyte abnormalities by the physician before implementing nutritional support can prevent death. Careful observation and monitoring by the nutritional support service can identify early signs of this syndrome. Open communication between all healthcare team members may be crucial to the patient's survival. All healthcare workers need to be knowledgeable about the hazards associated with refeeding the malnourished patient.

Summary

Stress is defined as any condition that threatens the body's equilibrium. Because the physical and emotional aspects of the self are closely related, it is difficult to separate the effects of mental from physical stress. Mental stress has been shown to have an impact on nitrogen and calcium balance. The best insurance against unexpected stress is good nutrient stores developed from the previous consumption of a well-balanced diet.

The stress response has three well-defined phases, which are mediated by hormones: the ebb phase, the flow phase, and the recovery (or anabolic) phase. Hypermetabolism differs from starvation in that resting energy expenditure (REE) increases during hypermetabolism and decreases during a prolonged state of starvation. Major surgery, severe infections, fever, major burns, and severe trauma are all examples of hypermetabolic states. All of these conditions require a high-kilocalorie, high-protein diet.

Recently, the relationship between nutritional status and impaired respiratory function has been studied. Respiratory diseases can affect both food intake and nutrient utilization. Nutritional support can decrease catabolism of the respiratory muscles, improve immune function, minimize carbon dioxide production, and improve the likelihood of successfully weaning patients who are on mechanical respirators.

Refeeding a previously starved patient has some risks. Refeeding may increase the work of the cardiorespiratory system beyond its diminished capacity and cause congestive heart failure and respiratory failure. Refeeding syndrome is a series of metabolic reactions seen in some malnourished patients when they are re-fed. All healthcare workers have a responsibility to understand this syndrome. A team approach to refeeding the malnourished patient is necessary to prevent tragic complications.

CASE STUDY 21–1

Mr. X. is a 42-year-old man who was admitted to the intensive care unit (ICU) with a diagnosis of acute bronchitis. He has a known history of carbon dioxide retention and chronic obstructive pulmonary disease. Mr. X. is 5′11″ (180 cm), 140 pounds (63.6 kg), and has a medium body frame (HBW = 87.5%). He reports a recent 9-pound weight loss over a 3-week period. The patient is on a mechanical respirator. The physician's goal is to wean the patient from the ventilator as soon as possible. Mr. X. complains of fatigue, gas pains, anorexia, <u>dyspnea</u> (difficulty breathing), and early satiety. The patient consumed a cup of coffee and one slice of toast for breakfast before falling asleep. The physician has ordered a 50 percent fat high kilocalorie high protein diet.

NURSING CARE PLAN FOR MR. X.

Assessment

Subjective:
   Reports a 3-pound week loss over the last 3 weeks.
   Complains of fatigue, gas pains, anorexia, dyspnea, and early satiety.

Objective:
    87.5 percent HBW
    Observed low food intake
    Known history of COPD with carbon dioxide retention

Nursing Diagnosis

Nutrition, altered less than body requirements, related to poor food intake, recent weight loss, fatigue, gas pains, anorexia, dyspnea, and early satiety as evidenced by 87.5 percent HBW and known history of COPD and carbon dioxide retention.

Desired Outcome/Evaluation Criteria

1. States that good nutrition is important to independent respiration in one day.
2. Consumes an appropriate food intake in 3 days.
3. Maintains his weight during hospitalization.
4. Demonstrates progressive weight gain toward his healthy body weight over the next 3 months.

Nursing Actions/Interventions with Rationales in Italics

1. Stress the importance of the prescribed diet to independent respiration.
2. a) Consult with the dietitian to set a nutritional goal for the patient based on the patient's estimated energy expenditure using the Harris-Benedict formula, total energy requirements, and protein requirements.
    b) Promote a pleasant, relaxed environment, including socialization if possible at mealtime.
    c) Consult with the dietitian to provide a diet with modifications that meet the patient's needs such as:
        i) Texture and modification as necessary.
        ii) Avoidance of foods not tolerated due to questionable limited gastrointestinal tract motility such as gassy vegetables, spicy foods, milk products (secondary to lactase deficiency), etc.
        iii) In-between meal supplements that are acceptable to the patient.
        iv) Limitation of empty kilocalories.
        v) Meal size and volume limits.
    d) Monitor the patient's food intakes, i.e., kilocalorie count.
    e) Provide oral care before/after meals.
3. Weigh patient daily.
4. Instruct patient to weigh himself weekly.

Rationale

1. *Successful weaning to independent respiration is enhanced by good nutrition. Current thought is that good nutrition decreases respiratory muscle catabolism, fosters protein synthesis, and facilitates production of pulmonary phospholipids.*
2. a) *The pulmonary patient should not be over- or underfed. Determination of the patient's energy and protein requirements will provide baseline information to determine nutritional needs. Kilocalories and carbohydrates in excess will increase carbon dioxide retention. A deficiency of kilocalories and protein will increase catabolism of the respiratory muscles.*
    b) *Eating is both a social and biological experience. Kilocalorie intake will be greater if an attempt is made to provide a pleasant eating environment.*
    c) *Patients with pulmonary disease are often too tired to eat and may have*

gastrointestinal complaints. Small frequent meals, easily chewed foods, and reduction of empty kilocalories may assist in helping the patient to meet estimated kilocalorie and protein needs.

d) Documentation of food intake with subsequent analysis of protein and kilocalorie content will provide an objective measure of nursing care plan effectiveness. The results of the analysis can be used to provide feedback to the patient.

e) Oral care before meals encourages food consumption and after meals minimizes dental caries.

3. The best way to evaluate the effectiveness of nutritional therapy is to weigh the nonedematous patient. For this patient, weight gain will require a considerable effort, hence, an intermediate goal of weight maintenance is realistic.

4. The ultimate goal for this patient is anabolism with a weight gain. A slow progressive weight gain means the approach taken is working.

STUDY AIDS

Chapter Review Questions

1. Hypermetabolism differs from the catabolism seen during uncomplicated starvation in that:
   a. Resting energy expenditure increases during hypermetabolism and decreases during starvation.
   b. Protein requirements decrease during hypermetabolism and increase during starvation.
   c. Most hypermetabolic patients lose their ability to ingest food, whereas most patients with uncomplicated starvation do not.
   d. Both types of patients progress to stage three of the stress response in the same way.

2. Metabolic changes that occur during the period immediately following severe injury include:
   a. Hypoglycemia
   b. Negative nitrogen balance
   c. Decreased metabolic rate
   d. Decreased oxygen consumption

3. Patients who complain about excessive mental stress would benefit the most by counseling to:
   a. Supplement their diet with thiamin.
   b. Drink extra fluids.
   c. Eat a balanced diet.
   d. Increase their protein intake.

4. All but one of the following conditions increase a patient's resting energy expenditure. Identify the *exception*.
   a. Infection
   b. Chronic obstructive pulmonary disease
   c. Starvation
   d. Burn

5. Following surgery, the patient can usually eat orally:
   a. After he or she is fully awake
   b. After about 4 hours of intravenous therapy
   c. After the return of normal bowel sounds
   d. After blood pressure returns to normal

6. The burn patient's need for kilocalories relates directly to:
   a. The amount of protein eaten
   b. The total body surface area burned
   c. The volume of food tolerated
   d. Existing nutrient stores

7. An individual's best insurance against stress is:
   a. Avoiding stressful situations
   b. Routine use of vitamins and minerals formulated for stress
   c. Adequate nutrient stores developed from the consumption of a well-balanced diet
   d. A high-protein diet

8. Fever increases resting energy expenditure:
   a. 7 percent for each degree above 98.6°F
   b. 10 percent for each degree above 98.6°F
   c. 14 percent for each degree above normal
   d. 21 percent for each degree above normal

9. Malnutrition is commonly seen in patients with pulmonary disease, for all except one of the following reasons. Identify the *exception*.
   a. Many of these patients have a decreased food intake.
   b. Many of these patients expend more kilocalories to breathe.
   c. Many of these patients have impaired gastrointestinal tract function.
   d. Many of these patients have an extraordinary ability to fight infection.

10. Experts advocate the following when refeeding a malnourished patient:
    a. Immediately pushing kilocalories and protein to replenish lost stores
    b. Progressing the rate, volume, and concentration of a tube feeding as rapidly as possible
    c. Full participation of all members of the healthcare team to manage commonly seen metabolic abnormalities
    d. Correction of the hyperphosphatemia seen during the refeeding of a malnourished patient

NCLEX-Style Quiz

Situation One

Mr. X is suffering from second- and third-degree burns over 40 percent of his body. His physician has decided to use topical agents and leave the wound open to air.

1. In the first 30 to 40 days postburn, the nurse is planning nutritional support. The best supplemental feedings for the patient would use:
   a. A modular feeding with a kilocalorie:nitrogen ratio of 150:1
   b. A modular feeding with a kilocalorie:nitrogen ratio of 300:1
   c. A polymeric (complete nutritional) supplement that is acceptable to the patient
   d. High-kilocalorie desserts such as apple pie, cake, and ice cream

Situation Two

Mrs. J. is an alcoholic who has previously reported that she has not eaten "food" for at least the last 3 months. She stated that her sole source of kilocalories had been in the form of alcohol. She was just recently transferred to the unit in which you work after treatment for alcohol withdrawal on another unit. The physician has ordered a high-kilocalorie, high-protein diet. So far, she has eaten 100 percent of the three high-kilocalorie, high-protein trays she has received while on your unit. While reviewing the patient's laboratory values, you notice her serum phosphorus, magnesium, and calcium levels are decreased.

2. As the nurse responsible for Mrs. Jones, you should:
   a. Contact the patient's physician and notify him or her of the recently obtained depressed laboratory values.
   b. Encourage the patient to continue to eat the high-kilocalorie, high-protein diet as ordered.
   c. Offer the patient a 500-kilocalorie polymeric supplement sent up from the Dietary Department, which was previously ordered by the physician.
   d. Follow the physician's orders and wait for the physician to notice the depressed laboratory values.

3. Mrs. Jones's depressed *phosphorus values* may be related to:
   a. A movement of phosphorus into the extracellular space
   b. A total compartmental depletion of phosphorus
   c. A lack of phosphorus in the patient's present dietary intake
   d. A movement of phosphorus into the intracellular space

Situation Three

Mr. C. is a heavy smoker. He was recently admitted to your unit with carbon dioxide retention and a diagnosis of chronic obstructive pulmonary disease. He complains of gas pains.

4. His diet should include all except the following:
   a. A high-fat complete nutritional supplement
   b. Broccoli, onions, peas, melons, and cabbage
   c. Six small meals
   d. Custard, hot cooked cereals, bananas, ground meats, and mashed potatoes

---

CLINICAL CALCULATION 21–1

Calculation of kilocaloric Need for Both a Male and a Female Patient

MALE PATIENT

Energy Need = REE × Activity Factor × Stress Factor

Step 1: Use the following Harris-Benedict formula to calculate the male patient's resting energy expenditure:

$$REE = 66 + (13.7 \times \text{weight in kilograms}) + (5 \times \text{height in centimeters}) - (6.8 \times \text{age})$$

Step 2: Multiply an activity factor by the patient's REE (from Table 21–2).

Step 3: Multiply the answer obtained in step 2 by the appropriate stress factor (Table 21–3).

FEMALE PATIENT

Energy Need = REE × Activity Factor × Stress Factor

Step 1: Use the following Harris-Benedict formula to calculate the female patient's resting energy expenditure:

$$REE = 655 + (9.6 \times \text{weight in kilograms}) + (1.7 \times \text{height in centimeters}) - (4.7 \times \text{age})$$

Step 2: Multiply an activity factor by the patient's REE (Table 24–2):

REE × Activity Factor

Step 3: Multiply the answer obtained in step 2 by the appropriate stress factor (from Table 21—3):

REE × Activity Factor × Stress Factor

EXAMPLE CALCULATION

Assume you need to estimate the kilocalorie need of a 154-pound (70-kilogram) male who is 5 feet 5 inches (165 centime-

Box continued on next page

CLINICAL CALCULATION 21-1 *(continued)*

Calculation of kilocaloric Need for Both a Male and Female
Patient

---

ters) tall and 25 years old. Assume he is confined to bed and has
a fractured long bone.

Sample calculation for step 1:

70-kilogram male who is 165 centimeters tall and 25 years old

$$REE = 66 + (13.7 \times 70) + (5 \times 165) - (6.8 \times 25)$$

$$REE = 66 + 959 + 825 - 170$$

$$REE = 1680$$

Sample calculation for step 2:

REE × Activity Factor

1680 × 1.2

2016

Sample calculation for step 3:

Answer from step 2 × Stress Factor

2016 × 1.35

2721.6 = patients's estimated energy need

BIBLIOGRAPHY

Alfin-Slater, RB (ed): Nutrition and the MD: Refeeding in the Setting of Chronic
Protein-Calorie Malnutrition, Vol 17 no. 3, March,1991

American Dietetic Association: Suggested Guidelines for Nutrition Management of
the Critically Ill Patient. Bronson-Adatto C, ed. The American Dietetic Association, Chicago, 1984.

Bassili, HR and Dietel, M: Effect of Nutritional Support on Weaning Patients Off
Mechanical Ventilators. JPEN 5:161–163, 1981.

Brown, SE and Light, RW: What is Now Known about Protein-Energy Depletion:
When COPD Patients are Malnourished. J Respir Dis: May, 1983.

Bullock, BL and Rosendahl, PP: Pathophysiology: Adaptations and Alterations in
Function, ed 3. JB Lippincott, Philadelphia, 1992.

Cerra, FB: Branched-chain amino acids and stress staging. Current concepts in nutritional support. Biomedical Information Corp, New York, 1993.

Cerra, FB: Pocket Manual of Surgical Nutrition. CV Mosby, St Louis, 1984.

Guthrie, H: Introductory Nutrition, ed 5. CV Mosby, St Louis, 1984.

Hamilton, EM, Whitney, EN, and Sizer, FS: Nutrition: Concepts and Controversies.
ed 3. West, St Paul, 1985.

Henningfield MF: Specialized Elemental Nutrition with Glutamine. Ross Laboratories Division of Abbott Laboratories. Columbus, OH, 1991.

Hui, YH: Human Nutrition and Diet Therapy. Wadsworth Health Sciences Division,
Monterey, CA, 1983.

Juskelis, D: Starvation in Patients: Guidelines for Refeeding. Registered Dietitian Clinical Interactions. Norwich Eaton Pharmaceuticals, Inc. 11:2, 1991.

LaQuatra, IL and Gerlach, MJ: Nutrition in Clinical Nursing. Delmar, Albany, NY, 1990.

Lacey, JM and Wilmore, DW: Is Glutamine a conditional essential amino acid? Nutrition Reviews 48(8):297, 1990.

Larca, L and Greenbaum, DM: Effectiveness of Intensive Nutritional Regimens in Patients Who Fail to Wean from Mechanical Ventilators. Crit Care Med 10:297–300, 1982.

McCauley, K and Weaver, TE: Cardiac and Pulmonary Diseases: Nursing Implications. Nurs Clin North Am 18:81, 1983.

National Research Council: Recommended Dietary Allowances, ed 10. National Academy Press, Washington DC, 1989.

Robinson, CH and Weigley, ES: Basic Nutrition and Diet Therapy. Macmillan, New York, 1989.

Simko, MD, Cowell, C, and Gilbride, JA: Nutritional Assessment: A Comprehensive Guide for Planning Intervention. Aspen Systems, Rockville, MD, 1984.

Solomon, SM and Kirby, DF: The Refeeding Syndrome: A Review JPEN 14:90–97, Jan/Feb, 1991.

Suitor, CW and Crowley MF: Nutrition: Principles and Applications in Health Promotion, ed 2. JB Lippincott. Philadelphia, 1984.

Thomas, CL (ed): Taber's Cyclopedic Medical Dictionary, ed 17. FA Davis, Philadelphia, 1993.

The University of Michigan Medical Center: Parenteral and Enteral Nutrition Manual, ed 4. Ann Arbor, 1986.

Vandenbergh, E, van de Woestijne, KP, and Gyselen A: Weight changes in the terminal stages of chronic obstructive pulmonary disease: Relation to respiratory function and prognosis. Am Rev Respir Dis 95:556, 1967.

National Center for Health Statistics: Vital and health statistics, data from the national health survey. Characteristics of persons with diabetes, United States 1964–1965. National Center for Health Statistics, Series 10, No 40. Washington, DC: Public Health Service, 1967.

Young, EA: The effect of intraluminal nutrients on gastrointestinal mucosa. In Roche, AF (ed): The Gastrointestinal Response to Injury, Starvation, and Enteral Nutrition. Report of the Eighth Ross Conference on Medical Research. Ross Laboratories, Columbus, OH 1988.

Zeman, FJ: Clinical Nutrition and Dietetics. Collamore Press DC Heath, Lexington, MA, 1983.

Chapter Outline

Key Terms

As a study aid, each key term is followed by the page number where the term is defined in the chapter. Terms that appear in **boldface** or <u>underscored</u> in the chapter text are located in the glossary.

Chapter Twenty-Two

Diet in HIV and AIDS

Learning Objectives

After completing this chapter, the student should be able to:

1. Define AIDS and HIV and list transmittal routes for the virus.
2. List nutrition-related complications seen in patients infected with HIV and for each complication describe interventions to improve nutritional status.
3. Discuss why malnutrition is commonly seen in these patients.
4. Describe why each patient with AIDS needs an individualized nutritional assessment.

663

*A*cquired immune deficiency syndrome (AIDS) is a life-threatening disease and a major public health issue. Investigators have discovered that a virus called the **human immunodeficiency virus** (HIV) causes AIDS. The impact of this virus on our society is and will continue to be devastating. This chapter discusses the prevention, diagnosis, and treatment of HIV infection. The course of acquired immune deficiency syndrome is often complicated by malnutrition. For this reason, a major portion of this chapter is devoted to the nutritional care of the patient infected with the human immunodeficiency virus.

HUMAN IMMUNODEFICIENCY VIRUS

The human immunodeficiency virus attacks both the immune system and the nervous system. **Immune** refers to resistance to or protection against a specified disease. When the AIDS virus enters the bloodstream, it begins to attack one type of white blood cell called the T-lymphocyte, or T cell. As is the case with viruses generally, the HIV lives within the cell and conscripts its DNA—reprograms it, in effect—to reproduce the virus. Figure 22–1 diagrams this process. Loss of T-lymphocyte function leaves an individual susceptible to infections and certain forms of cancers. Evidence shows that the AIDS virus may also attack the nervous system, causing damage to the brain.

ACQUIRED IMMUNE DEFICIENCY SYNDROME

AIDS is a disease complex characterized by a collapse of the body's natural immunity against disease. Every part of the human body may be affected. The disease is progressive but runs an unpredictable course with periods of remission. AIDS is diagnosed by finding certain indicator opportunistic diseases such as infection, tumor, wasting, or dementia. The Centers for Disease Control have published a specific list of infections and cancers that are used to diagnose AIDS. This list is constantly being reviewed and revised as more information is gathered on the course of this disease. The World Health Organization defines AIDS more simply (Table 22–1).

No Known Cure

Presently, most researchers believe the invariable outcome of AIDS is death. At this time, there is no cure and no vaccine to prevent this disease, although researchers continue to search for both.

Signs and Symptoms

Once the human immunodeficiency virus enters the body, the affected person may be without any signs or symptoms of disease or may develop AIDS.

The HIV-infected individual may develop an acute flu-like illness, with symptoms appearing in about 2 to 6 weeks after exposure to the virus. After this phase, the individual may be <u>asymptomatic</u> (without symptoms) for years. Most HIV-infected persons have no symptoms and are not even aware

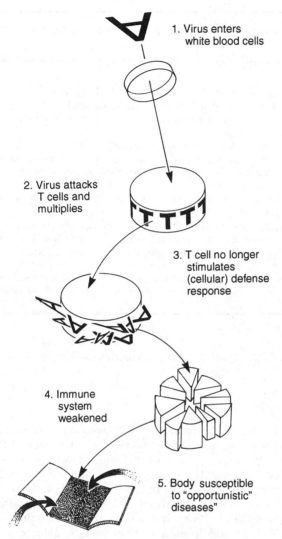

1. Virus enters
white blood cells

2. Virus attacks
T cells and
multiplies

3. T cell no longer
stimulates
(cellular) defense
response

4. Immune
system
weakened

5. Body susceptible
to "opportunistic"
diseases"

FIGURE 22–1. Diagram of AIDS virus entering the bloodstream. (From Koop CE: Surgeon General's Report on Acquired Immune Deficiency Syndrome, US Public Health Service, Washington DC. publication number HE 20.9002: AC, 1987.

that they are infected. The danger lies in their ability to infect other people unknowingly. Some people remain well for years after infection with the HIV virus. Magic Johnson played on the United States Olympic basketball team after testing positive for the virus.

THE EPIDEMIC

The AIDS epidemic is a public health concern not only in the United States but also worldwide. Epidemic means the occurence in a region of an illness clearly in excess of normal expectancy. To protect ourselves and others from this deadly disease, we must take appropriate action based on

---

TABLE 22–1 *World Health Organization's Case Definition of Adult AIDS**

Major Signs
  Weight loss of greater than 10 percent of body weight
  Chronic diarrhea of greater than 1 month's duration
  Fever of greater than 1 month's duration, either intermittent or constant
Minor Signs
  Persistent cough for greater than 1 month
  General pruritic dermatitis (severe itching due to inflammation of the skin)
  Recurrent herpes zoster (recurrent infectious disease caused by the
    varicella-zoster virus)
  Oropharyngeal candidiasis (infection of the throat with any species of
    Candida)
  Chronic progressive and disseminated herpes simplex infections (an acute
    infectious disease caused by the herpes simplex virus Type I)
  Generalized lymphadenopathy (disease of the lymph nodes)

---

*AIDS in an adult is diagnosed if at least two major and one minor signs are present in the absence of a known cause of immunosuppression, such as cancer or severe malnutrition.

---

knowledge of prevalence and transmittal routes. This is discussed in the following sections.

AIDS Worldwide

The World Health Organization has endeavored to collect information on the number of reported cases of AIDS. This has been difficult because reporting in many countries is unreliable and the definitions used to identify AIDS vary. Collectively, 180 countries have reported almost 300,000 cases. These numbers are believed to be underreported, and the World Health Organization estimates that perhaps 600,000 cases have already occurred worldwide (Mann et al., 1988). It is estimated that 50 million to 100 million persons worldwide could develop AIDS in the next 2 decades (Cross, 1992).

AIDS in the United States

The number of people estimated to be infected with the AIDS virus in the United States is about 1.5 million. It is difficult to predict the number of people who will develop AIDS because symptoms may take as long as 9 years to appear. As of October 31, 1990, 154,917 cases of AIDS have been reported to the Centers for Disease Control.

Transmittal Routes

The human immunodeficiency virus is not easily transmissible. Evidence indicates that the AIDS virus is spread through blood and body fluids. Direct contact of blood to blood or of virus to mucous membrane must occur for disease transmittal. In practical terms, there are three transmittal routes: bloodborne, perinatal, and sexual.

Bloodborne Route

HIV may be transmitted by exposure to contaminated blood or blood products through transfusion, sharing of drug apparatus, and injuries to health-care workers from needles and other sharp objects. Intravenous drug abusers often share needles and other equipment for drug injection. This practice can result in a minute amount of blood from an infected person being injected into the bloodstream of the next user. In addition, cases of AIDS have been linked with receipt of blood products from HIV-infected donors, acupuncture treatments performed with improperly sterilized needles, and receipt of transplanted organs from a person later discovered to have been HIV infected.

NEEDLE-STICK INJURIES   To prevent needle-stick injuries, needles should not be:

- Recapped,
- Purposely bent or broken by hand,
- Removed from disposable syringes, or
- Otherwise manipulated by hand.

Guidelines for disposal of syringes, needles, scalpel blades, and other sharp objects include:

- Placing them in a puncture-resistant container located as close to the area of use as is practical, and
- Placing large-bore reusable needles in a puncture-resistant container for transport to the processing area.

Perinatal Transmission

Most children with AIDS contract the virus from their <u>infected</u> mothers through blood-to-blood transmission prior to or at birth (New York State Department of Health, 1987). Breast-feeding has been implicated in transmission, since HIV has been isolated from breast milk (Durham and Cohen, 1991). In the United States, the Centers for Disease Control advise HIV-positive women against breast-feeding. On the other hand, in developing countries, breast-feeding is still currently being advocated by the World Health Organization because of the concern about infant morbidity and mortality due to poor sanitation.

Sexual Transmission

The most likely way to become infected with the human immunodeficiency virus is to have intimate sexual contact with an infected individual's blood, semen, and possibly vaginal secretions. The virus enters a person's bloodstream through the rectum, vagina, or penis. Small tears in the surface lining of the vagina or rectum may occur during insertion of the penis, fingers, or other objects, thus opening an avenue for entrance of the virus directly into the blood stream. Both homosexual and heterosexual persons are at risk for AIDS. The only people not at risk of infection by this route are couples who have maintained mutually faithful monogamous relationships (only one continuing sexual partner) for at least 7 years. Celibate individuals are also not at risk.

AIDS: YOU CAN PROTECT YOURSELF

The best advice to avoid infection is to avoid direct contact with anyone's blood or body fluids. This involves practicing safer sexual behaviors and following universal precautions or body substance isolation procedures. People need to be advised to adopt safer sexual practices. As precautions to prevent sexual transmission have been described elsewhere (Durham and Cohen, 1991), we will not discuss this important subject here.

Universal Precautions or Body Substance Isolation

Universal precautions—A list of procedures developed by the Centers for Disease Control for when blood and other certain body fluids should be considered contaminated and treated as such.

In 1987, the Centers for Disease Control published recommendations for the prevention of HIV transmission, emphasizing the need to consider all patients as potentially infected with HIV and/or other bloodborne pathogens. **Universal precautions** means that every patient and every patient's blood and certain body fluids should be considered contaminated and treated as such. **Body substance isolation** is used when *all* body fluids should be considered contaminated and treated as such. Body substance isolation is thus more comprehensive than universal precautions. Whether universal precautions or body substance isolation procedures are followed in a given facility varies.

Clinical Application 22–1 discusses the myth of risk via casual contact.

DIAGNOSIS AND TREATMENT

Body substance isolation—A situation in which all body fluids are considered contaminated and treated as such by all healthcare workers.

This section of the chapter describes screening for HIV, symptoms of HIV infection, treatment, and prognosis.

CLINICAL APPLICATION 22–1

No Risk of AIDS from Casual Contact

The majority of infected people contracted the virus through intimate sexual contact. Intimate sexual contact *does not* include sneezing, coughing, eating or drinking from common utensils, or merely being around an infected person. No cases have been found where AIDS has been transmitted through casual (nonsexual) contact with a household member, relative, co-worker, or friend.

The Centers for Disease Control performed a survey in the late 1980s on the general public's perception of transmission routes for the HIV infection. Nearly 50 percent of those questioned said they believed it was possible to get AIDS by eating in a restaurant where the cook or waiter has the disease (Gershoff, 1990). Most experts believe it is impossible to become infected with the virus that causes AIDS by eating or drinking food touched by cooks, waiters, or anyone else who is infected. You must have intimate sexual contact with a food handler or share a needle with him or her or come in contact with the infected food handler's blood to become infected.

Test Screening

A blood test can detect antibodies to the human immunodeficiency virus. The presence of HIV antibodies in the bloodstream means that a person has been exposed to the virus and can be assumed to be infected. The newly infected individual develops antibodies about 3 weeks to 6 months after exposure to the virus. Consequently, antibodies to HIV take a *minimum* of 3 weeks following exposure to the virus before they can be found in the blood. However, this time frame is not absolute; a negative test does not always mean that the person is free of infection. False-positive results also occur. In rare situations, there is viral infection without the formation of antiviral antibodies.

Complications of HIV Infection

AIDS is characterized by weakness, anorexia, diarrhea, weight loss, fever, and a decreased white blood cell count, or **leukopenia**. Commonly occurring problems associated with AIDS include opportunistic infections, gastrointestinal dysfunction, tumors, AIDS dementia complex (ADC), and organ dysfunction.

Leukopenia— Abnormal decrease in the number of white blood corpuscles, usually below 5000 per cubic millimeter.

Opportunistic Infections

Parasitic, bacterial, viral, and fungal organisms are everywhere in our environment. The healthy person's immune system keeps these organisms in check and under control. AIDS places the patient at high risk for certain infections, called **opportunistic infections**. Some of the infections these patients develop were rarely seen in the United States before the onset of the AIDS epidemic. We will discuss three opportunistic infections commonly seen in AIDS patients: thrush, tuberculosis, and pneumocystis pneumonia.

Opportunistic infection—An infection that occurs due to the opportunity afforded by the altered physiological state of an individual.

THRUSH   A physical assessment may show signs of **thrush**, which include a thick whitish coating on the tongue or in the throat, which may be accompanied by sore throat. Thrush is a fungal infection that can cause oral ulcers, frequent fevers, and gastrointestinal inflammation.

Thrush—An infection caused by the organism *Candida albicans* that is characterized by the formation of white patches and ulcers in the mouth and throat.

TUBERCULOSIS   Tuberculosis (TB) is spread from person to person through tiny airborne particles. By sharing surroundings with a person who has active pulmonary TB, a susceptible person may inhale the disease-producing particles. Fortunately, most people who have inhaled these particles never become contagious or develop active TB. Even a healthy immune system cannot kill all the particles. HIV infection weakens the body's immune system and makes it more likely that the individual who has inhaled TB-related particles will develop active TB.

PNEUMOCYSTIS PNEUMONIA   Pneumonia, characterized by shortness of breath, fatigue, and anorexia, is also seen in these patients. About 60 percent of AIDS patients are infected with one type of pneumonia-causing organism called *Pneumocystis carinii*, hence the name **pneumocystis pneumonia**. The organisms take up residence in the person's lungs, causing progressively worsening breathing problems, eventually leading to death.

Pneumocystis pneumonia—A type of pneumonia frequently seen in AIDS patients; caused by the organism *Pneumocystis carinii*.

Gastrointestinal Dysfunction

The gastrointestinal tract is a common site for expression of HIV-related symptoms. The patient may feel pain in the mouth or esophagus due to the growth of opportunistic infections. The patient may have difficulty swallowing because of open lesions or sores. Both the small and large intestine are commonly affected by AIDS. The enzymes necessary for digestion and absorption in the wall of the small intestine may be lacking or present in insufficient amounts. Malabsorption may occur with diarrhea. Gut failure may follow. The medications these patients receive to control their infections also contribute to the gastrointestinal dysfunction.

AIDS Dementia Complex

AIDS dementia complex (ADC)— A central nervous system disorder caused by the HIV virus.

AIDS dementia complex (ADC) is the most common HIV-caused central nervous system illness associated with AIDS. It is estimated that at least 40 to 50 percent of adults with AIDS have some neurological dysfunction (Boor and Strother, 1989). Experts believe ADC frequently is misdiagnosed as Alzheimer's disease in persons over 50 (Scharnhorst, 1992). This dysfunction is usually chronic and progressive. Early symptoms of ADC are difficulty in concentration, slowness in thinking and response, and memory impairment. Behavioral symptoms include social withdrawal, apathy, and personality changes. Such symptoms may be interpreted solely as a psychiatric disorder. Motor symptoms include clumsiness of gait, difficulty with fine motor movements, and poor balance and coordination.

Tumors

Kaposi's sarcoma—A type of cancer related to the immunocompromised state that accompanies AIDS; multiple areas of cell proliferation occur initially in the skin and eventually in other body sites.

Kaposi's sarcoma is the most frequently seen malignancy among AIDS patients. The most common manifestation of Kaposi's sarcoma is single or multiple lesions appearing on the lower extremities, especially of the feet and ankles. These open areas appear reddish, purple, or brown. Treatment consist of radiation, surgery, and/or chemotherapy.

Organ Dysfunction

AIDS affects many organs in the body, leading to organ dysfunction. Diseases of the gallbladder, liver, and kidneys are seen in some AIDS patients. Cholecystitis, inflammation of the gallbladder, can occur in conjunction with certain opportunistic infections seen in AIDS victims. Hepatomegaly, or an enlarged liver, is frequently seen with pain, fever, and abnormal liver function tests, especially alkaline phosphatase (Kotler, 1989). Pancreatitis, inflammation of the pancreas, has also been noted in some infected patients. AIDS can lead to end-stage renal disease within weeks.

Clearly, AIDS is a disease with many complications. Ongoing research has yet to discover a cure for this terrible disease.

Treatment

Treatment for AIDS is still in its infancy. A variety of new medications show some promise of killing or inhibiting the activity of the HIV virus. No drug is available to cure AIDS. Most treatment is directed at the specific

CLINICAL APPLICATION 22–2
Drug Treatment for AIDS

Drugs used to treat the opportunistic infections and tumors in AIDS patients are the same ones used for other patients. Side effects and their treatments are similar regardless of the cause of the patient's immunosuppression.

Only one drug, zidovudine (Retrovir, AZT), has a specific action on the AIDS virus. This drug interferes with the virus's ability to transform the cell's RNA into its own DNA. Although not a cure, zidovudine has been shown to prolong the lives of AIDS patients. The major side effects of zidovudine are those affecting the bone marrow. About 25 percent of patients receiving zidovudine develop leukopenia (decreased white blood cells), thrombocytopenia (decreased platelets for blood clotting), or anemia. Although nutritional therapy can assist in the control of these side effects, the definitive treatment is replacement of the missing blood components through transfusion.

infections or cancers that attack HIV-infected people. Clinical Application 22–2 discusses drug treatment for AIDS. Realistically, healthcare intervention can only suppress most infections for these patients, not cure them.

Prevention and Counseling

Notification of a positive HIV test finding creates a crisis for the individual. The person who has had pretest counseling is more prepared and likely to cope better. Counseling the individual on how best to fight the virus is important; for example, the HIV-positive individual needs to receive all current immunizations to boost his or her immunity. Negative behaviors that interfere with wellness and reduce immunity should be discouraged. Adequate rest, good nutrition, and exercise all can improve general good health and should be encouraged. Alcohol, smoking, and illegal drug use should be discouraged.

Prognosis

Prognosis— Expected outcome

Most patients want to know what is going to happen to them. Currently, only general guidelines are available. The only estimates are from the date of the infection, and most patients do not know when they became infected. Ten years after acquiring HIV, 50 percent of all persons will have AIDS, and another 30 percent will have some signs or symptoms (Boor and Strother, 1989). Patients with Kaposi's sarcoma who have very low immune function have an average life expectancy of 1 to 1 $\frac{1}{2}$ years. Some of these patients, those who can tolerate treatment, live as long as 2 years.

NUTRITION AND HIV INFECTION

Nutritional management is both a preventive and a therapeutic treatment in HIV infection. A malnourished patient has a limited ability to fight infection. Well-nourished individuals infected with the HIV virus are better able to offer some resistance to opportunistic infections and tolerate the side effects of treatment. Good nutritional status may influence response to medications by decreasing the incidence of adverse drug reactions, providing available raw materials for reactions evoked by medications, and supporting organ functions. Some experts believe that the most effective medical intervention involves the prevention, early identification, and early treatment of enteric infections and malabsorption. Keeping AIDS patients well nourished is often a challenge because of their numerous medical complications. Dietary modifications are frequently indicated for many of these patients.

Nutrition and Immunity

The function of the immune system is to protect the body against foreign invasion. Foreign invaders include viruses, bacteria, tumor cells, fungi, and transplant material. Studies have shown that a deficiency of almost any nutrient affects a cell's ability to fight infection and handle foreign invaders. Therefore, malnutrition by itself can produce an immune deficiency. Many experts believe that malnutrition aggravates AIDS and may suppress any residual immune function. Deficiencies of iron, zinc, pyridoxine, folic acid, and vitamins B_{12}, C, and A are associated with immunological changes (Cunningham-Rundles, 1982). The malnourished patient with AIDS has minimal internal resources to fight opportunistic infections.

Malnutrition among AIDS Patients

Malnutrition causes a number of physiological alterations that may lead to decreased resistance to infection. For example, malnutrition can cause increased gut permeability, which allows more alien material to be absorbed into the body. Malnutrition may also result in decreased intestinal secretions. Some of these secretions are necessary for the proper digestion and absorption of food. Malnutrition may also cause a change in intestinal flora. This may affect the utilization of nutrients. Malnutrition may lead to hormonal imbalances and decreased tissue repair (Scrimshaw, Taylor, and Gordon, 1990). The body ceases to replace and repair tissue because it lacks the raw materials to do so. A well-balanced diet is essential to optimal immune function.

Malabsorption

Diarrhea and malabsorption are probably the major nutrition-related problems occurring in AIDS patients. Mucosal atrophy and decreased digestive enzyme activity contribute to the malabsorption seen among persons with AIDS. Carbohydrate malabsorption and steatorrhea are frequently seen in AIDS patients with diarrhea. Gastrointestinal problems such as diarrhea may occur in children with HIV infection due to disaccharide intolerance, rather than to enteric infection with known pathogens (Koo, 1991). Malabsorption of fat, simple sugars, and vitamin B_{12} is known to occur in patients with intestinal infections.

Other factors may contribute to the diarrhea seen in these patients. Malnutrition can cause a decrease in pancreatic secretions, decreased levels of the enzymes found in the walls of the small intestine (lactase, sucrase, maltase), villous atrophy, and decreased absorptive surfaces (Resler, 1988). A low serum albumin level may cause diarrhea. Side effects of medication therapy may be related to malabsorption. For example, bacterial overgrowth may occur with long-term anti-infective therapy.

Initially, dietary treatment involves identification of the cause of the diarrhea and a determination of which nutrients the patient cannot absorb. The concentration of hydrogen in the breath can be measured after oral lactose or sucrose administration to determine if the patient is intolerant to either of these sugars. An elevated breath hydrogen implies intolerance, since the hydrogen is primarily a product of metabolism of these sugars by colon bacteria. Fecal microbiologic evaluations and intestinal biopsies are used to determine absorptive capability. In some patients infected with HIV, malabsorption of sucrose, maltose, lactose, and fat has been documented, even in the absence of diarrhea.

Patients with a form of carbohydrate intolerance may benefit from either a lactose-restricted diet or a disaccharide-free diet. A disaccharide-free diet is indicated for severe intolerance to sugar. Sucrose needs to be broken down into glucose and fructose (lactose into glucose and galactose; maltose into glucose and glucose) before absorption is possible. A disaccharide-free diet excludes most fruits and vegetables and many starches and is nutritionally inadequate. Vitamin C will be deficient and daily supplementation is recommended. Some of these patients may tolerate a small amount of sugar, but they usually need assistance in understanding their tolerance level. A lactose-free diet may be sufficient for patients who are deficient only in lactase.

A low-fat diet may be necessary to control steatorrhea. In cases of a severe fat intolerance, medium-chain triglycerides are more readily absorbed. Clinical Application 22–3 discusses several ways medium-chain triglycerides can be incorporated into table foods.

Several additional meal-planning tips are suggested to promote the patient's well-being and control the malabsorption. (1) Fluids should be encouraged to maintain hydration when large fluid volume is lost in stools. (2) Yogurt and other foods that contain the *Lactobacillus acidophilus* culture may be helpful if bacteria overgrowth is a problem secondary to long-term anti-infective use. (3) Small frequent meals make best use of a limited absorptive capacity of the gut. (4) A multivitamin supplement is indicated to

---

CLINICAL APPLICATION 22–3
Incorporating Medium-Chain Triglyceride Oil into Table Foods

Medium-chain triglyceride (MCT) oil can replace vegetable oil in most recipes with satisfactory results. The easiest ways to introduce MCT oil in food preparation are in salad dressings, blended with milk (pretreated with lactase enzyme if necessary) or fruit juices, and in sauteed foods. MCT oil can be used to make cookies, bread, pancakes, French toast, muffins, and pie crusts. MCT oil is made by Mead-Johnson and can usually be purchased from a pharmacy.

increase the amount of vitamin available for absorption. (5) An elemental formula for medical use or parenteral nutrition may be necessary during severe bouts of malabsorption. An elemental formula for medical use contains partially digested nutrients. Promising studies have shown that patients experienced increased weight gain and good tolerance when this type of formula was given at home (Trujillo et al., 1992).

In some situations, the malabsorption is highly resistant to any treatment. Nutritional therapy goals should be those that maximize patient comfort. Fiber-containing supplements or foods high in fiber may be beneficial for decreasing diarrhea; eliminating caffeine intake also may help control it. The benefits of overly restricting the patient's diet may not suffice to offset the resulting loss in patient comfort in an incurable situation.

Increased Nutritional Requirements

Patients with AIDS have moderate to severe metabolic stress similar to that found in other critically ill patients (Trujillo et al., 1992). Fever and infection increase kilocalorie, protein, and certain mineral and vitamin requirements. Dietitians frequently use the Harris-Benedict equation and multiply by appropriate stress and activity factors to determine kilocaloric requirements (see Chapter 21). Protein requirements should reflect a 150:1 kilocalorie-to-nitrogen ratio (McCorkindale, 1990) if the patient shows signs of hypermetabolism.

Decreased Food Intake

Anorexia can be a major problem for many patients with AIDS. A poor food intake may be the result of fever, respiratory infections, drug side effects, gastrointestinal complications, oral and esophageal pain, and emotional stress. Patients with ADC may experience mechanical problems with eating. Some drugs used in these patients, such as bactrim and pentamine, may cause nausea, vomiting, and taste changes that decrease the desire to eat (Resler, 1988). Daily interaction with the patient to encourage food intake is particularly important when the person is feeling relatively well.

Nutritional Care in AIDS

Manifestations of the HIV virus vary greatly from one patient to another. Therefore, the nutritional care must be tailored to each patient's unique set of symptoms. Quality nutritional care starts with screening.

Screening

Screening HIV-infected patients for nutritional problems is a crucial component of quality patient care. Early indicators of decreased nutritional status include decreases in body weight, percent body fat, and BMI (body mass index) (McCorkindale, 1990). All patients infected with the HIV virus should have an assessment made of their recent food intake. An effort should be made to correct all nutritional deficiencies as soon as possible. This intervention will help support response to treatment of opportunistic infections and improve patient strength and comfort.

Planning Nutrient Delivery

In keeping with the general principle, "if the gut works, use it," every effort should be made to feed the patient orally. The anorexia commonly seen in AIDS patients can sometimes be resolved by changing the meal plan. Try offering smaller, frequent feedings. Serving food cold or at room temperature may help some patients consume more kilocalories. Modification of seasonings and kilocaloric density may also improve intake. Modification of texture may assist the patient with poor chewing ability or oral lesions.

The Centers for Disease Control recommend the use of regular dishware for patients with bloodborne diseases. Because AIDS is not transmitted through food, food handling, or dishes, regular dishes and utensils may be used without risk (Centers for Disease Control, 1985). This means an isolation setup is not necessary. Historically, an isolation setup included only disposable dishware, a cardboard tray, and plastic utensils. Disposable dishware compounds the patient's feelings of social isolation. Regular dishware provides better quality food at appropriate temperatures and allows the food to appear more appetizing. Many healthcare institutions require all workers to wear protective gloves when handling soiled dishes.

If the patient is unable to consume sufficient nutrients in the form of table foods, supplemental feedings and/or other enteral feedings should be considered. The type of malnutrition should influence the food and supplements offered. The dietitian usually determines the kind of supplement the patient should be offered. For example, if the patient's protein status is adequate but the patient has an energy deficit, a carbohydrate and/or fat supplement may be the best choice. In such a situation the patient's serum albumin level would be normal but the patient still may be losing weight. On the other hand, if the patient's albumin is low but his or her body weight is stable, a protein supplement would be preferable. (Of course, water balance also influences body weight, so this example is necessarily an oversimplification.) The point is that not all supplemental feedings are equally desirable at any given stage of illness. Patients are encouraged to consume particular nutrients based on individual assessment data.

If the patient is unable to consume sufficient nutrients orally and the gut is working, a tube feeding may be considered. If the gut is not functioning properly, PPN or TPN may be considered. The goal with these patients should always be to prolong living, not to prolong dying. A patient has the right to refuse any alternate feeding route offered.

Monitoring

Periodic evaluation of the patient is necessary to ensure that adequate nutrients are being consumed. Body weight and nutritional intake should be monitored frequently. Body mass index and percent body fat should be monitored every few weeks. Throughout this process, healthcare workers should maintain a supportive, nonjudgmental approach, which is the key to establishing a trusting relationship.

Patient Teaching

Nutritional education is an important part of total patient care. All AIDS patients need instruction on food safety since low immune-system functioning makes them much more susceptible to foodborne illnesses (see Chapter 12). This will minimize the likelihood of opportunistic infection. Instructions on dietary modifications and the use of supplemental feedings are also indicated. Many of these patients need instruction on the importance of good nutrition and how to prepare nutrient-dense meals. An assessment of the patient's knowledge level and understanding of the individualized meal plan is appropriate.

Follow-up Care

The nutritional status of a patient often depends on appropriate follow-up care. A referral to a community agency, home healthcare program, outpatient clinic, or a dietitian should be made to provide continuity of care.

Summary

The AIDS epidemic is worldwide. Known transmittal routes include blood-to-blood, perinatal, and sexual contact. As healthcare professionals we can all protect ourselves from AIDS by using extreme care when handling blood and equipment that has been in contact with blood, and as private individuals by practicing safer sexual behaviors. The human immunodeficiency virus attacks the immune system and leaves its victims defenseless against opportunistic infections. AIDS is a disease with many clinical complications. Nutritional management is both a preventive and a therapeutic treatment in patients infected with the human immunodeficiency virus. Increased nutrient needs, decreased food intake, and impaired nutrient absorption contribute to the malnutrition seen in AIDS patients.

A case study and a sample plan of care appear below. Both are designed to show you how the information you have studied in this chapter can be used in nursing practice.

CASE STUDY 22–1

Ms. S. is a 30-year-old white woman who acquired HIV from her drug-abusing husband and subsequently infected their son in utero. She could not believe the test results when she was first told. Now she is seeking nutritional information to allow her to maximize her own chance for a quality life and her son's chance to survive infancy. Her knowledge of basic nutrition is good.

NURSING CARE PLAN FOR MS. S. AND HER SON

Assessment

Subjective

  Lack of information on relationship of nutrition to AIDS
  Concrete goals established

Objective: HIV-positive tests, both mother and infant

Nursing Diagnosis

  Knowledge deficit, related to AIDS progression/inhibition, as evidenced by verbal statements

Desired Outcome/Evaluation Criteria

Patient will verbalize areas in which nutrition could affect AIDS development

Nursing Actions/Interventions with Rationales in Italics

1. Reinforce need for regular, balanced meals. *The stress of receiving this diagnosis may impede use of previously learned information.*
2. Instruct Ms. S. to keep home environment clean, especially kitchen, bathrooms, and basements where molds and fungi could thrive. *Organisms that are harmless to persons with normal immune systems can cause opportunistic infections in HIV-infected persons.*
3. Teach patient to monitor herself and her son for changes in health related to food intake or digestion. *Discovering beginning malabsorption problems would permit treatment before malnutrition becomes apparent.*

STUDY AIDS

Chapter Review Questions

1. AIDS is transmitted through:
   a. Casual contact with dishes and utensils handled by an AIDS patient
   b. Casual contact with an infected person's saliva or sputum
   c. Intimate contact with an infected person's blood or semen
   d. An unknown mechanism

2. Which of the following patients does the Centers for Disease Control recommend be regarded as potentially infected with the HIV virus?
   a. Homosexual males
   b. Bisexual males
   c. Heterosexual females
   d. Everyone

3. Which of the following conditions appears much more frequently in AIDS-infected persons than in those without AIDS?
   a. Emphysema and tuberculosis
   b. Kaposi's sarcoma and pneumocystis pneumonia
   c. Thrush and typhoid fever
   d. Viral pneumonia and pancreatitis

4. The major nutrition-related problems in AIDS patients are:
   a. Diarrhea and malabsorption
   b. Financial and housing related
   c. Swallowing difficulties and general weakness
   d. Social ostracism and unclean surroundings

5. If a disaccharide-free diet is required, the patient will receive limited amounts of:
   a. Eggs and poultry
   b. Fruits and grains
   c. Milk and cheese
   d. Organ meats and saturated fats

6. Medium-chain triglyceride (MCT) oil can be used in salad dressing and baked goods to:
   a. Provide easier digestion of fats
   b. Increase the kilocaloric intake
   c. Act as a lubricant for swallowing difficulties
   d. Reduce serum triglyceride levels

7. Which of the following diet modifications is designed to compensate for the limited absorptive capacity of the gut in AIDS patients?
   a. Giving yogurt or buttermilk regularly
   b. Forcing fluids
   c. Offering small, frequent meals
   d. Cooking foods thoroughly

8. Put the following types of feedings in the recommended order to be started.
   1. Oral
   2. Total parenteral nutrition
   3. Tube feeding
       a.   1, 2, 3
       b.   1, 3, 2
       c.   2, 3, 1
       d.   3, 2, 1

9. A person who is HIV positive should use good hygiene to decrease the risk of:
   a. Rare tumors
   b. Malabsorption problems
   c. Renal failure
   d. Opportunistic infections

10. If a person with AIDS suffers from anemia related to treatment with zidovudine, in addition to his or her receiving blood therapy, which of the following nutrients should be available to the body when the bone marrow recovers function?
    a. Vitamin B_{12} and folic acid
    b. Iron and zinc
    c. Protein and vitamin C
    d. All of the above

NCLEX-Style Quiz

Mr. M. is a white man, 5 feet 8 inches tall, with advanced AIDS. His male companion died of AIDS 1 year ago. Mr. M. lives alone in an urban apartment. He has been losing weight steadily; he now weighs 118 pounds. Mr. M. has found it difficult to shop for groceries due to progressive weakness and chronic diarrhea.

1. Which of the following interventions would be most appropriate at this stage?
   a. Referral to a social service agency for a friendly visitor
   b. Arranging for Meals on Wheels service
   c. Obtaining a dietitian's recommendation for supplemental feedings
   d. Suggesting to the physician that tube feeding be started

2. If Mr. M.'s serum albumin level is normal, his diet should be modified to include more:
   a. Meat and potatoes
   b. Eliminating all fats from the diet
   c. Removing all dietary carbohydrate
   d. Removing lactose from the diet

3. Mr. M. develops pneumocystis pneumonia. In addition to monitoring nutrient intake, the nurse now would suggest which of the following interventions?
   a. Eating slowly and remaining upright after eating
   b. Encouraging fluids with meals
   c. Staying away from other people who might catch the pneumonia
   d. All of the above

4. If Mr. M. becomes anemic before the pneumonia is resolved, which of the following signs should alert the nurse to the need for closer supervision of the patient?
   a. Complaints of nausea and loss of appetite
   b. Increased bitter taste to foods
   c. Forgetfulness and sleepiness
   d. Appearance of white patches in his mouth

BIBLIOGRAPHY

Beisel, WR, et al: Single-nutrient effects on immunological functions. JAMA 245:53, 1981.

Boor, PA and Strother, LM (eds): A Physician's Guide AIDS-HIV in Michigan. Michigan State Medical Society, East Lansing, MI, 1989, p 43.

Centers for Disease Control. AIDS due to HIV-2 Infection: New Jersey. MMWR 37:33, 1988.

Centers for Disease Control: Recommendations for preventing transmission of infection with human T-lymphotropic virus type III/Lymphadenopathy-associated virus in the workplace. MMWR 34:682, 1985.

Cross, EW: AIDS: Legal implications for managers, J Am Diet Assoc 92(1):74, 1992.

Cunningham-Rundles, S: Effects of nutritional status on immunologic function. Am J Clin Nutr 35:1202, 1982.

Durham, JD and Cohen, FL (eds): The Person with AIDS: Nursing Perspectives. Springer, New York. 1991, p 21.

Dworkin, B: Gastrointestinal manifestations of the acquired immunodeficiency syndrome: A review of 22 cases. Am J Gastroenterol 80:774, 1985.

Gershoff, SN (ed): Tufts University Diet and Nutrition Letter: Tufts University Diet and Nutrition Letter. New York, November, 1990, p 2.

Gillin, JS: Malabsorption and mucosal abnormalities of the small intestine in the acquired immunodeficiency syndrome. Ann Intern Med 102:619, 1985.

Koo MB: Disaccharide intolerance in children with HIV. Nutrition and the MD 17(8):5, 1991.

Koop CE: Surgeon General's Report on Acquired Immune Deficiency Syndrome. US Public Health Service, Pub. No. HE 20, 9002: AC, 1987. Washington, DC.

Kotler, DP: Intestinal and hepatic manifestations of AIDS. Adv Inter Med 34:43, 1989.

Kotler, DP, Wang, J, and Pierson, RN: Body composition studies in patients with acquired immunodeficiency syndrome. Am J Clin Nutr 42:1255, 1985.

Kotler, DP, et al: Enteropathy associated with acquired immunodeficiency syndrome: An update. Ann Intern Med 101:421, 1984.

Lutgen, L: AIDS in the workplace: Fighting fear with facts and policy. Personnel 64(11):53, 1987.

Mann, JM, et al: The international epidemiology of AIDS. Scientific American 259(4):82, 1988.

McCorkindale, C: Nutrition status of HIV-infected patients during early disease stages. J Am Diet Assoc 90:1236, 1990.

New York State Department of Health: 100 Questions and Answers About Acquired Immune Deficiency Syndrome. New York State Department of Health, Albany, 1987, p 9.

Resler, SS: Nutrition care of AIDS patients. J Am Diet Assoc 88:828, 1988.

Rosenberg, IH, Solomons, NW, and Schneider, OO: Malabsorption associated with diarrhea and intestinal infections. Am J Clin Nutr 30:1248, 1977.

Scharnhorst, S: AIDS dementia complex in the elderly. Nurse Pract 17(8):41, 1992.

Scrimshaw, NS, Taylor, JE, and Gordon, JE: Interactions of nutrition and infection. Nutrition Reviews 48: 402, 1990.

Trujillo, EB, et al: Assessment of nutritional status, nutrient intake, and nutrition support in AIDS patients. J Am Diet Assoc 92:477, 1992.

US Department of Health and Human Services Public Health Service. Centers for Disease Control: TB: The HIV Connection, Atlanta, p. 1. Pub. No. HE 20. 7302: T79, 1991.

Nutritive Values of Foods

Foods, approximate measures, units, and weight (weight of edible portion only)		Water	Food energy	Pro- tein	Fat	Fatty Acids		
						Satu- rated	Mono- unsatu- rated	Poly- unsatu- rated
		Per- cent	*Cal- ories*	*Grams*	*Grams*	*Grams*	*Grams*	*Grams*
BEVERAGES	*Grams*							
Alcoholic:								
Beer:								
Regular- - - - - - - - - - - -	12 fl oz- - - - - - - -	360	92	150	1	0	0.0	0.0	0
Light- - - - - - - - - - - - -	12 fl oz- - - - - - - -	355	95	95	1	0	0.0	0.0	0.0
Gin, rum, vodka, whiskey:								
86-proof- - - - - - - - - - -	1½ fl oz- - - - - - - -	42	64	105	0	0	0.0	0.0	0.0
Wines:								
Dessert- - - - - - - - - - - -	3½ fl oz- - - - - - - -	103	77	140	Tr	0	0.0	0.0	0.0
Table:								
Red- - - - - - - - - - - -	3½ fl oz- - - - - - - -	102	88	75	Tr	0	0.0	0.0	0.0
White- - - - - - - - - -	3½ fl oz- - - - - - - -	102	87	80	Tr	0	0.0	0.0	0.0
Carbonated:[2]								
Club soda- - - - - - - - - - -	12 fl oz- - - - - - - -	355	100	0	0	0	0.0	0.0	0.0
Cola type:								
Regular- - - - - - - - - - - -	12 fl oz- - - - - - - -	369	89	160	0	0	0.0	0.0	0.0
Diet, artificially sweet-								
ened- - - - - - - - - - - -	12 fl oz- - - - - - - -	355	100	Tr	0	0	0.0	0.0	0.0
Ginger ale- - - - - - - - - - -	12 fl oz- - - - - - - -	366	91	125	0	0	0.0	0.0	0.0
Root beer- - - - - - - - - - -	12 fl oz- - - - - - - -	370	89	165	0	0	0.0	0.0	0.0
Coffee:								
Brewed- - - - - - - - - - - - -	6 fl oz- - - - - - - - -	180	100	Tr	Tr	Tr	Tr	Tr	Tr
Instant, prepared (2 tsp powder plus 6 fl oz								
water)- - - - - - - - - - - -	6 fl oz- - - - - - - - -	182	99	Tr	Tr	Tr	Tr	Tr	Tr
Fruit drinks, noncarbonated:								
Canned:								
Fruit punch drink- - - - -	6 fl oz- - - - - - - - -	190	88	85	Tr	0	0.0	0.0	0.0
Grape drink- - - - - - - - -	6 fl oz- - - - - - - - -	187	86	100	Tr	0	0.0	0.0	0.0
Pineapple-grapefruit juice drink- - - - - - - -	6 fl oz- - - - - - - - -	187	87	90	Tr	Tr	Tr	Tr	Tr
Fruit juices. See type under Fruits and Fruit Juices.								
Milk beverages. See Dairy Products								
Tea:								
Brewed- - - - - - - - - - - - -	8 fl oz- - - - - - - - -	240	100	Tr	Tr	Tr	Tr	Tr	Tr
Instant, powder, prepared:								
Unsweetened (1 tsp powder plus 8 fl oz								
water)- - - - - - - - - - -	8 fl oz- - - - - - - - -	241	100	Tr	Tr	Tr	Tr	Tr	Tr
Sweetened (3 tsp powder plus 8 fl oz water)- - -	8 fl oz- - - - - - - - -	262	91	85	Tr	Tr	Tr	Tr	Tr
DAIRY PRODUCTS								
Cheese:								
Natural:								
Blue- - - - - - - - - - - - -	1 oz- - - - - - - - - -	28	42	100	6	8	5.3	2.2	0.2

(Tr indicates nutrient present in trace amounts.)

Nutrients in Indicated Quantity

Cho-les-terol	Carbo-hydrate	Calcium	Phos-phorus	Iron	Potas-sium	Sodium	Vitamin A value		Thiamin	Ribo-flavin	Niacin	Ascorbic acid
							(IU)	(RE)				
Milli-grams	Grams	Milli-grams	Milli-grams	Milli-grams	Milli-grams	Milli-grams	Inter-national units	Retinol equiva-lents	Milli-grams	Milli-grams	Milli-grams	Milli-grams
0	13	14	50	0.1	115	18	0	0	0.02	0.09	1.8	0
0	5	14	43	0.1	64	11	0	0	0.03	0.11	1.4	0
0	Tr	Tr	Tr	Tr	1	Tr	0	0	Tr	Tr	Tr	0
0	8	8	9	0.2	95	9	(1)	(1)	0.01	0.02	0.2	0
0	3	8	18	0.4	113	5	(1)	(1)	0.00	0.03	0.1	0
0	3	9	14	0.3	83	5	(1)	(1)	0.00	0.01	0.1	0
0	0	18	0	Tr	0	78	0	0	0.00	0.00	0.0	0
0	41	11	52	0.2	7	18	0	0	0.00	0.00	0.0	0
0	Tr	14	39	0.2	7	[3]32	0	0	0.00	0.00	0.0	0
0	32	11	0	0.1	4	29	0	0	0.00	0.00	0.0	0
0	42	15	0	0.2	4	48	0	0	0.00	0.00	0.0	0
0	Tr	4	2	Tr	124	2	0	0	0.00	0.02	0.4	0
0	1	2	6	0.1	71	Tr	0	0	0.00	0.03	0.6	0
0	22	15	2	0.4	48	15	20	2	0.03	0.04	Tr	[4]61
0	26	2	2	0.3	9	11	Tr	Tr	0.01	0.01	Tr	[4]64
0	23	13	7	0.9	97	24	60	6	0.06	0.04	0.5	[4]110
0	Tr	0	2	Tr	36	1	0	0	0.00	0.03	Tr	0
0	1	1	4	Tr	61	1	0	0	0.00	0.02	0.1	0
0	22	1	3	Tr	49	Tr	0	0	0.00	0.04	0.1	0
21	1	150	110	0.1	73	396	200	65	0.01	0.11	0.3	0

Nutritive Values of Foods *(Continued)*

Foods, approximate measures, units, and weight (weight of edible portion only)		Water	Food energy	Pro-tein	Fat	Fatty Acids		
						Satu-rated	Mono-unsatu-rated	Poly-unsatu-rated
		Per-cent	*Cal-ories*	*Grams*	*Grams*	*Grams*	*Grams*	*Grams*
DAIRY PRODUCTS—Con.		*Grams*						
Camembert (3 wedges per 4-oz container)- - - - -	1 wedge- - - - - - - -	38	52	115	8	9	5.8	2.7	0.3
Cheddar:									
Cut pieces- - - - - - - -	1 oz - - - - - - - - -	28	37	115	7	9	6.0	2.7	0.3
	1 in³- - - - - - - - - -	17	37	70	4	6	3.6	1.6	0.2
Shredded- - - - - - - - -	1 cup - - - - - - - - -	113	37	455	28	37	23.8	10.6	1.1
Cottage (curd not pressed down):									
Lowfat (2%)- - - - - - -	1 cup - - - - - - - - -	226	79	205	31	4	2.8	1.2	0.1
Uncreamed (cottage cheese dry curd, less than ½% fat)- - - - -	1 cup - - - - - - - - -	145	80	125	25	1	0.4	0.2	Tr
Cream- - - - - - - - - - - - -	1 oz- - - - - - - - - -	28	54	100	2	10	6.2	2.8	0.4
Feta- - - - - - - - - - - - - -	1 oz - - - - - - - - - -	28	55	75	4	6	4.2	1.3	0.2
Mozzarella, made with:									
Whole milk- - - - - - - -	1 oz- - - - - - - - - -	28	54	80	6	6	3.7	1.9	0.2
Parmesan, grated:									
Tablespoon- - - - - - - -	1 tbsp- - - - - - - -	5	18	25	2	2	1.0	0.4	Tr
Ounce- - - - - - - - - - -	1 oz- - - - - - - - - -	28	18	130	12	9	5.4	2.5	0.2
Provolone- - - - - - - - - -	1 oz- - - - - - - - - -	28	41	100	7	8	4.8	2.1	0.2
Ricotta, made with:									
Whole milk- - - - - - - -	1 cup - - - - - - - - -	246	72	430	28	32	20.4	8.9	0.9
Part skim milk- - - - -	1 cup - - - - - - - - -	246	74	340	28	19	12.1	5.7	0.6
Swiss- - - - - - - - - - - - -	1 oz- - - - - - - - - -	28	37	105	8	8	5.0	2.1	0.3
Pasteurized process cheese:									
American- - - - - - - - - -	1 oz- - - - - - - - - -	28	39	105	6	9	5.6	2.5	0.3
Swiss- - - - - - - - - - - - -	1 oz- - - - - - - - - -	28	42	95	7	7	4.5	2.0	0.2
Pasteurized process cheese food, American- - - - -	1 oz- - - - - - - - - -	28	43	95	6	7	4.4	2.0	0.2
Cream, sweet:									
Half-and-half (cream and milk)- - - - - - - - - - - -	1 cup - - - - - - - - -	242	81	315	7	28	17.3	8.0	1.0
	1 tbsp- - - - - - - - -	15	81	20	Tr	2	1.1	0.5	0.1
Light, coffee, or table- - - -	1 cup - - - - - - - - -	240	74	470	6	46	28.8	13.4	1.7
	1 tbsp- - - - - - - - -	15	74	30	Tr	3	1.8	0.8	0.1
Whipping, unwhipped (vol-ume about double when whipped):									
Light- - - - - - - - - - - - -	1 tbsp- - - - - - - - -	15	64	45	Tr	5	2.9	1.4	0.1
Heavy- - - - - - - - - - - - -	1 tbsp- - - - - - - - -	15	58	50	Tr	6	3.5	1.6	0.2
Whipped topping, (pressur-ized)- - - - - - - - - - - - -	1 tbsp- - - - - - - - -	3	61	10	Tr	1	0.4	0.2	Tr
Cream, sour- - - - - - - - - - -	1 tbsp- - - - - - - - -	12	71	25	Tr	3	1.6	0.7	0.1
Cream products, imitation (made with vegeta-ble fat):									

(Tr indicates nutrient present in trace amounts.)

Nutrients in Indicated Quantity

Cholesterol	Carbohydrate	Calcium	Phosphorus	Iron	Potassium	Sodium	Vitamin A value (IU)	Vitamin A value (RE)	Thiamin	Riboflavin	Niacin	Ascorbic acid
Milligrams	Grams	Milligrams	Milligrams	Milligrams	Milligrams	Milligrams	International units	Retinol equivalents	Milligrams	Milligrams	Milligrams	Milligrams
27	Tr	147	132	0.1	71	320	350	96	0.01	0.19	0.2	0
30	Tr	204	145	0.2	28	176	300	86	0.01	0.11	Tr	0
18	Tr	123	87	0.1	17	105	180	52	Tr	0.06	Tr	0
119	1	815	579	0.8	111	701	1,200	342	0.03	0.42	0.1	0
19	8	155	340	0.4	217	918	160	45	0.05	0.42	0.3	Tr
10	3	46	151	0.3	47	19	40	12	0.04	0.21	0.2	0
31	1	23	30	0.3	34	84	400	124	Tr	0.06	Tr	0
25	1	140	96	0.2	18	316	130	36	0.04	0.24	0.3	0
22	1	147	105	0.1	19	106	220	68	Tr	0.07	Tr	0
4	Tr	69	40	Tr	5	93	40	9	Tr	0.02	Tr	0
22	1	390	229	0.3	30	528	200	49	0.01	0.11	0.1	0
20	1	214	141	0.1	39	248	230	75	0.01	0.09	Tr	0
124	7	509	389	0.9	257	207	1,210	330	0.03	0.48	0.3	0
76	13	669	449	1.1	307	307	1,060	278	0.05	0.46	0.2	0
26	1	272	171	Tr	31	74	240	72	0.01	0.10	Tr	0
27	Tr	174	211	0.1	46	406	340	82	0.01	0.10	Tr	0
24	1	219	216	0.2	61	388	230	65	Tr	0.08	Tr	0
18	2	163	130	0.2	79	337	260	62	0.01	0.13	Tr	0
89	10	254	230	0.2	314	98	1,050	259	0.08	0.36	0.2	2
6	1	16	14	Tr	19	6	70	16	0.01	0.02	Tr	Tr
159	9	231	192	0.1	292	95	1,730	437	0.08	0.36	0.1	2
10	1	14	12	Tr	18	6	110	27	Tr	0.02	Tr	Tr
17	Tr	10	9	Tr	15	5	170	44	Tr	0.02	Tr	Tr
21	Tr	10	9	Tr	11	6	220	63	Tr	0.02	Tr	Tr
2	Tr	3	3	Tr	4	4	30	6	Tr	Tr	Tr	0
5	1	14	10	Tr	17	6	90	23	Tr	0.02	Tr	Tr

Nutritive Values of Foods *(Continued)*

Foods, approximate measures, units, and weight (weight of edible portion only)		Water	Food energy	Pro-tein	Fat	Fatty Acids		
						Satu-rated	Mono-unsatu-rated	Poly-unsatu-rated
		Grams	Per-cent	Cal-ories	Grams	Grams	Grams	Grams	Grams
DAIRY PRODUCTS—Con.								
Sweet:								
Creamers:								
Powdered- - - - - - - -	1 tsp- - - - - - - - - -	2	2	10	Tr	1	0.7	Tr	Tr
Whipped topping:								
Frozen- - - - - - - - - - -	1 cup- - - - - - - - -	75	50	240	1	19	16.3	1.2	0.4
	1 tbsp- - - - - - - - -	4	50	15	Tr	1	0.9	0.1	Tr
	1 tbsp- - - - - - - - -	12	75	20	Tr	2	1.6	0.2	0.1
Ice cream. See Milk desserts, frozen.								
Ice milk. See Milk desserts, frozen.								
Milk:								
Fluid:								
Whole (3.3% fat)- - - - -	1 cup - - - - - - - - -	244	88	150	8	8	5.1	2.4	0.3
Lowfat (2%):								
No milk solids added-	1 cup- - - - - - - - -	244	89	120	8	5	2.9	1.4	0.2
Lowfat (1%):								
No milk solids added-	1 cup- - - - - - - - -	244	90	100	8	3	1.6	0.7	0.1
Nonfat (skim):								
No milk solids added-	1 cup- - - - - - - - -	245	91	85	8	Tr	0.3	0.1	Tr
Buttermilk- - - - - - - - -	1 cup- - - - - - - - -	245	90	100	8	2	1.3	0.6	0.1
Canned:								
Evaporated:								
Whole milk- - - - - - -	1 cup- - - - - - - - -	252	74	340	17	19	11.6	5.9	0.6
Skim milk- - - - - - - -	1 cup- - - - - - - - -	255	79	200	19	1	0.3	0.2	Tr
Dried:								
Nonfat, instantized:								
Envelope, 3.2 oz, net wt.[6]- - - - - - - - - - -	1 envelope- - - - - -	91	4	325	32	1	0.4	0.2	Tr
Milk beverages:								
Chocolate milk (commer-cial):								
Regular- - - - - - - - - - - -	1 cup - - - - - - - - -	250	82	210	8	8	5.3	2.5	0.3
Lowfat (2%)- - - - - - - -	1 cup - - - - - - - - -	250	84	180	8	5	3.1	1.5	0.2
Cocoa and chocolate-flavored beverages:								
Eggnog (commercial)- - - -	1 cup- - - - - - - - -	254	74	340	10	19	11.3	5.7	0.9
Malted milk:								
Chocolate:								
Powder								
Prepared (8 oz whole milk plus ¾ powder)- - - - - - -	1 serving- - - - - -	265	81	235	9	9	5.5	2.7	0.4
Shakes, thick:								
Chocolate- - - - - - - - - -	10-oz container- -	283	72	335	9	8	4.8	2.2	0.3
Vanilla- - - - - - - - - - - -	10-oz container- -	283	74	315	11	9	5.3	2.5	0.3

(Tr indicates nutrient present in trace amounts.)

Nutrients in Indicated Quantity

Cholesterol	Carbohydrate	Calcium	Phosphorus	Iron	Potassium	Sodium	Vitamin A value		Thiamin	Riboflavin	Niacin	Ascorbic acid
							(IU)	(RE)				
Milligrams	Grams	Milligrams	Milligrams	Milligrams	Milligrams	Milligrams	International units	Retinol equivalents	Milligrams	Milligrams	Milligrams	Milligrams
0	1	Tr	8	Tr	16	4	Tr	Tr	0.00	Tr	0.0	0
0	17	5	6	0.1	14	19	[b]650	[b]65	0.00	0.00	0.0	0
0	1	Tr	Tr	Tr	1	1	[b]30	[b]3	0.00	0.00	0.0	0
1	1	14	10	Tr	19	6	Tr	Tr	Tr	0.02	Tr	Tr
33	11	291	228	0.1	370	120	310	76	0.09	0.40	0.2	2
18	12	297	232	0.1	377	122	500	139	0.10	0.40	0.2	2
10	12	300	235	0.1	381	123	500	144	0.10	0.41	0.2	2
4	12	302	247	0.1	406	126	500	149	0.09	0.34	0.2	2
9	12	285	219	0.1	371	257	80	20	0.08	0.38	0.1	2
74	25	657	510	0.5	764	267	610	136	0.12	0.80	0.5	5
9	29	738	497	0.7	845	293	1,000	298	0.11	0.79	0.4	3
17	47	1,120	896	0.3	1,552	499	[7]2,160	[7]646	0.38	1.59	0.8	5
31	26	280	251	0.6	417	149	300	73	0.09	0.41	0.3	2
17	26	284	254	0.6	422	151	500	143	0.09	0.41	0.3	2
149	34	330	278	0.5	420	138	890	203	0.09	0.48	0.3	4
34	29	304	265	0.5	500	168	330	80	0.14	0.43	0.7	2
30	60	374	357	0.9	634	314	240	59	0.13	0.63	0.4	0
33	50	413	326	0.3	517	270	320	79	0.08	0.55	0.4	0

Nutritive Values of Foods *(Continued)*

Foods, approximate measures, units, and weight (weight of edible portion only)		Water	Food energy	Pro-tein	Fat	Satu-rated	Mono-unsatu-rated	Poly-unsatu-rated
							Fatty Acids	
	Grams	Per-cent	Cal-ories	Grams	Grams	Grams	Grams	Grams
DAIRY PRODUCTS—Con.								
Milk desserts, frozen:								
Ice cream, vanilla:								
Regular (about 11% fat):								
Hardened- - - - - - - - 1 cup- - - - - - - - -	133	61	270	5	14	8.9	4.1	0.5
3 fl oz- - - - - - - - -	50	61	100	2	5	3.4	1.6	0.2
Soft serve (frozen cus-								
tard)- - - - - - - - - - 1 cup- - - - - - - - -	173	60	375	7	23	13.5	6.7	1.0
Rich (about 16% fat),								
hardened- - - - - - - - 1 cup- - - - - - - - -	148	59	350	4	24	14.7	6.8	0.9
Ice milk, vanilla:								
Hardened (about								
4% fat)- - - - - - - - - 1 cup- - - - - - - - -	131	69	185	5	6	3.5	1.6	0.2
Soft serve (about								
3% fat)- - - - - - - - - 1 cup- - - - - - - - -	175	70	225	8	5	2.9	1.3	0.2
Sherbert (about 2% fat)- - 1 cup- - - - - - - - -	193	66	270	2	4	2.4	1.1	0.1
Yogurt:								
With added milk solids:								
Made with lowfat milk:								
Fruit-flavored[8]- - - - - 8-oz container- - -	227	74	230	10	2	1.6	0.7	0.1
Plain- - - - - - - - - - - - 8-oz container- - -	227	85	145	12	4	2.3	1.0	0.1
Made with nonfat milk- 8-oz container- - -	227	85	125	13	Tr	0.3	0.1	Tr
EGGS								
Eggs, large (24 oz per dozen):								
Raw:								
Whole, without shell - - 1 egg - - - - - -	50	75	75	6.3	5	1.5	1.6	0.7
White - - - - - - - - - - 1 white - - - - - -	33	88	15	3	Tr	0.0	0.0	0.0
Yolk - - - - - - - - - 1 yolk - - - - - -	16	48	57	2.8	5	1.6	2.0	0.7
Cooked:								
Fried in margarine - - - 1 egg - - - - - -	46	68	91	6	7	1.9	2.8	1.2
Hard-cooked, shell								
removed - - - - - - 1 egg - - - - - -	50	75	77	6	5.3	1.6	2.0	0.7
Poached - - - - - - - - 1 egg - - - - - -	50	74	74	6	5	1.5	1.9	0.7
Scrambled (milk added)								
in margarine. Also								
omelet - - - - - - 1 egg - - - - - -	64	73	101	6.7	7.5	2.2	2.9	1.3
FATS AND OILS								
Butter (4 sticks per lb):								
Tablespoon (⅛ stick)- - - - 1 tbsp- - - - - - - - -	14	16	100	Tr	11	7.1	3.3	0.4
Pat (1 in square, ⅓ in high;								
90 per lb)- - - - - - - - - - - 1 pat- - - - - - - - -	5	16	35	Tr	4	2.5	1.2	0.2
Fats, cooking (vegetable								
shortenings)- - - - - - - - - 1 tbsp- - - - - - - - -	13	0	115	0	13	3.3	5.8	3.4
Lard- - - - - - - - - - - - - - - - 1 tbsp- - - - - - - - -	13	0	115	0	13	5.1	5.9	1.5
Margarine:								
Imitation (about 40% fat),								
soft- - - - - - - - - - - 1 tbsp- - - - - - - - -	14	58	50	Tr	5	1.1	2.2	1.9

(Tr indicates nutrient present in trace amounts.)

Nutrients in Indicated Quantity

Cholesterol	Carbohydrate	Calcium	Phosphorus	Iron	Potassium	Sodium	Vitamin A value (IU)	Vitamin A value (RE)	Thiamin	Riboflavin	Niacin	Ascorbic acid
Milligrams	Grams	Milligrams	Milligrams	Milligrams	Milligrams	Milligrams	International units	Retinol equivalents	Milligrams	Milligrams	Milligrams	Milligrams
59	32	176	134	0.1	257	116	540	133	0.05	0.33	0.1	1
22	12	66	51	Tr	96	44	200	50	0.02	0.12	0.1	Tr
153	38	236	199	0.4	338	153	790	199	0.08	0.45	0.2	1
88	32	151	115	0.1	221	108	900	219	0.04	0.28	0.1	1
18	29	176	129	0.2	265	105	210	52	0.08	0.35	0.1	1
13	38	274	202	0.3	412	163	175	44	0.12	0.54	0.2	1
14	59	103	74	0.3	198	88	190	39	0.03	0.09	0.1	4
10	43	345	271	0.2	442	133	100	25	0.08	0.40	0.2	1
14	16	415	326	0.2	531	159	150	36	0.10	0.49	0.3	2
4	17	452	355	0.2	579	174	20	5	0.11	0.53	0.3	2
213	0.6	25	89	0.7	60	61	260	97	0.03	0.25	Tr	0
0	Tr	4	4	Tr	45	50	0	0	Tr	0.09	Tr	0
213	Tr	23	81	0.7	16	7	310	97	0.05	0.11	Tr	0
211	0.6	25	89	0.7	61	162	320	114	0.03	0.24	Tr	0
212	0.6	25	86	0.6	63	62	260	84	0.03	0.5	Tr	0
212	0.6	25	89	0.7	60	61	260	95	0.03	0.2	Tr	0
215	2.2	44	104	0.7	84	171	350	119	0.03	0.27	Tr	Tr
31	Tr	3	3	Tr	4	[9]116	[10]430	[10]106	Tr	Tr	Tr	0
11	Tr	1	1	Tr	1	[9]41	[10]150	[10]38	Tr	Tr	Tr	0
0	0	0	0	0.0	0	0	0	0	0.00	0.00	0.0	0
12	0	0	0	0.0	0	0	0	0	0.00	0.00	0.0	0
0	Tr	2	2	0.0	4	[11]134	[12]460	[12]139	Tr	Tr	Tr	Tr

Nutritive Values of Foods *(Continued)*

Foods, approximate measures, units, and weight (weight of edible portion only)		Water	Food energy	Pro-tein	Fat	Fatty Acids		
						Satu-rated	Mono-unsatu-rated	Poly-unsatu-rated
		Per-cent	Cal-ories					
FATS AND OILS—Con.	Grams			Grams	Grams	Grams	Grams	Grams
Regular (about 80% fat):								
Hard (4 sticks per lb):								
Tablespoon (⅛ stick)-	1 tbsp- - - - - - - -	14	16	100	Tr	11	2.2	5.0	3.6
Pat (1 in square, ⅓ in								
high; 90 per lb)- - - -	1 pat- - - - - - - -	5	16	35	Tr	4	0.8	1.8	1.3
Soft- - - - - - - - - - - - -	1 tbsp- - - - - - - -	14	16	100	Tr	11	1.9	4.0	4.8
Spread (about 60% fat):								
Hard (4 sticks per lb):								
Tablespoon (⅛ stick)-	1 tbsp- - - - - - - -	14	37	75	Tr	9	2.0	3.6	2.5
Pat (1 in square, ⅓ in								
high; 90 per lb)- - - -	1 pat- - - - - - - -	5	37	25	Tr	3	0.7	1.3	0.9
Soft- - - - - - - - - - - - -	8-oz container- - -	227	37	1,225	1	138	29.1	71.5	31.3
	1 tbsp- - - - - - - -	14	37	75	Tr	9	1.8	4.4	1.9
Oils, salad or cooking:								
Canola - - - - - - - - -	1 tbsp - - - - - -	14	0	120	0	14	0.8	8.0	4.0
Corn- - - - - - - - - - - - - -	1 tbsp- - - - - - - -	14	0	125	0	14	1.8	3.4	8.2
Olive- - - - - - - - - - - - -	1 tbsp- - - - - - - -	14	0	125	0	14	1.9	10.3	1.2
Peanut- - - - - - - - - - - - -	1 tbsp- - - - - - - -	14	0	125	0	14	2.4	6.5	4.5
Safflower- - - - - - - - - - -	1 tbsp- - - - - - - -	14	0	125	0	14	1.3	1.7	10.4
Soybean oil, hydrogenated								
(partially hardened)- - -	1 tbsp- - - - - - - -	14	0	125	0	14	2.1	6.0	5.3
Soybean-cottonseed oil								
blend, hydrogenated- - -	1 tbsp- - - - - - - -	14	0	125	0	14	2.5	4.1	6.7
Sunflower- - - - - - - - - - - -	1 tbsp- - - - - - - -	14	0	125	0	14	1.4	2.7	9.2
Salad dressings:								
Commercial:								
Blue cheese- - - - - - - -	1 tbsp- - - - - - - -	15	32	75	1	8	1.5	1.8	4.2
French:								
Regular- - - - - - - - - -	1 tbsp- - - - - - - -	16	35	85	Tr	9	1.4	4.0	3.5
Low calorie- - - - - - -	1 tbsp- - - - - - - -	16	75	25	Tr	2	0.2	0.3	1.0
Italian:								
Regular- - - - - - - - - -	1 tbsp- - - - - - - -	15	34	80	Tr	9	1.3	3.7	3.2
Low calorie- - - - - - -	1 tbsp- - - - - - - -	15	86	5	Tr	Tr	Tr	Tr	Tr
Mayonnaise:								
Regular- - - - - - - - - -	1 tbsp- - - - - - - -	14	15	100	Tr	11	1.7	3.2	5.8
Imitation- - - - - - - - -	1 tbsp- - - - - - - -	15	63	35	Tr	3	0.5	0.7	1.6
Mayonnaise type- - - - -	1 tbsp- - - - - - - -	15	40	60	Tr	5	0.7	1.4	2.7
Tartar sauce- - - - - - - -	1 tbsp- - - - - - - -	14	34	75	Tr	8	1.2	2.6	3.9
Thousand island:								
Regular- - - - - - - - - -	1 tbsp- - - - - - - -	16	46	60	Tr	6	1.0	1.3	3.2
Low calorie- - - - - - -	1 tbsp- - - - - - - -	15	69	25	Tr	2	0.2	0.4	0.9
Prepared from home recipe:								
Cooked type[13]- - - - - - -	1 tbsp- - - - - - - -	16	69	25	1	2	0.5	0.6	0.3
FISH AND SHELLFISH								
Clams:								
Raw, meat only- - - - - - -	3 oz- - - - - - - - - -	85	82	65	11	1	0.3	0.3	0.3
Canned, drained solids- - -	3 oz- - - - - - - - - -	85	77	85	13	2	0.5	0.5	0.4
Crabmeat, canned- - - - - - -	1 cup- - - - - - - -	135	77	135	23	3	0.5	0.8	1.4

(Tr indicates nutrient present in trace amounts.)

Nutrients in Indicated Quantity

Cholesterol	Carbohydrate	Calcium	Phosphorus	Iron	Potassium	Sodium	Vitamin A value (IU)	Vitamin A value (RE)	Thiamin	Riboflavin	Niacin	Ascorbic acid
Milligrams	Grams	Milligrams	Milligrams	Milligrams	Milligrams	Milligrams	International units	Retinol equivalents	Milligrams	Milligrams	Milligrams	Milligrams
0	Tr	4	3	Tr	6	[11]132	[12]460	[12]139	Tr	0.01	Tr	Tr
0	Tr	1	1	Tr	2	[11]47	[12]170	[1]50	Tr	Tr	Tr	Tr
0	Tr	4	3	0.0	5	[11]151	[12]460	[12]139	Tr	Tr	Tr	Tr
0	0	3	2	0.0	4	[11]139	[12]460	[12]139	Tr	Tr	Tr	Tr
0	0	1	1	0.0	1	[11]50	[12]170	[1]50	Tr	Tr	Tr	Tr
0	0	47	37	0.0	68	[11]2,256	[12]7,510	[12]2,254	0.02	0.06	Tr	Tr
0	0	3	2	0.0	4	[11]139	[12]460	[12]139	Tr	Tr	Tr	Tr
0	0	0	0	0.0	0	0	0	0	0	0	0	0
0	0	0	0	0.0	0	0	0	0	0.00	0.00	0.0	0
0	0	0	0	0.0	0	0	0	0	0.00	0.00	0.0	0
0	0	0	0	0.0	0	0	0	0	0.00	0.00	0.0	0
0	0	0	0	0.0	0	0	0	0	0.00	0.00	0.0	0
0	0	0	0	0.0	0	0	0	0	0.00	0.00	0.0	0
0	0	0	0	0.0	0	0	0	0	0.00	0.00	0.0	0
0	0	0	0	0.0	0	0	0	0	0.00	0.00	0.0	0
3	1	12	11	Tr	6	164	30	10	Tr	0.02	Tr	Tr
0	1	2	1	Tr	2	188	Tr	Tr	Tr	Tr	Tr	Tr
0	2	6	5	Tr	3	306	Tr	Tr	Tr	Tr	Tr	Tr
0	1	1	1	Tr	5	162	30	3	Tr	Tr	Tr	Tr
0	2	1	1	Tr	4	136	Tr	Tr	Tr	Tr	Tr	Tr
8	Tr	3	4	0.1	5	80	40	12	0.00	0.00	Tr	0
4	2	Tr	Tr	0.0	2	75	0	0	0.00	0.00	0.0	0
4	4	2	4	Tr	1	107	30	13	Tr	Tr	Tr	0
4	1	3	4	0.1	11	182	30	9	Tr	Tr	0.0	Tr
4	2	2	3	0.1	18	112	50	15	Tr	Tr	Tr	0
2	2	2	3	0.1	17	150	50	14	Tr	Tr	Tr	0
9	2	13	14	0.1	19	117	70	20	0.01	0.02	Tr	Tr
43	2	59	138	2.6	154	102	90	26	0.09	0.15	1.1	9
54	2	47	116	3.5	119	102	90	26	0.01	0.09	0.9	3
135	1	61	246	1.1	149	1,350	50	14	0.11	0.11	2.6	0

Nutritive Values of Foods *(Continued)*

Foods, approximate measures, units, and weight (weight of edible portion only)		Water	Food energy	Pro- tein	Fat	Fatty Acids Satu- rated	Mono- unsatu- rated	Poly- unsatu- rated
		Per- cent	Cal- ories					
FISH AND SHELLFISH—Con.	Grams			Grams	Grams	Grams	Grams	Grams
Fish sticks, frozen, reheated, (stick, 4 by 1 by ½ in)- -	1 fish stick- - - - -	28	52	70	6	3	0.8	1.4	0.8
Flounder or Sole, baked, with lemon juice:									
With butter- - - - - - - - -	3 oz- - - - - - - - - -	85	73	120	16	6	3.2	1.5	0.5
With margarine- - - - - - -	3 oz- - - - - - - - - -	85	73	120	16	6	1.2	2.3	1.9
Without added fat- - - - - -	3 oz- - - - - - - - - -	85	78	80	17	1	0.3	0.2	0.4
Haddock, breaded, fried[14]- - -	3 oz- - - - - - - - - -	85	61	175	17	9	2.4	3.9	2.4
Halibut, broiled, with butter and lemon juice- - - - - -	3 oz- - - - - - - - - -	85	67	140	20	6	3.3	1.6	0.7
Herring, pickled- - - - - - - -	3 oz- - - - - - - - - -	85	59	190	17	13	4.3	4.6	3.1
Ocean perch, breaded, fried[14]	1 fillet- - - - - - - -	85	59	185	16	11	2.6	4.6	2.8
Oysters:									
Raw, meat only (13–19 me- dium Selects)- - - - - - - -	1 cup- - - - - - - - -	240	85	160	20	4	1.4	0.5	1.4
Breaded, fried[14]- - - - - - - -	1 oyster- - - - - - -	45	65	90	5	5	1.4	2.1	1.4
Salmon:									
Canned (pink), solids and liquid- - - - - - - - - - - - -	3 oz- - - - - - - - - -	85	71	120	17	5	0.9	1.5	2.1
Baked (red)- - - - - - - - - - -	3 oz- - - - - - - - - -	85	67	140	21	5	1.2	2.4	1.4
Smoked- - - - - - - - - - - - -	3 oz- - - - - - - - - -	85	59	150	18	8	2.6	3.9	0.7
Sardines, Atlantic, canned in oil, drained solids- - - - -	3 oz- - - - - - - - - -	85	62	175	20	9	2.1	3.7	2.9
Scallops, breaded, frozen, re- heated- - - - - - - - - - - - -	6 scallops- - - - - -	90	59	195	15	10	2.5	4.1	2.5
Shrimp:									
Canned, drained solids- - -	3 oz- - - - - - - - - -	85	70	100	21	1	0.2	0.2	0.4
French fried (7 medium)[16]-	3 oz- - - - - - - - - -	85	55	200	16	10	2.5	4.1	2.6
Trout, broiled, with butter and lemon juice- - - - - - - - -	3 oz- - - - - - - - - -	85	63	175	21	9	4.1	2.9	1.6
Tuna, canned, drained solids:									
Oil pack, chunk light- - - -	3 oz- - - - - - - - - -	85	61	165	24	7	1.4	1.9	3.1
Water pack, solid white- -	3 oz- - - - - - - - - -	85	63	135	30	1	0.3	0.2	0.3
Tuna salad[17]- - - - - - - - - - -	1 cup- - - - - - - - -	205	63	375	33	19	3.3	4.9	9.2
FRUITS AND FRUIT JUICES									
Apples:									
Raw:									
Unpeeled, without cores:									
2¾-in diam. (about 3 per lb with cores)- -	1 apple- - - - - - -	138	84	80	Tr	Tr	0.1	Tr	0.1
3¼-in diam. (about 2 per lb with cores)- -	1 apple- - - - - - -	212	84	125	Tr	1	0.1	Tr	0.2
Dried, sulfured- - - - - - -	10 rings- - - - - - -	64	32	155	1	Tr	Tr	Tr	0.1
Apple juice, bottled or canned[19]- - - - - - - - - - -	1 cup- - - - - - - - -	248	88	115	Tr	Tr	Tr	Tr	0.1
Applesauce, canned:									
Sweetened- - - - - - - - - -	1 cup- - - - - - - - -	255	80	195	Tr	Tr	0.1	Tr	0.1

(Tr indicates nutrient present in trace amounts.)

Nutrients in Indicated Quantity

Cho-les-terol	Carbo-hydrate	Calcium	Phos-phorus	Iron	Potas-sium	Sodium	Vitamin A value		Thiamin	Ribo-flavin	Niacin	Ascorbic acid
							(IU)	(RE)				
Milli-grams	Grams	Milli-grams	Milli-grams	Milli-grams	Milli-grams	Milli-grams	Inter-national units	Retinol equiva-lents	Milli-grams	Milli-grams	Milli-grams	Milli-grams
26	4	11	58	0.3	94	53	20	5	0.03	0.05	0.6	0
68	Tr	13	187	0.3	272	145	210	54	0.05	0.08	1.6	1
55	Tr	14	187	0.3	273	151	230	69	0.05	0.08	1.6	1
59	Tr	13	197	0.3	286	101	30	10	0.05	0.08	1.7	1
75	7	34	183	1.0	270	123	70	20	0.06	0.10	2.9	0
62	Tr	14	206	0.7	441	103	610	174	0.06	0.07	7.7	1
85	0	29	128	0.9	85	850	110	33	0.04	0.18	2.8	0
66	7	31	191	1.2	241	138	70	20	0.10	0.11	2.0	0
120	8	226	343	15.6	290	175	740	223	0.34	0.43	6.0	24
35	5	49	73	3.0	64	70	150	44	0.07	0.10	1.3	4
34	0	[15]167	243	0.7	307	443	60	18	0.03	0.15	6.8	0
60	0	26	269	0.5	305	55	290	87	0.18	0.14	5.5	0
51	0	12	208	0.8	327	1,700	260	77	0.17	0.17	6.8	0
85	0	[15]371	424	2.6	349	425	190	56	0.03	0.17	4.6	0
70	10	39	203	2.0	369	298	70	21	0.11	0.11	1.6	0
128	1	98	224	1.4	104	1,955	50	15	0.01	0.03	1.5	0
168	11	61	154	2.0	189	384	90	26	0.06	0.09	2.8	0
71	Tr	26	259	1.0	297	122	230	60	0.07	0.07	2.3	1
55	0	7	199	1.6	298	303	70	20	0.04	0.09	10.1	0
48	0	17	202	0.6	255	468	110	32	0.03	0.10	13.4	0
80	19	31	281	2.5	531	877	230	53	0.06	0.14	13.3	6
0	21	10	10	0.2	159	Tr	70	7	0.02	0.02	0.1	8
0	32	15	15	0.4	244	Tr	110	11	0.04	0.03	0.2	12
0	42	9	24	0.9	288	[18]56	0	0	0.00	0.10	0.6	2
0	29	17	17	0.9	295	7	Tr	Tr	0.05	0.04	0.2	[20]2
0	51	10	18	0.9	156	8	30	3	0.03	0.07	0.5	[20]4

Nutritive Values of Foods *(Continued)*

Foods, approximate measures, units, and weight (weight of edible portion only)		Water	Food energy	Pro-tein	Fat	Fatty Acids		
						Satu-rated	Mono-unsatu-rated	Poly-unsatu-rated
		Grams	Per-cent	Cal-ories	Grams	Grams	Grams	Grams	Grams

Foods, approximate measures, units, and weight		Grams	Per-cent	Cal-ories	Grams	Grams	Grams	Grams	Grams
FRUITS AND FRUIT JUICES — Con.									
Unsweetened- - - - - - - - -	1 cup- - - - - - - -	244	88	105	Tr	Tr	Tr	Tr	Tr
Apricots:									
Raw, without pits (about 12 per lb with pits)- - - - -	3 apricots- - - - - -	106	86	50	1	Tr	Tr	0.2	0.1
Canned (fruit and liquid):									
Heavy syrup pack- - - - -	3 halves- - - - - - -	85	78	70	Tr	Tr	Tr	Tr	Tr
Juice pack- - - - - - - - -	3 halves- - - - - - -	84	87	40	1	Tr	Tr	Tr	Tr
Dried:									
Uncooked (28 large or 37 medium halves per cup)- - - - - - - - - - - - -	1 cup- - - - - - - - -	130	31	310	5	1	Tr	0.3	0.1
Cooked, unsweetened, fruit and liquid- - - - - - - - -	1 cup- - - - - - - - -	250	76	210	3	Tr	Tr	0.2	0.1
Apricot nectar, canned- - - - -	1 cup- - - - - - - - -	251	85	140	1	Tr	Tr	0.1	Tr
Avocados, raw, whole, without skin and seed:									
California (about 2 per lb with skin and seed)- - - -	1 avocado- - - - - -	173	73	305	4	30	4.5	19.4	3.5
Florida (about 1 per lb with skin and seed)- - - - - - -	1 avocado- - - - - -	304	80	340	5	27	5.3	14.8	4.5
Bananas, raw, without peel:									
Whole (about 2½ per lb with peel)- - - - - - - - - -	1 banana- - - - - - -	114	74	105	1	1	0.2	Tr	0.1
Sliced- - - - - - - - - - - - - - -	1 cup- - - - - - - - -	150	74	140	2	1	0.3	0.1	0.1
Blackberries, raw- - - - - - - -	1 cup- - - - - - - - -	144	86	75	1	1	0.2	0.1	0.1
Blueberries:									
Raw- - - - - - - - - - - - - - - -	1 cup- - - - - - - -	145	85	80	1	1	Tr	0.1	0.3
Frozen, sweetened- - - - - -	10-oz container- -	284	77	230	1	Tr	Tr	0.1	0.2
	1 cup- - - - - - - - -	230	77	185	1	Tr	Tr	Tr	0.1
Cantaloup. See Melons.									
Cherries:									
Sour, red, pitted, canned, water pack- - - - - - - - - -	1 cup- - - - - - - - -	244	90	90	2	Tr	0.1	0.1	0.1
Sweet, raw, without pits and stems- - - - - - - - - - - - -	10 cherries- - - - -	68	81	50	1	1	0.1	0.2	0.2
Cranberry juice cocktail, bottled, sweetened- - - - - -	1 cup- - - - - - - - -	253	85	145	Tr	Tr	Tr	Tr	0.1
Cranberry sauce, sweetened, canned, strained- - - - - - -	1 cup- - - - - - - - -	277	61	420	1	Tr	Tr	0.1	0.2
Dates:									
Whole, without pits- - - - -	10 dates- - - - - - -	83	23	230	2	Tr	0.1	0.1	Tr
Figs, dried- - - - - - - - - - - -	10 figs- - - - - - - - -	187	28	475	6	2	0.4	0.5	1.0
Fruit cocktail, canned, fruit and liquid:									
Heavy syrup pack- - - - - -	1 cup- - - - - - - - -	255	80	185	1	Tr	Tr	Tr	0.1
Juice pack- - - - - - - - - - -	1 cup- - - - - - - - -	248	87	115	1	Tr	Tr	Tr	Tr

(Tr indicates nutrient present in trace amounts.)

Nutrients in Indicated Quantity

Cholesterol	Carbohydrate	Calcium	Phosphorus	Iron	Potassium	Sodium	Vitamin A value (IU)	Vitamin A value (RE)	Thiamin	Riboflavin	Niacin	Ascorbic acid
Milligrams	*Grams*	*Milligrams*	*Milligrams*	*Milligrams*	*Milligrams*	*Milligrams*	*International units*	*Retinol equivalents*	*Milligrams*	*Milligrams*	*Milligrams*	*Milligrams*
0	28	7	17	0.3	183	5	70	7	0.03	0.06	0.5	[20]3
0	12	15	20	0.6	314	1	2,770	277	0.03	0.04	0.6	11
0	18	8	10	0.3	119	3	1,050	105	0.02	0.02	0.3	3
0	10	10	17	0.3	139	3	1,420	142	0.02	0.02	0.3	4
0	80	59	152	6.1	1,791	13	9,410	941	0.01	0.20	3.9	3
0	55	40	103	4.2	1,222	8	5,910	591	0.02	0.08	2.4	4
0	36	18	23	1.0	286	8	3,300	330	0.02	0.04	0.7	[20]2
0	12	19	73	2.0	1,097	21	1,060	106	0.19	0.21	3.3	14
0	27	33	119	1.6	1,484	15	1,860	186	0.33	0.37	5.8	24
0	27	7	23	0.4	451	1	90	9	0.05	0.11	0.6	10
0	35	9	30	0.5	594	2	120	12	0.07	0.15	0.8	14
0	18	46	30	0.8	282	Tr	240	24	0.04	0.06	0.6	30
0	20	9	15	0.2	129	9	150	15	0.07	0.07	0.5	19
0	62	17	20	1.1	170	3	120	12	0.06	0.15	0.7	3
0	50	14	16	0.9	138	2	100	10	0.05	0.12	0.6	2
0	22	27	24	3.3	239	17	1,840	184	0.04	0.10	0.4	5
0	11	10	13	0.3	152	Tr	150	15	0.03	0.04	0.3	5
0	38	8	3	0.4	61	10	10	1	0.01	0.04	0.1	[21]108
0	108	11	17	0.6	72	80	60	6	0.04	0.06	0.3	6
0	61	27	33	1.0	541	2	40	4	0.07	0.08	1.8	0
0	122	269	127	4.2	1,331	21	250	25	0.13	0.16	1.3	1
0	48	15	28	0.7	224	15	520	52	0.05	0.05	1.0	5
0	29	20	35	0.5	236	10	760	76	0.03	0.04	1.0	7

Nutritive Values of Foods *(Continued)*

Foods, approximate measures, units, and weight (weight of edible portion only)		Water	Food energy	Pro-tein	Fat	Fatty Acids		
						Satu-rated	Mono-unsatu-rated	Poly-unsatu-rated
FRUITS AND FRUIT JUICES — Con.	Grams	Per-cent	Cal-ories	Grams	Grams	Grams	Grams	Grams
Grapefruit:								
Raw, without peel, membrane and seeds (3¾-in diam., 1 lb 1 oz, whole, with refuse)- - - - - - - - ½ grapefruit- - - -	120	91	40	1	Tr	Tr	Tr	Tr
Canned, sections with syrup)- - - - - - - - - - - - 1 cup- - - - - - - - -	254	84	150	1	Tr	Tr	Tr	0.1
Grapefruit juice:								
Raw- - - - - - - - - - - - - - - 1 cup- - - - - - - - -	247	90	95	1	Tr	Tr	Tr	0.1
Canned:								
Unsweetened- - - - - - - - 1 cup- - - - - - - - -	247	90	95	1	Tr	Tr	Tr	0.1
Frozen concentrate, unsweetened								
Diluted with 3 parts water by volume- - - - - - - - - 1 cup- - - - - - - - -	247	89	100	1	Tr	Tr	Tr	0.1
Grapes, European type (adherent skin), raw:								
Thompson Seedless- - - - - 10 grapes- - - - - -	50	81	35	Tr	Tr	0.1	Tr	0.1
Tokay and Emperor, seeded types- - - - - - - - - - - - - - 10 grapes- - - - - -	57	81	40	Tr	Tr	0.1	Tr	0.1
Grape juice:								
Canned or bottled- - - - - - 1 cup- - - - - - - - -	253	84	155	1	Tr	0.1	Tr	0.1
Kiwifruit, raw, without skin (about 5 per lb with skin)- 1 kiwifruit- - - - - -	76	83	45	1	Tr	Tr	0.1	0.1
Lemons, raw, without peel and seeds (about 4 per lb with peel and seeds)- - - - - - - - 1 lemon- - - - - - -	58	89	15	1	Tr	Tr	Tr	0.1
Lemon juice:								
Raw- - - - - - - - - - - - - - - 1 cup- - - - - - - - -	244	91	60	1	Tr	Tr	Tr	Tr
Canned or bottled, unsweetened- - - - - - - - - - - - - - 1 cup- - - - - - - - -	244	92	50	1	1	0.1	Tr	0.2
	1 tbsp- - - - - - - -	15	92	5	Tr	Tr	Tr	Tr	Tr
Lime juice:								
Raw- - - - - - - - - - - - - - - 1 cup- - - - - - - - -	246	90	65	1	Tr	Tr	Tr	0.1
Canned, unsweetened- - - - 1 cup- - - - - - - - -	246	93	50	1	1	0.1	0.1	0.2
Mangos, raw, without skin and seed (about 1½ per lb with skin and seed)- - - - 1 mango- - - - - - -	207	82	135	1	1	0.1	0.2	0.1
Melons, raw, without rind and cavity contents:								
Cantaloup, orange-fleshed (5-in diam., 2⅓ lb, whole, with rind and cavity contents)- - - - - - - - - - - - ½ melon- - - - - - -	267	90	95	2	1	0.1	0.1	0.3
Honeydew (6½-in diam., 5¼ lb, whole, with rind and cavity contents)- - - - - - ⅒ melon- - - - - - -	129	90	45	1	Tr	Tr	Tr	0.1

(Tr indicates nutrient present in trace amounts.)

Nutrients in Indicated Quantity

Cho-les-terol	Carbo-hydrate	Calcium	Phos-phorus	Iron	Potas-sium	Sodium	Vitamin A value		Thiamin	Ribo-flavin	Niacin	Ascorbic acid
							(IU)	(RE)				
Milli-grams	Grams	Milli-grams	Milli-grams	Milli-grams	Milli-grams	Milli-grams	Inter-national units	Retinol equiva-lents	Milli-grams	Milli-grams	Milli-grams	Milli-grams
0	10	14	10	0.1	167	Tr	[22]10	[22]1	0.04	0.02	0.3	41
0	39	36	25	1.0	328	5	Tr	Tr	0.10	0.05	0.6	54
0	23	22	37	0.5	400	2	20	2	0.10	0.05	0.5	94
0	22	17	27	0.5	378	2	20	2	0.10	0.05	0.6	72
0	24	20	35	0.3	336	2	20	2	0.10	0.05	0.5	83
0	9	6	7	0.1	93	1	40	4	0.05	0.03	0.2	5
0	10	6	7	0.1	105	1	40	4	0.05	0.03	0.2	6
0	38	23	28	0.6	334	8	20	2	0.07	0.09	0.7	[20]Tr
0	11	20	30	0.3	252	4	130	13	0.02	0.04	0.4	74
0	5	15	9	0.3	80	1	20	2	0.02	0.01	0.1	31
0	21	17	15	0.1	303	2	50	5	0.07	0.02	0.2	112
0	16	27	22	0.3	249	[22]51	40	4	0.10	0.02	0.5	61
0	1	2	1	Tr	15	[23]3	Tr	Tr	0.01	Tr	Tr	4
0	22	22	17	0.1	268	2	20	2	0.05	0.02	0.2	72
0	16	30	25	0.6	185	[23]39	40	4	0.08	0.01	0.4	16
0	35	21	23	0.3	323	4	8,060	806	0.12	0.12	1.2	57
0	22	29	45	0.6	825	24	8,610	861	0.10	0.06	1.5	113
0	12	8	13	0.1	350	13	50	5	0.10	0.02	0.8	32

Nutritive Values of Foods *(Continued)*

Foods, approximate measures, units, and weight (weight of edible portion only)		Water	Food energy	Pro-tein	Fat	Fatty Acids		
						Satu-rated	Mono-unsatu-rated	Poly-unsatu-rated
		Grams	Per-cent	Cal-ories	Grams	Grams	Grams	Grams	Grams

FRUITS AND FRUIT JUICES — **Con.**		Grams	Per-cent	Cal-ories	Grams	Grams	Grams	Grams	Grams
Nectarines, raw, without pits (about 3 per lb with pits)	1 nectarine- - - - -	136	86	65	1	1	0.1	0.2	0.3
Oranges, raw:									
Whole, without peel and seeds (2⅝-in diam., about 2½ per lb, with peel and seeds)- - - - - - - - - - - -	1 orange- - - - - - -	131	87	60	1	Tr	Tr	Tr	Tr
Orange juice:									
Raw, all varieties- - - - - - -	1 cup- - - - - - - - -	248	88	110	2	Tr	0.1	0.1	0.1
Canned, unsweetened- - - -	1 cup- - - - - - - - -	249	89	105	1	Tr	Tr	0.1	0.1
Chilled- - - - - - - - - - - - - -	1 cup- - - - - - - - -	249	88	110	2	1	0.1	0.1	0.2
Frozen concentrate:									
Diluted with 3 parts water by volume- - - - - - - - -	1 cup- - - - - - - - -	249	88	110	2	Tr	Tr	Tr	Tr
Orange and grapefruit juice, canned- - - - - - - - - - - - - -	1 cup- - - - - - - - -	247	89	105	1	Tr	Tr	Tr	Tr
Papayas, raw, ½-in cubes- - -	1 cup- - - - - - - - -	140	86	65	1	Tr	0.1	0.1	Tr
Peaches:									
Raw: Whole, 2½-in diam., peeled, pitted (about 4 per lb with peels and pits)- - - - - - - - - - -	1 peach- - - - - - - -	87	88	35	1	Tr	Tr	Tr	Tr
Canned, fruit and liquid:									
Heavy syrup pack- - - - -	1 half- - - - - - - - -	81	79	60	Tr	Tr	Tr	Tr	Tr
Juice pack- - - - - - - - - -	1 half- - - - - - - -	77	87	35	Tr	Tr	Tr	Tr	Tr
Dried:									
Uncooked- - - - - - - - - - -	1 cup- - - - - - - - -	160	32	380	6	1	0.1	0.4	0.6
Cooked, unsweetened, fruit and liquid- - - - -	1 cup- - - - - - - - -	258	78	200	3	1	0.1	0.2	0.3
Frozen, sliced, sweetened-	10-oz container- -	284	75	265	2	Tr	Tr	0.1	0.2
	1 cup- - - - - - - - -	250	75	235	2	Tr	Tr	0.1	0.2
Pears:									
Raw, with skin, cored:									
Bartlett, 2½-in diam. (about 2½ per lb with cores and stems)- - - -	1 pear- - - - - - - - -	166	84	100	1	1	Tr	0.1	0.2
Bosc, 2½-in diam. (about 3 per lb with cores and stems)- - - - - - - - - - -	1 pear- - - - - - - - -	141	84	85	1	1	Tr	0.1	0.1
D'Anjou, 3-in diam. (about 2 per lb with cores and stems)- - - -	1 pear- - - - - - - - -	200	84	120	1	1	Tr	0.2	0.2
Canned, fruit and liquid:									
Heavy syrup pack- - - - -	1 half- - - - - - - - -	79	80	60	Tr	Tr	Tr	Tr	Tr
Juice pack- - - - - - - - - -	1 half- - - - - - - - -	77	86	40	Tr	Tr	Tr	Tr	Tr
Pineapple:									
Raw, diced- - - - - - - - - - -	1 cup- - - - - - - - -	155	87	75	1	1	Tr	0.1	0.2

(Tr indicates nutrient present in trace amounts.)

Nutrients in Indicated Quantity

Cho-les-terol	Carbo-hydrate	Calcium	Phos-phorus	Iron	Potas-sium	Sodium	Vitamin A value		Thiamin	Ribo-flavin	Niacin	Ascorbic acid
							(IU)	(RE)				
Milli-grams	Grams	Milli-grams	Milli-grams	Milli-grams	Milli-grams	Milli-grams	Inter-national units	Retinol equiva-lents	Milli-grams	Milli-grams	Milli-grams	Milli-grams
0	16	7	22	0.2	288	Tr	1,000	100	0.02	0.06	1.3	7
0	15	52	18	0.1	237	Tr	270	27	0.11	0.05	0.4	70
0	26	27	42	0.5	496	2	500	50	0.22	0.07	1.0	124
0	25	20	35	1.1	436	5	440	44	0.15	0.07	0.8	86
0	25	25	27	0.4	473	2	190	19	0.28	0.05	0.7	82
0	27	22	40	0.2	473	2	190	19	0.20	0.04	0.5	97
0	25	20	35	1.1	390	7	290	29	0.14	0.07	0.8	72
0	17	35	12	0.3	247	9	400	40	0.04	0.04	0.5	92
0	10	4	10	0.1	171	Tr	470	47	0.01	0.04	0.9	6
0	16	2	9	0.2	75	5	270	27	0.01	0.02	0.5	2
0	9	5	13	0.2	99	3	290	29	0.01	0.01	0.4	3
0	98	45	190	6.5	1,594	11	3,460	346	Tr	0.34	7.0	8
0	51	23	98	3.4	826	5	510	51	0.01	0.05	3.9	10
0	68	9	31	1.1	369	17	810	81	0.04	0.10	1.9	[21]268
0	60	8	28	0.9	325	15	710	71	0.03	0.09	1.6	[21]236
0	25	18	18	0.4	208	Tr	30	3	0.03	0.07	0.2	7
0	21	16	16	0.4	176	Tr	30	3	0.03	0.06	0.1	6
0	30	22	22	0.5	250	Tr	40	4	0.04	0.08	0.2	8
0	15	4	6	0.2	51	4	Tr	Tr	0.01	0.02	0.2	1
0	10	7	9	0.2	74	3	Tr	Tr	0.01	0.01	0.2	1
0	19	11	11	0.6	175	2	40	4	0.14	0.06	0.7	24

Nutritive Values of Foods *(Continued)*

Foods, approximate measures, units, and weight (weight of edible portion only)		Water	Food energy	Pro-tein	Fat	Fatty Acids		
						Satu-rated	Mono-unsatu-rated	Poly-unsatu-rated
		Per-cent	Cal-ories					
FRUITS AND FRUIT JUICES—Con.	Grams			Grams	Grams	Grams	Grams	Grams
Canned, fruit and liquid:								
Heavy syrup pack:								
Slices----------- 1 slice--------	58	79	45	Tr	Tr	Tr	Tr	Tr
Juice pack:								
Slices----------- 1 slice--------	58	84	35	Tr	Tr	Tr	Tr	Tr
Pineapple juice, unsweetened,								
canned-------------- 1 cup--------	250	86	140	1	Tr	Tr	Tr	0.1
Plantains, without peel:								
Cooked, boiled, sliced---- 1 cup--------	154	67	180	1	Tr	0.1	Tr	0.1
Plums, without pits:								
Raw:								
2⅛-in diam. (about 6½ per								
lb with pits)------ 1 plum--------	66	85	35	1	Tr	Tr	0.3	0.1
1½-in diam. (about 15 per								
lb with pits)------- 1 plum--------	28	85	15	Tr	Tr	Tr	0.1	Tr
Canned, purple, fruit and liquid:								
Heavy syrup pack----- 3 plums--------	133	76	120	Tr	Tr	Tr	0.1	Tr
Juice pack---------- 3 plums--------	95	84	55	Tr	Tr	Tr	Tr	Tr
Prunes, dried:								
Uncooked----------- 4 extra large or 5 large prunes---	49	32	115	1	Tr	Tr	0.2	0.1
Cooked, unsweetened, fruit and liquid----------- 1 cup--------	212	70	225	2	Tr	Tr	0.3	0.1
Prune juice, canned or bottled------------ 1 cup--------	256	81	180	2	Tr	Tr	0.1	Tr
Raisins, seedless:								
Cup, not pressed down--- 1 cup--------	145	15	435	5	1	0.2	Tr	0.2
Packet, ½ oz (1½ tbsp)--- 1 packet-------	14	15	40	Tr	Tr	Tr	Tr	Tr
Raspberries:								
Raw---------------- 1 cup--------	123	87	60	1	1	Tr	0.1	0.4
Frozen, sweetened------ 10-oz container--	284	73	295	2	Tr	Tr	Tr	0.3
Rhubarb, cooked, added sugar--------- 1 cup--------	240	68	280	1	Tr	Tr	Tr	0.1
Strawberries:								
Raw, capped, whole----- 1 cup--------	149	92	45	1	1	Tr	0.1	0.3
Frozen, sweetened, sliced- 10-oz container--	284	73	275	2	Tr	Tr	0.1	0.2
1 cup--------	255	73	245	1	Tr	Tr	Tr	0.2
Tangerines:								
Raw, without peel and seeds (2⅜-in diam., (about 4 per lb, with peel and seeds)- 1 tangerine-----	84	88	35	1	Tr	Tr	Tr	Tr
Watermelon, raw, without rind and seeds:								
Piece (4 by 8 in wedge with rind and seeds; ¹⁄₁₆ of 32⅝-lb melon, 10 by 16 in)-- 1 piece--------	482	92	155	3	2	0.3	0.2	1.0

(Tr indicates nutrient present in trace amounts.)

Nutrients in Indicated Quantity

Cholesterol	Carbohydrate	Calcium	Phosphorus	Iron	Potassium	Sodium	Vitamin A value		Thiamin	Riboflavin	Niacin	Ascorbic acid
							(IU)	(RE)				
Milligrams	Grams	Milligrams	Milligrams	Milligrams	Milligrams	Milligrams	International units	Retinol equivalents	Milligrams	Milligrams	Milligrams	Milligrams
0	12	8	4	0.2	60	1	10	1	0.05	0.01	0.2	4
0	9	8	3	0.2	71	1	20	2	0.06	0.01	0.2	6
0	34	43	20	0.7	335	3	10	1	0.14	0.06	0.6	27
0	48	3	43	0.9	716	8	1,400	140	0.07	0.08	1.2	17
0	9	3	7	0.1	114	Tr	210	21	0.03	0.06	0.3	6
0	4	1	3	Tr	48	Tr	90	9	0.01	0.03	0.1	3
0	31	12	17	1.1	121	25	340	34	0.02	0.05	0.4	1
0	14	10	14	0.3	146	1	960	96	0.02	0.06	0.4	3
0	31	25	39	1.2	365	2	970	97	0.04	0.08	1.0	2
0	60	49	74	2.4	708	4	650	65	0.05	0.21	1.5	6
0	45	31	64	3.0	707	10	10	1	0.04	0.18	2.0	10
0	115	71	141	3.0	1,089	17	10	1	0.23	0.13	1.2	5
0	11	7	14	0.3	105	2	Tr	Tr	0.02	0.01	0.1	Tr
0	14	27	15	0.7	187	Tr	160	16	0.04	0.11	1.1	31
0	74	43	48	1.8	324	3	170	17	0.05	0.13	0.7	47
0	75	348	19	0.5	230	2	170	17	0.04	0.06	0.5	8
0	10	21	28	0.6	247	1	40	4	0.03	0.10	0.3	84
0	74	31	37	1.7	278	9	70	7	0.05	0.14	1.1	118
0	66	28	33	1.5	250	8	60	6	0.04	0.13	1.0	106
0	9	12	8	0.1	132	1	770	77	0.09	0.02	0.1	26
0	35	39	43	0.8	559	10	1,760	176	0.39	0.10	1.0	46

Nutritive Values of Foods *(Continued)*

Foods, approximate measures, units, and weight (weight of edible portion only)			Water	Food energy	Pro-tein	Fat	Fatty Acids		
							Satu-rated	Mono-unsatu-rated	Poly-unsatu-rated
GRAIN PRODUCTS		Grams	Per-cent	Cal-ories	Grams	Grams	Grams	Grams	Grams
Bagels, plain or water,									
enriched, 3½-in diam.[24]	1 bagel	68	29	200	7	2	0.3	0.5	0.7
Barley, pearled, light,									
uncooked	1 cup	200	11	700	16	2	0.3	0.2	0.9
Biscuits, baking powder, 2-in diam. (enriched flour, vegetable shortening):									
From home recipe	1 biscuit	28	28	100	2	5	1.2	2.0	1.3
Breadcrumbs, enriched:									
Soft. See White bread.									
Breads:									
Boston brown bread, canned, slice, 3¼ in by ½ in[25]	1 slice	45	45	95	2	1	0.3	0.1	0.1
Cracked-wheat bread (¾ enriched wheat flour, ¼ cracked wheat flour):[25]									
Slice (18 per loaf)	1 slice	25	35	65	2	1	0.2	0.2	0.3
French or vienna bread, enriched:[25]									
Slice:									
French, 5 by 2½ by 1 in	1 slice	35	34	100	3	1	0.3	0.4	0.5
Vienna, 4¾ by 4 by ½ in	1 slice	25	34	70	2	1	0.2	0.3	0.3
Italian bread, enriched:									
Slice, 4½ by 3¼ by ¾ in	1 slice	30	32	85	3	Tr	Tr	Tr	0.1
Mixed grain bread, enriched:[25]									
Slice (18 per loaf)	1 slice	25	37	65	2	1	0.2	0.2	0.4
Oatmeal bread, enriched:[25]									
Slice (18 per loaf)	1 slice	25	37	65	2	1	0.2	0.4	0.5
Pita bread, enriched, white, 6½-in diam.	1 pita	60	31	165	6	1	0.1	0.1	0.4
Pumpernickel (⅔ rye flour, ⅓ enriched wheat flour):[25]									
Slice, 5 by 4 by ⅜ in	1 slice	32	37	80	3	1	0.2	0.3	0.5
Raisin bread, enriched:[25]									
Slice (18 per loaf)	1 slice	25	33	65	2	1	0.2	0.3	0.4
Rye bread, light (⅔ enriched wheat flour, ⅓ rye flour):[25]									
Slice, 4¾ by 3¾ by 7/16 in	1 slice	25	37	65	2	1	0.2	0.3	0.3
Wheat bread, enriched:[25]									
Slice (18 per loaf)	1 slice	25	37	65	2	1	0.2	0.4	0.3

(Tr indicates nutrient present in trace amounts.)

Nutrients in Indicated Quantity

Cho-les-terol	Carbo-hydrate	Calcium	Phos-phorus	Iron	Potas-sium	Sodium	Vitamin A value (IU)	(RE)	Thiamin	Ribo-flavin	Niacin	Ascorbic acid
Milli-grams	Grams	Milli-grams	Milli-grams	Milli-grams	Milli-grams	Milli-grams	Inter-national units	Retinol equiva-lents	Milli-grams	Milli-grams	Milli-grams	Milli-grams
0	38	29	46	1.8	50	245	0	0	0.26	0.20	2.4	0
0	158	32	378	4.2	320	6	0	0	0.24	0.10	6.2	0
Tr	13	47	36	0.7	32	195	10	3	0.08	0.08	0.8	Tr
3	21	41	72	0.9	131	113	[26]0	[26]0	0.06	0.04	0.7	0
0	12	16	32	0.7	34	106	Tr	Tr	0.10	0.09	0.8	Tr
0	18	39	30	1.1	32	203	Tr	Tr	0.16	0.12	1.4	Tr
0	13	28	21	0.8	23	145	Tr	Tr	0.12	0.09	1.0	Tr
0	17	5	23	0.8	22	176	0	0	0.12	0.07	1.0	0
0	12	27	55	0.8	56	106	Tr	Tr	0.10	0.10	1.1	Tr
0	12	15	31	0.7	39	124	0	0	0.12	0.07	0.9	0
0	33	49	60	1.4	71	339	0	0	0.27	0.12	2.2	0
0	16	23	71	0.9	141	177	0	0	0.11	0.17	1.1	0
0	13	25	22	0.8	59	92	Tr	Tr	0.08	0.15	1.0	Tr
0	12	20	36	0.7	51	175	0	0	0.10	0.08	0.8	0
0	12	32	47	0.9	35	138	Tr	Tr	0.12	0.08	1.2	Tr

Nutritive Values of Foods *(Continued)*

Foods, approximate measures, units, and weight (weight of edible portion only)		Water	Food energy	Pro-tein	Fat	Fatty Acids		
						Satu-rated	Mono-unsatu-rated	Poly-unsatu-rated
		Per-cent	Cal-ories					
GRAIN PRODUCTS—Con.	*Grams*	*cent*	*ories*	*Grams*	*Grams*	*Grams*	*Grams*	*Grams*
Wheat bread, enriched:[25]								
Slice (18 per loaf)----- 1 slice---------	25	37	65	2	1	0.3	0.4	0.2
Whole-wheat bread:[25]								
Slice (16 per loaf)----- 1 slice---------	28	38	70	3	1	0.4	0.4	0.3
Breakfast cereals:								
Hot type, cooked:								
Corn, (hominy) grits:								
Regular and quick,								
enriched-------- 1 cup---------	242	85	145	3	Tr	Tr	0.1	0.2
Instant, plain------ 1 pkt---------	137	85	80	2	Tr	Tr	Tr	0.1
Cream of Wheat®:								
Regular, quick,								
instant--------- 1 cup---------	244	86	140	4	Tr	0.1	Tr	0.2
Mix'n Eat, plain---- 1 pkt---------	142	82	100	3	Tr	Tr	Tr	0.1
Malt-O-Meal®------- 1 cup---------	240	88	120	4	Tr	Tr	Tr	0.1
Oatmeal or rolled oats:								
Regular, quick, instant,								
nonfortified------ 1 cup---------	234	85	145	6	2	0.4	0.8	1.0
Ready to eat:								
All-Bran® (about								
⅓ cup)--------- 1 oz----------	28	3	70	4	1	0.1	0.1	0.3
Cap'n Crunch® (about ¾								
cup)----------- 1 oz----------	28	3	120	1	3	1.7	0.3	0.4
Cheerios®　(about　1¼								
cup)----------- 1 oz----------	28	5	110	4	2	0.3	0.6	0.7
Corn　Flakes　(about　1¼								
cup):								
Kellogg's®-------- 1 oz----------	28	3	110	2	Tr	Tr	Tr	Tr
40% Bran Flakes:								
Kellogg's®　(about　¾								
cup)----------- 1 oz----------	28	3	90	4	1	0.1	0.1	0.3
Post® (about ⅔ cup)- 1 oz----------	28	3	90	3	Tr	0.1	0.1	0.2
Froot Loops® (about 1								
cup)----------- 1 oz----------	28	3	110	2	1	0.2	0.1	0.1
Golden Grahams®								
(about ¾ cup)----- 1 oz----------	28	2	110	2	1	0.7	0.1	0.2
Grape-Nuts®　(about　¼								
cup)----------- 1 oz----------	28	3	100	3	Tr	Tr	Tr	0.1
Honey　Nut　Cheerios®								
(about ¾ cup)----- 1 oz----------	28	3	105	3	1	0.1	0.3	0.3
Lucky Charms® (about 1								
cup)----------- 1 oz----------	28	3	110	3	1	0.2	0.4	0.4
Nature Valley® Granola								
(about ⅓ cup)----- 1 oz----------	28	4	125	3	5	3.3	0.7	0.7
100% Natural Cereal								
(about ¼ cup)----- 1 oz----------	28	2	135	3	6	4.1	1.2	0.5

(Tr indicates nutrient present in trace amounts.)

Nutrients in Indicated Quantity

Cholesterol	Carbohydrate	Calcium	Phosphorus	Iron	Potassium	Sodium	Vitamin A value (IU)	Vitamin A value (RE)	Thiamin	Riboflavin	Niacin	Ascorbic acid
							International units	Retinol equivalents				
Milligrams	Grams	Milligrams	Milligrams	Milligrams	Milligrams	Milligrams			Milligrams	Milligrams	Milligrams	Milligrams
0	12	32	27	0.7	28	129	Tr	Tr	0.12	0.08	0.9	Tr
0	13	20	74	1.0	50	180	Tr	Tr	0.10	0.06	1.1	Tr
0	31	0	29	[27]1.5	53	[28]0	[29]0	[29]0	[27]0.24	[27]0.15	[27]2.0	0
0	18	7	16	[27]1.0	29	343	0	0	[27]0.18	[27]0.08	[27]1.3	0
0	29	[30]54	[31]43	[30]10.9	46	[31,32]5	0	0	[30]0.24	[30]0.07	[31]1.5	0
0	21	[30]20	[30]20	[30]8.1	38	241	[30]1,250	[30]376	[30]0.43	[30]0.28	[30]5.0	0
0	26	5	[30]24	[30]9.6	31	[33]2	0	0	[30]0.48	[30]0.24	[30]5.8	0
0	19	178		1.6	131	[34]2	40	4	0.26	0.05	0.3	0
0	21	23	264	[30]4.5	350	320	[30]1,250	[30]375	[30]0.37	[30]0.43	[30]5.0	[30]15
0	23	5	36	[27]7.5	37	213	40	4	[27]0.50	[27]0.55	[27]6.6	0
0	20	48	134	[30]4.5	101	307	[30]1,250	[30]375	[30]0.37	[30]0.43	[30]5.0	[30]15
0	24	1	18	[30]1.8	26	351	[30]1,250	[30]375	[30]0.37	[30]0.43	[30]5.0	[30]15
0	22	14	139	[30]8.1	180	264	[30]1,250	[30]375	[30]0.37	[30]0.43	[30]5.0	0
0	22	12	179	[30]4.5	151	260	[30]1,250	[30]375	[30]0.37	[30]0.43	[30]5.0	0
0	25	3	24	[30]4.5	26	145	[30]1,250	[30]375	[30]0.37	[30]0.43	[30]5.0	[30]15
Tr	24	17	41	[30]4.5	63	346	[30]1,250	[30]375	[30]0.37	[30]0.43	[30]5.0	[30]15
0	23	11	71	1.2	95	197	[30]1,250	[30]375	[30]0.37	[30]0.43	[30]5.0	0
0	23	20	105	[30]4.5	99	257	[30]1,250	[30]375	[30]0.37	[30]0.43	[30]5.0	[30]15
0	23	32	79	[30]4.5	59	201	[30]1,250	[30]375	[30]0.37	[30]0.43	[30]5.0	[30]15
0	19	18	89	0.9	98	58	20	2	0.10	0.05	0.2	0
Tr	18	49	104	0.8	140	12	20	2	0.09	0.15	0.6	0

Nutritive Values of Foods *(Continued)*

Foods, approximate measures, units, and weight (weight of edible portion only)		Water	Food energy	Pro-tein	Fat	Fatty Acids		
						Satu-rated	Mono-unsatu-rated	Poly-unsatu-rated
		Per-cent	Cal-ories					
GRAIN PRODUCTS—Con.	Grams	cent	ories	Grams	Grams	Grams	Grams	Grams
Product 19® (about ¾ cup)- - - - - - - - - 1 oz- - - - - - - - - -	28	3	110	3	Tr	Tr	Tr	0.1
Raisin Bran:								
Kellogg's® (about ¾ cup)- - - - - - - - - - - 1 oz- - - - - - - - -	28	8	90	3	1	0.1	0.1	0.3
Post® (about ½ cup)- 1 oz- - - - - - - - - -	28	9	85	3	1	0.1	0.1	0.3
Rice Krispies® (about 1 cup)- - - - - - - - - - 1 oz- - - - - - - - -	28	2	110	2	Tr	Tr	Tr	0.1
Shredded Wheat (about ⅔ cup)- - - - - - - - - 1 oz- - - - - - - - - -	28	5	100	3	1	0.1	0.1	0.3
Special K® (about 1⅓ cup)- - - - - - - - - - - 1 oz- - - - - - - - -	28	2	110	6	Tr	Tr	Tr	Tr
Super Sugar Crisp® (about ⅞ cup)- - - - - 1 oz- - - - - - - - - -	28	2	105	2	Tr	Tr	Tr	0.1
Sugar Frosted Flakes, Kellogg's® (about ¾ cup)- - - - - - - - - - - 1 oz- - - - - - - - - -	28	3	110	1	Tr	Tr	Tr	Tr
Sugar Smacks® (about ¾ cup)- - - - - - - - - - - 1 oz- - - - - - - - - -	28	3	105	2	1	0.1	0.1	0.2
Total® (about 1 cup)- - 1 oz- - - - - - - - -	28	4	100	3	1	0.1	0.1	0.3
Trix® (about 1 cup)- - - 1 oz- - - - - - - - -	28	3	110	2	Tr	0.2	0.1	0.1
Wheaties® (about 1 cup)- - - - - - - - - 1 oz- - - - - - - - -	28	5	100	3	Tr	0.1	Tr	0.2
Buckwheat flour, light, sifted	1 cup- - - - - - - - -	98	12	340	6	1	0.2	0.4	0.4
Bulgur, uncooked- - - - - - -	1 cup- - - - - - - - -	170	10	600	19	3	1.2	0.3	1.2
Cakes prepared from cake mixes with enriched flour:[35]								
Angelfood:								
Piece, 1/12 of cake- - - - - - 1 piece- - - - - - - -	53	38	125	3	Tr	Tr	Tr	0.1
Coffeecake, crumb:								
Piece, ⅙ of cake- - - - - 1 piece- - - - - - - -	72	30	230	5	7	2.0	2.8	1.6
Devil's food with chocolate frosting:								
Piece, 1/16 of cake- - - - - - 1 piece- - - - - - - -	69	24	235	3	8	3.5	3.2	1.2
Cupcake, 2½-in diam.- - 1 cupcake- - - - - -	35	24	120	2	4	1.8	1.6	0.6
Gingerbread:								
Piece, ⅑ of cake- - - - - - 1 piece- - - - - - - -	63	37	175	2	4	1.1	1.8	1.2
Yellow with chocolate frosting:								
Piece, 1/16 of cake- - - - - - 1 piece- - - - - - - -	69	26	235	3	8	3.0	3.0	1.4
Cakes prepared from home recipes using enriched flour:								
Carrot, with cream cheese frosting:[36]								
Piece, 1/16 of cake- - - - - - 1 piece- - - - - - - -	96	23	385	4	21	4.1	8.4	6.7

(Tr indicates nutrient present in trace amounts.)

Nutrients in Indicated Quantity

Cholesterol	Carbohydrate	Calcium	Phosphorus	Iron	Potassium	Sodium	Vitamin A value		Thiamin	Riboflavin	Niacin	Ascorbic acid
							(IU)	(RE)				
Milligrams	Grams	Milligrams	Milligrams	Milligrams	Milligrams	Milligrams	International units	Retinol equivalents	Milligrams	Milligrams	Milligrams	Milligrams
0	24	3	40	[30]18.0	44	325	[30]5,000	[30]1,501	[30]1.50	[30]1.70	[30]20.0	[30]60
0	21	10	105	[303]3.5	147	207	[30]960	[30]288	[30]0.28	[30]0.34	[303]3.9	0
0	21	13	119	[304]4.5	175	185	[30]1,250	[30]375	[30]0.37	[30]0.43	[30]5.0	0
0	25	4	34	[30]1.8	29	340	[30]1,250	[30]375	[30]0.37	[30]0.43	[30]5.0	[30]15
0	23	11	100	1.2	102	3	0	0	0.07	0.08	1.5	0
Tr	21	8	55	[304]4.5	49	265	[30]1,250	[30]375	[30]0.37	[30]0.43	[30]5.0	[30]15
0	26	6	52	[30]1.8	105	25	[30]1,250	[30]375	[30]0.37	[30]0.43	[30]5.0	0
0	26	1	21	[30]1.8	18	230	[30]1,250	[30]375	[30]0.37	[30]0.43	[30]5.0	[30]15
0	25	3	31	[30]1.8	42	75	[30]1,250	[30]375	[30]0.37	[30]0.43	[30]5.0	[30]15
0	22	48	118	[30]18.0	106	352	[30]5,000	[30]1,501	[30]1.50	[30]1.70	[30]20.0	[30]60
0	25	6	19	[304]4.5	27	181	[30]1,250	[30]375	[30]0.37	[30]0.43	[30]5.0	[30]15
0	23	43	98	[304]4.5	106	354	[30]1,250	[30]375	[30]0.37	[30]0.43	[30]5.0	[30]15
0	78	11	86	1.0	314	2	0	0	0.08	0.04	0.4	0
0	129	49	575	9.5	389	7	0	0	0.48	0.24	7.7	0
0	29	44	91	0.2	71	269	0	0	0.03	0.11	0.1	0
47	38	44	125	1.2	78	310	120	32	0.14	0.15	1.3	Tr
37	40	41	72	1.4	90	181	100	31	0.07	0.10	0.6	Tr
19	20	21	37	0.7	46	92	50	16	0.04	0.05	0.3	Tr
1	32	57	63	1.2	173	192	0	0	0.09	0.11	0.8	Tr
36	40	63	126	1.0	75	157	100	29	0.08	0.10	0.7	Tr
74	48	44	62	1.3	108	279	140	15	0.11	0.12	0.9	1

Nutritive Values of Foods *(Continued)*

Foods, approximate measures, units, and weight (weight of edible portion only)		Water	Food energy	Pro-tein	Fat	Fatty Acids Satu-rated	Mono-unsatu-rated	Poly-unsatu-rated
		Per-cent	Cal-ories	Grams	Grams	Grams	Grams	Grams
GRAIN PRODUCTS—Con.	Grams							
Fruitcake, dark:[36]								
Piece, 1/32 of cake,								
2/3-in arc- - - - - - - - - 1 piece- - - - - - - -	43	18	165	2	7	1.5	3.6	1.6
Plain sheet cake:[37]								
Without frosting:								
Piece, 1/9 of cake- - - - - 1 piece- - - - - - - -	86	25	315	4	12	3.3	5.0	2.8
With uncooked white frosting:								
Piece, 1/9 of cake- - - - - 1 piece- - - - - - - -	121	21	445	4	14	4.6	5.6	2.9
Pound:[38]								
Slice, 1/17 of loaf- - - - - - 1 slice- - - - - - - - -	30	22	120	2	5	1.2	2.4	1.6
Cakes, commercial, made with enriched flour:								
Pound:								
Slice, 1/17 of loaf- - - - - - 1 slice- - - - - - - - -	29	24	110	2	5	3.0	1.7	0.2
Snack cakes:								
Devil's food with creme filling (2 small cakes per pkg)- - - - - - - - - 1 small cake- - - -	28	20	105	1	4	1.7	1.5	0.6
Sponge with creme filling (2 small cakes per pkg) 1 small cake- - - -	42	19	155	1	5	2.3	2.1	0.5
White with white frosting:								
Piece, 1/16 of cake- - - - - - 1 piece- - - - - - - -	71	24	260	3	9	2.1	3.8	2.6
Yellow with chocolate frost-ing:								
Piece, 1/16 of cake- - - - - - 1 piece- - - - - - - -	69	23	245	2	11	5.7	3.7	0.6
Cheesecake:								
Piece, 1/12 of cake- - - - - - 1 piece- - - - - - - -	92	46	280	5	18	9.9	5.4	1.2
Cookies made with enriched flour:								
Brownies with nuts:								
Commercial, with frost-ing, 1½ by 1¾ by ⅞ in- 1 brownie- - - - - -	25	13	100	1	4	1.6	2.0	0.6
From home recipe, 1¾ by 1¾ by ⅞ in[36]- - - - - - - 1 brownie- - - - - -	20	10	95	1	6	1.4	2.8	1.2
Chocolate chip:								
Commercial, 2¼-in diam., ⅜ in thick- - - - 4 cookies- - - - - - -	42	4	180	2	9	2.9	3.1	2.6
From home recipe, 2⅓-in diam.[25]- - - - - - - - - - 4 cookies- - - - - - -	40	3	185	2	11	3.9	4.3	2.0
From refrigerated dough, 2¼-in diam., ⅜ in thick 4 cookies- - - - - - -	48	5	225	2	11	4.0	4.4	2.0
Oatmeal with raisins, 2⅝-in diam., ¼ in thick- - - - 4 cookies- - - - - - -	52	4	245	3	10	2.5	4.5	2.8
Peanut butter cookie, from home recipe, 2⅝-in diam.[25]- - - - - - - - - - 4 cookies- - - - - - -	48	3	245	4	14	4.0	5.8	2.8

(Tr indicates nutrient present in trace amounts.)

Nutrients in Indicated Quantity

Cholesterol	Carbohydrate	Calcium	Phosphorus	Iron	Potassium	Sodium	Vitamin A value		Thiamin	Riboflavin	Niacin	Ascorbic acid
							(IU)	(RE)				
Milligrams	Grams	Milligrams	Milligrams	Milligrams	Milligrams	Milligrams	International units	Retinol equivalents	Milligrams	Milligrams	Milligrams	Milligrams
20	25	41	50	1.2	194	67	50	13	0.08	0.08	0.5	16
61	48	55	88	1.3	68	258	150	41	0.14	0.15	1.1	Tr
70	77	61	91	1.2	74	275	240	71	0.13	0.16	1.1	Tr
32	15	20	28	0.5	28	96	200	60	0.05	0.06	0.5	Tr
64	15	8	30	0.5	26	108	160	41	0.06	0.06	0.5	0
15	17	21	26	1.0	34	105	20	4	0.06	0.09	0.7	0
7	27	14	44	0.6	37	155	30	9	0.07	0.06	0.6	0
3	42	33	99	1.0	52	176	40	12	0.20	0.13	1.7	0
38	39	23	117	1.2	123	192	120	30	0.05	0.14	0.6	0
170	26	52	81	0.4	90	204	230	69	0.03	0.12	0.4	5
14	16	13	26	0.6	50	59	70	18	0.08	0.07	0.3	Tr
18	11	9	26	0.4	35	51	20	6	0.05	0.05	0.3	Tr
5	28	13	41	0.8	68	140	50	15	0.10	0.23	1.0	Tr
18	26	13	34	1.0	82	82	20	5	0.06	0.06	0.6	0
22	32	13	34	1.0	62	173	30	8	0.06	0.10	0.9	0
2	36	18	58	1.1	90	148	40	12	0.09	0.08	1.0	0
22	28	21	60	1.1	110	142	20	5	0.07	0.07	1.9	0

Nutritive Values of Foods *(Continued)*

Foods, approximate measures, units, and weight (weight of edible portion only)		Water	Food energy	Pro-tein	Fat	Fatty Acids		
						Satu-rated	Mono-unsatu-rated	Poly-unsatu-rated
		Grams	Per-cent	Cal-ories	Grams	Grams	Grams	Grams	Grams

Foods	measure	Grams	Per-cent	Cal-ories	Grams	Grams	Grams	Grams	Grams
GRAIN PRODUCTS—Con.									
Sandwich type (chocolate or vanilla), 1¾-in diam., ⅜ in thick- - - -	4 cookies- - - - - - -	40	2	195	2	8	2.0	3.6	2.2
Shortbread:									
Commercial- - - - - - - - -	4 small cookies- - -	32	6	155	2	8	2.9	3.0	1.1
Sugar cookie, from refriger-ated dough, 2½-in diam., ¼ in thick- - - -	4 cookies- - - - - - -	48	4	235	2	12	2.3	5.0	3.6
Vanilla wafers, 1¾-in diam., ¼ in thick- - - - - - - -	10 cookies- - - - - -	40	4	185	2	7	1.8	3.0	1.8
Corn chips- - - - - - - - - - - -	1-oz package- - - -	28	1	155	2	9	1.4	2.4	3.7
Cornmeal:									
Whole-ground, unbolted, dry form- - - - - - - - - -	1 cup- - - - - - - - -	122	12	435	11	5	0.5	1.1	2.5
Bolted (nearly whole-grain), dry form- - - - -	1 cup- - - - - - - - -	122	12	440	11	4	0.5	0.9	2.2
Degermed, enriched:									
Dry form- - - - - - - - - -	1 cup- - - - - - - - -	138	12	500	11	2	0.2	0.4	0.9
Crackers:[39]									
Cheese:									
Plain, 1 in square- - - - -	10 crackers- - - - -	10	4	50	1	3	0.9	1.2	0.3
Sandwich type (peanut butter)- - - - - - - - - - -	1 sandwich- - - - -	8	3	40	1	2	0.4	0.8	0.3
Graham, plain, 2½ in square- - - - - - -	2 crackers- - - - - -	14	5	60	1	1	0.4	0.6	0.4
Melba toast, plain- - - - - -	1 piece- - - - - - - -	5	4	20	1	Tr	0.1	0.1	0.1
Rye wafers, whole-grain, 1⅞ by 3½ in- - - - - - - - - -	2 wafers- - - - - - -	14	5	55	1	1	0.3	0.4	0.3
Saltines[40]- - - - - - - - - - - -	4 crackers- - - - - -	12	4	50	1	1	0.5	0.4	0.2
Snack-type, standard- - - -	1 round cracker- -	3	3	15	Tr	1	0.2	0.4	0.1
Wheat, thin- - - - - - - - - -	4 crackers- - - - - -	8	3	35	1	1	0.5	0.5	0.4
Whole-wheat wafers- - - - -	2 crackers- - - - - -	8	4	35	1	2	0.5	0.6	0.4
Croissants, made with enriched flour, 4½ by 4 by 1¾ in- - - - - - - - - - - - - -	1 croissant- - - - -	57	22	235	5	12	3.5	6.7	1.4
Danish pastry, made with enriched flour:									
Plain without fruit or nuts:									
Round piece, about 4¼-in diam., 1 in high- - - - -	1 pastry- - - - - - -	57	27	220	4	12	3.6	4.8	2.6
Fruit, round piece- - - - - -	1 pastry- - - - - - -	65	30	235	4	13	3.9	5.2	2.9
Doughnuts, made with enriched flour:									
Cake type, plain, 3¼-in diam., 1 in high- - - - - -	1 doughnut- - - - -	50	21	210	3	12	2.8	5.0	3.0
Yeast-leavened, glazed, 3¾-in diam., 1¼ in high- - -	1 doughnut- - - - -	60	27	235	4	13	5.2	5.5	0.9

(Tr indicates nutrient present in trace amounts.)

Nutrients in Indicated Quantity

Cho-les-terol	Carbo-hydrate	Calcium	Phos-phorus	Iron	Potas-sium	Sodium	Vitamin A value (IU)	Vitamin A value (RE)	Thiamin	Ribo-flavin	Niacin	Ascorbic acid
Milli-grams	Grams	Milli-grams	Milli-grams	Milli-grams	Milli-grams	Milli-grams	Inter-national units	Retinol equiva-lents	Milli-grams	Milli-grams	Milli-grams	Milli-grams
0	29	12	40	1.4	66	189	0	0	0.09	0.07	0.8	0
27	20	13	39	0.8	38	123	30	8	0.10	0.09	0.9	0
29	31	50	91	0.9	33	261	40	11	0.09	0.06	1.1	0
25	29	16	36	0.8	50	150	50	14	0.07	0.10	1.0	0
0	16	35	52	0.5	52	233	110	11	0.04	0.05	0.4	1
0	90	24	312	2.2	346	1	620	62	0.46	0.13	2.4	0
0	91	21	272	2.2	303	1	590	59	0.37	0.10	2.3	0
0	108	8	137	5.9	166	1	610	61	0.61	0.36	4.8	0
6	6	11	17	0.3	17	112	20	5	0.05	0.04	0.4	0
1	5	7	25	0.3	17	90	Tr	Tr	0.04	0.03	0.6	0
0	11	6	20	0.4	36	86	0	0	0.02	0.03	0.6	0
0	4	6	10	0.1	11	44	0	0	0.01	0.01	0.1	0
0	10	7	44	0.5	65	115	0	0	0.06	0.03	0.5	0
4	9	3	12	0.5	17	165	0	0	0.06	0.05	0.6	0
0	2	3	6	0.1	4	30	Tr	Tr	0.01	0.01	0.1	0
0	5	3	15	0.3	17	69	Tr	Tr	0.04	0.03	0.4	0
0	5	3	22	0.2	31	59	0	0	0.02	0.03	0.4	0
13	27	20	64	2.1	68	452	50	13	0.17	0.13	1.3	0
49	26	60	58	1.1	53	218	60	17	0.16	0.17	1.4	Tr
56	28	17	80	1.3	57	233	40	11	0.16	0.14	1.4	Tr
20	24	22	111	1.0	58	192	20	5	0.12	0.12	1.1	Tr
21	26	17	55	1.4	64	222	Tr	Tr	0.28	0.12	1.8	0

Nutritive Values of Foods *(Continued)*

Foods, approximate measures, units, and weight (weight of edible portion only)		Water	Food energy	Pro-tein	Fat	Fatty Acids Satu-rated	Mono-unsatu-rated	Poly-unsatu-rated
	Grams	Per-cent	Cal-ories	Grams	Grams	Grams	Grams	Grams
GRAIN PRODUCTS—Con.								
English muffins, plain,								
enriched- - - - - - - - - - -	1 muffin- - - - - - -	57	42	140	5	1	0.3	0.2	0.3
Toasted- - - - - - - - - - - - -	1 muffin- - - - - - -	50	29	140	5	1	0.3	0.2	0.3
French toast, from home								
recipe- - - - - - - - - - - - - - -	1 slice- - - - - - - - -	65	53	155	6	7	1.6	2.0	1.6
Macaroni, enriched, cooked (cut lengths, elbows, shells):								
Firm stage (hot)- - - - - - -	1 cup- - - - - - - - -	130	64	190	7	1	0.1	0.1	0.3
Tender stage:								
Cold- - - - - - - - - - - - -	1 cup- - - - - - - - -	105	72	115	4	Tr	0.1	0.1	0.2
Hot- - - - - - - - - - - - - -	1 cup- - - - - - - - -	140	72	155	5	1	0.1	0.1	0.2
Muffins made with enriched flour, 2½-in diam., 1½ in high:								
From home recipe:								
Blueberry[35]- - - - - - - - -	1 muffin- - - - - - -	45	37	135	3	5	1.5	2.1	1.2
Bran[36]- - - - - - - - - - - - -	1 muffin- - - - - - -	45	35	125	3	6	1.4	1.6	2.3
Corn (enriched, de-germed cornmeal and flour)[35]- - - - - - - - - - -	1 muffin- - - - - - -	45	33	145	3	5	1.5	2.2	1.4
From commercial mix (egg and water added):								
Blueberry- - - - - - - - - -	1 muffin- - - - - - -	45	33	140	3	5	1.4	2.0	1.2
Bran- - - - - - - - - - - - - -	1 muffin- - - - - - -	45	28	140	3	4	1.3	1.6	1.0
Corn- - - - - - - - - - - - - -	1 muffin- - - - - - -	45	30	145	3	6	1.7	2.3	1.4
Noodles (egg noodles), enriched, cooked- - - - - - -	1 cup- - - - - - - - -	160	70	200	7	2	0.5	0.6	0.6
Noodles, chow mein, canned	1 cup- - - - - - - - -	45	11	220	6	11	2.1	7.3	0.4
Pancakes, 4-in diam.:								
Buckwheat, from mix (with buckwheat and enriched flours), egg and milk added- - - - -	1 pancake- - - - - -	27	58	55	2	2	0.9	0.9	0.5
Plain:								
From home recipe using enriched flour- - - - - -	1 pancake- - - - - -	27	50	60	2	2	0.5	0.8	0.5
From mix (with enriched flour), egg, milk, and oil added- - - - - - - - - - - -	1 pancake- - - - - -	27	54	60	2	2	0.5	0.9	0.5
Piecrust, made with enriched flour and vegetable short-ening, baked:								
From home recipe, 9-in diam.- - - - - - - - - - - - -	1 pie shell- - - - - -	180	15	900	11	60	14.8	25.9	15.7
From mix, 9-in diam.- - - -	Piecrust for 2-crust pie- - - - - - - -	320	19	1,485	20	93	22.7	41.0	25.0

(Tr indicates nutrient present in trace amounts.)

Nutrients in Indicated Quantity

Cholesterol	Carbohydrate	Calcium	Phosphorus	Iron	Potassium	Sodium	Vitamin A value		Thiamin	Riboflavin	Niacin	Ascorbic acid
							(IU)	(RE)				
Milligrams	Grams	Milligrams	Milligrams	Milligrams	Milligrams	Milligrams	International units	Retinol equivalents	Milligrams	Milligrams	Milligrams	Milligrams
0	27	96	67	1.7	331	378	0	0	0.26	0.19	2.2	0
0	27	96	67	1.7	331	378	0	0	0.23	0.19	2.2	0
112	17	72	85	1.3	86	257	110	32	0.12	0.16	1.0	Tr
0	39	14	85	2.1	103	1	0	0	0.23	0.13	1.8	0
0	24	8	53	1.3	64	1	0	0	0.15	0.08	1.2	0
0	32	11	70	1.7	85	1	0	0	0.20	0.11	1.5	0
19	20	54	46	0.9	47	198	40	9	0.10	0.11	0.9	1
24	19	60	125	1.4	99	189	230	30	0.11	0.13	1.3	3
23	21	66	59	0.9	57	169	80	15	0.11	0.11	0.9	Tr
45	22	15	90	0.9	54	225	50	11	0.10	0.17	1.1	Tr
28	24	27	182	1.7	50	385	100	14	0.08	0.12	1.9	0
42	22	30	128	1.3	31	291	90	16	0.09	0.09	0.8	Tr
50	37	16	94	2.6	70	3	110	34	0.22	0.13	1.9	0
5	26	14	41	0.4	33	450	0	0	0.05	0.03	0.6	0
20	6	59	91	0.4	66	125	60	17	0.04	0.05	0.2	Tr
16	9	27	38	0.5	33	115	30	10	0.06	0.07	0.5	Tr
16	8	36	71	0.7	43	160	30	7	0.09	0.12	0.8	Tr
0	79	25	90	4.5	90	1,100	0	0	0.54	0.40	5.0	0
0	141	131	272	9.3	179	2,602	0	0	1.06	0.80	9.9	0

Nutritive Values of Foods *(Continued)*

Foods, approximate measures, units, and weight (weight of edible portion only)		Water	Food energy	Pro- tein	Fat	Satu- rated	Fatty Acids Mono- unsatu- rated	Poly- unsatu- rated
		Per- cent	Cal- ories	Grams	Grams	Grams	Grams	Grams
GRAIN PRODUCTS—Con.	Grams							
Pies, piecrust made with enriched flour, vegetable shortening, 9-in diam.:								
Apple:								
Piece, ⅙ of pie- - - - - - - 1 piece- - - - - - - -	158	48	405	3	18	4.6	7.4	4.4
Blueberry:								
Piece, ⅙ of pie- - - - - - - 1 piece- - - - - - - -	158	51	380	4	17	4.3	7.4	4.6
Cherry:								
Piece, ⅙ of pie- - - - - - - 1 piece- - - - - - - -	158	47	410	4	18	4.7	7.7	4.6
Creme:								
Piece, ⅙ of pie- - - - - - - 1 piece- - - - - - - -	152	43	455	3	23	15.0	4.0	1.1
Custard:								
Piece, ⅙ of pie- - - - - - - 1 piece- - - - - - - -	152	58	330	9	17	5.6	6.7	3.2
Lemon meringue:								
Piece, ⅙ of pie- - - - - - - 1 piece- - - - - - - -	140	47	355	5	14	4.3	5.7	2.9
Peach:								
Piece, ⅙ of pie- - - - - - - 1 piece- - - - - - - -	158	48	405	4	17	4.1	7.3	4.4
Pecan:								
Piece, ⅙ of pie- - - - - - - 1 piece- - - - - - - -	138	20	575	7	32	4.7	17.0	7.9
Pumpkin:								
Piece, ⅙ of pie- - - - - - - 1 piece- - - - - - - -	152	59	320	6	17	6.4	6.7	3.0
Pies, fried:								
Apple- - - - - - - - - - - - - - 1 pie - - - - - - - - - -	85	43	255	2	14	5.8	6.6	0.6
Cherry- - - - - - - - - - - - - - 1 pie - - - - - - - - - -	85	42	250	2	14	5.8	6.7	0.6
Popcorn, popped:								
Air-popped, unsalted- - - - 1 cup- - - - - - - - -	8	4	30	1	Tr	Tr	0.1	0.2
Popped in vegetable oil, salted- - - - - - - - - - - - - 1 cup- - - - - - - - -	11	3	55	1	3	0.5	1.4	1.2
Sugar syrup coated- - - - - - 1 cup- - - - - - - - -	35	4	135	2	1	0.1	0.3	0.6
Pretzels, made with enriched flour:								
Stick 2¼ in long- - - - - - - 10 pretzels- - - - - -	3	3	10	Tr	Tr	Tr	Tr	Tr
Twisted, dutch 2¾ by 2⅝ in- - - - - - - - - 1 pretzel- - - - - - -	16	3	65	2	1	0.1	0.2	0.2
Twisted, thin, 3¼ by 2¼ by ¼ in- - - - - - - - - - - - 10 pretzels- - - - - -	60	3	240	6	2	0.4	0.8	0.6
Rice:								
Brown, cooked, served hot- 1 cup- - - - - - - - -	195	70	230	5	1	0.3	0.3	0.4
White enriched:								
Commercial varieties, all types:								
Cooked, served hot - - - 1 cup- - - - - - - - -	205	73	225	4	Tr	0.1	0.1	0.1
Instant, ready-to-serve, hot- - - - - - - - - - - - - 1 cup- - - - - - - - -	165	73	180	4	0	0.1	0.1	0.1
Parboiled:								
Cooked, served hot - - - 1 cup- - - - - - - - -	175	73	185	4	Tr	Tr	Tr	0.1

(Tr indicates nutrient present in trace amounts.)

Nutrients in Indicated Quantity

Cho-les-terol	Carbo-hydrate	Calcium	Phos-phorus	Iron	Potas-sium	Sodium	Vitamin A value		Thiamin	Ribo-flavin	Niacin	Ascorbic acid
							(IU)	(RE)				
Milli-grams	Grams	Milli-grams	Milli-grams	Milli-grams	Milli-grams	Milli-grams	Inter-national units	Retinol equiva-lents	Milli-grams	Milli-grams	Milli-grams	Milli-grams
0	60	13	35	1.6	126	476	50	5	0.17	0.13	1.6	2
0	55	17	36	2.1	158	423	140	14	0.17	0.14	1.7	6
0	61	22	40	1.6	166	480	700	70	0.19	0.14	1.6	0
8	59	46	154	1.1	133	369	210	65	0.06	0.15	1.1	0
169	36	146	172	1.5	208	436	350	96	0.14	0.32	0.9	0
143	53	20	69	1.4	70	395	240	66	0.10	0.14	0.8	4
0	60	16	46	1.9	235	423	1,150	115	0.17	0.16	2.4	5
95	71	65	142	4.6	170	305	220	54	0.30	0.17	1.1	0
109	37	78	105	1.4	243	325	3,750	416	0.14	0.21	1.2	0
14	31	12	34	0.9	42	326	30	3	0.09	0.06	1.0	1
13	32	11	41	0.7	61	371	190	19	0.06	0.06	0.6	1
0	6	1	22	0.2	20	Tr	10	1	0.03	0.01	0.2	0
0	6	3	31	0.3	19	86	20	2	0.01	0.02	0.1	0
0	30	2	47	0.5	90	Tr	30	3	0.13	0.02	0.4	0
0	2	1	3	0.1	3	48	0	0	0.01	0.01	0.1	0
0	13	4	15	0.3	16	258	0	0	0.05	0.04	0.7	0
0	48	16	55	1.2	61	966	0	0	0.19	0.15	2.6	0
0	50	23	142	1.0	137	0	0	0	0.18	0.04	2.7	0
0	50	21	57	1.8	57	0	0	0	0.23	0.02	2.1	0
0	40	5	31	1.3	0	0	0	0	0.21	0.02	1.7	0
0	41	33	100	1.4	75	0	0	0	0.19	0.02	2.1	0

Nutritive Values of Foods *(Continued)*

Foods, approximate measures, units, and weight (weight of edible portion only)		Water	Food energy	Pro-tein	Fat	Fatty Acids		
						Satu-rated	Mono-unsatu-rated	Poly-unsatu-rated
		Per-cent	*Cal-ories*					
GRAIN PRODUCTS—Con.	*Grams*	*cent*	*ories*	*Grams*	*Grams*	*Grams*	*Grams*	*Grams*
Rolls, enriched:								
Commercial:								
Dinner, 2½-in diam., 2 in high- - - - - - - - - - 1 roll- - - - - - - -	28	32	85	2	2	0.5	0.8	0.6
Frankfurter and ham-burger (8 per 11½-oz pkg.)- - - - - - - - - - - - 1 roll- - - - - - - -	40	34	115	3	2	0.5	0.8	0.6
Hard, 3¾-in diam., 2 in high- - - - - - - - - - 1 roll- - - - - - - -	50	25	155	5	2	0.4	0.5	0.6
Hoagie or submarine, 11½ by 3 by 2½ in- - - 1 roll- - - - - - - -	135	31	400	11	8	1.8	3.0	2.2
From home recipe:								
Dinner, 2½-in diam., 2 in high- - - - - - - - - - - - 1 roll- - - - - - - -	35	26	120	3	3	0.8	1.2	0.9
Spaghetti, enriched, cooked:								
Firm stage, "al dente," served hot- - - - - - - - - - 1 cup- - - - - - - -	130	64	190	7	1	0.1	0.1	0.3
Tortillas, corn- - - - - - - - - - 1 tortilla- - - - - - -	30	45	65	2	1	0.1	0.3	0.6
Waffles, made with enriched flour, 7-in diam.:								
From home recipe- - - - - - 1 waffle- - - - - - - -	75	37	245	7	13	4.0	4.9	2.6
From mix, egg and milk added- - - - - - - - - - - - - 1 waffle- - - - - - - -	75	42	205	7	8	2.7	2.9	1.5
Wheat flours:								
All-purpose or family flour, enriched:								
Sifted, spooned- - - - - - - 1 cup- - - - - - - - -	115	12	420	12	1	0.2	0.1	0.5
Cake or pastry flour, enriched, sifted, spooned- - - - - - - - - - - 1 cup- - - - - - - -	96	12	350	7	1	0.1	0.1	0.3
Self-rising, enriched, unsifted, spooned- - - - 1 cup- - - - - - - - -	125	12	440	12	1	0.2	0.1	0.5
Whole-wheat, from hard wheats, stirred- - - - - 1 cup- - - - - - - - -	120	12	400	16	2	0.3	0.3	1.1
LEGUMES, NUTS, AND SEEDS								
Almonds, shelled:								
Slivered, packed- - - - - - - 1 cup - - - - - - - -	135	4	795	27	70	6.7	45.8	14.8
Whole- - - - - - - - - - - - - - 1 oz- - - - - - - - - -	28	4	165	6	15	1.4	9.6	3.1
Beans, dry:								
Cooked, drained:								
Black- - - - - - - - - - - - 1 cup- - - - - - - - -	171	66	225	15	1	0.1	0.1	0.5
Great Northern- - - - - - 1 cup - - - - - - - - -	180	69	210	14	1	0.1	0.1	0.6
Lima- - - - - - - - - - - - 1 cup- - - - - - - - -	190	64	260	16	1	0.2	0.1	0.5
Pea (navy)- - - - - - - - - 1 cup- - - - - - - - -	190	69	225	15	1	0.1	0.1	0.7
Pinto- - - - - - - - - - - - 1 cup- - - - - - - - -	180	65	265	15	1	0.1	0.1	0.5

(Tr indicates nutrient present in trace amounts.)

Nutrients in Indicated Quantity

Cholesterol	Carbohydrate	Calcium	Phosphorus	Iron	Potassium	Sodium	Vitamin A value		Thiamin	Riboflavin	Niacin	Ascorbic acid
							(IU)	(RE)				
Milligrams	Grams	Milligrams	Milligrams	Milligrams	Milligrams	Milligrams	International units	Retinol equivalents	Milligrams	Milligrams	Milligrams	Milligrams
Tr	14	33	44	0.8	36	155	Tr	Tr	0.14	0.09	1.1	Tr
Tr	20	54	44	1.2	56	241	Tr	Tr	0.20	0.13	1.6	Tr
Tr	30	24	46	1.4	49	313	0	0	0.20	0.12	1.7	0
Tr	72	100	115	3.8	128	683	0	0	0.54	0.33	4.5	0
12	20	16	36	1.1	41	98	30	8	0.12	0.12	1.2	0
0	39	14	85	2.0	103	1	0	0	0.23	0.13	1.8	0
0	13	42	55	0.6	43	1	80	8	0.05	0.03	0.4	0
102	26	154	135	1.5	129	445	140	39	0.18	0.24	1.5	Tr
59	27	179	257	1.2	146	515	170	49	0.14	0.23	0.9	Tr
0	88	18	100	5.1	109	2	0	0	0.73	0.46	6.1	0
0	76	16	70	4.2	91	2	0	0	0.58	0.38	5.1	0
0	93	331	583	5.5	113	1,349	0	0	0.80	0.50	6.6	0
0	85	49	446	5.2	444	4	0	0	0.66	0.14	5.2	0
0	28	359	702	4.9	988	15	0	0	0.28	1.05	4.5	1
0	6	75	147	1.0	208	3	0	0	0.06	0.22	1.0	Tr
0	41	47	239	2.9	608	1	Tr	Tr	0.43	0.05	0.9	0
0	38	90	266	4.9	749	13	0	0	0.25	0.13	1.3	0
0	49	55	293	5.9	1,163	4	0	0	0.25	0.11	1.3	0
0	40	95	281	5.1	790	13	0	0	0.27	0.13	1.3	0
0	49	86	296	5.4	882	3	Tr	Tr	0.33	0.16	0.7	0

Nutritive Values of Foods *(Continued)*

Foods, approximate measures, units, and weight (weight of edible portion only)		Water	Food energy	Pro-tein	Fat	Satu-rated	Mono-unsatu-rated	Poly-unsatu-rated
							Fatty Acids	
LEGUMES, NUTS, AND SEEDS—Con.	Grams	Per-cent	Cal-ories	Grams	Grams	Grams	Grams	Grams
Canned, solids and liquid:								
White with:								
Frankfurters (sliced)-	1 cup- - - - - - - - -	255	71	365	19	18	7.4	8.8	0.7
Pork and tomato									
sauce- - - - - - - - - -	1 cup- - - - - - - - -	255	71	310	16	7	2.4	2.7	0.7
Pork and sweet sauce-	1 cup- - - - - - - - -	255	66	385	16	12	4.3	4.9	1.2
Red kidney- - - - - - - - -	1 cup- - - - - - - - -	255	76	230	15	1	0.1	0.1	0.6
Black-eyed peas, dry, cooked									
(with residual cooking									
liquid)- - - - - - - - - - - - -	1 cup- - - - - - - - -	250	80	190	13	1	0.2	Tr	0.3
Brazil nuts, shelled- - - - - - -	1 oz- - - - - - - - - -	28	3	185	4	19	4.6	6.5	6.8
Carob flour- - - - - - - - - - - -	1 cup- - - - - - - - -	140	3	255	6	Tr	Tr	0.1	0.1
Cashew nuts, salted:									
Dry roasted- - - - - - - - - - -	1 oz- - - - - - - - - -	28	2	165	4	13	2.6	7.7	2.2
Roasted in oil- - - - - - - - -	1 oz- - - - - - - - - -	28	4	165	5	14	2.7	8.1	2.3
Chestnuts, European									
(Italian), roasted,									
shelled- - - - - - - - - - - - -	1 cup- - - - - - - - -	143	40	350	5	3	0.6	1.1	1.2
Chickpeas, cooked, drained-	1 cup- - - - - - - - -	163	60	270	15	4	0.4	0.9	1.9
Coconut:									
Raw:									
Piece, about 2 by									
2 by ½ in- - - - - - - - -	1 piece- - - - - - - -	45	47	160	1	15	13.4	0.6	0.2
Dried, sweetened,									
shredded- - - - - - - - -	1 cup- - - - - - - - -	93	13	470	3	33	29.3	1.4	0.4
Filberts (hazelnuts),									
chopped- - - - - - - - - - - -	1 oz- - - - - - - - - -	28	5	180	4	18	1.3	13.9	1.7
Lentils, dry, cooked- - - - - -	1 cup- - - - - - - - -	200	72	215	16	1	0.1	0.2	0.5
Macadamia nuts, roasted in									
oil, salted- - - - - - - - - - -	1 oz- - - - - - - - - -	28	2	205	2	22	3.2	17.1	0.4
Mixed nuts, with peanuts,									
salted:									
Dry roasted- - - - - - - - - -	1 oz- - - - - - - - - -	28	2	170	5	15	2.0	8.9	3.1
Roasted in oil- - - - - - - -	1 oz- - - - - - - - - -	28	2	175	5	16	2.5	9.0	3.8
Peanuts, roasted in oil,									
salted- - - - - - - - - - - - - -	1 oz- - - - - - - - - -	28	2	165	8	14	1.9	6.9	4.4
Peanut butter- - - - - - - - - -	1 tbsp- - - - - - - - -	16	1	95	5	8	1.4	4.0	2.5
Peas, split, dry, cooked- - - -	1 cup- - - - - - - - -	200	70	230	16	1	0.1	0.1	0.3
Pecans, halves- - - - - - - - -	1 oz- - - - - - - - - -	28	5	190	2	19	1.5	12.0	4.7
Pine nuts (pinyons), shelled-	1 oz- - - - - - - - - -	28	6	160	3	17	2.7	6.5	7.3
Pistachio nuts, dried, shelled	1 oz- - - - - - - - - -	28	4	165	6	14	1.7	9.3	2.1
Pumpkin and squash kernels,									
dry, hulled- - - - - - - - - - -	1 oz- - - - - - - - - -	28	7	155	7	13	2.5	4.0	5.9
Refried beans, canned- - - - -	1 cup- - - - - - - - -	290	72	295	18	3	0.4	0.6	1.4
Sesame seeds, dry, hulled- - -	1 tbsp- - - - - - - - -	8	5	45	2	4	0.6	1.7	1.9
Soybeans, dry, cooked,									
drained- - - - - - - - - - - - -	1 cup- - - - - - - - -	180	71	235	20	10	1.3	1.9	5.3

(Tr indicates nutrient present in trace amounts.)

Nutrients in Indicated Quantity

Cholesterol	Carbohydrate	Calcium	Phosphorus	Iron	Potassium	Sodium	Vitamin A value		Thiamin	Riboflavin	Niacin	Ascorbic acid
							(IU)	(RE)				
Milligrams	Grams	Milligrams	Milligrams	Milligrams	Milligrams	Milligrams	International units	Retinol equivalents	Milligrams	Milligrams	Milligrams	Milligrams
30	32	94	303	4.8	668	1,374	330	33	0.18	0.15	3.3	Tr
10	48	138	235	4.6	536	1,181	330	33	0.20	0.08	1.5	5
10	54	161	291	5.9	536	969	330	33	0.15	0.10	1.3	5
0	42	74	278	4.6	673	968	10	1	0.13	0.10	1.5	0
0	35	43	238	3.3	573	20	30	3	0.40	0.10	1.0	0
0	4	50	170	1.0	170	1	Tr	Tr	0.28	0.03	0.5	Tr
0	126	390	102	5.7	1,275	24	Tr	Tr	0.07	0.07	2.2	Tr
0	9	13	139	1.7	160	[41]181	0	0	0.06	0.06	0.4	0
0	8	12	121	1.2	150	[42]177	0	0	0.12	0.05	0.5	0
0	76	41	153	1.3	847	3	30	3	0.35	0.25	1.9	37
0	45	80	273	4.9	475	11	Tr	Tr	0.18	0.09	0.9	0
0	7	6	51	1.1	160	9	0	0	0.03	0.01	0.2	1
0	44	14	99	1.8	313	244	0	0	0.03	0.02	0.4	1
0	4	53	88	0.9	126	1	20	2	0.14	0.03	0.3	Tr
0	38	50	238	4.2	498	26	40	4	0.14	0.12	1.2	0
0	4	13	57	0.5	93	[43]74	Tr	Tr	0.06	0.03	0.6	0
0	7	20	123	1.0	169	[44]190	Tr	Tr	0.06	0.06	1.3	0
0	6	31	131	0.9	165	[44]185	10	1	0.14	0.06	1.4	Tr
0	5	24	143	0.5	199	[45]122	0	0	0.08	0.03	4.2	0
0	3	5	60	0.3	110	75	0	0	0.02	0.02	2.2	0
0	42	22	178	3.4	592	26	80	8	0.30	0.18	1.8	0
0	5	10	83	0.6	111	Tr	40	4	0.24	0.04	0.3	1
0	5	2	10	0.9	178	20	10	1	0.35	0.06	1.2	1
0	7	38	143	1.9	310	2	70	7	0.23	0.05	0.3	Tr
0	5	12	333	4.2	229	5	110	11	0.06	0.09	0.5	Tr
0	51	141	245	5.1	1,141	1,228	0	0	0.14	0.16	1.4	17
0	1	11	62	0.6	33	3	10	1	0.06	0.01	0.4	0
0	19	131	322	4.9	972	4	50	5	0.38	0.16	1.1	0

Nutritive Values of Foods *(Continued)*

Foods, approximate measures, units, and weight (weight of edible portion only)		Water	Food energy	Pro- tein	Fat	Fatty Acids		
						Satu- rated	Mono- unsatu- rated	Poly- unsatu- rated
		Per- cent	*Cal- ories*	*Grams*	*Grams*	*Grams*	*Grams*	*Grams*
LEGUMES, NUTS, AND SEEDS—Con.	*Grams*							
Soy products:								
Miso- - - - - - - - - - - - - - - 1 cup- - - - - - - - -	276	53	470	29	13	1.8	2.6	7.3
Tofu, piece 2½ by 2¾								
by 1 in- - - - - - - - - - - 1 piece- - - - - - - -	120	85	85	9	5	0.7	1.0	2.9
Sunflower seeds, dry, hulled- 1 oz- - - - - - - - - -	28	5	160	6	14	1.5	2.7	9.3
Tahini- - - - - - - - - - - - - - - 1 tbsp- - - - - - - - -	15	3	90	3	8	1.1	3.0	3.5
Walnuts:								
Black, chopped- - - - - - - - 1 oz- - - - - - - - - -	28	4	170	7	16	1.0	3.6	10.6
English or Persian, pieces								
or chips- - - - - - - - - - - - 1 oz- - - - - - - - - -	28	4	180	4	18	1.6	4.0	11.1
MEAT AND MEAT PRODUCTS								
Beef, cooked:[46]								
Cuts braised, simmered, or								
pot roasted:								
Relatively fat such as								
chuck blade:								
Lean and fat, piece, 2½								
by 2½ by ¾ in - - - 3 oz - - - - - -	85	46	222	25	13	4.8	5.7	0.5
Lean only - - - - - - 2.2 oz - - - - - -	62	53	170	19	9.5	3.9	4.2	0.3
Relatively lean, such as								
bottom round:								
Lean and fat, piece, 4⅛								
by 2¼ by ½ in - - - 3 oz - - - - - -	85	54	220	25	13	4.8	5.7	0.5
Lean only - - - - - - 2.8 oz - - - - - -	78	57	175	25	7.7	2.7	3.4	0.3
Ground beef, broiled, patty,								
3 by ⅝ in:								
Lean- - - - - - - - - - - - - - 3 oz- - - - - - - - - -	85	56	230	21	16	6.2	6.9	0.6
Regular- - - - - - - - - - - - 3 oz- - - - - - - - - -	85	54	245	20	18	6.9	7.7	0.7
Liver, fried, slice, 6½ by 2⅜								
by ⅜ in[47]- - - - - - - - 3 oz- - - - - - - - - -	85	56	185	23	7	2.5	3.6	1.3
Roast, oven cooked, no liq-								
uid added:								
Relatively fat, such as rib:								
Lean and fat, 2 pieces,								
4¼ by 2¼ by ¼ in - - 3 oz - - - - - -	85	46	324	19	27	11.4	12.1	0.9
Lean only - - - - - - 2.2 oz - - - - - -	61	57	150	17	8.5	3.6	3.7	0.3
Relatively lean, such as								
eye of round:								
Lean and fat, 2 pieces,								
2½ by 2½ by ⅜ in - - 3 oz- - - - - - - - - -	85	57	205	23	12	4.9	5.4	0.5
Lean only- - - - - - - - 2.6 oz- - - - - - - - -	75	63	135	22	5	1.9	2.1	0.2
Steak:								
Sirloin, broiled:								
Lean and fat, piece, 2½								
by 2½ by ¾ in - - - 3 oz - - - - - -	85	53	240	23	15	6.4	6.9	0.6
Lean only - - - - - - 2.5 oz - - - - - -	72	59	150	22	6	2.6	2.8	0.3
Beef, canned, corned - - - - 3 oz - - - - - -	85	59	2.3	23	13	5.3	5.1	0.5

(Tr indicates nutrient present in trace amounts.)

Nutrients in Indicated Quantity

Cho-les-terol	Carbo-hydrate	Calcium	Phos-phorus	Iron	Potas-sium	Sodium	Vitamin A value		Thiamin	Ribo-flavin	Niacin	Ascorbic acid
							(IU)	(RE)				
Milli-grams	Grams	Milli-grams	Milli-grams	Milli-grams	Milli-grams	Milli-grams	Inter-national units	Retinol equiva-lents	Milli-grams	Milli-grams	Milli-grams	Milli-grams
0	65	188	853	4.7	922	8,142	110	11	0.17	0.28	0.8	0
0	3	108	151	2.3	50	8	0	0	0.07	0.04	0.1	0
0	5	33	200	1.9	195	1	10	1	0.65	0.07	1.3	Tr
0	3	21	119	0.7	69	5	10	1	0.24	0.02	0.8	1
0	3	16	132	0.9	149	Tr	80	8	0.06	0.03	0.2	Tr
0	5	27	90	0.7	142	3	40	4	0.11	0.04	0.3	1
81	0	5	217	2.8	248	43	Tr	Tr	0.06	0.21	3.29	0
66	0	8	146	2.3	163	44	Tr	Tr	0.05	0.17	1.7	0
81	0	5	217	2.8	248	43	Tr	Tr	0.06	0.21	3.3	0
75	0	4	216	2.7	240	40	Tr	Tr	0.06	0.20	3.2	0
74	0	9	134	1.8	256	65	Tr	Tr	0.04	0.18	4.4	0
76	0	9	144	2.1	248	70	Tr	Tr	0.03	0.16	4.9	0
410	7	9	392	5.3	309	90	[46]30,690	[46]9,120	0.18	3.52	12.3	23
72	0	10	145	1.8	250	54	Tr	Tr	0.06	0.15	2.8	0
50	0	5	127	1.7	218	45	Tr	Tr	0.05	0.13	2.7	0
62	0	5	177	1.6	308	50	Tr	Tr	0.07	0.14	3.0	0
52	0	3	170	1.5	297	46	Tr	Tr	0.07	0.13	2.8	0
77	0	9	186	2.6	306	53	Tr	Tr	0.10	0.23	3.3	0
64	0	8	176	2.4	290	48	Tr	Tr	0.09	0.22	3.1	0
73	0	17	94	1.7	116	856	Tr	Tr	0.02	0.20	2.0	0

Nutritive Values of Foods *(Continued)*

Foods, approximate measures, units, and weight (weight of edible portion only)		Water	Food energy	Pro-tein	Fat	Fatty Acids		
						Satu-rated	Mono-unsatu-rated	Poly-unsatu-rated
	Grams	Per-cent	Cal-ories	Grams	Grams	Grams	Grams	Grams
MEAT AND MEAT PRODUCTS—Con.								
Beef, dried, chipped - - - - - - 2.5 oz - - - - - - - - -	72	48	145	24	4	1.8	2.0	0.2
Lamb, cooked:								
Chops, (3 per lb with bone):								
Arm, braised:								
Lean and fat - - - - - - 2.2 oz - - - - - - - - -	63	44	220	20	15	6.9	6.0	0.9
Lean only - - - - - - - - 1.7 oz - - - - - - - - -	48	49	135	17	7	2.9	2.6	0.4
Loin, broiled:								
Lean and fat - - - - - - 2.8 oz - - - - - - - - -	80	54	235	22	16	7.3	6.4	1.0
Lean only - - - - - - - - 2.3 oz - - - - - - - - -	64	61	140	19	6	2.6	2.4	0.4
Leg, roasted:								
Lean and fat, 2 pieces, 4⅛								
by 2¼ by ¼ in - - - - - 3 oz - - - - - - - - - -	85	59	205	22	13	5.6	4.9	0.8
Lean only - - - - - - - - - 2.6 oz - - - - - - - -	73	64	140	20	6	2.4	2.2	0.4
Rib, roasted:								
Lean and fat, 3 pieces, 2½								
by 2½ by ¼ in - - - - - 3 oz - - - - - - - - - -	85	47	315	18	26	12.1	10.6	1.5
Lean only - - - - - - - - - 2 oz - - - - - - - - - -	57	60	130	15	7	3.2	3.0	0.5
Pork, cured, cooked:								
Bacon:								
Regular - - - - - - - - - - - 3 medium slices - -	19	13	110	6	9	3.3	4.5	1.1
Canadian-style - - - - - - - 2 slices - - - - - - - -	46	62	85	11	4	1.3	1.9	0.4
Ham, light cure, roasted:								
Lean and fat, 2 pieces, 4⅛								
by 2¼ by ¼ in - - - - - - 3 oz - - - - - - - - - -	85	58	205	18	14	5.1	6.7	1.5
Lean only - - - - - - - - - 2.4 oz - - - - - - - -	68	66	105	17	4	1.3	1.7	0.4
Luncheon meat:								
Canned, spiced or un-spiced, slice, 3 by 2 by ½								
in - - - - - - - - - - - - - 2 slices - - - - - - - -	42	52	140	5	13	4.5	6.0	1.5
Cooked ham (8 slices per 8-oz pkg):								
Regular - - - - - - - - - 2 slices - - - - - - - -	57	65	105	10	6	1.9	2.8	0.7
Extra lean - - - - - - - - 2 slices - - - - - - - -	57	71	75	11	3	0.9	1.3	0.3
Pork, fresh, cooked:								
Chop, loin (cut 3 per lb with bone):								
Broiled:								
Lean and fat - - - - - - 3.1 oz - - - - - - - - -	87	50	275	24	19	7.0	8.8	2.2
Lean only - - - - - - - - 2.5 oz - - - - - - - - -	72	57	165	23	8	2.6	3.4	0.9
Pan fried:								
Lean and fat - - - - - - 3.1 oz - - - - - - - - -	89	45	335	21	27	9.8	12.5	3.1
Lean only - - - - - - - - 2.4 oz - - - - - - - - -	67	54	180	19	11	3.7	4.8	1.3
Ham (leg), roasted:								
Lean and fat, piece, 2½ by								
2½ by ¾ in - - - - - - 3 oz - - - - - - - - - -	85	53	250	21	18	6.4	8.1	2.0
Lean only - - - - - - - - - 2.5 oz - - - - - - - -	72	60	160	20	8	2.7	3.6	1.0

(Tr indicates nutrient present in trace amounts.)

Nutrients in Indicated Quantity

Cho-les-terol	Carbo-hydrate	Calcium	Phos-phorus	Iron	Potas-sium	Sodium	Vitamin A Value		Thiamin	Ribo-flavin	Niacin	Ascorbic acid
							(IU)	(RE)				
Milli-grams	Grams	Milli-grams	Milli-grams	Milli-grams	Milli-grams	Milli-grams	Inter-national units	Retinol equiva-lents	Milli-grams	Milli-grams	Milli-grams	Milli-grams
46	0	14	287	2.3	142	3,053	Tr	Tr	0.05	0.23	2.7	0
77	0	16	132	1.5	195	46	Tr	Tr	0.04	0.16	4.4	0
59	0	12	111	1.3	162	36	Tr	Tr	0.03	0.13	3.0	0
78	0	16	162	1.4	272	62	Tr	Tr	0.09	0.21	5.5	0
60	0	12	145	1.3	241	54	Tr	Tr	0.08	0.18	4.4	0
78	0	8	162	1.7	273	57	Tr	Tr	0.09	0.24	5.5	0
65	0	6	150	1.5	247	50	Tr	Tr	0.08	0.20	4.6	0
77	0	19	139	1.4	224	60	Tr	Tr	0.08	0.18	5.5	0
50	0	12	111	1.0	179	46	Tr	Tr	0.05	0.13	3.5	0
16	Tr	2	64	0.3	92	303	0	0	0.13	0.05	1.4	6
27	1	5	136	0.4	179	711	0	0	0.38	0.09	3.2	10
53	0	6	182	0.7	243	1,009	0	0	0.51	0.19	3.8	0
37	0	5	154	0.6	215	902	0	0	0.46	0.17	3.4	0
26	1	3	34	0.3	90	541	0	0	0.15	0.08	1.3	Tr
32	2	4	141	0.6	189	751	0	0	0.49	0.14	3.0	*16
27	1	4	124	0.4	200	815	0	0	0.53	0.13	2.8	*15
84	0	3	184	0.7	312	61	10	3	0.87	0.24	4.3	Tr
71	0	4	176	0.7	302	56	10	1	0.83	0.22	4.0	Tr
92	0	4	190	0.7	323	64	10	3	0.91	0.24	4.6	Tr
72	0	3	178	0.7	305	57	10	1	0.84	0.22	4.0	Tr
79	0	5	210	0.9	280	50	10	2	0.54	0.27	3.9	Tr
68	0	5	202	0.8	269	46	10	1	0.50	0.25	3.6	Tr

Nutritive Value of Foods *(Continued)*

Foods, approximate measures, units, and weight (weight of edible portion only)		Water	Food energy	Pro-tein	Fat	Fatty Acids		
						Satu-rated	Mono-unsatu-rated	Poly-unsatu-rated
		Per-cent	*Cal-ories*	*Grams*	*Grams*	*Grams*	*Grams*	*Grams*
MEAT AND MEAT PRODUCTS—Con.	*Grams*							
Rib, roasted:								
Lean and fat, piece, 2½ by								
¾ in - - - - - - - - - - 3 oz - - - - - - - - - -	85	51	270	21	20	7.2	9.2	2.3
Lean only - - - - - - - - - 2.5 oz - - - - - - - -	71	57	175	20	10	3.4	4.4	1.2
Shoulder cut, braised:								
Lean and fat, 3 pieces, 2½								
by 2½ by ¼ in - - - - 3 oz - - - - - - - - - -	85	47	295	23	22	7.9	10.0	2.4
Lean only - - - - - - - - - 2.4 oz - - - - - - - -	67	54	165	22	8	2.8	3.7	1.0
Sausages (See also Luncheon meats):								
Bologna, slice (8 per 8-oz								
pkg) - - - - - - - - - - - - 2 slices - - - - - - - -	57	54	180	7	16	6.1	7.6	1.4
Braunschweiger, slice (6 per								
6-oz pkg) - - - - - - - - - 2 slices - - - - - - - -	57	48	205	8	18	6.2	8.5	2.1
Brown and serve (10–11 per								
8-oz pkg), browned - - - 1 link - - - - - - - - -	13	45	50	2	5	1.7	2.2	0.5
Frankfurter (10 per 1-lb pkg), cooked (reheated) - - - - - - 1 beef frankfurter (2 oz ea) - - - -	57	31	184	6	17	6.8	8.2	0.6
Frankfurter - - - - - - - 1 turkey - - - - -	45	28	102	6	8.2	2.7	3.3	2.1
Pork link (16 per 1-lb pkg), cooked[60] - - - - - - - - - - 1 link - - - - - - - - -	13	45	50	3	4	1.4	1.8	0.5
Salami:								
Cooked type, slice (8 per								
8-oz pkg) - - - - - - - - - 2 slices - - - - - - - -	57	60	145	8	11	4.6	5.2	1.2
Dry type, slice (12 per								
4-oz pkg) - - - - - - - - - 2 slices - - - - - - - -	20	35	85	5	7	2.4	3.4	0.6
Sandwich spread (pork,								
beef) - - - - - - - - - - - - 1 tbsp - - - - - - - -	15	60	35	1	3	0.9	1.1	0.4
Vienna sausage (7 per 4-oz								
can) - - - - - - - - - - - - 1 sausage - - - - - -	16	60	45	2	4	1.5	2.0	0.3
Veal, medium fat, cooked, bone removed:								
Cutlet, 4⅛ by 2¼ by ½ in,								
braised or broiled - - - - 3 oz - - - - - - - - - -	85	60	185	23	9	4.1	4.1	0.6
Rib, 2 pieces, 4⅛ by 2¼ by ¼								
in, roasted - - - - - - - - - - 3 oz - - - - - - - - - -	85	55	230	23	14	6.0	6.0	1.0
MIXED DISHES AND FAST FOODS								
Mixed dishes:								
Chicken potpie, from home recipe, baked, piece, ⅓								
of 9-in diam. pie[61] - - - 1 piece - - - - - - - -	232	57	545	23	31	10.3	15.5	6.6
Chili con carne with beans,								
canned - - - - - - - - - - - 1 cup - - - - - - - - -	255	72	340	19	16	5.8	7.2	1.0
Chop suey with beef and pork, from home								
recipe - - - - - - - - - - - 1 cup - - - - - - - -	250	75	300	26	17	4.3	7.4	4.2

(Tr indicates nutrient present in trace amounts.)

Nutrients in Indicated Quantity

| Cho-les-terol | Carbo-hydrate | Calcium | Phos-phorus | Iron | Potas-sium | Sodium | Vitamin A value | | Thiamin | Ribo-flavin | Niacin | Ascorbic acid |
| | | | | | | | (IU) | (RE) | | | | |
Milli-grams	Grams	Milli-grams	Milli-grams	Milli-grams	Milli-grams	Milli-grams	Inter-national units	Retinol equiva-lents	Milli-grams	Milli-grams	Milli-grams	Milli-grams
69	0	9	190	0.8	313	37	10	3	0.50	0.24	4.2	Tr
56	0	8	182	0.7	300	33	10	2	0.45	0.22	3.8	Tr
93	0	6	162	1.4	286	75	10	3	0.46	0.26	4.4	Tr
76	0	5	151	1.3	271	68	10	1	0.40	0.24	4.0	Tr
31	2	7	52	0.9	103	581	0	0	0.10	0.08	1.5	*12
89	2	5	96	5.3	113	652	8,010	2,405	0.14	0.87	4.8	*6
9	Tr	1	14	0.1	25	105	0	0	0.05	0.02	0.4	0
27	1	0.03	47	0.8	90	584	0	0	0.02	0.06	1.4	14
39	0.7	48	70	0.8	84	454	170	17	0.18	0.08	1.9	0
11	Tr	4	24	0.2	47	168	0	0	0.10	0.03	0.6	Tr
37	1	7	66	1.5	113	607	0	0	0.14	0.21	2.0	*7
16	1	2	28	0.3	76	372	0	0	0.12	0.06	1.0	*5
6	2	2	9	0.1	17	152	10	1	0.03	0.02	0.3	0
8	Tr	2	8	0.1	16	152	0	0	0.01	0.02	0.3	0
109	0	9	196	0.8	258	56	Tr	Tr	0.06	0.21	4.6	0
109	0	10	211	0.7	259	57	Tr	Tr	0.11	0.26	6.6	0
56	42	70	232	3.0	343	594	7,220	735	0.32	0.32	4.9	5
28	31	82	321	4.3	594	1,354	150	15	0.08	0.18	3.3	8
68	13	60	248	4.8	425	1,053	600	60	0.28	0.38	5.0	33

Nutritive Values of Foods *(Continued)*

Foods, approximate measures, units, and weight (weight of edible portion only)			Water	Food energy	Pro-tein	Fat	Fatty Acids		
							Satu-rated	Mono-unsatu-rated	Poly-unsatu-rated
		Grams	Per-cent	Cal-ories	Grams	Grams	Grams	Grams	Grams
MIXED DISHES AND FAST FOODS—Con.									
Macaroni (enriched) and cheese:									
Canned[52]	1 cup	240	80	230	9	10	4.7	2.9	1.3
Quiche Lorraine, ⅛ of 8-in diam. quiche[51]	1 slice	176	47	600	13	48	23.2	17.8	4.1
Spaghetti (enriched) in to-mato sauce with cheese:									
Canned	1 cup	250	80	190	6	2	0.4	0.4	0.5
From home recipe	1 cup	250	77	260	9	9	3.0	3.6	1.2
Spaghetti (enriched) with meatballs and tomato sauce:									
From home recipe	1 cup	248	70	330	19	12	3.9	4.4	2.2
Fast food entrees:									
Cheeseburger:									
Regular	1 sandwich	112	46	300	15	15	7.3	5.6	1.0
4 oz patty	1 sandwich	194	46	525	30	31	15.1	12.2	1.4
Chicken, fried. See Poultry and Poultry Products.									
Enchilada	1 enchilada	230	72	235	20	16	7.7	6.7	0.6
English muffin, egg, cheese, and bacon	1 sandwich	138	49	360	18	18	8.0	8.0	0.7
Fish sandwich:									
Regular, with cheese	1 sandwich	140	43	420	16	23	6.3	6.9	7.7
Large, without cheese	1 sandwich	170	48	470	18	27	6.3	8.7	9.5
Hamburger:									
Regular	1 sandwich	98	46	245	12	11	4.4	5.3	0.5
4 oz patty	1 sandwich	174	50	445	25	21	7.1	11.7	0.6
Pizza, cheese, ⅛ of 15-in diam. pizza[51]	1 slice	120	46	290	15	9	4.1	2.6	1.3
Roast beef sandwich	1 sandwich	150	52	345	22	13	3.5	6.9	1.8
Taco	1 taco	81	55	195	9	11	4.1	5.5	0.8
POULTRY AND POULTRY PRODUCTS									
Chicken:									
Fried, flesh, with skin:[53]									
Batter dipped:									
Breast, ½ breast (5.6 oz with bones)	4.9 oz	140	52	365	35	18	4.9	7.6	4.3
Drumstick (3.4 oz with bones)	2.5 oz	72	53	195	16	11	3.0	4.6	2.7
Flour coated:									
Breast, ½ breast (4.2 oz with bones)	3.5 oz	98	57	220	31	9	2.4	3.4	1.9
Drumstick (2.6 oz with bones)	1.7 oz	49	57	120	13	7	1.8	2.7	1.6

(Tr indicates nutrient present in trace amounts.)

Nutrients in Indicated Quantity

Cholesterol	Carbohydrate	Calcium	Phosphorus	Iron	Potassium	Sodium	Vitamin A value (IU)	Vitamin A value (RE)	Thiamin	Riboflavin	Niacin	Ascorbic acid
Milligrams	Grams	Milligrams	Milligrams	Milligrams	Milligrams	Milligrams	International units	Retinol equivalents	Milligrams	Milligrams	Milligrams	Milligrams
24	26	199	182	1.0	139	730	260	72	0.12	0.24	1.0	Tr
285	29	211	276	1.0	283	653	1,640	454	0.11	0.32	Tr	Tr
3	39	40	88	2.8	303	955	930	120	0.35	0.28	4.5	10
8	37	80	135	2.3	408	955	1,080	140	0.25	0.18	2.3	13
89	39	124	236	3.7	665	1,009	1,590	159	0.25	0.30	4.0	22
44	28	135	174	2.3	219	672	340	65	0.26	0.24	3.7	1
104	40	236	320	4.5	407	1,224	670	128	0.33	0.48	7.4	3
19	24	97	198	3.3	653	1,332	2,720	352	0.18	0.26	Tr	Tr
213	31	197	290	3.1	201	832	650	160	0.46	0.50	3.7	1
56	39	132	223	1.8	274	667	160	25	0.32	0.26	3.3	2
91	41	61	246	2.2	375	621	110	15	0.35	0.23	3.5	1
32	28	56	107	2.2	202	463	80	14	0.23	0.24	3.8	1
71	38	75	225	4.8	404	763	160	28	0.38	0.38	7.8	1
56	39	220	216	1.6	230	699	750	106	0.34	0.29	4.2	2
55	34	60	222	4.0	338	757	240	32	0.40	0.33	6.0	2
21	15	109	134	1.2	263	456	420	57	0.09	0.07	1.4	1
119	13	28	259	1.8	281	385	90	28	0.16	0.20	14.7	0
62	6	12	106	1.0	134	194	60	19	0.08	0.15	3.7	0
87	2	16	228	1.2	254	74	50	15	0.08	0.13	13.5	0
44	1	6	86	0.7	112	44	40	12	0.04	0.11	3.0	0

Nutritive Values of Foods *(Continued)*

Foods, approximate measures, units, and weight (weight of edible portion only)		Water	Food energy	Pro- tein	Fat	Satu- rated	Mono- unsatu- rated	Poly- unsatu- rated
							Fatty Acids	
POULTRY AND POULTRY PRODUCTS—Con.	Grams	*Per- cent*	*Cal- ories*	Grams	Grams	Grams	Grams	Grams
Roasted, flesh only:								
Breast, ½ breast (4.2 oz with bones								
and skin)- - - - - - - - 3.0 oz- - - - - - - - -	86	65	140	27	3	0.9	1.1	0.7
Drumstick, (2.9 oz with								
bones and skin)- - - 1.6 oz- - - - - - - - -	44	67	75	12	2	0.7	0.8	0.6
Stewed, flesh only, light and dark meat, chopped								
or diced- - - - - - - - - 1 cup- - - - - - - - -	140	67	250	38	9	2.6	3.3	2.2
Chicken liver, cooked- - - - - 1 liver- - - - - - - - -	20	68	30	5	1	0.4	0.3	0.2
Duck, roasted, flesh only- - - ½ duck- - - - - - - -	221	64	445	52	25	9.2	8.2	3.2
Turkey, roasted, flesh only:								
Dark meat, piece, 2½ by 1⅝ by ¼ in- - - - - - - - - - - - 4 pieces- - - - - - - -	85	63	160	24	6	2.1	1.4	1.8
Light meat, piece, 4 by 2 by ¼ in- - - - - - - - - - - - - 2 pieces- - - - - - - -	85	66	135	25	3	0.9	0.5	0.7
Poultry food products:								
Turkey:								
Loaf, breast meat (8 slices per 6-oz pkg)- - - - - - 2 slices- - - - - - - -	42	72	45	10	1	0.2	0.2	0.1
Roast, boneless, frozen, seasoned, light and dark meat, cooked- - - 3 oz- - - - - - - - - -	85	68	130	18	5	1.6	1.0	1.4
SOUPS, SAUCES, AND GRAVIES								
Soups:								
Canned, condensed:								
Prepared with equal vol- ume of milk:								
Clam chowder, New England- - - - - - - - 1 cup- - - - - - - - -	248	85	165	9	7	3.0	2.3	1.1
Cream of chicken- - - - 1 cup- - - - - - - - -	248	85	190	7	11	4.6	4.5	1.6
Cream of mushroom- - 1 cup- - - - - - - - -	248	85	205	6	14	5.1	3.0	4.6
Tomato- - - - - - - - - - 1 cup- - - - - - - - -	248	85	160	6	6	2.9	1.6	1.1
Prepared with equal vol- ume of water:								
Bean with bacon- - - - 1 cup- - - - - - - -‘-	253	84	170	8	6	1.5	2.2	1.8
Beef broth, bouillon, consomme- - - - - - - 1 cup- - - - - - - - -	240	98	15	3	1	0.3	0.2	Tr
Beef noodle- - - - - - - 1 cup- - - - - - - - -	244	92	85	5	3	1.1	1.2	0.5
Chicken noodle- - - - - 1 cup- - - - - - - - -	241	92	75	4	2	0.7	1.1	0.6
Chicken rice- - - - - - - 1 cup- - - - - - - - -	241	94	60	4	2	0.5	0.9	0.4
Clam chowder, Man- hattan- - - - - - - - - 1 cup- - - - - - - - -	244	90	80	4	2	0.4	0.4	1.3
Cream of chicken- - - - 1 cup- - - - - - - - -	244	91	115	3	7	2.1	3.3	1.5
Cream of mushroom- - 1 cup- - - - - - - - -	244	90	130	2	9	2.4	1.7	4.2
Minestrone- - - - - - - - 1 cup- - - - - - - - -	241	91	80	4	3	0.6	0.7	1.1
Pea, green- - - - - - - - 1 cup- - - - - - - - -	250	83	165	9	3	1.4	1.0	0.4

(Tr indicates nutrient present in trace amounts.)

Nutrients in Indicated Quantity

Cho-les-terol	Carbo-hydrate	Calcium	Phos-phorus	Iron	Potas-sium	Sodium	Vitamin A value (IU)	(RE)	Thiamin	Ribo-flavin	Niacin	Ascorbic acid
Milli-grams	Grams	Milli-grams	Milli-grams	Milli-grams	Milli-grams	Milli-grams	Inter-national units	Retinol equiva-lents	Milli-grams	Milli-grams	Milli-grams	Milli-grams
73	0	13	196	0.9	220	64	20	5	0.06	0.10	11.8	0
41	0	5	81	0.6	108	42	30	8	0.03	0.10	2.7	0
116	0	20	210	1.6	252	98	70	21	0.07	0.23	8.6	0
126	Tr	3	62	1.7	28	10	3,270	983	0.03	0.35	0.9	3
197	0	27	449	6.0	557	144	170	51	0.57	1.04	11.3	0
72	0	27	173	2.0	246	67	0	0	0.05	0.21	3.1	0
59	0	16	186	1.1	259	54	0	0	0.05	0.11	5.8	0
17	0	3	97	0.2	118	608	0	0	0.02	0.05	3.5	840
45	3	4	207	1.4	253	578	0	0	0.04	0.14	5.3	0
22	17	186	156	1.5	300	992	160	40	0.07	0.24	1.0	3
27	15	181	151	0.7	273	1,047	710	94	0.07	0.26	0.9	1
20	15	179	156	0.6	270	1,076	150	37	0.08	0.28	0.9	2
17	22	159	149	1.8	449	932	850	109	0.13	0.25	1.5	68
3	23	81	132	2.0	402	951	890	89	0.09	0.03	0.6	2
Tr	Tr	14	31	0.4	130	782	0	0	Tr	0.05	1.9	0
5	9	15	46	1.1	100	952	630	63	0.07	0.06	1.1	Tr
7	9	17	36	0.8	55	1,106	710	71	0.05	0.06	1.4	Tr
7	7	17	22	0.7	101	815	660	66	0.02	0.02	1.1	Tr
2	12	34	59	1.9	261	1,808	920	92	0.06	0.05	1.3	3
10	9	34	37	0.6	88	986	560	56	0.03	0.06	0.8	Tr
2	9	46	49	0.5	100	1,032	0	0	0.05	0.09	0.7	1
2	11	34	55	0.9	313	911	2,340	234	0.05	0.04	0.9	1
0	27	28	125	2.0	190	988	200	20	0.11	0.07	1.2	2

Nutritive Values of Foods *(Continued)*

Foods, approximate measures, units, and weight (weight of edible portion only)		Water	Food energy	Pro-tein	Fat	Satu-rated	Mono-unsatu-rated	Poly-unsatu-rated
	Grams	Per-cent	Cal-ories	Grams	Grams	Grams	Grams	Grams
SOUPS, SAUCES, AND GRAVIES—Con.								
Tomato- - - - - - - - - 1 cup - - - - - - - -	244	90	85	2	2	0.4	0.4	1.0
Vegetable beef - - - - - 1 cup - - - - - - - -	244	92	80	6	2	0.9	0.8	0.1
Vegetarian - - - - - - - 1 cup - - - - - - - -	241	92	70	2	2	0.3	0.8	0.7
Dehydrated:								
Prepared with water:								
Chicken noodle - - - - 1 pkt (6-fl-oz) - - -	188	94	40	2	1	0.2	0.4	0.3
Onion - - - - - - - - - - 1 pkt (6-fl-oz) - - -	184	96	20	1	Tr	0.1	0.2	0.1
Tomato vegetable - - - 1 pkt (6-fl-oz) - - -	189	94	40	1	1	0.3	0.2	0.1
Sauces:								
From dry mix:								
Hollandaise, prepared with water - - - - - - - 1 cup - - - - - - - -	259	84	240	5	20	11.6	5.9	0.9
White sauce, prepared with milk - - - - - - - - 1 cup - - - - - - - -	264	81	240	10	13	6.4	4.7	1.7
From home recipe:								
White sauce, medium[55] - 1 cup - - - - - - - -	250	73	395	10	30	9.1	11.9	7.2
Ready to serve:								
Barbecue - - - - - - - - - 1 tbsp - - - - - - - -	16	81	10	Tr	Tr	Tr	0.1	0.1
Soy - - - - - - - - - - - - - 1 tbsp - - - - - - - -	18	68	10	2	0	0.0	0.0	0.0
SUGARS AND SWEETS								
Candy:								
Caramels, plain or choco-late - - - - - - - - - - - - 1 oz - - - - - - - - - -	28	8	115	1	3	2.2	0.3	0.1
Chocolate:								
Milk, plain - - - - - - - - 1 oz - - - - - - - - - -	28	1	145	2	9	5.4	3.0	0.3
Milk, with almonds - - - - 1 oz - - - - - - - - - -	28	2	150	3	10	4.8	4.1	0.7
Milk, with peanuts - - - - 1 oz - - - - - - - - - -	28	1	155	4	11	4.2	3.5	1.5
Milk, with rice cereal - - 1 oz - - - - - - - - - -	28	2	140	2	7	4.4	2.5	0.2
Semisweet, small pieces (60 per oz) - - - - - - - 1 cup or 6 oz - - - -	170	1	860	7	61	36.2	19.9	1.9
Sweet (dark) - - - - - - - 1 oz - - - - - - - - - -	28	1	150	1	10	5.9	3.3	0.3
Fudge, chocolate, plain - - - 1 oz - - - - - - - - - -	28	8	115	1	3	2.1	1.0	0.1
Gum drops - - - - - - - - - - 1 oz - - - - - - - - - -	28	12	100	Tr	Tr	Tr	Tr	0.1
Hard - - - - - - - - - - - - - 1 oz - - - - - - - - - -	28	1	110	0	0	0.0	0.0	0.0
Jelly beans - - - - - - - - - - 1 oz - - - - - - - - - -	28	6	105	Tr	Tr	Tr	Tr	0.1
Marshmallows - - - - - - - - 1 oz - - - - - - - - - -	28	17	90	1	0	0.0	0.0	0.0
Custard, baked - - - - - - - - 1 cup - - - - - - - -	265	77	305	14	15	6.8	5.4	0.7
Gelatin dessert prepared with gelatin dessert powder and water - - - - - - - - - - - - - - ½ cup - - - - - - - -	120	84	70	2	0	0.0	0.0	0.0
Honey, strained or extracted 1 cup - - - - - - - -	339	17	1,030	1	0	0.0	0.0	0.0
1 tbsp - - - - - - - -	21	17	65	Tr	0	0.0	0.0	0.0
Jams and preserves - - - - - - 1 tbsp - - - - - - - -	20	29	55	Tr	Tr	0.0	Tr	Tr
1 packet - - - - - - -	14	29	40	Tr	Tr	0.0	Tr	Tr
Jellies - - - - - - - - - - - - - - 1 tbsp - - - - - - - -	18	28	50	Tr	Tr	Tr	Tr	Tr
1 packet - - - - - - -	14	28	40	Tr	Tr	Tr	Tr	Tr
Popsicle, 3-fl-oz size - - - - - 1 popsicle - - - - - -	95	80	70	0	0	0.0	0.0	0.0

(Tr indicates nutrient present in trace amounts.)

Nutrients in Indicated Quantity

Cholesterol	Carbohydrate	Calcium	Phosphorus	Iron	Potassium	Sodium	Vitamin A value (IU)	Vitamin A value (RE)	Thiamin	Riboflavin	Niacin	Ascorbic acid
Milligrams	Grams	Milligrams	Milligrams	Milligrams	Milligrams	Milligrams	International units	Retinol equivalents	Milligrams	Milligrams	Milligrams	Milligrams
0	17	12	34	1.8	264	871	690	69	0.09	0.05	1.4	66
5	10	17	41	1.1	173	956	1,890	189	0.04	0.05	1.0	2
0	12	22	34	1.1	210	822	3,010	301	0.05	0.05	0.9	1
2	6	24	24	0.4	23	957	50	5	0.05	0.04	0.7	Tr
0	4	9	22	0.1	48	635	Tr	Tr	0.02	0.04	0.4	Tr
0	8	6	23	0.5	78	856	140	14	0.04	0.03	0.6	5
52	14	124	127	0.9	124	1,564	730	220	0.05	0.18	0.1	Tr
34	21	425	256	0.3	444	797	310	92	0.08	0.45	0.5	3
32	24	292	238	0.9	381	888	1,190	340	0.15	0.43	0.8	2
0	2	3	3	0.1	28	130	140	14	Tr	Tr	0.1	1
0	2	3	38	0.5	64	1,029	0	0	0.01	0.02	0.6	0
1	22	42	35	0.4	54	64	Tr	Tr	0.01	0.05	0.1	Tr
6	16	50	61	0.4	96	23	30	10	0.02	0.10	0.1	Tr
5	15	65	77	0.5	125	23	30	8	0.02	0.12	0.2	Tr
5	13	49	83	0.4	138	19	30	8	0.07	0.07	1.4	Tr
6	18	48	57	0.2	100	46	30	8	0.01	0.08	0.1	Tr
0	97	51	178	5.8	593	24	30	3	0.10	0.14	0.9	Tr
0	16	7	41	0.6	86	5	10	1	0.01	0.04	0.1	Tr
1	21	22	24	0.3	42	54	Tr	Tr	0.01	0.03	0.1	Tr
0	25	2	Tr	0.1	1	10	0	0	0.00	Tr	Tr	0
0	28	Tr	2	0.1	1	7	0	0	0.10	0.00	0.0	0
0	26	1	1	0.3	11	7	0	0	0.00	Tr	Tr	0
0	23	1	2	0.5	2	25	0	0	0.00	Tr	Tr	0
278	29	297	310	1.1	387	209	530	146	0.11	0.50	0.3	1
0	17	2	23	Tr	Tr	55	0	0	0.00	0.00	0.0	0
0	279	17	20	1.7	173	17	0	0	0.02	0.14	1.0	3
0	17	1	1	0.1	11	1	0	0	Tr	0.01	0.1	Tr
0	14	4	2	0.2	18	2	Tr	Tr	Tr	0.01	Tr	Tr
0	10	3	1	0.1	12	2	Tr	Tr	Tr	Tr	Tr	Tr
0	13	2	Tr	0.1	16	5	Tr	Tr	Tr	0.01	Tr	1
0	10	1	Tr	Tr	13	4	Tr	Tr	Tr	Tr	Tr	1
0	18	0	0	Tr	4	11	0	0	0.00	0.00	0.0	0

Nutritive Values of Foods *(Continued)*

Foods, approximate measures, units, and weight (weight of edible portion only)		Water	Food energy	Pro- tein	Fat	Fatty Acids		
						Satu- rated	Mono- unsatu- rated	Poly- unsatu- rated
SUGARS AND SWEETS— Con.		Grams	Per- cent	Cal- ories	Grams	Grams	Grams	Grams
Puddings:								
Canned:								
Vanilla- - - - - - - - - - -	5-oz can- - - - - - -	142	69	220	2	10	9.5	0.2	0.1
Dry mix, prepared with whole milk:								
Chocolate:								
Instant- - - - - - - - - - -	½ cup- - - - - - - - -	130	71	155	4	4	2.3	1.1	0.2
Regular (cooked)- - - -	½ cup- - - - - - - - -	130	73	150	4	4	2.4	1.1	0.1
Rice- - - - - - - - - - - - - -	½ cup- - - - - - - - -	132	73	155	4	4	2.3	1.1	0.1
Tapioca- - - - - - - - - - -	½ cup- - - - - - - - -	130	75	145	4	4	2.3	1.1	0.1
Vanilla:								
Instant- - - - - - - - - - -	½ cup- - - - - - - - -	130	73	150	4	4	2.2	1.1	0.2
Sugars:								
Brown, pressed down- - - -	1 cup- - - - - - - - -	220	2	820	0	0	0.0	0.0	0.0
White:								
Granulated- - - - - - - - -	1 cup- - - - - - - - -	200	1	770	0	0	0.0	0.0	0.0
	1 tbsp- - - - - - - - -	12	1	45	0	0	0.0	0.0	0.0
	1 packet- - - - - - -	6	1	25	0	0	0.0	0.0	0.0
Powdered, sifted, spooned into cup- - - -	1 cup- - - - - - - - -	100	1	385	0	0	0.0	0.0	0.0
Syrups:								
Chocolate-flavored syrup or topping:								
Thin type- - - - - - - - -	2 tbsp- - - - - - - - -	38	37	85	1	Tr	0.2	0.1	0.1
Fudge type- - - - - - - - -	2 tbsp- - - - - - - - -	38	25	125	2	5	3.1	1.7	0.2
Molasses, cane, blackstrap	2 tbsp- - - - - - - - -	40	24	85	0	0	0.0	0.0	0.0
Table syrup (corn and maple)- - - - - - - - - - -	2 tbsp- - - - - - - - -	42	25	122	0	0	0.0	0.0	0.0
VEGETABLES AND VEGETABLE PRODUCTS								
Alfalfa seeds, sprouted, raw-	1 cup- - - - - - - - -	33	91	10	1	Tr	Tr	Tr	0.1
Artichokes, globe or French, cooked, drained- - - - - - - -	1 artichoke- - - - -	120	87	55	3	Tr	Tr	Tr	0.1
Asparagus, green:								
Cooked, drained:								
From raw:								
Cuts and tips- - - - - -	1 cup- - - - - - - - -	180	92	45	5	1	0.1	Tr	0.2
Spears, ½-in diam. at base- - - - - - - - - - -	4 spears- - - - - - -	60	92	15	2	Tr	Tr	Tr	0.1
From frozen:								
Cuts and tips- - - - - -	1 cup- - - - - - - - -	180	91	50	5	1	0.2	Tr	0.3
Spears, ½-in diam. at base- - - - - - - - - - -	4 spears- - - - - - -	60	91	15	2	Tr	0.1	Tr	0.1
Canned, spears, ½-in diam. at base- - - - - - - - -	4 spears- - - - - - -	80	95	10	1	Tr	Tr	Tr	0.1
Bamboo shoots, canned, drained- - - - - - - - - - - - -	1 cup- - - - - - - - -	131	94	25	2	1	0.1	Tr	0.2

(Tr indicates nutrient present in trace amounts.)

Nutrients in Indicated Quantity

| Cho-les-terol | Carbo-hydrate | Calcium | Phos-phorus | Iron | Potas-sium | Sodium | Vitamin A value | | Thiamin | Ribo-flavin | Niacin | Ascorbic acid |
| | | | | | | | (IU) | (RE) | | | | |
Milli-grams	Grams	Milli-grams	Milli-grams	Milli-grams	Milli-grams	Milli-grams	Inter-national units	Retinol equiva-lents	Milli-grams	Milli-grams	Milli-grams	Milli-grams
1	33	79	94	0.2	155	305	Tr	Tr	0.03	0.12	0.6	Tr
14	27	130	329	0.3	176	440	130	33	0.04	0.18	0.1	1
15	25	146	120	0.2	190	167	140	34	0.05	0.20	0.1	1
15	27	133	110	0.5	165	140	140	33	0.10	0.18	0.6	1
15	25	131	103	0.1	167	152	140	34	0.04	0.18	0.1	1
15	27	129	273	0.1	164	375	140	33	0.04	0.17	0.1	1
0	212	187	56	4.8	757	97	0	0	0.02	0.07	0.2	0
0	199	3	Tr	0.1	7	5	0	0	0.00	0.00	0.0	0
0	12	Tr	Tr	Tr	Tr	Tr	0	0	0.00	0.00	0.0	0
0	6	Tr	Tr	Tr	Tr	Tr	0	0	0.00	0.00	0.0	0
0	100	1	Tr	Tr	4	2	0	0	0.00	0.00	0.0	0
0	22	6	49	0.8	85	36	Tr	Tr	Tr	0.02	0.1	0
0	21	38	60	0.5	82	42	40	13	0.02	0.08	0.1	0
0	22	274	34	10.1	1,171	38	0	0	0.04	0.08	0.8	0
0	32	1	4	Tr	7	19	0	0	0.00	0.00	0.0	0
0	1	11	23	0.3	26	2	50	5	0.03	0.04	0.2	3
0	12	47	72	1.6	316	79	170	17	0.07	0.06	0.7	9
0	8	43	110	1.2	558	7	1,490	149	0.18	0.22	1.9	49
0	3	14	37	0.4	186	2	500	50	0.06	0.07	0.6	16
0	9	41	99	1.2	392	7	1,470	147	0.12	0.19	1.9	44
0	3	14	33	0.4	131	2	490	49	0.04	0.06	0.6	15
0	2	11	30	0.5	122	[56]278	380	38	0.04	0.07	0.7	13
0	4	10	33	0.4	105	9	10	1	0.03	0.03	0.2	1

Nutritive Values of Foods *(Continued)*

Foods, approximate measures, units, and weight (weight of edible portion only)		Water	Food energy	Pro-tein	Fat	Fatty Acids		
						Satu-rated	Mono-unsatu-rated	Poly-unsatu-rated
VEGETABLES AND VEGETABLE PRODUCTS—Con.	Grams	Per-cent	Cal-ories	Grams	Grams	Grams	Grams	Grams
Beans:								
Lima, immature seeds, frozen, cooked, drained:								
Thick-seeded types (Fordhooks)- - - - - - 1 cup- - - - - - - - -	170	74	170	10	1	0.1	Tr	0.3
Thin-seeded types (baby limas)- - - - - - - - - - 1 cup- - - - - - - - -	180	72	190	12	1	0.1	Tr	0.3
Snap:								
Cooked, drained:								
From raw (cut and French style)- - - - - 1 cup- - - - - - - - -	125	89	45	2	Tr	0.1	Tr	0.2
From frozen (cut)- - - 1 cup- - - - - - - - -	135	92	35	2	Tr	Tr	Tr	0.1
Canned, drained solids (cut) 1 cup- - - - - - - - -	135	93	25	2	Tr	Tr	Tr	0.1
Beans, mature. See Beans, dry and Black-eyed peas, dry.								
Bean sprouts (mung):								
Raw- - - - - - - - - - - - - - - - 1 cup- - - - - - - - -	104	90	30	3	Tr	Tr	Tr	0.1
Beets:								
Cooked, drained:								
Diced or sliced- - - - - - - 1 cup- - - - - - - - -	170	91	55	2	Tr	Tr	Tr	Tr
Canned, drained solids, diced or sliced- - - - - - 1 cup- - - - - - - - -	170	91	55	2	Tr	Tr	Tr	0.1
Beet greens, leaves and stems, cooked, drained- - - - - - - - - 1 cup- - - - - - - - -	144	89	40	4	Tr	Tr	0.1	0.1
Black-eyed peas, immature seeds, cooked and drained:								
From raw- - - - - - - - - - - - 1 cup- - - - - - - - -	165	72	180	13	1	0.3	0.1	0.6
From frozen- - - - - - - - - - 1 cup- - - - - - - - -	170	66	225	14	1	0.3	0.1	0.5
Broccoli:								
Raw- - - - - - - - - - - - - - - - 1 spear- - - - - - - -	151	91	40	4	1	0.1	Tr	0.3
Cooked, drained:								
From raw:								
Spear, medium- - - - - 1 spear- - - - - - - -	180	90	50	5	1	0.1	Tr	0.2
Spears, cut into ½-in pieces- - - - - - - - - - 1 cup- - - - - - - - -	155	90	45	5	Tr	0.1	Tr	0.2
Brussels sprouts, cooked, drained:								
From frozen- - - - - - - - - - 1 cup- - - - - - - - -	155	87	65	6	1	0.1	Tr	0.3
Cabbage, common varieties:								
Raw, coarsely shredded or sliced- - - - - - - - - - - - - 1 cup- - - - - - - - -	70	93	15	1	Tr	Tr	Tr	0.1
Cooked, drained- - - - - - - 1 cup- - - - - - - - -	150	94	30	1	Tr	Tr	Tr	0.2
Cabbage, Chinese:								
Pak-choi, cooked, drained- 1 cup- - - - - - - - -	170	96	20	3	Tr	Tr	Tr	0.1
Pe-tsai, raw, 1-in pieces- - 1 cup- - - - - - - - -	76	94	10	1	Tr	Tr	Tr	0.1

(Tr indicates nutrient present in trace amounts.)

Nutrients in Indicated Quantity

Cho-les-terol	Carbo-hydrate	Calcium	Phos-phorus	Iron	Potas-sium	Sodium	Vitamin A value		Thiamin	Ribo-flavin	Niacin	Ascorbic acid
							(IU)	(RE)				
Milli-grams	Grams	Milli-grams	Milli-grams	Milli-grams	Milli-grams	Milli-grams	Inter-national units	Retinol equiva-lents	Milli-grams	Milli-grams	Milli-grams	Milli-grams
0	32	37	107	2.3	694	90	320	32	0.13	0.10	1.8	22
0	35	50	202	3.5	740	52	300	30	0.13	0.10	1.4	10
0	10	58	49	1.6	374	4	[57]830	[57]83	0.09	0.12	0.8	12
0	8	61	32	1.1	151	18	[58]710	[58]71	0.06	0.10	0.6	11
0	6	35	26	1.2	147	[59]339	[60]470	[60]47	0.02	0.08	0.3	6
0	6	14	56	0.9	155	6	20	2	0.09	0.13	0.8	14
0	11	19	53	1.1	530	83	20	2	0.05	0.02	0.5	9
0	12	26	29	3.1	252	[61]466	20	2	0.02	0.07	0.3	7
0	8	164	59	2.7	1,309	347	7,340	734	0.17	0.42	0.7	36
0	30	46	196	2.4	693	7	1,050	105	0.11	0.18	1.8	3
0	40	39	207	3.6	638	9	130	13	0.44	0.11	1.2	4
0	8	72	100	1.3	491	41	2,330	233	0.10	0.18	1.0	141
0	10	205	86	2.1	293	20	2,540	254	0.15	0.37	1.4	113
0	9	177	74	1.8	253	17	2,180	218	0.13	0.32	1.2	97
0	13	37	84	1.1	504	36	910	91	0.16	0.18	0.8	71
0	4	33	16	0.4	172	13	90	9	0.04	0.02	0.2	33
0	7	50	38	0.6	308	29	130	13	0.09	0.08	0.3	36
0	3	158	49	1.8	631	58	4,370	437	0.05	0.11	0.7	44
0	2	59	22	0.2	181	7	910	91	0.03	0.04	0.3	21

Nutritive Values of Foods *(Continued)*

Foods, approximate measures, units, and weight (weight of edible portion only)		Grams	Water Per-cent	Food energy Cal-ories	Pro-tein Grams	Fat Grams	Fatty Acids Satu-rated Grams	Mono-unsatu-rated Grams	Poly-unsatu-rated Grams
VEGETABLES AND VEGETABLE PRODUCTS—Con.									
Cabbage, red, raw, coarsely shredded or sliced- - - - -	1 cup- - - - - - - -	70	92	20	1	Tr	Tr	Tr	0.1
Cabbage, savoy, raw, coarsely shredded or sliced- - - - -	1 cup- - - - - - - -	70	91	20	1	Tr	Tr	Tr	Tr
Carrots:									
Raw, without crowns and tips, scraped:									
Whole, 7½ by 1⅛ in, or strips, 2½ to 3 in long-	1 carrot or 18 strips- - - - - - - -	72	88	30	1	Tr	Tr	Tr	0.1
Cooked, sliced, drained:									
From frozen- - - - - - - - -	1 cup- - - - - - - -	146	90	55	2	Tr	Tr	Tr	0.1
Canned, sliced, drained solids- - - - - - - - - - - -	1 cup- - - - - - - -	146	93	35	1	Tr	0.1	Tr	0.1
Cauliflower:									
Cooked, drained:									
From raw (flowerets)- - -	1 cup- - - - - - - -	125	93	30	2	Tr	Tr	Tr	0.1
From frozen (flowerets)-	1 cup- - - - - - - -	180	94	35	3	Tr	0.1	Tr	0.2
Celery, pascal type, raw:									
Stalk, large outer, 8 by 1½ in (at root end)- - - - - - - -	1 stalk- - - - - - - -	40	95	5	Tr	Tr	Tr	Tr	Tr
Collards, cooked, drained:									
From raw (leaves without stems)- - - - - - - - - - - - -	1 cup- - - - - - - -	190	96	25	2	Tr	0.1	Tr	0.2
Corn, sweet:									
Cooked, drained:									
From raw, ear 5 by 1¾ in- - - - - - - - - -	1 ear- - - - - - - - -	77	70	85	3	1	0.2	0.3	0.5
From frozen:									
Kernels- - - - - - - - - -	1 cup- - - - - - - -	165	76	135	5	Tr	Tr	Tr	0.1
Canned:									
Cream style- - - - - - - -	1 cup- - - - - - - -	256	79	185	4	1	0.2	0.3	0.5
Whole kernel, vacuum pack- - - - - - - - - - -	1 cup- - - - - - - -	210	77	165	5	1	0.2	0.3	0.5
Cowpeas. See Black-eyed peas.									
Cucumber, with peel, slices, ⅛ in thick (large, 2⅛-in diam.; small, 1¾-in diam.)- - - - -	6 large or 8 small slices- - - - - - - -	28	96	5	Tr	Tr	Tr	Tr	Tr
Dandelion greens, cooked, drained- - - - - - - - - - - - -	1 cup- - - - - - - -	105	90	35	2	1	0.1	Tr	0.3
Eggplant, cooked, steamed- -	1 cup- - - - - - - -	96	92	25	1	Tr	Tr	Tr	0.1
Endive, curly (including escarole), raw, small pieces- - - - - - - - - - - - - -	1 cup- - - - - - - -	50	94	10	1	Tr	Tr	Tr	Tr
Jerusalem-artichoke, raw, sliced- - - - - - - - - - - - - -	1 cup- - - - - - - -	150	78	115	3	Tr	0.0	Tr	Tr

(Tr indicates nutrient present in trace amounts.)

Nutrients in Indicated Quantity

Cholesterol	Carbohydrate	Calcium	Phosphorus	Iron	Potassium	Sodium	Vitamin A value (IU)	Vitamin A value (RE)	Thiamin	Riboflavin	Niacin	Ascorbic acid
Milligrams	Grams	Milligrams	Milligrams	Milligrams	Milligrams	Milligrams	International units	Retinol equivalents	Milligrams	Milligrams	Milligrams	Milligrams
0	4	36	29	0.3	144	8	30	3	0.04	0.02	0.2	40
0	4	25	29	0.3	161	20	700	70	0.05	0.02	0.2	22
0	7	19	32	0.4	233	25	20,250	2,025	0.07	0.04	0.7	7
0	12	41	38	0.7	231	86	25,850	2,585	0.04	0.05	0.6	4
0	8	37	35	0.9	261	[62]352	20,110	2,011	0.03	0.04	0.8	4
0	6	34	44	0.5	404	8	20	2	0.08	0.07	0.7	69
0	7	31	43	0.7	250	32	40	4	0.07	0.10	0.6	56
0	1	14	10	0.2	114	35	50	5	0.01	0.01	0.1	3
0	5	148	19	0.8	177	36	4,220	422	0.03	0.08	0.4	19
0	19	2	79	0.5	192	13	[63]170	[63]17	0.17	0.06	1.2	5
0	34	3	78	0.5	229	8	[63]410	[63]41	0.11	0.12	2.1	4
0	46	8	131	1.0	343	[64]730	[63]250	[63]25	0.06	0.14	2.5	12
0	41	11	134	0.9	391	[65]571	[63]510	[63]51	0.09	0.15	2.5	17
0	1	4	5	0.1	42	1	10	1	0.01	0.01	0.1	1
0	7	147	44	1.9	244	46	12,290	1,229	0.14	0.18	0.5	19
0	6	6	21	0.3	238	3	60	6	0.07	0.02	0.6	1
0	2	26	14	0.4	157	11	1,030	103	0.04	0.04	0.2	3
0	26	21	117	5.1	644	6	30	3	0.30	0.09	2.0	6

Nutritive Values of Foods *(Continued)*

Foods, approximate measures, units, and weight (weight of edible portion only)		Water	Food energy	Pro-tein	Fat	Fatty Acids Satu-rated	Mono-unsatu-rated	Poly-unsatu-rated
VEGETABLES AND VEGETABLE PRODUCTS—Con.	*Grams*	*Per-cent*	*Cal-ories*	*Grams*	*Grams*	*Grams*	*Grams*	*Grams*
Kale, cooked, drained:								
From raw, chopped- - - - -	1 cup- - - - - - - - -	130	91	40	2	1	0.1	Tr	0.3
From frozen, chopped- - - -	1 cup- - - - - - - - -	130	91	40	4	1	0.1	Tr	0.3
Kohlrabi, thickened bulb-like stems, cooked, drained, diced- - - - - - - - - - - - - -	1 cup- - - - - - - - -	165	90	50	3	Tr	Tr	Tr	0.1
Lettuce, raw:								
Butterhead, as Boston types:								
Head, 5-in diam- - - - -	1 head- - - - - - - -	163	96	20	2	Tr	Tr	Tr	0.2
Leaves- - - - - - - - - - -	1 outer or 2 inner leaves- - - - - - -	15	96	Tr	Tr	Tr	Tr	Tr	Tr
Crisphead, as iceberg:								
Head, 6-in diam- - - - -	1 head- - - - - - - -	539	96	70	5	1	0.1	Tr	0.5
Looseleaf (bunching varieties including romaine or cos), chopped or shredded pieces- - - - -	1 cup- - - - - - - - -	56	94	10	1	Tr	Tr	Tr	0.1
Mushrooms:								
Raw, sliced or chopped- - -	1 cup- - - - - - - - -	70	92	20	1	Tr	Tr	Tr	0.1
Cooked, drained- - - - - - -	1 cup- - - - - - - - -	156	91	40	3	1	0.1	Tr	0.3
Canned, drained solids- - -	1 cup- - - - - - - - -	156	91	35	3	Tr	0.1	Tr	0.2
Mustard greens, without stems and midribs, cooked, drained- - - - - - - - - - - - -	1 cup- - - - - - - - -	140	94	20	3	Tr	Tr	0.2	0.1
Okra pods, 3 by ⅝ in, cooked	8 pods- - - - - - - - -	85	90	25	2	Tr	Tr	Tr	Tr
Onions:								
Raw:								
Sliced- - - - - - - - - - - -	1 cup- - - - - - - - -	115	91	40	1	Tr	0.1	Tr	0.1
Cooked (whole or sliced), drained- - - - - - - - - -	1 cup- - - - - - - - -	210	92	60	2	Tr	0.1	Tr	0.1
Onions, spring, raw, bulb (⅜-in diam.) and white portion of top- - - - - - - - - - - - - -	6 onions- - - - - - -	30	92	10	1	Tr	Tr	Tr	Tr
Onion rings, breaded, par-fried, frozen, prepared- - -	2 rings- - - - - - - -	20	29	80	1	5	1.7	2.2	1.0
Parsley:								
Raw- - - - - - - - - - - - - - -	10 sprigs- - - - - - -	10	88	5	Tr	Tr	Tr	Tr	Tr
Parsnips, cooked (diced or 2 in lengths), drained- - - - - - -	1 cup- - - - - - - - -	156	78	125	2	Tr	0.1	0.2	0.1
Peas, edible pod, cooked, drained- - - - - - - - - - - - -	1 cup- - - - - - - - -	160	89	65	5	Tr	0.1	Tr	0.2
Peas, green:								
Canned, drained solids- - -	1 cup- - - - - - - - -	170	82	115	8	1	0.1	0.1	0.3
Frozen, cooked, drained- -	1 cup- - - - - - - - -	160	80	125	8	Tr	0.1	Tr	0.2
Peppers:								
Hot chili, raw- - - - - - - - -	1 pepper- - - - - - -	45	88	20	1	Tr	Tr	Tr	Tr

(Tr indicates nutrient present in trace amounts.)

Nutrients in Indicated Quantity

Cho-les-terol	Carbo-hydrate	Calcium	Phos-phorus	Iron	Potas-sium	Sodium	Vitamin A value		Thiamin	Ribo-flavin	Niacin	Ascorbic acid
							(IU)	(RE)				
Milli-grams	Grams	Milli-grams	Milli-grams	Milli-grams	Milli-grams	Milli-grams	Inter-national units	Retinol equiva-lents	Milli-grams	Milli-grams	Milli-grams	Milli-grams
0	7	94	36	1.2	296	30	9,620	962	0.07	0.09	0.7	53
0	7	179	36	1.2	417	20	8,260	826	0.06	0.15	0.9	33
0	11	41	74	0.7	561	35	60	6	0.07	0.03	0.6	89
0	4	52	38	0.5	419	8	1,580	158	0.10	0.10	0.5	13
0	Tr	5	3	Tr	39	1	150	15	0.01	0.01	Tr	1
0	11	102	108	2.7	852	49	1,780	178	0.25	0.16	1.0	21
0	2	38	14	0.8	148	5	1,060	106	0.03	0.04	0.2	10
0	3	4	73	0.9	259	3	0	0	0.07	0.31	2.9	2
0	8	9	136	2.7	555	3	0	0	0.11	0.47	7.0	6
0	8	17	103	1.2	201	663	0	0	0.13	0.03	2.5	0
0	3	104	57	1.0	283	22	4,240	424	0.06	0.09	0.6	35
0	6	54	48	0.4	274	4	490	49	0.11	0.05	0.7	14
0	8	29	33	0.4	178	2	0	0	0.07	0.01	0.1	10
0	13	57	48	0.4	319	17	0	0	0.09	0.02	0.2	12
0	2	18	10	0.6	77	1	1,500	150	0.02	0.04	0.1	14
0	8	6	16	0.3	26	75	50	5	0.06	0.03	0.7	Tr
0	1	13	4	0.6	54	4	520	52	0.01	0.01	0.1	9
0	30	58	108	0.9	573	16	0	0	0.13	0.08	1.1	20
0	11	67	88	3.2	384	6	210	21	0.20	0.12	0.9	77
0	21	34	114	1.6	294	[66]372	1,310	131	0.21	0.13	1.2	16
0	23	38	144	2.5	269	139	1,070	107	0.45	0.16	2.4	16
0	4	8	21	0.5	153	3	[67]4,840	[67]484	0.04	0.04	0.4	109

Nutritive Values of Foods *(Continued)*

Foods, approximate measures, units, and weight (weight of edible portion only)		Water	Food energy	Pro- tein	Fat	Fatty Acids		
						Satu- rated	Mono- unsatu- rated	Poly- unsatu- rated
VEGETABLES AND VEGETABLE PRODUCTS—Con.	Grams	Per- cent	Cal- ories	Grams	Grams	Grams	Grams	Grams
Sweet (about 5 per lb, whole), stem and seeds removed:								
Raw- - - - - - - - - - - - - -	1 pepper- - - - - - -	74	93	20	1	Tr	Tr	Tr	0.2
Cooked, drained- - - - - -	1 pepper- - - - - - -	73	95	15	Tr	Tr	Tr	Tr	0.1
Potatoes, cooked:								
Baked (about 2 per lb, raw):								
With skin- - - - - - - - - -	1 potato- - - - - - -	202	71	220	5	Tr	0.1	Tr	0.1
Flesh only- - - - - - - - -	1 potato- - - - - - -	156	75	145	3	Tr	Tr	Tr	0.1
Boiled (about 3 per lb, raw):								
Peeled after boiling- - - -	1 potato- - - - - - -	136	77	120	3	Tr	Tr	Tr	0.1
Peeled before boiling- - -	1 potato- - - - - - -	135	77	115	2	Tr	Tr	Tr	0.1
French fried, strip, 2 to 3½ in long, frozen:								
Oven heated- - - - - - - -	10 strips- - - - - - -	50	53	110	2	4	2.1	1.8	0.3
Fried in vegetable oil- - -	10 strips- - - - - - -	50	38	160	2	8	2.5	1.6	3.8
Potato products, prepared:								
Hashed brown, from frozen	1 cup- - - - - - - - -	156	56	340	5	18	7.0	8.0	2.1
Mashed:								
From home recipe:								
Milk added- - - - - - - -	1 cup- - - - - - - - -	210	78	160	4	1	0.7	0.3	0.1
Milk and margarine added- - - - - - - - - -	1 cup- - - - - - - - -	210	76	225	4	9	2.2	3.7	2.5
Potato salad, made with mayonnaise- - - - - -	1 cup- - - - - - - - -	250	76	360	7	21	3.6	6.2	9.3
Scalloped:								
From dry mix- - - - - - - -	1 cup- - - - - - - - -	245	79	230	5	11	6.5	3.0	0.5
Potato chips- - - - - - - - - - - -	10 chips- - - - - - -	20	3	105	1	7	1.8	1.2	3.6
Pumpkin:								
Cooked from raw, mashed-	1 cup- - - - - - - - -	245	94	50	2	Tr	0.1	Tr	Tr
Canned- - - - - - - - - - - - -	1 cup- - - - - - - - -	245	90	85	3	1	0.4	0.1	Tr
Radishes, raw, stem ends, rootlets cut off- - - - - - - -	4 radishes- - - - - -	18	95	5	Tr	Tr	Tr	Tr	Tr
Sauerkraut, canned, solids and liquid- - - - - - - - - - - -	1 cup- - - - - - - - -	236	93	45	2	Tr	0.1	Tr	0.1
Seaweed:								
Kelp, raw- - - - - - - - - - -	1 oz- - - - - - - - - -	28	82	10	Tr	Tr	0.1	Tr	Tr
Southern peas. See Black- eyed peas.								
Spinach:								
Raw, chopped- - - - - - - - -	1 cup- - - - - - - - -	55	92	10	2	Tr	Tr	Tr	0.1
Cooked, drained:								
From raw- - - - - - - - - -	1 cup- - - - - - - - -	180	91	40	5	Tr	0.1	Tr	0.2
Canned, drained solids- - -	1 cup- - - - - - - - -	214	92	50	6	1	0.2	Tr	0.4
Squash, cooked:								
Summer (all varieties), sliced, drained- - - - - -	1 cup- - - - - - - - -	180	94	35	2	1	0.1	Tr	0.2

(Tr indicates nutrient present in trace amounts.)

Nutrients in Indicated Quantity

Cholesterol	Carbohydrate	Calcium	Phosphorus	Iron	Potassium	Sodium	Vitamin A value		Thiamin	Riboflavin	Niacin	Ascorbic acid
							(IU)	(RE)				
Milligrams	Grams	Milligrams	Milligrams	Milligrams	Milligrams	Milligrams	International units	Retinol equivalents	Milligrams	Milligrams	Milligrams	Milligrams
0	4	4	16	0.9	144	2	[66]390	[66]39	0.06	0.04	0.4	[60]95
0	3	3	11	0.6	94	1	[70]280	[70]28	0.04	0.03	0.3	[71]81
0	51	20	115	2.7	844	16	0	0	0.22	0.07	3.3	26
0	34	8	78	0.5	610	8	0	0	0.16	0.03	2.2	20
0	27	7	60	0.4	515	5	0	0	0.14	0.03	2.0	18
0	27	11	54	0.4	443	7	0	0	0.13	0.03	1.8	10
0	17	5	43	0.7	229	16	0	0	0.06	0.02	1.2	5
0	20	10	47	0.4	366	108	0	0	0.09	0.01	1.6	5
0	44	23	112	2.4	680	53	0	0	0.17	0.03	3.8	10
4	37	55	101	0.6	628	636	40	12	0.18	0.08	2.3	14
4	35	55	97	0.5	607	620	360	42	0.18	0.08	2.3	13
170	28	48	130	1.6	635	1,323	520	83	0.19	0.15	2.2	25
27	31	88	137	0.9	497	835	360	51	0.05	0.14	2.5	8
0	10	5	31	0.2	260	94	0	0	0.03	Tr	0.8	8
0	12	37	74	1.4	564	2	2,650	265	0.08	0.19	1.0	12
0	20	64	86	3.4	505	12	54,040	5,404	0.06	0.13	0.9	10
0	1	4	3	0.1	42	4	Tr	Tr	Tr	0.01	0.1	4
0	10	71	47	3.5	401	1,560	40	4	0.05	0.05	0.3	35
0	3	48	12	0.8	25	66	30	3	0.01	0.04	0.1	(¹)
0	2	54	27	1.5	307	43	3,690	369	0.04	0.10	0.4	15
0	7	245	101	6.4	839	126	14,740	1,474	0.17	0.42	0.9	18
0	7	272	94	4.9	740	[72]683	18,780	1,878	0.03	0.30	0.8	31
0	8	49	70	0.6	346	2	520	52	0.08	0.07	0.9	10

Nutritive Values of Foods *(Continued)*

Foods, approximate measures, units, and weight (weight of edible portion only)		Water	Food energy	Pro-tein	Fat	Fatty Acids		
						Satu-rated	Mono-unsatu-rated	Poly-unsatu-rated
VEGETABLES AND VEGETABLE PRODUCTS—Con.	Grams	Per-cent	Cal-ories	Grams	Grams	Grams	Grams	Grams
Winter (all varieties), baked, cubes- - - - - - -	1 cup- - - - - - - - -	205	89	80	2	1	0.3	0.1	0.5
Sunchoke. See Jerusalem-artichoke.									
Sweet potatoes:									
Cooked (raw, 5 by 2 in; about 2½ per lb):									
Baked in skin, peeled- -	1 potato- - - - - - -	114	73	115	2	Tr	Tr	Tr	0.1
Boiled, without skin- - -	1 potato- - - - - - -	151	73	160	2	Tr	0.1	Tr	0.2
Candied, 2½ by 2-in piece-	1 piece- - - - - - - -	105	67	145	1	3	1.4	0.7	0.2
Canned:									
Solid pack (mashed)- - -	1 cup- - - - - - - - -	255	74	260	5	1	0.1	Tr	0.2
Vacuum pack, piece 2¾ by 1 in- - - - - - - - - - -	1 piece- - - - - - - -	40	76	35	1	Tr	Tr	Tr	Tr
Tomatoes:									
Raw, 2⅗-in diam. (3 per 12 oz pkg.)- - - - - - - - - - -	1 tomato- - - - - - -	123	94	25	1	Tr	Tr	Tr	0.1
Canned, solids and liquid-	1 cup- - - - - - - - -	240	94	50	2	1	0.1	0.1	0.2
Tomato juice, canned- - - - -	1 cup- - - - - - - - -	244	94	40	2	Tr	Tr	Tr	0.1
Tomato products, canned:									
Paste- - - - - - - - - - - - - -	1 cup- - - - - - - - -	262	74	220	10	2	0.3	0.4	0.9
Puree- - - - - - - - - - - - - -	1 cup- - - - - - - - -	250	87	105	4	Tr	Tr	Tr	0.1
Sauce- - - - - - - - - - - - - -	1 cup- - - - - - - - -	245	89	75	3	Tr	0.1	0.1	0.2
Turnips, cooked, diced- - - - -	1 cup- - - - - - - - -	156	94	30	1	Tr	Tr	Tr	0.1
Turnip greens, cooked, drained:									
From raw (leaves and stems)- - - - - - - - - - - -	1 cup- - - - - - - - -	144	93	30	2	Tr	0.1	Tr	0.1
From frozen (chopped)- - -	1 cup- - - - - - - - -	164	90	50	5	1	0.2	Tr	0.3
Vegetable juice cocktail, canned- - - - - - - - - - - - - -	1 cup- - - - - - - - -	242	94	45	2	Tr	Tr	Tr	0.1
Vegetables, mixed:									
Frozen, cooked, drained- -	1 cup- - - - - - - - -	182	83	105	5	Tr	0.1	Tr	0.1
Water chestnuts, canned- - -	1 cup- - - - - - - - -	140	86	70	1	Tr	Tr	Tr	Tr
MISCELLANEOUS ITEMS									
Baking powders for home use:									
Sodium aluminum sulfate:									
With monocalcium phos-phate monohydrate- -	1 tsp- - - - - - - - - -	3	2	5	Tr	0	0.0	0.0	0.0
Catsup- - - - - - - - - - - - - -	1 cup- - - - - - - - -	273	69	290	5	1	0.2	0.2	0.4
	1 tbsp- - - - - - - - -	15	69	15	Tr	Tr	Tr	Tr	Tr
Chili powder- - - - - - - - - - -	1 tsp- - - - - - - - - -	2.6	8	10	Tr	Tr	0.1	0.1	0.2
Chocolate:									
Bitter or baking- - - - - - -	1 oz- - - - - - - - - -	28	2	145	3	15	9.0	4.9	0.5
Semisweet, see Candy									
Cinnamon- - - - - - - - - - - - -	1 tsp- - - - - - - - - -	2.3	10	5	Tr	Tr	Tr	Tr	Tr
Curry powder- - - - - - - - - -	1 tsp- - - - - - - - - -	2	10	5	Tr	Tr	(¹)	(¹)	(¹)

(Tr indicates nutrient present in trace amounts.)

Nutrients in Indicated Quantity

Cho-les-terol	Carbo-hydrate	Calcium	Phos-phorus	Iron	Potas-sium	Sodium	Vitamin A value		Thiamin	Ribo-flavin	Niacin	Ascorbic acid
							(IU)	(RE)				
Milli-grams	Grams	Milli-grams	Milli-grams	Milli-grams	Milli-grams	Milli-grams	Inter-national units	Retinol equiva-lents	Milli-grams	Milli-grams	Milli-grams	Milli-grams
0	18	29	41	0.7	896	2	7,290	729	0.17	0.05	1.4	20
0	28	32	63	0.5	397	11	24,880	2,488	0.08	0.14	0.7	28
0	37	32	41	0.8	278	20	25,750	2,575	0.08	0.21	1.0	26
8	29	27	27	1.2	198	74	4,400	440	0.02	0.04	0.4	7
0	59	77	133	3.4	536	191	38,570	3,857	0.07	0.23	2.4	13
0	8	9	20	0.4	125	21	3,190	319	0.01	0.02	0.3	11
0	5	9	28	0.6	255	10	1,390	139	0.07	0.06	0.7	22
0	10	62	46	1.5	530	[73]391	1,450	145	0.11	0.07	1.8	36
0	10	22	46	1.4	537	[74]881	1,360	136	0.11	0.08	1.6	45
0	49	92	207	7.8	2,442	[75]170	6,470	647	0.41	0.50	8.4	111
0	25	38	100	2.3	1,050	[76]50	3,400	340	0.18	0.14	4.3	88
0	18	34	78	1.9	909	[77]1,482	2,400	240	0.16	0.14	2.8	32
0	8	34	30	0.3	211	78	0	0	0.04	0.04	0.5	18
0	6	197	42	1.2	292	42	7,920	792	0.06	0.10	0.6	39
0	8	249	56	3.2	367	25	13,080	1,308	0.09	0.12	0.8	36
0	11	27	41	1.0	467	883	2,830	283	0.10	0.07	1.8	67
0	24	46	93	1.5	308	64	7,780	778	0.13	0.22	1.5	6
0	17	6	27	1.2	165	11	10	1	0.02	0.03	0.5	2
0	1	58	87	0.0	5	329	0	0	0.00	0.00	0.0	0
0	69	60	137	2.2	991	2,845	3,820	382	0.25	0.19	4.4	41
0	4	3	8	0.1	54	156	210	21	0.01	0.01	0.2	2
0	1	7	8	0.4	50	26	910	91	0.01	0.02	0.2	2
0	8	22	109	1.9	235	1	10	1	0.01	0.07	0.4	0
0	2	28	1	0.9	12	1	10	1	Tr	Tr	Tr	1
0	1	10	7	0.6	31	1	20	2	0.01	0.01	0.1	Tr

Nutritive Values of Foods *(Continued)*

Foods, approximate measures, units, and weight (weight of edible portion only)		Water	Food energy	Pro-tein	Fat	Fatty Acids Satu-rated	Mono-unsatu-rated	Poly-unsatu-rated
	Grams	Per-cent	Cal-ories	Grams	Grams	Grams	Grams	Grams
MISCELLANEOUS ITEMS—Con.								
Garlic powder- - - - - - - - - - -	1 tsp- - - - - - - - -	2.8	6	10	Tr	Tr	Tr	Tr	Tr
Gelatin, dry- - - - - - - - - - - -	1 envelope- - - - - -	7	13	25	6	Tr	Tr	Tr	Tr
Mustard, prepared, yellow- -	1 tsp or individual								
	packet- - - - - - -	5	80	5	Tr	Tr	Tr	0.2	Tr
Olives, canned:									
Green- - - - - - - - - - - - - -	4 medium or 3								
	extra large- - - -	13	78	15	Tr	2	0.2	1.2	0.1
Ripe, Mission, pitted- - - -	3 small or 2 large-	9	73	15	Tr	2	0.3	1.3	0.2
Oregano- - - - - - - - - - - - - -	1 tsp- - - - - - - - -	1.5	7	5	Tr	Tr	Tr	Tr	0.1
Paprika- - - - - - - - - - - - - -	1 tsp- - - - - - - - -	2.1	10	5	Tr	Tr	Tr	Tr	0.2
Pepper, black- - - - - - - - - -	1 tsp- - - - - - - - -	2.1	11	5	Tr	Tr	Tr	Tr	Tr
Pickles, cucumber:									
Dill, medium, whole, 3¾ in long, 1¼-in diam.- - - - -	1 pickle- - - - - - - -	65	93	5	Tr	Tr	Tr	Tr	0.1
Fresh-pack, slices 1½-in diam., ¼ in thick- - - - - -	2 slices- - - - - - - -	15	79	10	Tr	Tr	Tr	Tr	Tr
Sweet, gherkin, small, whole, about 2½ in long, ¾-in diam.- - - - - - - - - -	1 pickle- - - - - - - -	15	61	20	Tr	Tr	Tr	Tr	Tr
Popcorn. See Grain Products									
Salt- - - - - - - - - - - - - - - -	1 tsp- - - - - - - - -	5.5	0	0	0	0	0.0	0.0	0.0
Vinegar, cider- - - - - - - - - -	1 tbsp- - - - - - - -	15	94	Tr	Tr	0	0.0	0.0	0.0
Yeast:									
Baker's, dry, active- - - - -	1 pkg- - - - - - - - -	7	5	20	3	Tr	Tr	0.1	Tr

(Tr indicates nutrient present in trace amounts.)

[1] Value not determined.

[2] Mineral content varies depending on water source.

[3] Blend of aspartame and saccharin; if only sodium saccharin is used, sodium is 75 mg; if only aspartame is used, sodium is 23 mg.

[4] With added ascorbic acid.

[5] Vitamin A value is largely from beta-carotene used for coloring.

[6] Yields 1 qt of fluid milk when reconstituted according to package directions.

[7] With added vitamin A.

[8] Carbohydrate content varies widely because of amount of sugar added and amount and solids content of added flavoring. Consult the label if more precise values for carbohydrate and calories are needed.

[9] For salted butter; unsalted butter contains 12 mg sodium per stick, 2 mg per tbsp, or 1 mg per pat.

[10] Values for vitamin are year-round average.

[11] For salted margarine.

[12] Based on average vitamin A content of fortified margarine. Federal specifications for fortified margarine require a minimum of 15,000 IU per pound.

[13] Fatty acid values apply to product made with regular margarine.

[14] Dipped in egg, milk, and breadcrumbs; fried in vegetable shortening.

[15] If bones are discarded, value for calcium will be greatly reduced.

[16] Dipped in egg, breadcrumbs, and flour; fried in vegetable shortening.

[17] Made with drained chunk light tuna, celery, onion, pickle relish, and mayonnaise-type salad dressing.

Nutrients in Indicated Quantity

Cho-les-terol	Carbo-hydrate	Calcium	Phos-phorus	Iron	Potas-sium	Sodium	Vitamin A value		Thiamin	Ribo-flavin	Niacin	Ascorbic acid
							(IU)	(RE)				
Milli-grams	Grams	Milli-grams	Milli-grams	Milli-grams	Milli-grams	Milli-grams	Inter-national units	Retinol equiva-lents	Milli-grams	Milli-grams	Milli-grams	Milli-grams
0	2	2	12	0.1	31	1	0	0	0.01	Tr	Tr	Tr
0	0	1	0	0.0	2	6	0	0	0.00	0.00	0.0	0
0	Tr	4	4	0.1	7	63	0	0	Tr	0.01	Tr	Tr
0	Tr	8	2	0.2	7	312	40	4	Tr	Tr	Tr	0
0	Tr	10	2	0.2	2	68	10	1	Tr	Tr	Tr	0
0	1	24	3	0.7	25	Tr	100	10	0.01	Tr	0.1	1
0	1	4	7	0.5	49	1	1,270	127	0.01	0.04	0.3	1
0	1	9	4	0.6	26	1	Tr	Tr	Tr	0.01	Tr	0
0	1	17	14	0.7	130	928	70	7	Tr	0.01	Tr	4
0	3	5	4	0.3	30	101	20	2	Tr	Tr	Tr	1
0	5	2	2	0.2	30	107	10	1	Tr	Tr	Tr	1
0	0	14	3	Tr	Tr	2,132	0	0	0.00	0.00	0.0	0
0	1	1	1	0.1	15	Tr	0	0	0.00	0.00	0.0	0
0	3	3	90	1.1	140	4	Tr	Tr	0.16	0.38	2.6	Tr

[18] Sodium bisulfite used to preserve color; unsulfited product would contain less sodium.

[19] Also applies to pasteurized apple cider.

[20] Without added ascorbic acid. For value with added ascorbic acid, refer to label.

[21] With added ascorbic acid.

[22] For white grapefruit; pink grapefruit have about 310 IU or 31 RE.

[23] Sodium benzoate and sodium bisulfite added as preservatives.

[24] Egg bagels have 44 mg cholesterol and 22 IU or 7 RE vitamin A per bagel.

[25] Made with vegetable shortening.

[26] Made with white cornmeal. If made with yellow cornmeal, value is 32 IU or 3 RE.

[27] Nutrient added.

[28] Cooked without salt. If salt is added according to label recommendations, sodium content is 540 mg.

[29] For white corn grits. Cooked yellow grits contain 145 IU or 14 RE.

[30] Value based on label declaration for added nutrients.

[31] For regular and instant cereal. For quick cereal, phosphorus is 102 mg and sodium is 142 mg.

[32] Cooked without salt. If salt is added according to label recommendations, sodium content is 390 mg.

[33] Cooked without salt. If salt is added according to label recommendations, sodium content is 324 mg.

[34] Cooked without salt. If salt is added according to label recommendations, sodium content is 374 mg.

[35] Excepting angelfood cake, cakes were made from mixes containing vegetable shortening and frostings were made with margarine.

[36] Made with vegetable oil.

(Footnotes continue on next page.)

[37] Cake made with vegetable shortening; frosting with margarine.
[38] Made with margarine.
[39] Crackers made with enriched flour except for rye wafers and whole-wheat wafers.
[40] Made with lard.
[41] Cashews without salt contain 21 mg sodium per cup or 4 mg per oz.
[42] Cashews without salt contain 22 mg sodium per cup or 5 mg per oz.
[43] Macadamia nuts without salt contain 9 mg sodium per cup or 2 mg per oz.
[44] Mixed nuts without salt contain 3 mg sodium per oz.
[45] Peanuts without salt contain 22 mg sodium per cup or 4 mg per oz.
[46] Outer layer of fat was removed to within approximately ½ inch of the lean. Deposits of fat within the cut were not removed.
[47] Fried in vegetable shortening.
[48] Value varies widely.
[49] Contains added sodium ascorbate. If sodium ascorbate is not added, ascorbic acid content is negligible.
[50] One patty (8 per pound) of bulk sausage is equivalent to 2 links.
[51] Crust made with vegetable shortening and enriched flour.
[52] Made with corn oil.
[53] Fried in vegetable shortening.
[54] If sodium ascorbate is added, product contains 11 mg ascorbic acid.
[55] Made with enriched flour, margarine, and whole milk.
[56] For regular pack; special dietary pack contains 3 mg sodium.
[57] For green varieties; yellow varieties contain 101 IU or 10 RE.
[58] For green varieties; yellow varieties contain 151 IU or 15 RE.
[59] For regular pack; special dietary pack contains 3 mg sodium.
[60] For green varieties; yellow varieties contain 142 IU or 14 RE.
[61] For regular pack; special dietary pack contains 78 mg sodium.
[62] For regular pack; special dietary pack contains 61 mg sodium.
[63] For yellow varieties; white varieties contain only a trace of vitamin A.
[64] For regular pack; special dietary pack contains 8 mg sodium.
[65] For regular pack; special dietary pack contains 6 mg sodium.
[66] For regular pack; special dietary pack contains 3 mg sodium.
[67] For red peppers; green peppers contain 350 IU or 35 RE.
[68] For green peppers; red peppers contain 4220 IU or 422 RE.
[69] For green peppers; red peppers contain 141 mg ascorbic acid.
[70] For green peppers; red peppers contain 2740 IU or 274 RE.
[71] For green peppers; red peppers contain 121 mg ascorbic acid.
[72] With added salt; if none is added, sodium content is 58 mg.
[73] For regular pack; special dietary pack contains 31 mg sodium.
[74] With added salt; if none is added, sodium content is 24 mg.
[75] With no added salt; if salt is added, sodium content is 2070 mg.
[76] With no added salt; if salt is added, sodium content is 998 mg.
[77] With salt added.

Adapted from Thomas, CL (ed): Taber's Cyclopedic Medical Dictionary, ed 16. FA Davis, Philadelphia, 1989.

Metropolitan Height and Weight Tables for Men and Women According to Frame, Ages 25–59

Men (Indoor Clothing†)

Height (in Shoes)*			Small Frame		Medium Frame		Large Frame	
Feet	Inches	Centimeters	Pounds	Kilograms	Pounds	Kilograms	Pounds	Kilograms
5	2	157.5	128–134	58.2–60.9	131–141	59.5–64.1	138–150	62.7–68.2
5	3	160.0	130–136	59.1–61.8	133–143	60.4–65.0	140–153	63.6–69.5
5	4	162.6	132–138	60.0–62.7	135–145	61.4–65.9	142–156	64.5–70.9
5	5	165.1	134–140	60.9–63.6	137–148	62.3–67.2	144–160	65.5–72.7
5	6	167.6	136–142	61.8–64.5	139–151	63.2–68.6	146–164	66.4–74.5
5	7	170.2	138–145	62.7–65.9	142–154	64.5–70.0	149–168	67.7–76.4
5	8	172.7	140–148	63.6–67.2	145–157	65.9–71.4	152–172	69.1–78.2
5	9	175.3	142–151	64.5–68.6	148–160	67.2–72.7	155–176	70.5–80.0
5	10	177.8	144–154	65.5–70.0	151–163	68.6–74.1	158–180	71.8–81.8
5	11	180.3	146–157	66.4–71.4	154–166	70.0–75.5	161–184	73.2–83.6
6	0	182.9	149–160	67.7–72.7	157–170	71.4–77.3	164–188	74.5–85.5
6	1	185.4	152–164	69.1–74.5	160–174	72.7–79.1	168–192	76.4–87.3
6	2	188.0	155–168	70.5–76.4	164–178	74.5–80.9	172–197	78.2–89.5
6	3	190.5	158–172	71.8–78.2	167–182	75.9–82.7	176–202	80.0–91.8
6	4	193.0	162–176	73.6–80.0	171–187	77.7–85.0	181–207	82.3–94.1

*Shoes with 1-inch heels.

†Allow 5 pounds.

Women (Indoor Clothing†)

Height (in Shoes)*			Small Frame		Medium Frame		Large Frame	
Feet	Inches	Centimeters	Pounds	Kilograms	Pounds	Kilograms	Pounds	Kilograms
4	10	147.3	102–111	46.4–50.0	109–121	49.5–55.0	118–131	53.6–59.5
4	11	149.9	103–113	46.8–51.4	111–123	50.0–55.9	102–134	54.5–60.9
5	0	152.4	104–115	47.3–52.3	113–126	51.4–57.2	122–137	55.5–62.3
5	1	154.9	106–118	48.2–53.6	115–129	52.3–58.6	125–140	56.8–63.6
5	2	157.5	108–121	49.1–55.0	118–132	53.6–60.0	128–143	58.2–65.0
5	3	160.0	111–124	50.5–56.4	121–135	55.0–61.4	131–147	59.5–66.8
5	4	162.6	114–127	51.8–57.7	124–138	56.4–62.7	134–151	60.9–68.6
5	5	165.1	117–130	53.2–59.0	127–141	57.7–64.1	137–155	62.3–70.5
5	6	167.6	120–133	54.5–60.5	130–144	59.0–65.5	140–159	63.6–72.3
5	7	170.2	123–136	55.9–61.8	133–147	60.5–66.8	143–163	65.0–74.1
5	8	172.7	126–139	57.3–63.2	136–150	61.8–68.2	146–167	66.4–75.9
5	9	175.3	129–142	58.6–64.5	139–153	63.2–69.5	149–170	67.7–77.3
5	10	177.8	132–145	60.0–65.9	142–156	64.6–70.9	152–173	69.1–78.6
5	11	180.3	135–148	61.4–67.3	145–159	65.9–72.3	155–176	70.5–80.0
6	0	182.9	138–151	62.7–73.6	148–162	67.3–73.6	158–179	71.8–81.4

*Shoes with 1-inch heels.

†Allow 3 pounds

Source of basic data: Build Study, 1979, Society of Actuaries and Association of Life Insurance Medical Directors of America, 1980. © 1983 Metropolian Life Insurance Company.

Note: The weights presented are those associated with the lowest mortality. They are not necessarily the weights at which people are healthiest, perform their jobs optimally, or even look their best. From Metropolitan Life, Warwick, RI, with permission.

Growth Charts for Boys and Girls, Ages 0 to 18

Growth charts, such as the eight that follow, are used to evaluate growth in infants and children. They are a valuable tool in the nutritional assessment. To plot a measurement on the percentile graph, follow these steps:

- Select the appropriate chart based on age, sex, and type of measurement.
- Locate the child's age on the top or bottom of the chart.
- Locate the child's weight (in pounds or kilograms), length (in inches or centimeters), or head circumference on the left- or right-hand side of the chart.
- Mark the chart where the age and weight, length, or head circumference lines intersect.

Each chart contains a series of curved lines that represent percentiles. For example, when a mark is on the 95th percentile line of weight for age, it means that only 5 children out of 100 (of the same age and sex) have a greater weight. A series of plot marks on a chart will show the pattern of growth for a particular child. If any marks appear above the 95th percentile or below the 5th percentile, you may want to report this to the physician. Rapid changes above the 75th percentile or below the 25th percentile may also be significant.

BOYS: BIRTH TO 36 MONTHS
PHYSICAL GROWTH
NCHS PERCENTILES*

NAME _____ RECORD # _____

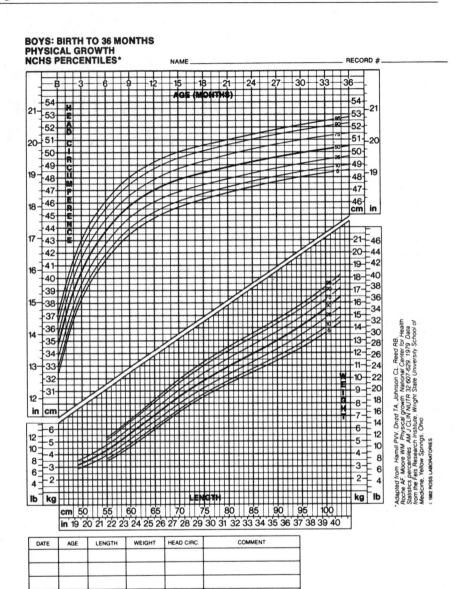

*Adapted from Hamil PVV, Drizd TA, Johnson CL, Reed RB, Roche AF, Moore WM. Physical growth: National Center for Health Statistics percentiles. AM J CLIN NUTR 32:607-629, 1979. Data from the Fels Research Institute. Wright State University School of Medicine, Yellow Springs, Ohio

© 1982 ROSS LABORATORIES

DATE	AGE	LENGTH	WEIGHT	HEAD CIRC.	COMMENT

**BOYS: BIRTH TO 36 MONTHS
PHYSICAL GROWTH
NCHS PERCENTILES***

NAME_____ RECORD #_____

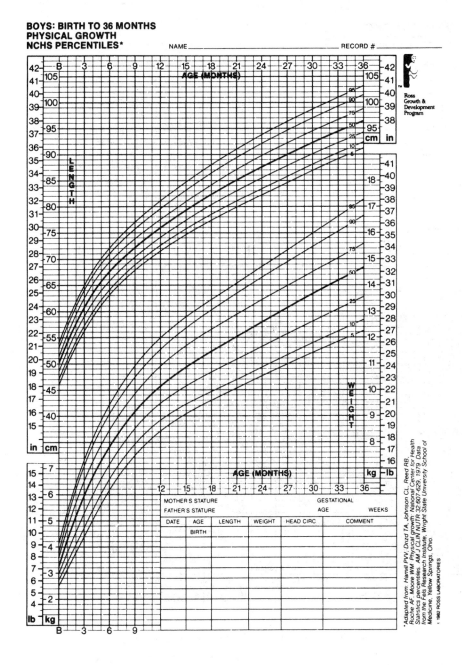

*Adapted from: Hamill PVV, Drizd TA, Johnson CL, Reed RB,
Roche AF, Moore WM: Physical growth: National Center for Health
Statistics percentiles. AM J CLIN NUTR 32:607-629, 1979. Data
from the Fels Research Institute, Wright State University School of
Medicine, Yellow Springs, Ohio.
© 1982 ROSS LABORATORIES*

**BOYS: PREPUBESCENT
PHYSICAL GROWTH
NCHS PERCENTILES***

NAME _____ RECORD # _____

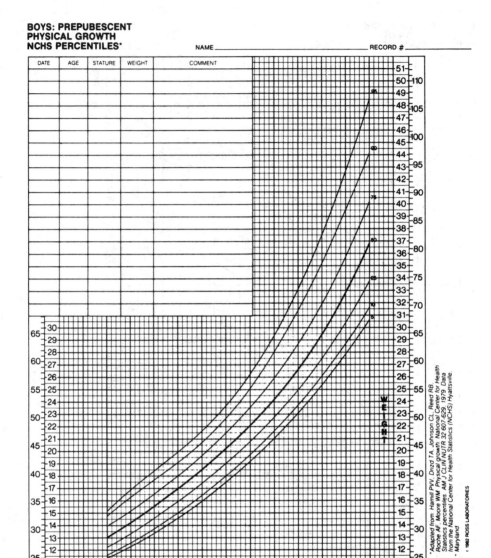

*Adapted from Hamill PVV, Drizd TA, Johnson CL, Reed RB
Roche AF, Moore WM Physical growth: National Center for Health
Statistics percentiles AM J CLIN NUTR 32:607-629, 1979 Data
from the National Center for Health Statistics (NCHS) Hyattsville.
- Maryland

© 1982 ROSS LABORATORIES

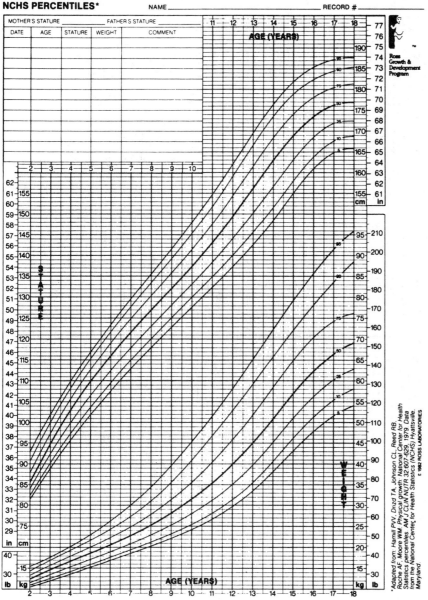

**BOYS: 2 TO 18 YEARS
PHYSICAL GROWTH
NCHS PERCENTILES***

NAME _____ RECORD # _____

GIRLS: BIRTH TO 36 MONTHS
PHYSICAL GROWTH
NCHS PERCENTILES*

NAME _____ RECORD # _____

*Adapted from Hamill PVV, Dnzd TA, Johnson CL, Reed RB, Roche AF, Moore WM. Physical growth: National Center for Health Statistics percentiles. AM J CLIN NUTR 32 607-629, 1979. Data from the Fels Research Institute, Wright State University School of Medicine, Yellow Springs, Ohio

© 1982 ROSS LABORATORIES

DATE	AGE	LENGTH	WEIGHT	HEAD CIRC	COMMENT

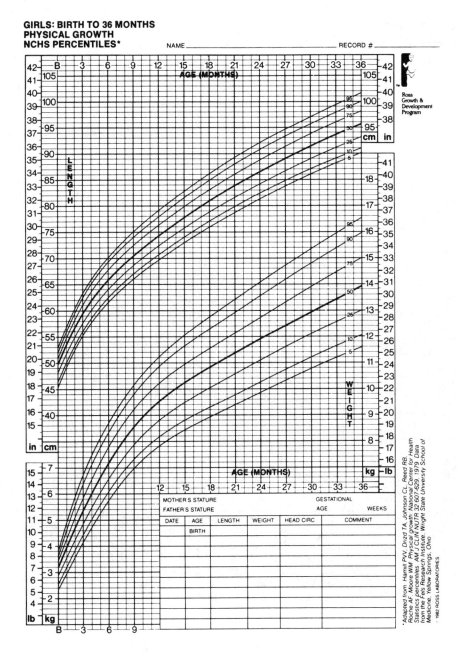

GIRLS: BIRTH TO 36 MONTHS
PHYSICAL GROWTH
NCHS PERCENTILES*

NAME _____ RECORD # _____

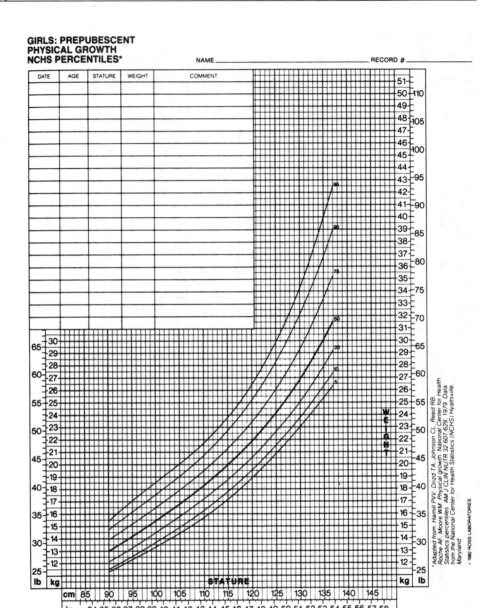

**GIRLS: PREPUBESCENT
PHYSICAL GROWTH
NCHS PERCENTILES***

GIRLS: 2 TO 18 YEARS
PHYSICAL GROWTH
NCHS PERCENTILES*

NAME _____ RECORD # _____

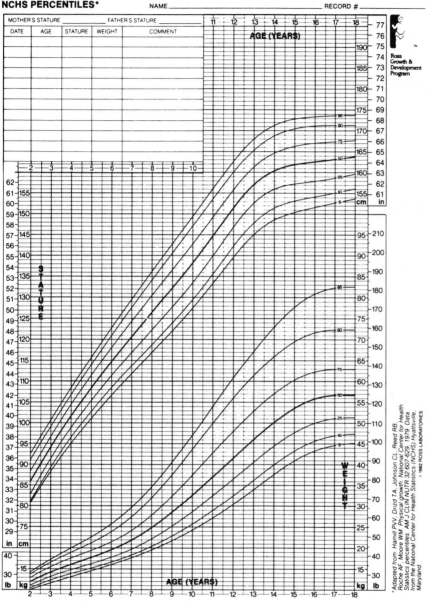

Adapted from Hamill PVV, Druzd TA, Johnson CL, Reed RB, Roche AF, Moore WM. Physical growth: National Center for Health Statistics percentiles. AM J CLIN NUTR 32:607-629, 1979. Data from the National Center for Health Statistics (NCHS) Hyattsville, Maryland

© 1982 ROSS LABORATORIES

Ross
Growth &
Development
Program

Food Frequency Questionnaire

Please indicate the number of times you eat/drink the following food/beverages by placing a check (√) in the appropriate column.

	Food	Daily	2×/Week	3×/Week	Other	Never	Comments
Milk and Milk Products	Whole-milk products						
	Skimmed milk products						
	Cheeses/cottage cheese						
	Ice cream/custards/ puddings						
Meat and Meat Substitutes	Beef						
	Pork						
	Cured meats						
	Chicken/turkey						
	Fish						
	Eggs/omelets						
	Egg substitutes						
	Legumes (peas, beans)						
	Peanut butter/nuts						
Fruits and Vegetables	Fresh fruits						
	Canned fruits						
	Fruit Juices						
	Vegetables						
	Vegetable juices						
Grains	Whole-grain breads/cereals						
	Other breads/cereals						
Snacks	Chips/snacks						
	Desserts						

Table continued on next page.

Food Frequency Questionnaire (*Continued*)

	Food	Daily	2×/Week	3×/Week	Other	Never	Comments
Simple Sugars	Sugar						
	Honey						
	Jam						
Beverages	Wine						
	Beer						
	Liquor						
	Coffee/tea						
	Regular pop or soda						
	Diet pop or soda						
Fats	Margarine						
	Butter						
	Lard						
	Oil, canola/olive/peanut						
	Oil, corn/safflower/soybean						
Other	Table salt						
	Gravies/sauces						

Appendix E

Recommended Dietary Allowances

Recommended Dietary Allowances (RDA), Revised 1989[a]

Age (Years)	Weight[b] (kg)	Weight[b] (lb)	Height[b] (cm)	Height[b] (inches)	Protein (g)	Fat-Soluble Vitamins Vitamin A (μg RE)[c]	Vitamin D[d] (μg)	Vitamin E (mg α-TE)[e]	Vitamin K (μg)	Water-Soluble Vitamins Vitamin C (mg)	Thiamin (mg)	Riboflavin (mg)	Niacin (mg NE)[f]	Vitamin B6 (mg)	Folate (μg)	Vitamin B12 (μg)	Minerals Calcium (mg)	Phosphorus (mg)	Magnesium (mg)	Iron (mg)	Zinc (mg)	Iodine (μg)	Selenium (μg)
Infants																							
0.0–0.5	6	13	60	24	13	375	7.5	3	5	30	0.3	0.4	5	0.3	25	0.3	400	300	40	6	5	40	10
0.5–1.0	9	20	71	28	14	375	10	4	10	35	0.4	0.5	6	0.6	35	0.5	600	500	60	10	5	50	15
Children																							
1–3	13	29	90	35	16	400	10	6	15	40	0.7	0.8	9	1.0	50	0.7	800	800	80	10	10	70	20
4–6	20	44	112	44	24	500	10	7	20	45	0.9	1.1	12	1.1	75	1.0	800	800	120	10	10	90	20
7–10	28	62	132	52	28	700	10	7	30	45	1.0	1.2	13	1.4	100	1.4	800	800	170	10	10	120	30
Males																							
11–14	45	99	157	62	45	1000	10	10	45	50	1.3	1.5	17	1.7	150	2.0	1200	1200	270	12	15	150	40
15–18	66	145	176	69	59	1000	10	10	65	60	1.5	1.8	20	2.0	200	2.0	1200	1200	400	12	15	150	50
19–24	72	160	177	70	58	1000	10	10	70	60	1.5	1.7	19	2.0	200	2.0	1200	1200	350	10	15	150	70
25–50	79	174	176	70	63	1000	5	10	80	60	1.5	1.7	19	2.0	200	2.0	800	800	350	10	15	150	70
51+	77	170	173	68	63	1000	5	10	80	60	1.2	1.4	15	2.0	200	2.0	800	800	350	10	15	150	70

Females																							
11–14	46	101	157	62	46	800	10	8	45	50	1.1	1.3	15	1.4	150	2.0	1200	1200	280	15	12	150	45
15–18	55	120	163	64	44	800	10	8	55	60	1.1	1.3	15	1.5	180	2.0	1200	1200	300	15	12	150	50
19–24	58	128	164	65	46	800	10	8	60	60	1.1	1.3	15	1.6	180	2.0	1200	1200	280	15	12	150	55
25–50	63	138	163	64	50	800	5	8	65	60	1.1	1.3	15	1.6	180	2.0	800	800	280	15	12	150	55
51+	65	143	160	63	50	800	5	8	65	60	1.0	1.2	13	1.6	180	2.0	800	800	280	10	12	150	55
Pregnant					60	800	10	10	65	70	1.5	1.6	17	2.2	400	2.2	1200	1200	320	30	15	175	65
Lactating																							
1st 6 months					65	1300	10	12	65	95	1.6	1.8	20	2.1	280	2.6	1200	1200	355	15	19	200	75
2nd 6 months					62	1200	10	11	65	90	1.6	1.7	20	2.1	260	2.6	1200	1200	340	15	16	200	75

a The allowances, expressed as average daily intakes over time, are intended to provide for individual variations among most normal persons as they live in the United States under usual environmental stresses. Diets should be based on a variety of common foods in order to provide other nutrients for which human requirements have been less well defined.

b Weights and heights of Reference Adults are actual medians for the US population of the designated age, as reported by NHANES II. The use of these figures does not imply that the height-to-weight ratios are ideal.

c Retinol equivalents. 1 retinol equivalent = 1 µg retinol or 6 µg β-carotene. See Clinical Calculation 6–1 to convert IU of vitamin A to retinol equivalents.

d As cholecalciferol. 10 µg cholecalciferol = 400 IU of vitamin D. See Clinical Calculation 6–2 to convert IU of vitamin D to mg of cholecalciferol.

e α-Tocopherol equivalents. 1 mg d-α tocopherol = 1 α-TE.

f 1 NE (niacin equivalent) is equal to 1 mg of niacin or 60 mg of dietary tryptophan.

Note: The Committee on Dietary Allowances has published a separate table showing energy allowances which appears as Table 8–4.

Source: From Recommended Dietary Allowances, © 1989, by the National Academy of Sciences, National Academy Press, Washington, DC, with permission.

Estimated Safe and Adequate Daily Dietary Intakes of Selected Vitamins and Minerals

Estimated Safe and Adequate Daily Dietary Intakes of Selected Vitamins and Minerals[a]

		Vitamins	
Category	Age (Years)	Biotin (μg)	Pantothenic Acid (mg)
Infants	0–0.5	10	2
	0.5–1	15	3
Children and adolescents	1–3	20	3
	4–6	25	3–4
	7–10	30	4–5
	11+	30–100	4–7
Adults		30–100	4–7

		Trace Elements[b]				
Category	Age (Years)	Copper (mg)	Manganese (mg)	Fluoride (mg)	Chromium (μg)	Molybdenum (μg)
Infants	0–0.5	0.4–0.6	0.3–0.6	0.1–0.5	10–40	15–30
	0.5–1	0.6–0.7	0.6–1.0	0.2–1.0	20–60	20–40
Children and	1–3	0.7–1.0	1.0–1.5	0.5–1.5	20–80	25–50
adolescents	4–6	1.0–1.5	1.5–2.0	1.0–2.5	30–120	30–75
	7–10	1.0–2.0	2.0–3.0	1.5–2.5	50–200	50–150
	11+	1.5–2.5	2.0–5.0	1.5–2.5	50–200	75–250
Adults		1.5–3.0	2.0–5.0	1.5–4.0	50–200	75–250

[a]Because there is less information on which to base allowances, these figures are not given in the main table of RDA and are provided here in the form of ranges of recommended intakes.

[b]Since the toxic levels for many trace elements may be only several times usual intakes, the upper levels for the trace elements given in this table should not be habitually exceeded.

Source: From Recommended Dietary Allowances, © 1989, by the National Academy of Sciences, National Academy Press, Washington, DC, with permission.

Estimated Sodium, Chloride, and Potassium Minimum Requirements of Healthy Persons

Estimated Sodium, Chloride, and Potassium Minimum Requirements of Healthy Persons[a]

Age	Weight (kg)[d]	Sodium (mg)[a,b]	Chloride (mg)[a,b]	Potassium (mg)[c]
Months				
0–5	4.5	120	180	500
6–11	8.9	200	300	700
Years				
1	11.0	225	350	1,000
2–5	16.0	300	500	1,400
6–9	25.0	400	600	1,600
10–18	50.0	500	750	2,000
>18[d]	70.0	500	750	2,000

[a]No allowance has been included for large, prolonged losses from the skin through sweat.

[b]There is no evidence that higher intakes confer any health benefit.

[c]Desirable intakes of potassium may considerably exceed these values (~3,500 mg for adults—see text).

[d]No allowance included for growth. Values for those below 18 years assume a growth rate at the 50th percentile reported by the National Center for Health Statistics (Hamill et al., 1979) and averaged for males and females. See text for information on pregnancy and lactation.

Source: From Recommended Dietary Allowances, © 1989, by the National Academy of Sciences, National Academy Press, Washington, DC, with permission.

Exchange Lists of the American Dietetic and Diabetic Associations, Revised 1989

The exchange lists are divided into six different basic groups: starch/breads, meat and meat substitutes (with three subcategories), vegetables, fruits, milk (with three subcategories), and fats. Each exchange list contains foods that are alike—each choice contains about the same amount of carbohydrate, protein, fat, and calories. The term *calorie*, which is used throughout, refers to kilocalories. Also included in this appendix are three other lists—combination foods, foods for occasional use, and free foods for diabetic and low-calorie diets. The following chart shows the amount of these nutrients in one serving from each exchange list.

Exchange List	Carbohydrate (Grams)	Protein (Grams)	Fat (Grams)	Calories
Starch/Bread	15	3	trace	80
Meat				
Lean	—	7	3	55
Medium-Fat	—	7	5	75
High-Fat	—	7	8	100
Vegetable	5	2	—	25
Fruit	15	—	—	60
Milk				
Skimmed	12	8	trace	90
Low-fat	12	8	5	120
Whole	12	8	8	150
Fat	—	—	5	45

STARCH/BREAD LIST

Contains 15 grams of carbohydrate, 3 grams of protein, and 80 calories.

Bread

Bagel	½ (1 oz)
Bread sticks, crisp 4"×½"	2 (⅔ oz)
Bun, hamburger or hotdog	½
Croutons, low-fat	1 cup
Dinner roll, small	1 (1 oz)
English muffin	½
Matzoth, 6" sq.	1
Pita, 6" across	½
Tortilla, 6" across	1
White, whole wheat, rye, etc.	1 slice

Crackers/Snacks

Animal crackers	8
Graham crackers 2½" sq.	3
Melba toast	5 pieces
Oyster crackers	20
Popcorn (popped, no fat added)	3 cups
Pretzels	25 sm, 3 twisted
Rye Krisp (2" × 3½")	4
Saltine-type	6
Whole wheat crackers, no fat added (crisp breads such as Finn, Kavli, Wasa)	2–4 pieces (¾ oz)

Cereal/Grains/Pasta

Bran cereals, conc., such as All Bran, Bran Buds	⅓ cup
Bran cereals, flaked, such as 40% Bran	½ cup
Bulgar (cooked)	½ cup
Cooked cereals	½ cup
Cornmeal (dry)	2½ Tbsp
Grape Nuts	3 Tbsp
Grits (cooked)	½ cup
Other ready-to-eat cereals (unsweetened)	¾ cup
Pasta (cooked)	½ cup
Puffed cereals	1½ cup

Rice, white or brown (cooked)	⅓ cup
Shredded wheat	½ cup

Other

Cornstarch	2 Tbsp.
Flour	2½ Tbsp
Pearl barley	1½ Tbsp
Tapioca, dry	2 Tbsp

Starchy Vegetables

Baked beans	¼ cup
Beans and peas (cooked) such as kidney, white northern, split	⅓ cup
Corn	½ cup
Corn-on-the-cob, 6" long	1
Lentils (cooked)	⅓ cup
Lima beans	½ cup
Peas, green	½ cup
Plantain	½ cup
Potato, baked	1 sm. (3 oz)
Potato, mashed	½ cup
Pumpkin	¾ cup
Squash, winter	½ cup
Succotash	½ cup
Yam, sweet potato (plain)	⅓ cup

Starches prepared with fat (Count as one starch/bread serving plus 1 fat)

Biscuit 2½" across	1
Chow mein noodles	½ cup
Cornbread, 2" cube	1 (2 oz)
Cracker, round, butter-type	6
French fried potatoes 2–3½" long	10 (1½ oz)
Pancake 4" across	2
Stuffing, bread (prepared)	¼ cup
Taco shell, 6" across	2
Whole-wheat crackers, fat added (such as Triscuits)	4–6 (1 oz)

MEAT AND MEAT SUBSTITUTES LIST

Contains 7 grams of protein and some fat. The amount of fat and calories depends on the type of meat or substitute chosen. The meat list is divided into three parts based on fat content. Make most choices from the first two lists. Meat should be weighed after cooking. They should be baked, broiled, grilled, microwaved, or roasted. Any fat used in cooking them should be subtracted from the fat allowed for the day.

Lean Meats and Meat Substitutes

Contain 7 grams protein, 3 grams of fat, and 55 calories

Beef: Lean beef such as round, sirloin, flank steak, tenderloin, chipped beef.	1 oz	Pork: Lean pork such as fresh ham; canned, cured, or boiled ham; Canadian bacon; tenderloin.	1 oz

MEAT AND MEAT SUBSTITUTES (*Continued*)

Veal: Any cut of veal except veal cutlets	1 oz	Cheese: Skimmed or part skimmed cheese such as:	
Poultry: Chicken, turkey, Cornish hen (no skin)	1 oz	Ricotta	¼ cup
		Mozzarella	1 oz
Fish: Any fresh or frozen crab, lobster, scallops, clams	2 oz	Diet cheese with 56–80 calories	
		Peanut butter	1 Tbsp
Tuna (canned in water)	¼ cup	Other: 86% fat-free luncheon meat	1 oz
Oysters	6 med		
Herring, uncreamed	1 oz	Egg (limit to 3/week)	1
Sardines (canned)	2 med	Tofu (2½" × 2¾" × 1")	4 oz
Wild Game: Venison, rabbit, squirrel, pheasant	1 oz.	Liver, heart, kidney, sweetbreads (high cholesterol)	1 oz
Cheese: Cottage cheese	¼ cup	*High-Fat Meats and Meat Substitutes*	
Diet cheese with less than 55 calories per ounce	1 oz.	Contain 7 grams of protein, 8 grams of fat, and 100 calories	
Parmesan	2 Tbsp	Beef: Most USDA prime cuts such as prime rib (restaurants may use prime cuts); corned beef	1 oz
Other: 95% fat-free luncheon meats	1 oz.		
Egg whites	3 whites		
Egg substitutes	¼ cup	Pork: Spareribs, ground pork, pork sausage	1 oz
Medium-Fat Meats and Meat Substitutes		Lamb: Patties, ground lamb	1 oz
Contain 7 grams of protein, 5 grams of fat, and 75 calories.		Fish: Any fried fish product	1 oz
Beef: Most beef products, including ground beef, any roast, steaks, meatloaf	1 oz	Cheese: All regular cheese such as American, bleu, Chedder, Colby, Swiss	1 oz
Pork: Most pork products, including chops, roasts, and cutlets	1 oz	Other: Lunch meats such as bologna, salami, pimento loaf	1 oz
Lamb: Most lamb products including, chops, leg, and roasts	1 oz	Sausage such as Polish, Italian	1 oz
		Knockwurst	1 oz
Veal: Cutlet (unbreaded)	1 oz	Bratwurst	1 frank
Poultry: Chicken w/skin; Domestic duck or goose (no skin); ground turkey	1 oz.	Frankfurter made with turkey or chicken (10/lb)	1 frank
		Counts as one high-fat meat plus 1 fat exchange:	
Fish: Tuna canned (in oil, drained)	¼ cup	Frankfurter, beef, pork or mix	1 frank
Salmon (canned)	¼ cup		

VEGETABLE LIST

Contains 5 grams of carbohydrate, 2 grams of protein, and 25 calories. Unless specified, the serving size for vegetables is ½ cup of cooked vegetable or vegetable juice or 1 cup of raw vegetables. Starchy vegetables are found on the Starch/Bread List. Free vegetables are found on the Free Food List.

Artichoke (½ med)	Carrots	Mushrooms, cooked	Summer squash, (crookneck)
Asparagus	Cauliflower	Okra	
Beans (green, wax, Italian)	Eggplant	Onions	Tomato (one large)
	Greens (collard, mustard, turnip)	Pea Pods	Tomato juice
Bean Sprouts		Peppers (green)	Turnips
Beets	Kohlrabi	Rutabaga	Vegetable juice cocktail
Broccoli	Leeks	Sauerkraut	Waterchestnuts
Brussel sprouts		Spinach, cooked	Zucchini, cooked
Cabbage, cooked			

FRUIT

Contains 15 grams of carbohydrates and 60 calories. Fruits may be fresh, dried, cooked, canned or frozen as long as no sugar is added. Rinsing syrup-packed fruits does not remove all added sugar!

Apple, 2″ across	1	Grape juice	⅓ cup
Apple juice/cider	½ cup	Guava, raw	1 medium
Applesauce	½ cup	Honeydew, melon, med.	⅛ melon
Apricots (fresh)	4 apricots	Kiwi, large	1
Apricots, canned	½ cup	Mandarin oranges	¾ cup
Apricots, dried	7 halves	Mango	½ sm
Banana (9″ long)	½	Nectarine, 1½″ across	1
Berries:		Orange, 2½″ across	1
Blackberries	¾ cup	Orange juice	½ cup
Blueberries	¾ cup	Orange sections	¾ cup
Boysenberries	1 cup	Papaya	¾ cup
Raspberries	1 cup	Peach, 2¾″ across	1
Strawberries	1¼ cup	Peaches, canned	½ cup
Cantaloupe, 5″ across	⅓ melon	Pear, fresh	½ large or 1 small
Cherries, large, raw	12 large	Pear, canned	½ cup
Cherries, canned	½ cup	Persimmons, med. native	2
Dates	2½ med	Pineapple, fresh	¾ cup
Figs, fresh, 2″ across	2	Pineapple juice	½ cup
Figs, dried	1½	Plums, 2″ across	2
Fruit cocktail	½ cup	Pomegranate, raw	½
Fresh fruit cup	½ cup	Prunes, dried	3 med
Grapefruit	½ medium	Prune juice	⅓ cup
Grapefruit juice	½ cup	Raisins	2 Tbsp
Grapefruit sections	¾ cup	Tangerine, 2½″ across	2
Grapes, small	15	Watermelon	1¼ cup

MILK LIST

Contains 12 grams carbohydrate, 8 grams protein, and may contain fat. The amount of fat and calories depends on the type of milk chosen.

Skim and Very Low-Fat Milk
Contains 12 grams carbohydrate, 8 grams protein, a trace of fat, and 80 calories.

Skimmed milk	1 cup
½% milk	1 cup
1% milk	1 cup
Low-fat buttermilk	1 cup
Evaporated skimmed milk	½ cup
Dry nonfat milk	⅓ cup
Plain nonfat yogurt	1 cup

Low-fat Milk
Contains 12 grams carbohydrate, 8 grams protein, 5 grams of fat, and 120 calories.

2% milk	1 cup
Plain low-fat yogurt (with added nonfat milk solids)	1 cup

Whole Milk
Contains 12 grams carbohydrate, 8 grams protein, 8 grams fat, and 150 calories.

Whole milk	1 cup
Evaporated whole milk	½ cup
Whole plain yogurt	1 cup

FAT LIST

Contains 5 grams of fat and 45 calories.

Unsaturated fats		Nuts and seeds:	
Avocado	⅛	Almonds	6
Margarine	1 tsp	Brazil nuts	2
Margarine, diet	2 tsp	Cashews	1 Tbsp

FAT (*Continued*)

Unsaturated fats (continued)

Nuts and seeds *(continued)*:

Macadamia	3
Peanuts	20 sm/10 large
Pistachio	20
Walnuts	2
Other nuts	1 Tbsp
Sunflower seeds	1 Tbsp
Pumpkin seeds (hulled)	2 tsp
Oils	1 tsp
Olives	10 sm/5 large

Salad dressing:

French, Italian, etc.	1 Tbsp
Mayonnaise	1 tsp
Mayonnaise, reduced calorie	2 tsp
Mayonnaise-type	2 tsp
Mayonnaise-type, reduced calorie	1 Tbsp
Reduced-calorie French, Italian, etc.	2 Tbsp
Low-calorie French, Italian, etc.	2 Tbsp = Free Food

Saturated Fats

Butter	1 tsp
Bacon	1 slice
Chitterlings	½ oz
Coconut	2 Tbsp

Cream

Half and half	2 Tbsp
Sour cream	2 Tbsp
Whipping cream	1 Tbsp
Whipped cream	2 Tbsp
Cream cheese	1 Tbsp
Nondairy coffee creamer, liquid	2 Tbsp
Nondairy coffee creamer, powdered	4 tsp
Salt pork	¼ oz

COMBINATION FOODS LIST

There are many foods that contain ingredients from more than one list. If a food you want to use is not found on the following list, ask your dietitian how to include it.

Casseroles, homemade	1 cup = 2 starch, 2 meat, 1 fat
Chili with beans, (canned)	1 cup = 2 starch, 2 meat, 2 fat
Cheese, thin crust	¼ of 10″ pizza = 2 starch, 1 meat, 1 fat
Chow mein (measure rice or noodles separately)	2 cups = 2 starch, 2 meat, 2 veg
Macaroni and cheese	1 cup = 2 starch, 1 meat, 2 fat

Soup:

Bean	1 cup = 1 starch 1 meat, 1 veg

Soup *(continued)*:

Chunky	10¾ oz can = 1 starch, 1 meat, 1 veg
Cream	1 cup = 1 starch, 1 fat
Vegetable or broth-based	1 cup = 1 starch
Spaghetti sauce with meat	1 cup = 2 meat, 2 veg
Sugar-free pudding	½ cup = 1 starch

When beans are used as a meat substitute:

Dried beans, peas, lentils	1 cup = 2 starch, 1 meat

FOODS FOR OCCASIONAL USE

Limit to one choice from this list once a week. Eat these foods with a meal; do not use them for a snack.

Cake:

Angel food	¹⁄₂₀ of 9″ cake = 1 starch
Plain, no icing	3″ sq. = 2 starch, 1 fat

Cookies:

Ginger snaps	3 = 1 starch
Vanilla wafers	6 = 1 starch, 1 fat
Other	2 sm(1¾″ across) = 1 starch, 1 fat

Frozen desserts:

Frozen fruit yogurt	⅓ cup = 1 starch
Ice cream, any flavor	½ cup = 1 starch, 2 fat
Ice milk, any flavor	½ cup = 1 starch, 1 fat
Sherbert, any flavor	¼ cup = 1 starch
Granola	¼ cup = 1 starch, 1 fat
Granola bar	1 small = 1 starch, 1 fat

FREE FOODS FOR DIABETIC AND LOW-CALORIE DIETS

"Free foods" are food or drink that provide less than 20 calories per serving. If no serving size is listed, any amount may be used; make 2–3 choices per day from those foods that have a specific serving size listed.

Boullion or broth without fat
Catsup, 1 Tbsp
Coffee; regular, flavored beans or decaffeinated
Club soda
Cranberries, unsweetened (½ cup)
Candy, hard, sugar free
Dietetic catsup
Flavoring extracts such as vanilla
Gelatin, sugar free
Gum, sugar free

Herbs
Horseradish
Hot pepper sauce
Jam/jelly, sugar free (2 tsp)
Lemon or lime (juice or rind)
Mustard
Nonstick pan spray
Pancake syrup, sugar free (1–2 Tbsp)
Pickles, dill, unsweetened
Pimento
Rhubarb, unsweetened (½ cup)

Sauces, meat, such as A-1
Salad dressing, low calorie (2 Tbsp)
Soy sauce
Salad greens (endive, escarole, lettuce, romaine, spinach)
Spices
Sugar substitutes
Sugar-free soft drinks
Taco sauce
Tea, regular, decaffeinated, herbal
Tonic water, sugar free

Vegetables (1 cup raw of only the following):
Cabbage
Celery
Chinese cabbage
Cucumber
Green onion
Hot peppers
Mushrooms
Radishes
Zucchini
Vinegar
Whipped topping (2 Tbsp)
Wine, when used in cooking (¼ cup)
Worcestershire sauce

The Exchange Lists are the basis of a meal planning system designed by a committee of the American Diabetes Association and The American Dietetic Association. While designed primarily for people with diabetes and others who must follow special diets, the Exchange Lists are based on principles of good nutrition that apply to everyone.

Source: Adapted from *Exchange Lists for Meal Planning* © 1989, American Diabetes Association, The American Dietetic Association.

Body Fat and Skinfolds of Adults and Children

The equivalent fat content, as a percentage of body weight, for a range of values for the sum of four skinfolds (biceps, triceps, subscapular, and suprailiac) of men and women of different ages.

TABLE A *Body Fat and Skinfolds of Men*

Skinfolds (mm)	Ages			
	17–29	30–39	40–49	50+
15	4.8	—	—	—
20	8.1	12.2	12.2	12.6
25	10.5	14.2	15.0	15.6
30	12.9	16.2	17.7	18.6
35	14.7	17.7	19.6	20.8
40	16.4	19.2	21.4	22.9
45	17.7	20.4	23.0	24.7
50	19.0	21.5	24.6	26.5
55	20.1	22.5	25.9	27.9
60	21.2	23.5	27.1	29.2
65	22.2	24.3	28.2	30.4
70	23.1	25.1	29.3	31.6
75	24.0	25.9	30.3	32.7
80	24.8	26.6	31.2	33.8
85	25.5	27.2	32.1	34.8
90	26.2	27.8	33.0	35.8
95	26.9	28.4	33.7	36.6
100	27.6	29.0	34.4	37.4
105	28.2	29.6	35.1	38.2
110	28.8	30.1	35.8	39.0
115	29.4	30.6	36.4	39.7
120	30.0	31.1	37.0	40.4
125	30.5	31.5	37.6	41.1
130	31.0	31.9	38.2	41.8
135	31.5	32.3	38.7	42.4
140	32.0	32.7	39.2	43.0
145	32.5	33.1	39.7	43.6
150	32.9	33.5	40.2	44.1

TABLE A *Body Fat and Skinfolds of Men (Continued)*

Skinfolds (mm)	Ages			
	17–29	30–39	40–49	50+
155	33.3	33.9	40.7	44.6
160	33.7	34.3	41.2	45.1
165	34.1	34.6	41.6	45.6
170	34.5	34.8	42.0	46.1
175	34.9	—	—	—
180	35.3	—	—	—
185	35.6	—	—	—
190	35.9	—	—	—
195	—	—	—	—
200	—	—	—	—
205	—	—	—	—
210	—	—	—	—

TABLE B *Body Fat and Skinfolds of Women*

Skinfolds (mm)	Ages			
	16–29	30–39	40–49	50+
15	10.5	—	—	—
20	14.1	17.0	19.8	21.4
25	16.8	19.4	22.2	24.0
30	19.5	21.8	24.5	26.6
35	21.5	23.7	26.4	28.5
40	23.4	25.5	28.2	30.3
45	25.0	26.9	29.6	31.9
50	26.5	28.2	31.0	33.4
55	27.8	29.4	32.1	34.6
60	29.1	30.6	33.2	35.7
65	30.2	31.6	34.1	36.7
70	31.2	32.5	35.0	37.7
75	32.2	33.4	35.9	38.7
80	33.1	34.3	36.7	39.6
85	34.0	35.1	37.5	40.4
90	34.8	35.8	38.3	41.2
95	35.6	36.5	39.0	41.9
100	36.4	37.2	39.7	42.6
105	37.1	37.9	40.4	43.3
110	37.8	38.6	41.0	43.9
115	38.4	39.1	41.5	44.5
120	39.0	39.6	42.0	45.1
125	39.6	40.1	42.5	45.7
130	40.2	40.6	43.0	46.2
135	40.8	41.1	43.5	46.7
140	41.3	41.6	44.0	47.2
145	41.8	42.1	44.5	47.7
150	42.3	42.6	45.0	48.2

TABLE B *Body Fat and Skinfolds of Women (Continued)*

Skinfolds (mm)	Ages			
	16–29	30–39	40–49	50+
155	42.8	43.1	45.4	48.7
160	43.3	43.6	45.8	49.2
165	43.7	44.0	46.2	49.6
170	44.1	44.4	46.6	50.0
175	—	44.8	47.0	50.4
180	—	45.2	47.4	50.8
185	—	45.6	47.8	51.2
190	—	45.9	48.2	51.6
195	—	46.2	48.5	52.0
200	—	46.5	48.8	52.4
205	—	—	49.1	52.7
210	—	—	49.4	53.0

In two thirds of the instances, the error was within +3.5% of the body-weight as fat for the women and ±5% for the men.

The relationship of skinfold thickness to body fat in children and individuals under 17 is addressed by The American Alliance for Health, Physical Education, Recreation and Dance in the publication *Lifetime Health Related Physical Fitness Test Manual*. They suggest that national percentile norms provide the best reference. They further suggest that the ideal is at the 50th percentile. Those below the 25th percentile should be encouraged to reduce amount of body fat, while those above the 90th percentile should not be encouraged to lose body fat.

TABLE C *Percentile Norms. Ages 6–18* for Sum of Triceps plus Subscapular Skinfolds (mm) for Boys*

Age	6	7	8	9	10	11	12	13	14	15	16	17
Percentile												
99	7	7	7	7	7	8	8	7	7	8	8	8
95	8	9	9	9	9	9	9	9	9	9	9	9
90	9	9	9	10	10	10	10	10	9	10	10	10
85	10	10	10	10	11	11	10	10	10	11	11	11
80	10	10	10	11	11	12	11	11	11	11	11	12
75	11	11	11	11	12	12	11	12	11	12	12	12
70	11	11	11	12	12	12	12	12	12	12	12	13
65	11	11	12	12	13	13	13	12	12	13	13	13
60	12	12	12	13	13	14	13	13	13	13	13	14
55	12	12	13	13	14	15	14	14	13	14	14	14
50	12	12	13	14	14	16	15	15	14	14	14	15
45	13	13	14	14	15	16	15	16	14	15	15	16
40	13	13	14	15	16	17	16	17	15	16	16	16
35	13	14	15	16	17	19	17	18	16	18	17	17
30	14	14	16	17	18	20	19	19	18	18	18	19

TABLE C *Percentile Norms. Ages 6–18* for Sum of Triceps plus Subscapular Skinfolds (mm) for Boys (Continued)*

Age	6	7	8	9	10	11	12	13	14	15	16	17
Percentile												
25	14	15	17	18	19	22	21	22	20	20	20	21
20	15	16	18	20	21	24	24	25	23	22	22	24
15	16	17	19	23	24	28	27	29	27	25	24	26
10	18	18	21	26	28	33	33	36	31	30	29	30
5	20	24	28	34	33	38	44	46	37	40	37	38

*The norms for age 17 may be used for age 18.

Source: Based on data from Johnston, F.E., Hamill, D.V., and Lemeshow, S.: (1) *Skinfold Thickness of Children 6–11 Years* (Series II, No. 120, 1972), and (2) *Skinfold Thickness of Youths 12–17 Years* (Series II, No. 132, 1974). US National Center for Health Statistics, US Department of HEW, Washington, DC.

TABLE D *Percentile Norms, Ages 6–18* for Sum of Triceps plus Subscapular Skinfolds (mm) for Girls*

Age	6	7	8	9	10	11	12	13	14	15	16	17
Percentile												
99	8	8	8	9	9	8	9	10	10	11	11	12
95	9	10	10	10	10	11	11	12	13	14	14	15
90	10	11	11	12	12	12	12	13	15	16	16	16
85	11	12	12	12	13	13	13	14	16	17	18	18
80	12	12	12	13	13	14	14	15	17	18	19	19
75	12	12	13	14	14	15	15	16	18	20	20	20
70	12	13	14	15	15	16	16	17	19	21	21	22
65	13	13	14	15	16	16	17	18	20	22	22	23
60	13	14	15	16	17	17	17	19	21	23	23	24
55	14	15	16	16	18	18	19	20	22	24	24	26
50	14	15	16	17	18	19	19	20	24	25	25	27
45	15	16	17	18	20	20	21	22	25	26	27	28
40	15	16	18	19	20	21	22	23	26	28	29	30
35	16	17	19	20	22	22	24	25	27	29	30	32
30	16	18	20	22	24	23	25	27	30	32	32	34
25	17	19	21	24	25	25	27	30	32	34	34	36
20	18	20	23	26	28	28	31	33	35	37	37	40
15	19	22	25	29	31	31	35	39	39	42	42	42
10	22	25	30	34	35	36	40	43	42	48	46	46
5	26	28	36	40	41	42	48	51	52	56	57	58

*The norms for age 17 may be used for age 18.

Source: Based on data from Johnston, F.E., Hamill, D.V. and Lemeshow, S: (1) *Skinfold Thickness of Children 6–11 Years* (Series II, No. 120, 1972), and (2) *Skinfold Thickness of Youths 12–17 Years* (Series II, No. 132, 1974). US National Center for Health Statistics, US Department of HEW, Washington, DC.

Tables from Lifetime Health Related Physical Fitness Test Manual, ADHPERD, Reston, VA., 1980. With permission of the American Alliance for Health, Physical Education, Recreation and Dance.

Subjective Data that May Suggest Nutritional Problems

This outline is intended to guide the nurse in ongoing nutritional assessment. Problem areas may be incorporated into the nursing care plan or referred to the dietitian or physician, as appropriate.

    I. Medical history
   II. Surgical history
  III. Medication/drug history
      A. Prescription
      B. Nonprescription, including caffeine, alcohol, nicotine
  IV. Height and weight
      A. Usual
      B. At age 25
      C. Recent gains/losses
         1. Intentional
            a. Methods used
         2. Unintentional
   V. Usual food intake
      A. Special diet
      B. Meal pattern
         1. Number of times per day
         2. Changes with day of week, work schedule
      C. On a typical day
         1. Amount of starches/breads
         2. Amount of vegetables (Vitamin A sources)
         3. Amount of fruits (Vitamin C sources)
         4. Amount of milk/cheese
         5. Amount of meat/fish/poultry/eggs
         6. Amount of fat/oils
         7. Amount of sugars/sweets
         8. Fluid intake
            a. Amount
            b. Kind
         9. Vitamin or mineral supplements
  VI. Food items avoided
      A. Allergies
         1. Monosodium glutamate

B. Intolerances
VII. Usual physical activity
    A. Occupational
    B. Recreational
VIII. Socioeconomic status
    A. Cultural background
        1. Food choices affected by
            a. Religious practices
            b. Education
        2. Travel in past month
        3. Attitudes and beliefs about food
    B. Financial status
        1. Income adequate for food
        2. Eligibility for assistance programs
            a. Willingness to participate
        3. Living arrangements
            a. Lives with ?
            b. Eats with ?
            c. Shopping and transporting ease
            d. Cooking and storing facilities
            e. Meals out
IX. Changes in nutritional status during past 12 months
    A. Appetite
    B. Taste
    C. Smell
X. Reproductive function
    A. Pregnant
    B. Nursing mother
    C. Intention to become pregnant
    D. Number and ages of children
XI. Skin and mucous membranes
    A. Changes in moisture, texture
    B. Difficulty healing
    C. Presence of ulcers/wounds
XII. Cardiovascular function
    A. Areas of swelling
    B. Fatigue
    C. Shortness of breath
    D. Cough, sputum
    E. Bleeding, bruising
XIII. Endocrine function
    A. Heat, cold intolerance
    B. Changes in amount of food or fluids consumed
XIV. Urinary function
    A. Changes in amount
    B. Character of urine
XV. Gastrointestinal function
    A. Oral cavity
        1. Caries
        2. Loose or missing teeth
        3. Removable bridges

   4. Dentures
      a. Use
      b. Fit
   5. Pain in teeth
   6. Problems chewing
   7. Last dental visit
B. Esophagus
   1. Problems swallowing
   2. Heartburn: frequency, severity, and treatment
C. Abdominal cavity
   1. Nausea: frequency, severity, and treatment
   2. Vomiting: frequency, severity, and treatment; whether self-induced
   3. Constipation: frequency, severity, and treatment
   4. Diarrhea: frequency, severity, and treatment
   5. Flatulence, gas pains
   6. Pain

How to Evaluate
Dietary Status

Reviewing a patient's reported intake or actual food consumption and comparing this to the Food Pyramid guide can assist in the identification of some nutrients that may be lacking in a person's diet. The table lists the recommended number of servings needed each day according to sex, age, and physiological state (breast-feeding or pregnant). The following method of comparing a patient's daily intake to the Food Pyramid is suggested:

1. Did the patient consume at least the recommended servings of grains for his or her sex, age, and physiological state? Nutrients supplied by this group include carbohydrate, thiamin, iron, and niacin. A person who does not eat enough grains may be deficient in these nutrients. In addition, this group supplies fiber.
2. Did the patient consume recommended servings of fruits? After counting the number of servings of fruits eaten, check for a reliable source of vitamin C. It is difficult for a patient to meet his or her vitamin C allowance without including fruits or some vegetables in the diet. Other nutrients in this group are fiber, iron, potassium, folic acid, carbohydrate, and other trace minerals. Remember, many fruits function as a scrub brush for the teeth and intestines. If an individual's diet is low in fruits ask about his or her dentation. The patient may avoid this fruit (especially raw) because of chewing problems. The patient may also have a problem with elimination.
3. Did the patient consume the recommended number of servings of vegetables? After counting the servings of vegetables, check for a reliable source of vitamin A. It is difficult for an individual to meet his or her vitamin A allowance without including some vegetables in the diet. Many of the comments listed under fruits also apply to the vegetable group such as: nutrients high in this group, fiber, potential dentation, and elimination problems if not part of the diet, etc.
4. Did the patient consume the appropriate amount of milk for his or her age, sex, and physiological state? If not, the diet may be lacking in calcium, vitamin D, and riboflavin. Double check for other reliable sources of calcium such as cheese and foods made with milk.
5. Did the patient consume the number of recommended servings from the meat group for his or her age and physiological state? If not, the diet may be lacking in protein, iron, and B-vitamins. Remember, the meat group also includes cheese, eggs, beans, and other protein-rich foods.

How Many Servings Do You Need Each Day?

	Women and Some Older Adults	Children, Teen Girls, Active Women, Most Men	Teen Boys and Active Men
Calorie level*	about 1,600	about 2,200	about 2,800
Bread group	6	9	11
Vegetable group	3	4	5
Fruit group	2	3	4
Milk group	**2–3	**2–3	**2–3
Meat group	2, for a total of 5 ounces	2, for a total of 6 ounces	3 for a total of 7 ounces

*These are the calorie levels if you choose low-fat, lean foods from the five major food groups and use foods from the fats, oils, and sweets group sparingly.

**Women who are pregnant or breast-feeding, teenagers, and young adults to age 24 need three servings.

Source: USDA: Food Guide Pyramid—A Guide to Good Eating. Consumer Information Center, Pueblo, Colorado.

Selected Religious Dietary Restrictions

Selected Religious Customs Which Affect Food Intake

Religion	Restricted Food and Beverages
Buddhism	1. All meat
Christian	1. Meat prohibited by some denominations on holy days such as Good Friday and Ash Wednesday 2. Alcoholic beverages by some denominations
Hinduism	1. Beef, pork, and some fowl
Moslem (Islam)	1. All pork and pork products 2. All meat must be slaughtered according to ritual letting of blood 3. Coffee and tea 4. All alcoholic beverages
Orthodox Jewish	1. All pork and pork products 2. All fish without scales and fins 3. Dairy products should not be eaten at the same meal that contains meat and meat products 4. All meat must be slaughtered and prepared according to Biblical ordinances. Since blood is forbidden as food, meat must be drained thoroughly. 5. Bakery products and prepared food mixtures must be prepared under acceptable Kosher standards. 6. Leavened bread and cake is forbidden during Passover
Seventh Day Adventist	1. All pork and pork products 2. Shellfish 3. All flesh foods (some members) 4. All dairy products and eggs (some members) 5. Blood 6. Highly spiced foods 7. Meat broths 8. All alcoholic beverages 9. Coffee and tea

Characteristic Eating Patterns of Selected Cultural Groups

Characteristic Eating Patterns of Selected Cultural Groups

Group	Grains and Starches	Fruits	Vegetables	Meat and Meat Substitutes	Milk and Milk Substitutes	To Decrease Fat
HISPANIC Mexican	Tortillas, corn products, potatoes, corn		Chili peppers, tomatoes, onions, beets, cabbage, pumpkins, string beans	Meat, poultry, eggs; pinto, calico, garbanzo beans	Cheese (milk seldom consumed)	Encourage: • Salsa as dip or topping • Baked corn tortillas, especially stuffed with chicken to make tamales, tostados, or enchiladas • Rice with chicken or beans • Reduced-fat cheeses Discourage: • Fried tortillas • Sour cream and regular cheese as toppings • Refried beans that are cooked in lard • Deep-fried dishes such as chimichangas
Puerto Rican	Platanos (starchy vegetable which looks like a large banana), Puerto Rican bread (resembles Italian bread), rice, viands (starchy vegetable whose roots and tubers are peeled, boiled, and eaten as a side dish)	Guava, canned peaches, pears, fruit cocktail, apples	Beets, eggplant, carrots, green beans, onions	Legumes (especially red kidney beans), eggs, pork, chicken, cod, fish, pigeon, peas, garbanzo beans	Milk seldom consumed, Flan (custard)	
Cuban	Rice		Green peppers, onions, tomatoes.	Black beans, pork, chicken, chorizo, (a highly seasoned sausage)	Milk seldom used	
ITALIAN	Pasta, yeast breads, starchy root vegetables		Green peppers, onions, tomatoes	Spiced sausages, fish, tomato-based meat sauces	Cheese (milk seldom consumed—high incidence of lactose intolerance in Italians)	Encourage: • Salad with no-fat dressing • Minestrone soup • Pasta with tomato or clam sauce • Grilled meat or seafood

	Breads/Starches	Fruits	Vegetables	Meats/Protein	Milk/Dairy	
SOUTHERN BLACK AMERICANS	Cornbread, biscuits, white bread, butter beans, corn, sweet potatoes, grits, rice, white potatoes, corn, yams	Melons, bananas, peaches	Kale, collards, and mustard greens, okra, tomatoes, cabbage, summer squash	Catfish, pork, (all parts), chicken, black-eyes peas, other dried beans and peas	Buttermilk, evaporated milk, ice cream (high incidence of lactose intolerance in blacks)	Discourage: • White sauces made with cream, butter, cheese • Breaded and fried meats and vegetables • Sausages and other fatty meats such as prosciutto (spiced ham)
ASIAN Southern China	Rice		Mushrooms, bean sprouts, Chinese greens, bok choy	Beef, pork, poultry, seafood	Limited except for ice cream	Encourage: • Baked fish and chicken • Steamed vegetables • Fresh melon • Grilled foods
Northern China	Wheat, millet seed used in noodles, bread, dumplings		Chinese greens, bamboo, alfalfa sprouts, bok choy	Beef, poultry, seafood, eggs, tofu, soy beans	None (high incidence of lactose intolerance among all Chinese)	Encourage: • Hot and sour soup; wonton soup • Steamed (not fried) dumplings • Lightly stir-fried chicken or seafood • Steamed whole fish • Steamed vegetables; steamed rice
Japanese	Rice, most other complex carbohydrates	All	All	Fish, beef, pork, eggs, poultry, shellfish, soybean products	None (high incidence of lactose intolerance among all Japanese)	Discourage: • Egg rolls • Crispy fried noodles • Fried rice • Deep-fried entrees • Spareribs • Tempura

Characteristic Eating Patterns of Selected Cultural Groups (Continued)

Group	Grains and Starches	Fruits	Vegetables	Meat and Meat Substitutes	Milk and Milk Substitutes	To Decrease Fat
MIDDLE EASTERN EUROPEAN	Pita bread		Grape leaves	Lamb, chicken, goat, legumes	Yogurt	Encourage: • Lean beef, pork, poultry • Broiled, poached, or steamed meats • Wine-and tomato-based sauces • Consommé Discourage: • Creamed soups and sauces • Sausages • Whole milk and whole-milk products • Fried potatoes • Sour cream
	Bulgar, dark breads, wheat breads, potatoes	All	All, especially, onions, carrots, beans	Beef, pork, poultry, fish, shellfish, eggs, sausages	All cheese and milk products	

The New Food Label

"The New Food Label," was developed by the federal government to provide up-to-date, easier-to-use nutrition information (see figures). A summary of many of the new food label features follows:

1. Standardized Format—Every label has the same layout and design and entitled "Nutrition Facts." Some very small packages may use a simplified format.
2. Serving Sizes—All serving sizes listed on similar products are stated in identical household and metric measures to allow comparison shopping.
3. Daily Values—The bottom half of the "Nutrition Facts" panel shows either the minimum or maximum levels of nutrients which should be consumed each day for a healthful diet. For example, the value listed for carbohydrates refers to the minimum level while the value for fat refers to the maximum level.
4. Percent Daily Values—The % daily values are based on a 2,000 kilocalorie diet and make judging the nutritional quality of a food easier.
5. Health Claims—The Food and Drug Administration allows only seven specific claims about the relationships between:
   - *fat and cancer risk*
   - *saturated fat and cholesterol and heart disease risk*
   - *calcium and osteoporosis risk*
   - *sodium and hypertension risk*
   - *fruits, vegetables, and grains that contain soluble fiber and heart disease risk*
   - *fruits and vegetables and cancer risk*
6. Descriptors—terms like "low," "high," and "free" must now meet legal definitions. Following is a list of key words and what they mean:
   Free: less than 0.5 grams of fat per serving and tiny or insignificant amounts of cholesterol, sodium, and sugar

   Low: 3 grams of fat (or less) per serving; also low in saturated fat, cholesterol, and/or kilocalories

   Lean: Less than 10 grams of fat, 4 grams of saturated fat, and 95 milligrams of cholesterol per serving. ("Lean" is not as lean as "Low")

   Extra Lean: 5 grams of fat, 2 grams of saturated fat, and 95 milligrams of cholesterol per serving; (Leaner than "Lean," "Extra Lean" is still not as lean as "Low.")

Light (Lite): $^1/_3$ fewer kilocalories or $^1/_2$ the fat of the original; no more than $^1/_2$ the sodium of the higher-sodium version

Cholesterol Free: Less than 2 milligrams of cholesterol and 2 grams (or less) of saturated fat per serving

High: A food "High" in a particular nutrient must contain 20% or more of the Daily Value for that nutrient

Good Source Of: One serving contains 10–19% of the Daily Value for a particular vitamin, mineral, or fiber.

7. Ingredients will be listed in descending order by weight, and now the list will be required on almost all foods, even standardized ones like mayonnaise and bread.

The New Food Label at a Glance

Descriptors: While descriptive terms like "low," "good source," and "free" have long been used on food labels, their meaning — and their usefulness in helping consumers plan a healthy diet — have been murky. Now FDA has set specific definitions for these terms, assuring shoppers that they can believe what they read on the package:
- free
- high
- light
- low
- more
- reduced
- good source
- less

For fish, meat and poultry:
- lean
- extra lean

Ingredients still will be listed in descending order by weight, and now the list will be required on almost all foods, even standardized ones like mayonnaise and bread.

Health claim message referred to on the front panel is shown here.

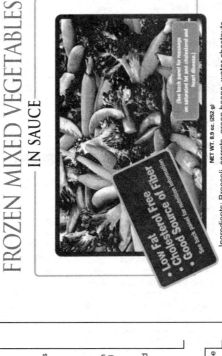

FROZEN MIXED VEGETABLES
— IN SAUCE —

- Low Fat Free
- Cholesterol of Fiber
- Good Source

NET WT. 8.9 oz. (252 g)

Ingredients: Broccoli, carrots, green beans, water chestnuts, soybean oil, milk solids, modified cornstarch, salt, spices.

"While many factors affect heart disease, diets low in saturated fat and cholesterol may reduce the risk of this disease."

Source: Food and Drug Administration 1993

Health Claims: For the first time, food labels will be allowed to carry information about the link between certain nutrients and specific diseases. For such a "health claim" to be made on a package, FDA must first determine that the diet-disease link is supported by scientific evidence. At this time, FDA is allowing seven specific claims about the relationships between:
- fat and cancer risk
- saturated fat and cholesterol and heart disease risk
- calcium and osteoporosis risk
- sodium and hypertension risk
- fruits, vegetables and grains that contain soluble fiber and heart disease risk
- fiber-containing grain products, fruits and vegetables and cancer risk
- fruits and vegetables and cancer risk.

The New Food Label at a Glance

The new food label will carry an up-to-date, easier-to-use nutrition information guide, to be required on almost all packaged foods (compared to about 60 percent of products up till now). The guide will serve as a key to help in planning a healthy diet.*

Serving sizes are now more consistent across product lines, stated in both household and metric measures, and reflect the amounts people actually eat.

New title signals that the label contains the newly required information.

Calories from fat are now shown on the label to help consumers meet dietary guidelines that recommend people get no more than 30 percent of their calories from fat.

Nutrition Facts

Serving Size 1/2 cup (114g)

Servings Per Container 4

Amount Per Serving

Calories 90   Calories from Fat 30

% Daily Value*

Total Fat 3g	**5%**
Saturated Fat 0g	**0%**
Cholesterol 0mg	**0%**
Sodium 300mg	**13%**
Total Carbohydrate 13g	**4%**
Dietary Fiber 3g	**12%**
Sugars 3g	
Protein 3g	

Vitamin A	80%	Vitamin C	60%
Calcium	4%	Iron	4%

* Percent Daily Values are based on a 2,000 calorie diet. Your daily values may be higher or lower depending on your calorie needs:

		Calories	2,000	2,500
Total Fat	Less than		65g	80g
Sat Fat	Less than		20g	25g
Cholesterol	Less than		300mg	300mg
Sodium	Less than		2,400mg	2,400mg
Total Carbohydrate			300g	375g
Fiber			25g	30g

Calories per gram:

Fat 9 • Carbohydrate 4 • Protein 4

The **list of nutrients** covers those most important to the health of today's consumers, most of whom need to worry about getting too much of certain items (fat, for example), rather than too few vitamins or minerals, as in the past.

% Daily Value shows how a food fits into the overall daily diet.

Daily Values are also something new. Some are maximums, as with fat (65 grams or less); others are minimums, as with carbohydrate (300 grams or more). The daily values for a 2,000- and 2,500-calorie diet must be listed on the label of larger packages. Individuals should adjust the values to fit their own calorie intake.

The label of larger packages must now tell the number of calories per gram of fat, carbohydrate, and protein.

* This label is only a sample. Exact specifications are in the final rules.
Source: Food and Drug Administration 1993

Calculation Aids

Weights and Measures

Linear (Length)
1 inch (in) = 2.54 centimeters (cm)
1 foot (ft) = 30.48 centimeters
39.37 inches = 1 meter (m)
Volume
1 liter (1) = 1.06 quarts (qt) or 0.85 imperial quart (Canada)
1 liter = 1000 milliliters (ml)
1 milliliter = 0.03 fluid ounces
1 gallon = 3.79 liters
1 quart = 0.95 liter or 32 fluid ounces
1 cup (c) = 8 fluid ounces
1 tablespoon (tbsp) = 15 milliliters
3 teaspoons (tsp) = 1 tablespoon
16 tablespoons = 1 cup
4 cups = 1 quart
Weight
1 ounce (oz) = approximately 28 grams (g)
16 ounces = 1 pound (lb)
1 pound = 454 grams
1 kilogram (kg) = 1000 grams or 2.2 pounds
1 gram = 1000 milligrams (mg)
1 milligram = 1000 micrograms (μg)
Temperature

Fahrenheit		*Celsius**
212°F	Boiling point	100°C
98.6°F	Body temperature	37°C
32°F	Freezing point	0°C

To convert Fahrenheit (F) temperature to Celsius (C):
°F = 9/5 C + 32.
To convert Celsius temperature to Fahrenheit:
°C = 5/9 (°F − 32).

*Also know as centigrade.

Conversion Factors

When You Know	Multiply by	To Find
Linear		
Inches	2.5	Centimeters
Feet	30	Centimeters
Miles	1.6	Kilometers
Volume		
Teaspoons	5	Milliliters
Tablespoons	15	Milliliters
Fluid ounces	30	Milliliters
Cups	0.24	Liters
Pints	0.47	Liters
Quarts	0.95	Liters
Weight		
Ounces	28	Grams
Pounds	0.45	Kilograms

Adapted from Stehman, ME: Pre-Nursing Reviews in Arithmetic, ed 2. FA Davis, Philadelphia, 1961.

Answers to Study Aids

CHAPTER ONE

Chapter Review Questions
    1. c 2. d 3. a 4. c 5. b
    6. d 7. a 8. c 9. c 10. a
NCLEX-Style Quiz
    1. b 2. a 3. b 4. c 5. b

CHAPTER TWO

Chapter Review Questions
    1. b 2. b 3. b 4. a 5. c
    6. c 7. b 8. d 9. d 10. c
NCLEX-Style Quiz
    1. c 2. d 3. a 4. c

CHAPTER THREE

Chapter Review Questions
    1. a 2. c 3. c 4. a 5. d
    6. b 7. c 8. c 9. d 10. c
NCLEX-Style Quiz
    1. d 2. b 3. b 4. c

CHAPTER FOUR

Chapter Review Questions
    1. d 2. c 3. a 4. a 5. d
    6. c 7. b 8. b 9. b 10. d
NCLEX-Style Quiz
    1. d 2. a 3. c 4. c 5. a

CHAPTER FIVE

Chapter Review Questions
    1. d 2. a 3. a 4. c 5. d
    6. b 7. b 8. c 9. d 10. c
NCLEX-Style Quiz
    1. b 2. d 3. a

CHAPTER SIX

Chapter Review Questions
    1. a 2. c 3. d 4. b 5. d
    6. b 7. a 8. d 9. c 10. a

NCLEX-Style Quiz
    1. d 2. b 3. a 4. d 5. a

CHAPTER SEVEN

Chapter Review Questions
    1. b 2. c 3. b 4. c 5. a
    6. d 7. c 8. c 9. a 10. c
NCLEX-Style Quiz
    1. b 2. c 3. d 4. a 5. b

CHAPTER EIGHT

Chapter Review Questions
    1. b 2. a 3. a 4. c 5. a
    6. c 7. d 8. b 9. c 10. d
NCLEX-Style Quiz
    1. d 2. d 3. a 4. b

CHAPTER NINE

Chapter Review Questions
    1. a 2. d 3. c 4. c 5. b
    6. a 7. d 8. a 9. b 10. c
NCLEX-Style Quiz
    1. a 2. b 3. d 4. c 5. b

CHAPTER TEN

Chapter Review Questions
    1. c 2. b 3. b 4. d 5. c
    6. c 7. b 8. d 9. b 10. a
NCLEX-Style Quiz
    1. c 2. b 3. b 4. d 5. c

CHAPTER ELEVEN

Chapter Review Questions
    1. c 2. b 3. d 4. b 5. a
    6. d 7. a 8. d 9. c 10. a
NCLEX-Style Quiz
    1. c 2. b 3. b 4. c 5. a

CHAPTER TWELVE

Chapter Review Questions
1. b   2. a   3. c   4. d   5. a
6. d   7. c   8. a   9. b   10. d
NCLEX-Style Quiz
1. b   2. d   3. c   4. b

CHAPTER THIRTEEN

Chapter Review Questions
1. c   2. b   3. a   4. c   5. a
6. d   7. d   8. b   9. d   10. a
NCLEX-Style Quiz
1. c   2. c   3. a   4. c

CHAPTER FOURTEEN

Chapter Review Questions
1. b   2. e   3. b   4. c   5. a
6. d   7. c   8. a   9. d   10. a
NCLEX-Style Quiz
1. d   2. b   3. c   4. c   5. a

CHAPTER FIFTEEN

Chapter Review Questions
1. d   2. a   3. c   4. b   5. d
6. a   7. b   8. d   9. b   10. b
NCLEX-Style Quiz
1. a   2. a   3. c   4. c

CHAPTER SIXTEEN

Chapter Review Questions
1. b   2. b   3. c   4. c   5. a
6. d   7. c   8. a   9. b   10. a
NCLEX-Style Quiz
1. c   2. c   3. a   4. d   5. b

CHAPTER SEVENTEEN

Chapter Review Questions
1. a   2. c   3. c   4. b   5. d
6. d   7. b   8. c   9. a   10. d
NCLEX-Style Quiz
1. a   2. b   3. d   4. d   5. c

CHAPTER EIGHTEEN

Chapter Review Questions
1. b   2. b   3. d   4. a   5. c
6. a   7. b   8. a   9. c   10. d
NCLEX-Style Quiz
1. c   2. b   3. b   4. a   5. b

CHAPTER NINETEEN

Chapter Review Questions
1. d   2. c   3. a   4. d   5. b
6. a   7. d   8. b   9. b   10. d
NCLEX-Style Quiz
1. a   2. b   3. c   4. b   5. a

CHAPTER TWENTY

Chapter Review Questions
1. d   2. c   3. d   4. b   5. a
6. b   7. d   8. c   9. d   10. a
NCLEX-Style Quiz
1. c   2. b   3. a   4. d

CHAPTER TWENTY-ONE

Chapter Review Questions
1. a   2. b   3. c   4. c   5. c
6. b   7. c   8. a   9. d   10. d
NCLEX-Style Quiz
1. c   2. a   3. d   4. b

CHAPTER TWENTY-TWO

Chapter Review Questions
1. c   2. d   3. b   4. a   5. b
6. b   7. c   8. b   9. d   10. d
NCLEX-Style Quiz
1. b   2. b   3. a   4. c

GLOSSARY

Commonly used terms and terms that appear either **boldface** or <u>underscored</u> in the chapter can be found in this glossary. After each definition, the chapter or chapters in which the term is either introduced or discussed extensively are identified numerically in parentheses.

Abdominal obesity—Excess body fat located between the chest and pelvis. (15)

Absorption—The movement of the end products of digestion from the gastrointestinal tract into the blood and/or lymphatic system. (5)

Acetone—A ketone body found in urine, which can be due to the excessive breakdown of stored body fat. (2)

Acetonemia (Ketonemia)—Large amounts of acetone in the blood. (16)

Acetylcholine—A chemical necessary to the transmission of nervous impulses. (6)

Acetyl CoA—Important intermediate by-product in metabolism formed from the breakdown of glucose, fatty acids, and certain amino acids. (5)

Achalasia—Failure of the gastrointestinal muscle fibers to relax where one part joins another. (19)

Acidosis—Condition that results when the pH of the blood falls below 7.35; may be caused by diarrhea, uremia, diabetes mellitus, respiratory depressions, and certain drug therapies. (9)

Achlorhydria—Absence of free hydrochloric acid in the stomach. (11)

Acquired immune deficiency syndrome (AIDS)—A disease complex caused by a virus that attacks the immune system and causes neurological disease and permits opportunistic infections and malignancies. (22)

Acute illness—A sickness characterized by rapid onset, severe symptoms, and a short course. (13)

Acute renal failure—Condition that occurs suddenly, in which the kidneys are unable to perform essential functions; usually temporary. (18)

Adaptive thermogenesis—The adjustment in energy expenditure the body makes to a large increase or decrease in kilocalorie intake of several days' duration. (8)

Additive—A substance added to food to increase its flavor, shelf life, and/or characteristics such as texture, color, and aroma. (12)

Adipose cells—Cells in the human body that store fat. (3)

Adipose tissue—Tissue containing masses of fat cells. (3)

Adolescence—Time from the onset of puberty until full growth is reached. (10)

ADP (adenosine diphosphate)—A substance present in all cells involved in energy metabolism. Energy is released when molecules of ATP, another compound in cells, release a phosphoric acid chain and become ADP. The opposite chemical reaction of adding the third phosphoric acid group to ADP requires much energy. (5, 8)

Adrenal glands—Small organs on the superior surface of the kidneys that secrete many hormones, including epinephrine (adrenalin). (6)

Aerobic exercise—Training methods such as running or swimming that require continuous inspired oxygen. (8)

Afferent arteriole—Small blood vessel by which blood enters the glomerulus (functional unit of the kidney). (18)

Aflatoxin—A naturally occurring food contaminant produced by some strains of *Aspergillus* molds found especially on peanuts and peanut products. (12)

AIDS dementia complex (ADC)—A central nervous system disorder caused by the human immunodeficiency virus. (22)

Albumin—A plasma protein responsible for much of the colloidal osmotic pressure of the blood. (9)

Aldosterone—An adrenocorticoid hormone that increases sodium and water retention by the kidneys. (9, 18)

Alimentary canal—The digestive tube extending from the mouth to the anus. (5)

Alkaline phosphatase—An enzyme found in highest concentration in the liver, biliary tract epithelium, and bones; enzyme levels are elevated in liver, bone, and biliary disease. (12)

Alkalosis—Condition that results when the pH of the blood rises above 7.45; may be caused by vomiting, nasogastric suctioning, or hyperventilation. (7)

Alpha-tocopherol equivalent (α-TE)—The measure of vitamin E; one milligram of alpha-tocopherol equivalent equals 1.5 of the older measure, International Units. (6)

Allergen—A substance that provokes an allergic response. (10)

Allergy—State of abnormal, individual hypersensitivity to a substance. (10)

Amenorrhea—Cessation of menstruation. (15)

Amino acids—Organic compounds that are the building blocks of protein; also the end products of protein digestion. (4, 5)

Amniotic fluid—Albuminous liquid that surrounds and protects the fetus throughout pregnancy. (10)

Amylase—A class of enzymes that splits starches; for example, salivary amylase, pancreatic amylase. (5)

Anabolic phase—The third and last phase of stress; characterized by the building up of body tissue and nutrient stores; also called recovery phase. (21)

Anabolism—The building up of body compounds or tissues by the synthesis of more complex substances from simpler ones; the constructive phase of metabolism. (4, 8)

Anaerobic exercise—A form of physical activity such as weight lifting or sprinting that does not rely on continuous inspired oxygen. (8)

Anastomosis—The surgical connection between tubular structures. (19)

Anemia—Condition of less-than-normal values for red blood cells or hemoglobin, or both; result is decreased effectiveness in oxygen transport (6, 7)

Angina pectoris—Severe pain and a sense of constriction about the heart caused by lack of oxygen to the heart muscle. (17)

Angiotensin II—End product of complex reaction in response to low blood pressure; effect is vasoconstriction and aldosterone secretion. (9)

Anion—An ion with a negative charge. (9)

Antagonist—A substance that counteracts the action of another substance. (6)

Anthropometry—The science of measuring the human body. (1)

Anti-insulin antibodies (AIAs)—A protein found to be elevated in persons with insulin-dependent diabetes mellitus. (16)

Anorexia nervosa—A mental disorder characterized by a 25 percent loss of usual body weight, an intense fear of becoming obese, and self-starvation. (15)

Anthropometric measurements—Physical measurements of the human body such as height, weight, and skinfold thickness; used to determine body composition and growth. (1)

Antibody—A specific protein developed in the body in response to a substance that the body senses to be foreign. (4)

Antidiuretic hormone (ADH)—Hormone formed in the hypothalamus and released from the posterior pituitary in response to blood that is too concentrated; effect is return of water to the bloodstream by the kidney. (9, 18)

Antineoplastic—A drug or other agent that prevents the development, growth, or proliferation of malignant cells. (14)

Antioxidant—A substance that prevents or inhibits the uptake of oxygen; in the body, antioxidants prevent tissue damage from unstable molecules; in food, antioxidants prevent deterioration; vitamins A, C, and E and selenium are antioxidants. (6, 12)

Anuria—A total lack of urine output. (18)

Apoferritin—A protein found in intestinal mucosal cells that combines with iron to form ferritin; it is always found attached to iron in the body. (7)

Appetite—A strong desire for food or for a pleasant sensation, based on previous experience, that causes one to seek food for the purpose of tasting and enjoying. (8)

Ariboflavinosis—Condition arising from a deficiency of riboflavin in the diet. (6)

Arteriosclerosis—A group of cardiovascular diseases characterized by the thickening, hardening, and loss of elasticity of the walls of the arteries. (17)

Ascites—Accumulation of serous fluid in the peritoneal (abdominal) cavity. (9)

Ascorbic acid—Vitamin C; ascorbic literally means "without scurvy." (6)

Ash—The residue that remains after an item is burned; usually refers to the mineral content of the human body. (1)

Aspergillus—Genus of molds that produce aflatoxins. (12)

Aspiration—The state whereby a substance has been drawn into the nose, throat, or lungs. (13)

Asymptomatic—Without symptoms. (22)

Atherosclerosis—A form of arteriosclerosis characterized by the deposits of fatty material inside the arteries; ninth leading cause of death and major factor contributing to heart disease. (17)

Atom—Smallest particle of an element that has all the properties of the element. An atom consists of the nucleus, which contains protons (positively charged particles), neutrons (particles with no electrical charge), and surrounding electrons (negatively charged particles). (2)

ATP (adenosine triphosphate)—Compound in cells, especially muscle cells, that stores energy; when needed, enzymes break off one phosphoric acid group, which releases energy for muscle contraction. (5, 8)

Atrophy—Decrease in size of a normally developed organ or tissue. (21)

Autoimmune disease—A disorder in which the body produces an immunologic response against itself. (16)

Autonomy—Achieving independence; the psychosocial developmental task of the toddler. (10)

Avidin—Protein in raw egg white that inhibits the B-vitamin biotin. (6)

Bacteria—Single-celled microorganisms that lack a true nucleus; may be either harmless to humans or disease producing. (2)

Balanced diet—One that contains all the essential nutrients in required amounts. (1)

Barium enema—Series of x-ray studies of the colon used to demonstrate the presence and location of polyps, tumors, diverticula, or positional abnormalities. The patient is first administered an enema containing a radio-opaque substance (barium) that enhances the visualization when the film is exposed. (13)

Beta-endorphin—Chemical released in the brain during exercise that produces a state of relaxation. (8)

Beriberi—Disease caused by deficiency of vitamin B_1 (thiamin). (6)

Bicarbonate—Any salt containing the HCO_3 anion; blood bicarbonate is a measure of alkali (base) reserve of the body; bicarbonate of soda is sodium bicarbonate ($NaHCO_3$). (9)

Bile—Yellow secretion of the liver that alkalinizes the intestine and breaks large fat globules into smaller ones to facilitate enzyme digestive action. (5)

Binging—Eating to excess; eating from 5,000 to 20,000 kilocalories per day. (15)

Biotin—B-complex vitamin widely available in foods. (6)

Bladder—A body organ, also called the urinary bladder, that receives urine from the kidneys and discharges it through the urethra. (5)

Blood pressure—Force exerted against the walls of blood vessels by the pumping action of the heart. (17)

Blood urea nitrogen (BUN)—The amount of nitrogen present in the blood as urea, often elevated in renal disorders; may be referred to as serum urea nitrogen (SUN). (11)

Body image—The mental image a person has of himself or herself. (15)

Body substance isolation—A situation in which all body fluids should be considered contaminated and treated as such by all healthcare workers. (22)

Bolus—A mass of food that is ready to be swallowed. (5)

Bolus feeding—Giving a 4- to 6-hour volume of a tube feeding within a few minutes. (13)

Bomb calorimeter—A device used to measure the energy content of food. (8)

Botulism—An often fatal form of food intoxication caused by the ingestion of food containing poisonous toxins produced by the microorganism *Clostridium botulinum.* (12)

Bowman's capsule—The cup-like top of an individual nephron; functions as a filter in the formation of urine. (18)

Brewer's yeast—Unicellular fungus used in brewing beer and baking bread; good source of vitamin B complex. (6)

Buffer—A substance that can react to offset excess acid or excess alkali (base) in a solution; blood buffers include carbonic acid, bicarbonate, phosphates, and proteins, including hemoglobin. (9)

Bulimia—Excessive food intake followed by extreme methods, such as self-induced vomiting and the use of laxatives, to rid the body of the foods eaten. (2, 15)

Cachexia—State of malnutrition and wasting seen in chronic conditions such as cancer, AIDS, malaria, tuberculosis, and pituitary disease. (20)

Calcidiol—inactive form of vitamin D produced by the liver. (6)

Calcification—Process in which tissue becomes hardened with calcium deposits. (18)

Calcitriol—The activated form of vitamin D, 1,25-dihydroxycholecalciferol. (6, 18)

Calcitonin—Hormone produced by the C cells of the thyroid gland that slows bone resorption when serum calcium levels are high. (7)

Calorie—A measurement unit of energy; unit equaling the amount of heat required to raise the temperature of 1 gram of water 1 degree Celsius; laypersons' term for kilocalorie. (8)

Campylobacter—Flagellated, gram-negative bacteria; important cause of diarrheal illnesses. (12)

Capillary—A tiny blood vessel that brings the blood into intimate relationship with the tissue cells. (5)

Carbohydrate—Any of a group of organic compounds, including sugar, starch, and cellulose, that contains only carbon, oxygen, and hydrogen. (2)

Carbonic acid—Aqueous solution of carbon dioxide; carbon dioxide in solution or in blood is carbonic acid. (8)

Carcinogen—Any substance or agent that causes the development of or increases the risk of cancer. (6)

Carcinoma—A malignant neoplasm that occurs in epithelial tissue. (20)

Cardiac arrhythmia—Irregular heartbeat. (17)

Cardiac output—The amount of blood discharged per minute from the left or right ventricle of the heart. (18)

Cardiac sphincter—Smooth muscle band at the lower end of the esophagus; prevents reflux of stomach contents. (5)

Cardiomyopathy—Disease of heart muscle; may be primary due to unknown cause or secondary to another cardiac disorder or systemic disease. (7)

Carotene—Yellow pigment in vegetables; precursor of vitamin A. (6)

Carotenemia—Excess carotene in the blood, producing yellow skin but not discoloring the whites of the eyes. (7)

Caseinate—A derivative of casein, is the principal protein in milk. (13)

Catabolism—The breaking down of body compounds or tissues into simpler substances; the destructive phase of metabolism (4, 8)

Catalyst—A substance that speeds up a chemical reaction without entering into or being changed by the reaction. (4)

Cataract—Clouding of the lens of the eye. (11)

Cation—An ion with a positive charge. (9)

Cecum—The first portion of the large intestine. (5)

Celiac disease (gluten-sensitive enteropathy)—An intolerance to dietary gluten, which damages the intestine and produces diarrhea and malabsorption. (5, 19)

Cell—The smallest functional unit of structure in all plants and animals. (5)

Cellular immunity—Delayed immune response produced by T-lymphocytes, which mature in the thymus gland; examples of this type of response are rejection of transplanted organs and some autoimmune diseases. (20)

Cerebrovascular accident (CVA)—An abnormal condition in which the brain's blood vessels are occluded by an embolus or hemorrhage, resulting in damaged brain tissue; stroke. (17)

Chelating agent—A chemical compound that binds metallic ions into a ring structure, inactivating them; used to remove poisonous metals from the body. (7)

Chemical digestion—Digestive process that involves the splitting of complex molecules into simpler forms. (5)

Chemical reaction—The process of combining or breaking down substances to obtain different substances. (5)

Chlorophyll—The green plant pigment necessary for the manufacture of carbohydrates. (2)

Cholecalciferol—Vitamin D_3, formed when the skin is exposed to sunlight; further processed by the liver and kidneys. (6)

Cholecystitis—Inflammation of the gallbladder. (19)

Cholecystokinin—A hormone secreted by the duodenum; stimulates contraction of the gallbladder (releases bile) and the secretion of pancreatic juice. (5)

Cholelithiasis—The presence of gallstones. (19)

Cholesterol—A fat-like substance made in the human body and found in foods of animal origin; associated with an increased risk of heart disease. (3, 16)

Chronic illness—A sickness persisting for a long period that shows little change or a slow progression over time. (13)

Chronic obstructive pulmonary disease (COPD)—A group of chronic diseases with a common characteristic of chronic airflow obstruction. (21)

Chronic renal failure—An irreversible condition in which the kidneys cannot perform vital functions. (18)

Chvostek's sign—Spasm of facial muscles following a tap over the facial nerve in front of the ear; indication of tetany. (7)

Chylomicron—A lipoprotein that carries triglycerides in the bloodstream after meals. (5)

Chyme—The mixture of partly digested food and digestive secretions found in the stomach and small intestine during digestion of a meal. (5)

Chymotrypsin—A protein-splitting enzyme produced by the pancreas; active in the intestine. (5)

Cirrhosis—Chronic disease of the liver in which functioning cells degenerate and are replaced by fibrosed connective tissue. (19)

Claviceps purpurea—A parasitic fungus from which the drug ergot is obtained; produces mycotoxins that can cause death. (12)

Clostridium botulinum—An anaerobic (grows without air) organism that produces a poisonous toxin, the cause of botulism. (12)

Clostridium perfringens—A bacterium that produces a poisonous toxin which causes a food intoxication; the symptoms are generally mild and of short duration and include intestinal disorders. (12)

Coenzyme—A substance that combines with an enzyme to activate it. (6)

Cognitive—Referring to or associated with the act of knowing. (15)

Colectomy—Surgical removal of part or all of the colon. (19)

Collagen—Fibrous insoluble protein found in connective tissue. (6)

Collecting tubule—The last segment of the renal tubule; follows the distal convoluted tubule. Several nephrons usually share a single collecting tubule. (18)

Colloidal osmotic pressure—Pressure produced by plasma and cellular proteins. (9)

Colon—The large intestine from the end of the small intestine to the rectum. (5)

Colostomy—Surgical procedure in which an opening to the large intestine is constructed on the abdomen. (19)

Complete protein—A protein containing all eight (nine for infants) essential amino acids that humans need; usually found in animal sources such as milk, meat, eggs, and fish. (4)

Complex carbohydrate—A carbohydrate composed of many molecules of $C_6H_{12}O_6$ joined together; polysaccharide; includes starch, glycogen, and fiber. (2)

Compound—Two or more elements united chemically in specific proportions. (8)

Compound fat—Substance obtained when one of the fatty acids joined to the glycerol molecule is replaced by another molecule, such as a protein. (3)

Congestive heart failure (CHF)—Condition resulting from the failure of the heart to maintain adequate blood circulation; due to complex reactive mechanisms, fluid is retained in the body's tissues. (17)

Constipation—Infrequent passage of hard, dry feces. (11)

Contamination iron—Iron that leaches from cookware into the food; in special circumstances, can become hazardous. (7)

Continuous feeding—On an ongoing basis. (13)

Continuous ambulatory peritoneal dialysis (CAPD)—A form of self-dialysis in which the dialysate is allowed to remain in the abdominal cavity for 4 to 6 hours before replacement. (18)

Contraindication—Any circumstance under which treatment should not be given. (13)

Coronary heart disease (CHD)—Disease resulting from the decreased flow of blood through the coronary arteries to the heart muscle. (17)

Coronary occlusion—Blockage of one or more branches of the coronary arteries, which supply the heart muscle with oxygen and nutrients. (17)

Creatinine—Nonprotein nitrogenous end product of creatine metabolism; because creatinine is excreted by the kidneys, serum creatinine levels are used to detect and monitor renal disease and to estimate muscle protein reserves (7, 19)

Cretinism—A congenital condition resulting from a lack of thyroid secretions characterized by a stunted and malformed body and arrested mental development. (7)

Crohn's disease—Inflammatory disease appearing in any area of the bowel, in which diseased areas can be found alternating with healthy tissue. (19)

Cross-contamination—The spreading of a disease-producing organism from one food, person, or object to another food, person, or object. (12)

Crystalluria—The presence of crystals in the urine; may be caused by the administration of sulfonamides. (14)

Cyanocobalamin—Vitamin B_{12}; essential for proper blood formation. (6)

Cyclical variation—A recurring series of events during a specified period. (1)

Cystic fibrosis—Hereditary disease often affecting the lungs and pancreas in which glandular secretions are abnormally thick. (19)

Cystitis—Inflammation of the bladder. (18)

Daily food guide—Tool used to assist consumers in making informed food choices. (1)

Deamination—Metabolic process whereby nitrogen is removed from an amino acid. (4)

Deciliter—100 milliliters or 100 cubic centimeters.

Decubitus ulcer—A pressure sore on the lower back, such as a bedsore. (16)

Delusion—False belief that is firmly maintained despite obvious proof to the contrary. (6)

Dementia—The impairment of intellectual function that usually is progressive and interferes with normal social and occupational activities. (1)

Dental caries—The gradual decay and disintegration of the teeth; a dental cavity is a hole in a tooth caused by dental caries. (2)

Dental plaque—Colorless and transparent gummy mass of microorganisms that grows on the teeth, predisposing them to decay. (2)

Deoxyribonucleic acid (DNA)—Protein substance in the cell nucleus that directs all the cell's activities, including reproduction. (4)

Desirable body weight—A person's body weight as compared with the 1959 Desirable Height/Weight Table. (15)

Development—Process of changing to a mature individual; involves psychosocial and physical aspects, often including an increase in size. (10)

Dextrose—Another name for the simple sugar glucose. (2)

Diabetes mellitus—Disease caused by insufficient insulin secretion by the pancreas or insulin resistance by body tissues causing excess glucose in the blood and deranged carbohydrate, fat, and protein metabolism. (16)

Diabetic neuropathy—Group of diseases affecting all types of nerves.

Diacetic acid—A ketone body found in the urine, which can be due to the excessive breakdown of stored body fat. (2)

Diagnostic—Relating to scientific and skillful methods to establish the cause and nature of a sick person's illness. (13)

Dialysate—In renal failure, the fluid used to remove or deliver compounds or electrolytes that the failing kidney cannot excrete or retain in proper concentrations. (18)

Dialysis—The process of diffusing blood across a semipermeable membrane to remove toxic materials and to maintain fluid, electrolyte, and acid-base balance in cases of impaired kidney function or absence of the kidneys. (18)

Dialysis dementia—A neurological disturbance seen in patients who have been on dialysis for a number of years. (18)

Diastolic pressure—Pressure exerted against the arteries between heart beats; the lower number of a blood pressure reading. (17)

Dietary recall, 24-hour—Description of what a person has eaten for the previous 24 hours. (1)

Dietary status—Description of what a person has been eating. (1)

Digestion—The process by which food is broken down mechanically and chemically in the gastrointestinal tract into forms simple enough for intestinal absorption. (5)

Diglyceride—Two fatty acids joined to a glycerol molecule. (3)

Disaccharide—A simple sugar composed of two units of $C_6H_{12}O_6$ joined together; examples include sucrose, lactose, and maltose. (2)

Disulfide linkage—Specific chemical bond joining amino acids; in hair, skin, and nails, holds amino acids in their distinct shapes. (7)

Diverticulitis—Inflammation of a diverticulum. (19)

Diverticulosis—Presence of one or more diverticula. (19)

Diverticulum—A sac or pouch in the walls of a tubular organ; pl., diverticula. (19)

Double bond—A type of chemical connection in which, for example, a fatty acid has two neighboring carbon atoms, each lacking one hydrogen atom. (3)

Duct—A structural tube designed to allow secretions to move from one body part to another body part. (5, 18)

Dumping syndrome—A condition in which the contents of the stomach empty too rapidly into the duodenum; mostly occurs in patients who have had gastric resections. (19)

Duodenum—The first part of the small intestine. (5)

Dyspnea—Difficulty breathing. (21)

Ebb phase—The first phase in the stress response; the body reduces blood pressure, cardiac output, body temperature, and oxygen consumption to meet increased demands. (21)

Eclampsia—An obstetrical emergency involving hypertension, edema, proteinuria, and convulsions appearing after the 20th week of pregnancy. (10)

Edema—The accumulation of excessive amounts of fluid in interstitial spaces. (9)

Edentulous—The state of having no teeth. (11, 13)

Efferent arteriole—Small blood vessel by which blood leaves the nephron. (18)

Electrocardiogram (ECG)—A graphic record produced by an electrocardiograph that shows the electrical activity of the heart. (9)

Electroencephalogram (EEG)—The record obtained from an electroencephalograph that shows the electrical activity of the brain. (9)

Electrolyte—An element or compound that when dissolved in water separates (dissociates) into ions that are capable of conducting an electrical current; acids, bases, and salts are common electrolytes. (9)

Element—A substance that cannot be separated into simpler parts by ordinary means. (2)

Elemental or "predigested" formula—Formula that contains either partially or totally predigested nutrients. (13)

Embolus—A circulating mass of undissolved matter in a blood or lymphatic vessel; may be composed of tissues, fat globules, air bubbles, clumps of bacteria, or foreign bodies, including pieces of medical devices. (17)

Embryo—A developing infant in the prenatal period between the second and eighth weeks inclusive. (10)

Empty kilocalories—Refers to a food that contains kilocalories and almost no other nutrients. (8)

Emulsification—The physical breaking up of fat into tiny droplets. (5)

Emulsifier—A molecule that attracts both water- and fat-soluble molecules. (12)

Emulsion—One liquid evenly distributed in a second liquid with which it usually does not mix. (3)

End-stage renal failure—A state in which the kidneys have lost most or all their ability to maintain internal homeostasis and produce urine. (18)

Energy—The capacity to do work. (1)

Energy balance—A situation in which kilocaloric intake equals kilocaloric output. (8)

Energy expenditure—The amount of fuel the body uses for a specified period. (8)

Energy nutrients—The chemical substances in food that are able to supply fuel; refers collectively to carbohydrate, fat, and protein. (1)

Energy imbalance—Situation in which kilocalories eaten do not equal the number of kilocalories used for energy. (15)

Enrichment—The addition of nutrients previously present in a food but removed during food processing or lost during storage. (2)

Enteral tube feeding—The feeding of a formula by tube into the gastrointestinal tract. (13)

Enteric-coated—A type of drug preparation designed to dissolve in the intestine rather than in the stomach. (14)

Enzyme—Complex protein produced by living cells that acts as a catalyst. (5)

Epidemic—Occurrence in a region of more than the expected number of cases of a communicable disease. (22)

Epigastric region—Central region of the abdomen above the umbilicus. (19)

Epinephrine—Hormone of the adrenal gland; produces the fight-or-flight response. (21)

Epithelial tissue—A type of tissue that forms the outer layer of skin and lines body surfaces opening to the outside; functions include protection, absorption, and secretion. (6, 10)

Ergocalciferol—Vitamin D_2, formed by the action of sunlight on plants. (6)

Ergot poisoning—Poisoning resulting from excessive use of the drug ergot or from the ingestion of grain or grain products infected with the *Claviceps purpurea* fungus. (12)

Erikson, Erik—Psychologist who devised a theory of human development consisting of eight stages of life, each with a psychosocial developmental task to be mastered. (10)

Erosion—Destruction of the surface of a tissue, either on the external surface of the body or internally. (19)

Erythropoietin—Hormone released by the kidney to stimulate red blood cell production. (18)

Esophageal reflux—Regurgitation of the stomach contents into the esophagus. (19)

Esophagostomy—A surgical opening in the esophagus. (13)

Esophagus—A muscular canal extending from the mouth to the stomach. (5)

Essential amino acid—One of the nine amino acids that cannot be manufactured by the human body; must be obtained from food or artificial feeding. (4)

Essential (primary) hypertension—Elevated blood pressure that develops without apparent cause. (17)

Essential nutrient—A substance found in food that must be present in the diet because the human body lacks the ability to manufacture it in sufficient amounts for optimal health. (1)

Evaporative water loss—Insensible water loss through the skin. (9)

Exchange—A defined quantity of food on the American Dietetic and Diabetic Associations' food exchange list or on another, similar, exchange list. (1)

Exchange lists—A food guide developed by the American Dietetic and Diabetic Associations; often used in clinical practice to aid in meal planning. (1)

Excretion—The elimination of waste products from the body in feces, urine, exhaled air, and perspiration. (5)

Exogenous—Outside the body. (16)

External muscle layer—Muscle layer of the alimentary canal. (5)

External water loss—Water lost to the outside of the body. (9)

Extracellular fluid—Fluid found between the cells and within the blood and lymph vessels. (9)

Extrinsic factor—Vitamin B_{12}, necessary for proper red blood cell development. (6)

Failure to thrive (FTT)—Medical diagnosis for infants who fail to gain weight appropriately or who lose weight. (10, 15)

Fasting—The state of having had no food or fluid enterally or no parenteral nutrition. (13)

Fasting blood sugar (FBS)—Blood glucose measured in the fasting state; normal values are 70 to 110 mg per deciliter. (16)

Fatty acid—Part of the structure of a fat. (3)

Fatty liver—Accumulation of lipids in the liver cells; may be reversible if the cause, of which there are many, is removed. (19)

Ferric iron—Oxidized iron, which is less absorbable from the gastrointestinal tract than ferrous iron; abbreviated Fe^{3+}. (7)

Ferritin—An iron-phosphorus-protein complex formed in the intestinal mucosa by the union of ferric iron with apoferritin; the form in which iron is stored in the tissues mainly in liver, spleen, and bone marrow cells. (7)

Ferrous iron—The more absorbable form of iron for humans; abbreviated Fe^{2+}. (7)

Fetal alcohol syndrome (FAS)—A condition characterized by mental and physical abnormalities in an infant caused by the mother's consumption of alcohol during pregnancy. (10)

Fetus—The human child in utero from the third month until birth; also applicable to the later stages of gestation of other animals. (10)

Fiber, dietary—Material in foods, mostly from plants, that the human body cannot break down or digest. (2)

Fibrin—Insoluble protein formed from fibrinogen by the action of thrombin; forms the meshwork of a blood clot. (7)

Fibrinogen—Protein in blood essential to the clotting process; also called Factor I; see fibrin. (7)

Filtration—The process of removing particles from a solution by allowing the liquid portion to pass through a membrane or other partial barrier. (18)

Flatus—Gas in the digestive tract, averaging 400 to 1200 milliliters per day. (19)

Flow phase—The second phase in the stress response; marked by pronounced hormonal changes. (21)

Fluorosis—Condition due to excessive prolonged intake of fluoride; tissues affected are teeth and bones. (7)

Folic acid—B-complex vitamin necessary for DNA formation and proper red blood cell formation. (6)

Food—Any material that provides the nutrients necessary to maintain growth and physical well-being. (1)

Food acceptance record—A checklist that indicates food items accepted or rejected by the patient; see Table 13–1 for an example. (13)

Food allergy—Sensitivity to a food that does not cause a negative reaction in most people. (5)

Food frequency—A usual food intake or a description of what an individual usually eats during a typical day; see Appendix D for a food frequency questionnaire. (1)

Food infection—One acquired through contact with food or water contaminated with disease-producing microorganisms. (12)

Food intoxication—An illness caused by the consumption of a food in which bacteria have produced a poisonous toxin. (14)

Food Pyramid—Food guide commonly used to evaluate a person's dietary status and to educate patients about food choices; food is divided into six groups: each contains foods of similar nutritional content. (1)

Food record—A diary of a person's self-reported food intake. (1)

Free radicals—Atoms or molecules that have lost an electron and vigorously pursue its replacement; in doing so, free radicals can damage normal cell constituents. (6)

Fructose—A monosaccharide found in fruits and honey; a simple sugar. (2)

Fundus—Larger part of a hollow organ; the part of the stomach above its attachment to the esophagus. (19)

Galactose—A monosaccharide derived mainly from the breakdown of the sugar in milk, lactose; a simple sugar. (2)

Galactosemia—Lack of an enzyme needed to metabolize galactose. (10)

Gallbladder—A pear-shaped organ on the underside of the liver that concentrates and stores bile. (5)

Gastric bypass—A surgical procedure that routes food around the stomach. (15)

Gastric lipase—An enzyme in the stomach that aids in the digestion of fats. (6)

Gastric stapling—A surgical procedure on the stomach to induce weight loss by reducing the size of the stomach; also known as gastroplasty. (15)

Gastrin—A hormone secreted by the gastric mucosa; stimulates the secretion of gastric juice. (5)

Gastritis—Inflammation of the stomach. (19)

Gastrostomy—A surgical opening in the stomach. (16)

Gene—Basic unit of heredity; occupies a specific location on a specific chromosome. (4)

Generativity—The seventh of Erikson's developmental stages, in which the middle-aged adult guides the next generation. (11)

Generic name—The name given to a drug by its original developer; usually the same as the official name given to it by the Food and Drug Administration. (14)

Genetic susceptibility—The likelihood of an individual developing a given trait as determined by heredity. (2)

Geriatrics—The branch of medicine involved in the study and treatment of diseases of the elderly. (12)

Gestation—The time from fertilization of the ovum until birth; in humans the length of gestation is usually 38 to 42 weeks. (10)

Gestational diabetes (GDM)—Hyperglycemia and altered carbohydrate, protein, and fat metabolism related to the increased demands of pregnancy. (16)

Globin—The simple protein portion of hemoglobin. (4)

Glomerular filtrate—The fluid that has been passed through the glomerulus. (18)

Glomerular filtration rate (GFR)—An index of kidney function; the amount of filtrate formed each minute in all the nephrons of both kidneys. (18)

Glomerulonephritis—Inflammation of the glomeruli. (18)

Glomerulus—The network of capillaries inside Bowman's capsule. (18)

Glucagon—A hormone secreted by the alpha cells of the pancreas; increases the concentration of glucose in the blood. (4, 16)

Gluconeogenesis—The production of glucose from noncarbohydrate sources such as amino acids and glycerol. (16, 21)

Glucose—A monosaccharide (simple sugar) commonly called the blood sugar; the same as dextrose. (2)

Glucose tolerance factor (GTF)—Organic compound containing chromium, which enhances the action of insulin, facilitating the uptake of glucose by the body's cells. (7)

Glucose tolerance test—A test of blood and urine after the patient receives a concentrated dose of glucose; used to diagnose abnormalities of glucose metabolism. (16)

Gluteal-femoral obesity—Excess body fat centered around an individual's buttocks, hips, and thighs. (15)

Gluten—A type of protein found in wheat, rye, oats, and barley. (5)

Gluten-sensitive enteropathy (celiac disease)—An intestinal disorder caused by an abnormal response following the consumption of gluten. (5)

Glycemic index—A measure of how much the blood glucose level increases following consumption of a food that contains a given amount of carbohydrate. (16)

Glycerol—The backbone of a fat molecule. (3)

Glycogen—The form in which carbohydrate is stored in liver and muscle. (2)

Glycogenolysis—The breakdown of glycogen (16, 21)

Glycosuria—Glucose in the urine. (16)

Glycosylated hemoglobin—Hemoglobin to which a glucose group is attached; in diabetes mellitus, if the blood glucose level has not been controlled over the previous 120 days, the glycosylated hemoglobin level is elevated. (16)

Goiter—Enlargement of the thyroid gland hypofunction, characterized by pronounced swelling in the neck. (7)

Goitrogens—Substances that block the absorption of iodine, thereby causing goiter; found in cabbage, rutabaga, and turnips. (7)

Gout—A hereditary metabolic disease that is a form of acute arthritis and is marked by inflammation of the joints. (18)

Growth—Progressive increase in size of living organism. (10)

"Gut" failure—Impaired absorption due to structural damage to the small intestine; symptoms include diarrhea, malabsorption, and unsuccessful absorption of oral food. (5)

Harris-Benedict equation—A formula commonly used to estimate resting energy expenditure in a stressed patient. (21)

Health—A state of complete physical, mental, and social well-being, not just the absence of disease or infirmity. (1)

Hematocrit—Percent of total blood volume that is red blood cells; normals are 40 to 54 percent for men; 37 to 47 percent for women. (7)

Hematuria—blood in the urine. (18)

Heme—The iron-containing portion of the hemoglobin molecule. (6)

Heme iron—Iron bound to hemoglobin and myoglobin in meat, fish, and poultry; 10 to 30 percent of the iron in these foods is absorbed. (7)

Hemochromatosis—A disease of iron metabolism in which iron accumulates in the tissues (7)

Hemodialysis—A method for cleansing the blood of wastes by circulating blood through a machine that contains tubes made of synthetic semipermeable membranes. (18)

Hemoglobin—The iron-carrying pigment of the red blood cells; carries oxygen from the lungs to the tissues. (7)

Hemolysis—Rupture of red blood cells releasing hemoglobin into the plasma; causes include bacterial toxins, chemicals, inappropriate medications, vitamin E deficiency. (6)

Hemolytic anemia—An abnormal reduction in the number of red blood cells due to hemolysis. (6)

Hemosiderin—An iron oxide–protein compound derived from hemoglobin; a secondary storage form of iron. (7)

Hemosiderosis—Condition resulting from excess deposits of hemosiderin, especially in the liver and spleen; caused by destruction of red blood cells, which occurs in diseases such as hemolytic anemia, pernicious anemia, and chronic infection. (7)

Heparin—A chemical, found naturally in many tissues, that inhibits blood clotting by preventing the conversion of prothrombin to thrombin; also given as an anticoagulant medication. (7)

Hepatic portal circulation—A subdivision of the vascular system in which blood from the digestive organs and spleen circulates through the liver before returning to the heart. (5)

Hepatitis—Inflammation of the liver, caused by viruses, drugs, alcohol, or toxic substances. (19)

Hiatal hernia—A protrusion of part of the stomach into the chest cavity. (19)

High-density lipoprotein (HDL)—A plasma protein that carries fat in the bloodstream to the tissues or to the liver to be excreted; elevated blood levels are associated with a decreased risk of heart disease. (16)

High-fructose corn syrup (HFCS)—A common food additive used as a sweetener; made from fructose. (2)

Hives (urticaria)—Sudden swelling and itching of skin or mucous membranes, often caused by allergies; if the respiratory tract is involved, may be life-threatening. (10)

Homeostasis—Tendency toward balance in the internal environment of the body, achieved by automatic monitoring and regulating mechanisms. (8)

Hormone—A substance produced by cells of the body that is released into the bloodstream and carried to target sites to regulate the activity of other cells and organs. (3, 6)

Human immunodeficiency virus (HIV)—The virus that causes AIDS. (22)

Humoral immunity—Development of antibodies to specific antigens by the B-lymphocytes, some of which retain the ability to recognize the antigen if it is encountered again; basis of immunizations. (20)

Humulin—Exact duplicate of human insulin manufactured by altering bacterial DNA. (16)

Hunger—The sensation resulting from a lack of food, characterized by dull or acute pain around the lower part of the chest. (15)

Hydrochloric acid (HCl)—Strong acid secreted by the stomach that aids in protein digestion. (5)

Hydrogenation—The process of adding hydrogen to a fat to make it more highly saturated. (3)

Hydrolysis—A chemical reaction that splits a substance into simpler compounds by the addition of water. (5)

Hydrostatic pressure—The pressure created by the pumping action of the heart on the fluid in the blood vessels. (9)

Hyperalimentation—Another name for total parenteral nutrition. (13)

Hyperbilirubinemia—Excessive bilirubin in the blood; bilirubin is produced by the breakdown of red blood cells. (6)

Hypercalcemia—A serum calcium level that is too high; in adults, more than 5.5 milliequivalents per liter. (7)

Hypercholesterolemia—Excessive cholesterol in the blood. (6)

Hyperglycemia—An elevated level of glucose in the blood; fasting value above 110 or 120 milligrams per deciliter, depending on measuring technique used. (16)

Hyperglycemic hyperosmolar nonketotic syndrome (HHNS)—Life-threatening complication of NIDDM characterized by blood glucose levels greater than 600 milligrams per deciliter, absence of or slight ketosis, profound cellular dehydration, and electrolyte imbalances. (16)

Hyperkalemia—Excessive potassium in the blood; greater than 5.0 milliequivalents per liter in adults. (7)

Hyperlipoproteinemia—Increased lipoproteins and lipids in the blood. (17)

Hypermetabolism—An abnormal increase in the rate at which fuel or kilocalories are burned. (21)

Hyponatremia—An excess of sodium in the blood; greater than 145 milliequivalents per liter in adults. (7, 9)

Hyperparathyroidism—Excessive secretion of parathyroid hormone, causing changes in the bones, kidney, and gastrointestinal tract. (7)

Hyperphosphatemia—Excessive amount of phosphates in the blood; in adults, greater than 4.7 milligrams per deciliter. (7)

Hypertension—Blood pressure above normal, usually more than 140/90 on three successive occasions. (10, 17)

Hypertensive kidney disease—A condition in which vascular or glomerular lesions cause hypertension but not total renal failure. (17)

Hyperthyroidism—Oversecretion of thyroid hormones, which increases the metabolic rate above normal. (7)

Hypertonic—A solution that contains more particles and exerts more osmotic pressure than the plasma. (9)

Hypervitaminosis—Condition caused by excessive intake of vitamins. (6)

Hypocalcemia—A depressed level of calcium in the blood; less than 4.5 mEq per liter in adults. (7)

Hypoglycemia—A depressed level of glucose in the blood; less than 60 milligrams per deciliter. (16)

Hypokalemia—Potassium depletion in the circulating blood; less than 3.5 milliequivalents per liter in adults. (7, 9, 17)

Hyponatremia—Too little sodium per volume of blood; less than 135 milliequivalents per liter in adults. (7, 9)

Hypophosphatemia—Too little phosphates per volume of blood; in adults, less than 2.4 milligrams per deciliter. (7)

Hypothalamus—A portion of the brain that helps to regulate water balance, thirst, body temperature, carbohydrate and fat metabolism, and sleep. (9)

Hypothyroidism—Undersecretion of thyroid hormones; reduces the metabolic rate. (7)

Hypotonic—A solution that contains fewer particles and exerts less osmotic pressure than the plasma does. (9)

Iatrogenic malnutrition—Excessive or deficit intake of one or more nutrients induced by the oversight or omissions of healthcare workers. (13)

Ideal body weight—A person's weight as compared with the 1943 Height/Weight Tables. (15)

Identity—The fifth developmental task in Erikson's theory, in which the adolescent decides on an appropriate role. (10)

Ileocecal valve—The valve between the ileum and cecum. (5)

Ileostomy—Surgical procedure in which an opening to the small intestine (ileum) is constructed on the abdomen. (19)

Ileum—The lower portion of the small intestine. (10)

Ileus—An intestinal obstruction or paralysis. (18, 21)

Immune—Produced by, involved in, or concerned with resistance or protection against a specified disease. (22)

Immune system—The organs in the body responsible for fighting off substances interpreted as foreign. (22)

Immunity—The state of being protected from a particular disease, especially an infectious disease. (4)

Immunoglobulin—Blood proteins with known antibody activity; five classes of immunoglobulins have been identified. (4)

Impaired glucose tolerance (IGT)—A type of classification for hyperglycemia; for persons who have a glucose intolerance but do not meet the criteria for classification as having diabetes. (10)

Immunosuppressive agent—Medication that interferes with the body's ability to fight infection. (12)

Incidence—The frequency of occurrence of any event or condition over a given time and in relation to the population in which it occurs. (15)

Incomplete protein—Protein lacking one or more of the essential amino acids that humans need; found primarily in plant sources such as grains and vegetables; gelatin is an animal product but is an incomplete protein. (4)

Incubation period—The time it takes to show disease symptoms after exposure to the offending organism. (12)

Indication—A circumstance that indicates when a treatment should or can be used. (13)

Indoles—Compounds found in vegetables of the cruciferous family that activate enzymes to destroy carcinogens. (20)

Industry—The fourth stage of development in Erikson's theory in which the school-age child learns to work effectively. (10)

Initiation—The first step in the cell's becoming cancerous, when physical forces, chemicals, or biological agents permanently alter the cell's DNA. (20)

Initiative—The third stage of development in Erikson's theory, in which the preschooler learns to set and achieve goals. (10)

Insensible water loss—Water that is lost invisibly through the lungs and skin. (9)

Insoluble—Incapable of being dissolved. (2)

Insulin—Hormone secreted by the beta cells of the pancreas in response to an elevated blood glucose level. (5)

Insulin-dependent diabetes mellitus (IDDM)—Type I diabetes; persons with this disorder must take insulin to survive. (16)

Insulin resistance—A disorder characterized by elevated levels of both glucose and insulin; thought to be related to a lack of insulin receptors. (16)

Intact feeding—A feeding consisting of nutrients that have not been predigested. (13)

Intact or "polymeric" formula—An oral or enteral feeding that contains all the essential nutrients in a specified volume. (13)

Integrity—The final stage of Erikson's theory of psychosocial development, in which the older adult learns to look back on his or her life as worthwhile. (11)

Intermittent peritoneal dialysis—Method of dialysis treatment in which the dialysate remains in a patient's abdominal cavity for about 30 minutes and then drains from the body by gravity. (18)

Intermittent feeding—Giving a 4- to 6-hour volume of a tube feeding over 20 to 30 minutes. (16)

International Unit (IU)—Individually scaled measure of vitamins A, D, and E agreed to by a committee of scientists; largely replaced by finer measures. (6)

Interstitial fluid—Extracellular fluid located between the cells. (9)

Intimacy—The sixth stage of development in Erikson's theory, in which the young adult builds reciprocal, caring relationships. (11)

Intracellular fluid—Fluid located within the cells. (9)

Intravascular fluid—Fluid found in the blood and lymph vessels. (9)

Intravenous—Through a vein. (2, 7, 13)

Intrinsic factor—Specific protein-binding factor secreted by the stomach, necessary for the absorption of vitamin B_{12}. (6)

Invisible fat—Dietary fats that cannot be seen easily; hidden fats in foods such as baked goods, peanut butter, emulsified milk, and so forth. (3)

Ion—an atom or group of atoms carrying an electrical charge; an ion with a positive charge is called a cation; an ion with a negative charge is called an anion. (9)

Ionic bond—A chemical bond formed between atoms by the loss and gain of electrons. (10)

Iron-deficiency anemia—Anemia due to a greater demand on the stored iron than can be supplied; causes include inadequate iron intake, malabsorption, and chronic or acute blood loss. (7, 10)

Irrigation—Flushing water through a tube or cavity. (13)

Irritable bowel syndrome—Diarrhea, or alternating constipation-diarrhea with no discernible organic cause. (19)

Islet cell antibody—A protein found to be elevated in a person with insulin-dependent diabetes mellitus. (16)

Islets of Langerhans—Clusters of cells in the pancreas including alpha, beta, and delta cells; alpha cells produce glucagon, beta cells produce insulin, and delta cells produce somatostatin. (16)

Isotonic—A solution that has the same osmotic pressure as blood plasma. (9, 13)

Jaundice—Yellowing of skin, whites of eyes, and mucous membranes due to excessive bilirubin in the blood; causes may be obstructed bile duct, liver disease, or hemolysis of red blood cells. (6)

Jejunoileal bypass—A surgical procedure that removes a portion of the small intestine, bypassing about 90 percent of it. (15)

Jejunostomy—A surgical opening in the jejunum. (13)

Jejunum—The second portion of the small intestine. (5)

Kaposi's sarcoma—A type of cancer often related to the immunocompromised state that accompanies AIDS; characterized by multiple areas of cell proliferation, initially in the skin and eventually in other body sites. (22)

Kilocaloric density—The kilocalories contained in a given volume of a food. (8)

Kilocalorie:nitrogen ratios—A mathematical relationship expressed as the number of kilocalories per gram of nitrogen provided in a feeding. (21)

Keto acid—Amino acid residue left after deamination. (4)

Ketoacidosis—Acidosis due to an excess of ketone bodies. (16)

Ketone bodies—Compounds such as acetone and diacetic acid that are formed when fat is metabolized incompletely. (2)

Ketonuria—The presence of ketone bodies in the urine. (16)

Ketosis—The physical state of the human body with ketones elevated in the blood and present in the urine; one example is diabetic ketoacidosis. (2, 21)

Kilocalorie—A measurement unit of energy; the amount of heat required to raise 1 kilogram of water 1 degree Celsius; often referred to as calories by the general public. (8)

Kilojoule—A measurement unit of energy; one kilocalorie equals 4.184 kilojoules. (8)

Krebs cycle—A complicated series of reactions that results in the release of energy from carbohydrates, fats, and proteins; also known as the TCA (tricarboxylic acid) cycle. (5)

Kussmaul respirations—Pattern of rapid and deep breathing due to the body's attempt to correct metabolic acidosis by eliminating carbon dioxide through the lungs. (16)

Kwashiorkor—Severe protein deficiency in child after weaning; symptoms include edema, pigmentation changes, impaired growth and development, and liver pathology. (4, 9)

Kyphosis—exaggerated thoracic curvature of spine; humpback. (11)

Lactase—An intestinal enzyme that converts lactose into glucose and galactose. (5)

Lacteal—The central lymph vessel in each villus. (5)

Lactose—A disaccharide found mainly in milk and milk products. (3)

Large intestine—The part of the alimentary canal that extends from the small intestine to the anus. (5)

LCAT deficiency—A lack of LCAT, an enzyme that transports cholesterol from the tissues to the liver for removal from the body. (18)

Legumes—Plants that have nitrogen-fixing bacteria in their roots; a good alternative to meat as a protein source; examples are dried beans, lentils. (4)

Lesion—Area of diseased or injured tissue. (18)

Leukopenia—Abnormal decrease in the number of white blood corpuscles; usually below 5000 per cubic millimeter. (22)

Life expectancy—The probable number of years that persons of a given age may be expected to live. (11)

Linoleic acid—An essential fatty acid. (3)

Lipectomy—The surgical procedure in which fat tissue is removed through a vacuum hose. (15)

Lipid—Any one of a group of fats or fat-like substances that are insoluble in water; includes true fats (fatty acids and glycerol), lipoids, and sterols. (3)

Lipoid—Substances resembling fats, but containing other groups than glycerol and fatty acids that make up true fats; phospholipids for one. (3)

Lipolysis—The breakdown of adipose tissue for energy (16, 21)

Lipoprotein—Combination of a protein with lipid components such as cholesterol, phospholipids, and triglycerides. (3, 4, 5, 10, 17)

Lipoprotein lipase—An enzyme that breaks down chylomicrons. (17)

Liver—A digestive organ that aids in the metabolism of all the energy nutrients, screens toxic substances from the blood, manufactures blood proteins, and performs many other important functions. (5)

Loop of Henle—The segment of the renal tubule that follows the proximal convoluted tubule. (18)

Low-density lipoprotein (LDL)—A plasma protein containing more cholesterol and triglycerides than protein; elevated blood levels are associated with increased risk of heart disease. (17)

Luminal effect—Drug-induced changes within the intestine that affect the absorption of nutrients and drugs without altering the intestine. (14)

Lymph—A body fluid collected from the interstitial fluid all over the body and returned to the bloodstream via the lymphatic vessels. (5)

Lymphatic system—All the structures involved in the transportation of lymph from the tissues to the bloodstream. (5)

Lysine—Amino acid often lacking in grains. (4)

Macrocytic anemia—Anemia in which the red blood cells are larger than normal; also found in folic acid deficiency; one characteristic of pernicious anemia. (6, 18)

Malabsorption—Inadequate movement of digested food from the small intestine into the blood or lymphatic system. (5)

Malnutrition—Poor nutrition; results when the body's cells receive either an excess or a deficiency of one or more nutrients. (1)

Maltase—An intestinal enzyme that converts maltose into glucose. (5)

Maltose—A disaccharide produced when starches are broken down by the body into simpler units; two units of glucose joined together. (3)

Marasmus—Malnutrition due to a protein and kilocalorie deficit. (4, 15)

Mastication—The process of chewing. (5)

Mechanical digestion—The digestive process that involves the physical breaking down of food into smaller pieces. (5)

Megadose—Dose providing 10 times the recommended dietary allowance or more. (6)

Megaloblastic anemia—Anemia characterized by the formation of large immature red blood cells that cannot carry oxygen properly; caused by folic acid deficiency. (6)

Menadione—Synthetic, water-soluble vitamin K; also called vitamin K_3. (6)

Menaquinone—Vitamin K that is synthesized by intestinal bacteria; also called vitamin K_2. (6)

Metabolism—The sum of all physical and chemical changes that take place in the body; the two fundamental processes involved are anabolism and catabolism. (6, 9)

Metastasis—The "seeding" of cancer cells to distant sites of the body; spread via blood and lymph vessels or by spilling into a body cavity. (20)

Methionine—Amino acid often lacking in legumes. (4)

Microgram—One-millionth of a gram or one-thousandth of a milligram; abbreviated mcg or μg. (6)

Micronize—To pulverize a substance into very tiny particles. (14)

Microvilli—Microscopic, hairlike rodlets (resembling bristles on a brush) covering the edge of each villus. (5)

Mildly obese—Twenty to 40 percent overweight; 120 to 140 percent healthy body weight. (15)

Milliequivalent—Unit of measure used for determining the concentration of electrolytes in solution; expressed as milliequivalents per liter. (9)

Milling—The process of grinding grain into flour. (2)

Milliosmole—Unit of measure for osmotic activity. (9)

Mineral—An inorganic element or compound occurring in nature; in the body, minerals help regulate bodily functions and are essential to good health. (7)

Mixed malnutrition—The result of a deficiency or excess of more than one nutrient. (15)

Moderately obese—Forty-one to 100 percent overweight; 141 to 200 percent healthy body weight.

Modular supplement—A nutritional supplement that contains a limited number of nutrients, usually only one. (13)

Mold—Any of a group of parasitic or other organisms living on decaying matter; fungi. (12)

Molecule—The smallest quantity into which a substance may be divided without loss of its characteristics. (2)

Monoamine oxidase inhibitor (MAO inhibitor)—A class of antidepressant drugs that may have critical interactions with foods. (14)

Monoglyceride—One fatty acid joined to a glycerol molecule. (3)

Monosaccharide—A simple sugar composed of one unit of $C_6H_{12}O_6$; examples include glucose, fructose, and galactose. (2)

Monounsaturated fat—A lipid in which the majority of fatty acids contain one carbon-to-carbon double bond. (3)

Morbidity—The state of being diseased; number of cases of disease in relation to population. (13)

Mortality—The death rate; number of deaths per unit of population. (11)

Motility—Power to move spontaneously. (11)

Mucosal effect—Drug-induced changes within the intestine that affect the absorption of drugs or nutrients by damaging the tissues. (14)

Mucus—A thick fluid secreted by the mucous membranes and glands. (5)

Mucosa—A mucous membrane that lines body cavities. (5)

Muscular dystrophy—A disease characterized by wasting away of skeletal muscle with replacement of muscle cells by fat and connective tissue; most forms are genetic but one form is associated with a vitamin E deficiency. (6)

Mycotoxin—A substance produced by mold growing in food that can cause illness or death when ingested by humans or animals. (12)

Myelin sheath—Fatty covering surrounding the long appendages of some nerves; serves to increase the transmission speed of impulses. (6)

Myocardium—The heart muscle. (18)

Myocardial infarction (MI)—Area of dead heart muscle; usually the result of coronary occlusion. (17)

Myoglobin—A protein located in muscle tissue that contains and stores oxygen. (7)

Myxedema—A condition that occurs in older children and adults, resulting from hypofunction of the thyroid gland characterized by a drying and thickening of the skin and slowing of physical and mental activity. (8)

Narcolepsy—A chronic condition consisting of recurrent attacks of drowsiness and sleep. (14)

Nasoduodenal tube (ND tube)—A tube inserted via the nose into the duodenum. (13)

Nasogastric tube (NG tube)—A tube inserted via the nose into the stomach. (13)

Nasojejunal tube (NJ tube)—A tube inserted via the nose into the jejunum. (13)

Neoplasm—A new and abnormal formation of tissue (tumor) that grows at the expense of the healthy organism. (20)

Nephritis—General term for inflammation of the kidneys. (18)

Nephron—The structural and functional unit of the kidney. (18)

Nephrosclerosis—A hardening of the renal arteries; may be caused by arteriosclerosis of the kidney arteries. (18)

Nephrotic syndrome—The end result of a variety of diseases that cause the abnormal passage of plasma proteins into the urine. (18)

Neuropathy—Any disease of the nerves. (16)

Niacin—A B-vitamin that functions as a coenzyme in the production of energy from glucose; obtained from meat or produced from the amino acid tryptophan, present in milk, eggs, and meat; also called nicotinic acid. (6)

Niacin equivalent (NE)—Measure of niacin activity; equal to 1 milligram of preformed niacin or 60 milligrams of tryptophan. (6)

Night blindness—Vision that is slow to adapt to dim light; caused by vitamin A deficiency or hereditary factors, or, in the elderly, by poor circulation. (6)

Nitrogen—Colorless, odorless, tasteless gas forming about 80 percent of the earth's air. (4)

Nitrogen balance—The difference between the amount of nitrogen ingested and that excreted each day; when intake is greater, a positive balance exists; when intake is less, a negative balance exists. (4)

Nitrogen-fixing bacteria—Organisms that absorb nitrogen from the air, which, upon the death of the bacteria, is released for legume plants to use in the anabolism of protein. (4)

Nomogram—A chart that shows a relationship between numerical values. (15)

Nonessential—In nutrition, refers to a chemical substance or nutrient the body can manufacture. (1)

Nonessential amino acid—Any amino acid that can be synthesized by the body. (4)

Nonheme iron—Iron that is not bound to hemoglobin or myoglobin; all the iron in plant sources. (7)

Noninsulin-dependent diabetes mellitus (NIDDM)—Type II diabetes; insulin resistance commonly occurs; although some persons with this disorder take insulin, it is not necessary for their long-term survival. (16)

Nursing-bottle syndrome—A condition in which an infant has many dental caries caused by drinking milk or other sweet liquids during sleep. (2)

Nutrient—Chemical substance supplied by food that the body needs for growth, maintenance, and/or repair. (1)

Nutrient density—The concentration of nutrients in a given volume of food compared with the food's kilocalorie content. (9)

Nutrition—The science of food and its relationship to humans. (1)

Nutrition support service—A team service for patients on enteral and parenteral feedings which assesses, monitors, and counsels these patients. (13)

Nutritional assessment—The evaluation of a patient's nutritional status based on a physical examination, anthropometric measurements, laboratory data, and food intake information. (1)

Nutritional status—Refers to the condition of the body as it relates to the intake and use of nutrients. (1)

Obesity—Excessive amount of fat on the body; obesity for women is a fat content greater than 33 percent; obesity for men is a fat content greater than 24 percent. (15)

Obligatory excretion—Minimum amount of urine production necessary to keep waste products in solution, amounting to 400 to 600 milliliters per day. (9)

Oliguria—A decreased output of urine. (18)

Oncogene—A gene found in tumor cells making the host cells susceptible to initiation and promotion by carcinogens. (20)

Opportunistic infection—An infection that occurs due to the opportunity afforded by the altered physiological state of an individual. (22)

Opsin—A protein that combines with vitamin A to form rhodopsin, a chemical in the retina necessary for vision. (6)

Optic nerve—The second cranial nerve, which transmits impulses for the sense of sight. (6)

Oral cavity—The cavity in the skull bounded by the mouth, palate, cheeks, and tongue. (6)

Organ—Somewhat independent body part having specific functions. Examples: stomach, liver. (5)

Osmolality—Number of dissolved particles per volume of liquid. (9)

Osmosis—The movement of water across a semipermeable cell membrane from an area with fewer particles to one with more particles. (9)

Osmotic pressure—The pressure that develops when a concentrated solution is separated from a less concentrated solution by a semipermeable membrane; only water crosses the membrane. (9)

Osteoblasts—Bone cells that build bone. (7)

Osteoclasts—Bone cells that break down bone. (7)

Osteodystrophy—Defective bone formation. (18)

Osteomalacia—Adult form of rickets. (6)

Osteoporosis—A loss of bone mass. (7, 11)

Ostomy—A surgically formed opening to permit passage of urine or bowel contents to the outside. (13)

Overnutrition—The result of an excess of one or more nutrients in the diet. (1)

Overweight—Ten to 20 percent above healthy body weight; 110 to 120 percent healthy body weight. (15)

Ovum—The egg cell, which, after fertilization by a sperm cell, develops into a new individual. (10)

Oxalates—Salts of oxalic acid found in some plant foods; bind with the calcium in the plant, making it unavailable to the body. (7, 12, 18)

Oxidation—The process in which a substance is combined with oxygen. (5)

Oxytocin—A hormone produced by the posterior pituitary gland in the brain; effects are uterine contractions and release of milk. (10)

Pancreas—An abdominal gland that secretes enzymes important in the digestion of carbohydrates, fats, and proteins; also secretes the hormones insulin and glucagon. (5)

Pancreatic lipase—An enzyme produced by the pancreas; used in fat digestion. (5)

Pancreatitis—Inflammation of the pancreas. (19)

Pantothenic acid—A B-complex vitamin found in almost all foods; deficiencies from lack of food have not been documented. (6)

Paralytic ileus—A temporary cessation of peristalsis that may cause an intestinal obstruction. (21)

Paralytic shellfish poisoning—Disease caused by the consumption of poisonous clams, oysters, mussels, or scallops. (12)

Parasite—An organism that lives within, upon, or at the expense of a living host. (14)

Parathyroid hormone—Hormone secreted by the parathyroid glands; regulates calcium and phosphorus metabolism in the body. (7)

Parenteral feeding—A feeding administered by any route other than the gastrointestinal tract. (13)

Parotid glands—One of the salivary glands of the mouth, located just below and in front of the ears; the mumps virus causes infectious parotitis. (6)

Patient care conference—A meeting which includes all healthcare team members and may include the patient or a significant other to review and update the patient's nursing care plan. (13)

Pellagra—Deficiency disease due to lack of niacin and tryptophan; characterized by the so-called three Ds: dermatitis, diarrhea, and dementia. (6)

Pepsin—An enzyme secreted in the stomach that begins protein digestion. (5)

Pepsinogen—The antecedent of pepsin; activated by hydrochloric acid, a component of gastric juice. (5)

Peptidases—Enzymes that assist in the digestion of protein by reducing the smaller molecules to single amino acids. (5)

Peptide bond—Chemical bond that links two amino acids in a protein molecule. (4)

Perforated ulcer—Condition in which an ulcer penetrates completely through the stomach or intestinal wall, spilling the organ's contents into the peritoneal cavity. (19)

Periodontal disease—Any disorder of the supporting structures of the teeth. (11)

Peripheral parenteral nutrition (PPN)—An intravenous feeding via a vein away from the center of the body. (13)

Peristalsis—A wave-like movement that propels food along the alimentary canal. (5)

Peritoneal dialysis—Method of removing waste products from the blood by injecting the flushing solution into a patient's abdomen and using the patient's peritoneum as the semipermeable membrane. (18)

Peritoneum—The membrane that covers the internal abdominal organs and lines the abdominal cavity. (18)

Peritonitis—Inflammation of the peritoneal cavity. (19)

Pernicious anemia—Inadequate red blood cell formation due to lack of intrinsic factor from the stomach, which is required for the absorption of vitamin B_{12}. (6)

Pesticides—A chemical used to kill insects or rodents. (12)

Petechiae—Pinpoint, flat, round, red lesions caused by intradermal or submucosal hemorrhage. (6)

pH—A scale representing the relative acidity or alkalinity of a solution; a value of 7 is neutral, less than 7 is acidic and greater than 7 is alkaline. (9)

Pharynx—The muscular passage between the oral cavity and the esophagus. (5)

Phenylalanine—Essential amino acid, which is indigestible if a person lacks a particular enzyme. Accumulation of phenylalanine in the blood can lead to mental retardation. (4)

Phenylketonuria (PKU)—Hereditary disease caused by the body's failure to convert phenylalanine to tyrosine because of a defective enzyme. (5)

Phospholipid—An organic compound in the lipid group composed of one glycerol, two fatty acids, and one phosphate molecule; examples include lecithin and myelin. (7)

Photosynthesis—Process by which plants containing chlorophyll are able to manufacture carbohydrates from carbon dioxide and water using the sun's energy. (2)

Phylloquinone—Vitamin K_1, found in foods. (6)

Phytic acid—A substance found in grains that forms an insoluble complex with calcium; phytates. (7)

Pica—The craving to eat nonfood substances such as clay and starch. (10)

Placenta—The organ in the uterus through which the unborn child exchanges carbon dioxide for oxygen and wastes for nourishment; lay term is afterbirth. (10)

Pneumocystis pneumonia—A type of pneumonia frequently seen in AIDS patients; caused by the organism *Pneumocystis carinii*. (22)

Polydipsia—Excessive thirst. (16)

Polymer—A natural or synthetic substance formed by combining two or more molecules of the same substance. (2)

Polypeptide—A chain of amino acids linked by peptide bonds that form proteins. (4)

Polyphagia—Excessive appetite. (16)

Polysaccharide—Complex carbohydrates composed of many units of $C_6H_{12}O_6$ joined together; examples important in nutrition include starch, glycogen, and fiber. (2)

Polyunsaturated fat—A fat in which the majority of fatty acids contain more than one carbon-to-carbon double bond; intake is associated with a decreased risk of heart disease. (3)

Polyuria—Excessive urination. (16)

Positive feedback cycle—Situation in which a condition provokes a response that worsens the condition. Example: low blood pressure due to a failing heart stimulates the kidney to save sodium and water. (17)

Precursor—A substance from which another substance is derived. (6)

Preeclampsia—Hypertension, edema, and proteinuria, appearing after the 20th week of pregnancy. (10)

Preformed vitamin—A vitamin already in a complete state in ingested foods, as opposed to a provitamin, which requires conversion in the body to be in a complete state. (6)

Pregnancy-induced hypertension (PIH)—A potentially life-threatening disorder that may develop after the 20th week of pregnancy; includes preeclampsia and eclampsia. (10)

Pressure ulcer—Tissue breakdown from external force impairing circulation.

Prevalence—The likelihood of an occurrence taking place within a population group. (15)

Primary malnutrition—A nutrient deficiency due to poor food choices or a lack of nutritious food to eat. (15)

Principle of complementarity—Combining incomplete-protein foods so that each supplies the amino acids lacking in the other. (4)

Prognosis—Expected outcome. (22)

Promotion—The second step in a cell turning cancerous, through the action of environmental substances on the altered, initiated gene. (20)

Prostaglandins—Long-chain, unsaturated fatty acids mostly synthesized in the body from arachidonic acid; have hormone-like effects. (3)

Protein—Nutrient necessary for building body tissue; composed of carbon, hydrogen, oxygen, and nitrogen (and sometimes with sulfur, phosphorus, or iron); amino acids represent the basic structure of proteins. (4, 5)

Protein binding sites—Various sites in the body tissues to which drugs may become attached, rendering the drug temporarily inactive. (14)

Proteinuria—Protein in the urine. (10, 18)

Protein-calorie malnutrition (PCM)—Condition in which the person's diet lacks both protein and kilocalories. (4)

Prothrombin—A protein essential to the blood-clotting process; manufactured by the liver using vitamin K. (6)

Protocol—A description of steps to be followed when performing a procedure or providing care for a particular condition. (13)

Provitamin—Inactive substance that the body converts to an active vitamin. (6)

Provitamin A—Carotene. (6)

Proximal convoluted tubule—The first segment of the renal tubule. (18)

Psychosis—Severe mental disturbance with personality derangement and loss of contact with reality. (6)

Psychology—The science of mental processes and their effects upon behavior. (15)

Psychosocial development—The maturing of an individual in relationships with others and within himself or herself. (10)

Ptyalin—A salivary enzyme that breaks down starch and glycogen to maltose and a small amount of glucose; also known as salivary amylase. (5)

Puberty—The period of life at which the physical ability to reproduce is attained. (10)

Pulmonary—Concerning or involving the lungs. (21)

Pulmonary edema—The accumulation of fluid in the lungs. (17)

Purging—The intentional clearing of food out of the human body by vomiting, and/or using enemas, laxatives, and/or diuretics. (15)

Purines—One of the end products of the digestion of some nitrogen-containing compounds. (18)

Pyelonephritis—An inflammation of the central portion of the kidney. (18)

Pyloric sphincter—The sphincter muscle guarding the opening between the stomach and small intestine. (5)

Pyridoxine—Coenzyme in the synthesis and catabolism of amino acids; also called vitamin B_6. (5)

Pyruvate—An intermediate in the metabolism of energy nutrients. (5)

Quality assurance—A planned and systematic program for evaluating the quality and appropriateness of services rendered. (13)

Radiologist—Physician with special training in diagnostic imaging and radiation treatments. (13)

Rancid—Term used to describe a deteriorated fat that has an offensive odor and taste caused by the partial breakdown of its structure. (3)

Rate—The speed or frequency of an event per unit of time. (15)

Rebound scurvy—Vitamin C deficiency produced in a person following cessation of megadosing due to a habitually lessened rate of absorption. (6)

Recessive trait—One that requires two recessive genes for the trait, one from each parent, for the trait to be expressed (to be manifested) in the individual. (19)

Recommended dietary allowance(s)—RDA(s); the levels of essential nutrients that, on the basis of scientific knowledge, are judged by the Food and Nutrition Board of the National Research Council to be adequate to meet the known nutrient needs of practically all healthy persons. (1)

Rectum—The lower part of the large intestine. (5)

Refeeding syndrome—A series of metabolic reactions seen in some malnourished patients when re-fed; characterized by congestive heart failure and respiratory failure. (21)

Regurgitate—To cause to flow backward, as with an infant "spitting up." (13)

Renal—Pertaining to the kidney. (9, 18)

Renal corpuscle—Refers collectively to both Bowman's capsule and the glomerulus. (18)

Renal exchange lists—A specialized type of exchange list for patients with kidney disease who require restriction of one or more of the following: protein, sodium, phosphorus, and potassium. (18)

Renal osteodystrophy—Defective bone development caused by phosphorus retention, a low or normal serum calcium level, and increased parathyroid activity. (18)

Renal pelvis—A structure inside the kidney that receives urine from the collecting tubules. (18)

Renal threshold—The blood glucose level at which glucose begins to spill into the urine. (16)

Renal tubule—The second major portion of the nephron; appears rope-like. (18)

Renin—An enzyme produced by the kidney that catalyzes the conversion of angiotensinogen to angiotensin I. (9)

Rennin—An enzyme that coagulates milk. (5)

Residue—Trace amount of any substance in a product at the time of sale; substance remaining in the bowel after absorption. (12, 19)

Respiration—The exchange of oxygen and carbon dioxide between a living organism and the environment. (21)

Respirator—A machine used to assist respiration. (21)

Respiratory acidosis—Blood pH less than 7.35 caused by pulmonary disease, characterized by a retention of carbon dioxide. (18)

Respiratory alkalosis—Blood pH greater than 7.45 caused by pulmonary disease, characterized by a loss of carbon dioxide. (18)

Resting energy expenditure (REE)—the amount of fuel the human body uses at rest for a specified period of time; often used interchangeably with basal metabolic rate (BMR). (8)

Retina—Inner lining of eyeball that contains light-sensitive nerve cells; corresponds to film in camera. (6)

Retinol—The chemical name for preformed vitamin A. (6)

Retinol equivalents (RE)—A measure of vitamin A activity which considers both preformed vitamin A (retinol) and its precursor (carotene); 1 RE equals 3.3 International Units from animal foods and 10 International Units from plant foods; 1 RE corresponds to 1 microgram of retinol. (6)

Retinopathy—Any disorder of the retina. (16)

Retrolental fibroplasia (RLF)—A disease of the vessels of the retina present in premature infants; often caused by exposure to high postnatal oxygen concentration. (10)

Rhodopsin—Light-sensitive protein in the retina that contains vitamin A; also called visual purple. (6)

Riboflavin—Coenzyme in the metabolism of protein; also called vitamin B_2. (6)

Ribonucleic acid (RNA)—A substance in the cell nucleus that controls protein synthesis in all living cells. (5)

Rickets—Disease caused by a deficiency of vitamin D that affects the young during the period of skeletal growth, resulting in bones that are abnormally shaped and weak. (6)

Rooting reflex—The infant's natural response to a stroke on its cheek, which turns the head toward that side to nurse. (10)

Rugae—Folds of mucosa of organs such as the stomach. (5)

Salivary amylase—An enzyme that initiates the breakdown of starch in the mouth. (5)

Salivary glands—The glands that secrete saliva into the mouth. (5)

Salmonella—A genus of bacteria responsible for many cases of foodborne illness. (12)

Salmonellosis—A bacterial infection manifested by the sudden onset of headache, abdominal pain, diarrhea, nausea, and vomiting. Fever is almost always present. Contaminated food is the predominant method of transmission. (12)

Sarcoma—A malignant neoplasm that occurs in connective tissue such as muscle or bone. (20)

Satiety—The feeling of satisfaction after eating. (3, 10, 15)

Saturated fat—A fat in which the majority of fatty acids contain no carbon-to-carbon double bonds. (3)

Scurvy—Disease due to deficiency of vitamin C marked by bleeding problems and later, by bony skeleton changes. (6)

Seasonal variation—Refers to differences during spring, summer, fall, and winter. (1)

Sebaceous gland—Oil-secreting gland of the skin; most sebaceous glands have a hair follicle associated with them. (3)

Secondary diabetes—A World Health Organization (WHO) classification for diabetes when the hyperglycemia occurs as a result of a second disorder. (16)

Secondary hypertension—High blood pressure that develops as the result of another condition. (17)

Secondary malnutrition—A nutrient deficiency due to improper absorption and distribution of nutrients. (15)

Secretin—A hormone that stimulates the production of bile by the liver and the secretion of sodium bicarbonate juice by the pancreas. (5)

Self-monitoring of blood glucose (SMBG)—A procedure that persons with diabetes follow to test their own blood glucose levels. (16)

Sensible water loss—Visible water loss through perspiration, urine, and feces. (9)

Sepsis—A condition in which disease-producing organisms are present in the blood. (21)

Serosa—A serous membrane that covers internal organs and lines body cavities. (5)

Serotonin—A body chemical that assists the transmission of nerve impulses; it produces constriction of blood vessels and is thought to be related to sleep. (6)

Severely obese—Greater than 100 percent overweight; also expressed as greater than 201 percent healthy body weight. (15)

Shelf life—The duration of time a product can remain in storage without deterioration. (4)

Shigella—Organisms causing intestinal disease; spread by fecal-oral transmission from a patient or carrier via direct contact or indirectly by contaminated food. (12)

Simple carbohydrate—Composed of one or two units of $C_6H_{12}O_6$; includes the monosaccharides (glucose, fructose, and galactose) and the disaccharides (sucrose, lactose, and maltose). (2)

Simple fat—Lipids that consist of fatty acids or a simple filler such as a hydroxyl (OH) molecule joined to glycerol. (3)

Small intestine—The part of the alimentary canal between the stomach and the large intestine, where most absorption of nutrients occurs. (5)

Solubility—The ability of one substance to dissolve into another in solution. (2)

Soluble—Able to be dissolved. (2)

Solute—The substance that is dissolved in a solvent. (9)

Solvent—A liquid holding another substance in solution. (9)

Somatostatin—A hormone produced by the delta cells of the islets of Langerhans that inhibits both the release of insulin and the production of glucagon. (16)

Sphincter—A circular band of muscles that constricts a passage. (5)

Spore—A form assumed by some bacteria that is highly resistant to heat, drying, and chemicals. (12)

Sprue—Chronic form of malabsorption syndrome affecting the small intestine; subcategories: tropical and nontropical. (5)

Staphylococcus aureus—One of the most common species bacteria, which produce a poisonous toxin. The main reservoir is nose and throat discharge. Food can act as a vehicle for transmission, so proper handwashing is an essential means of control. (12)

Starches—Polysaccharides; many units of $C_6H_{12}O_6$ joined together; complex carbohydrates. (3)

Steatorrhea—The presence of greater than normal amounts of fat in the stool, producing foul-smelling, bulky excrement. (5)

Sterol—Substance related to fats and belonging to the lipoids; for example, cholesterol. (3)

Stimulus control—The identification of cues that precede a behavior and rearranging daily activities to avoid such cues. (15)

Stoma—A surgically created opening in the abdominal wall. (19)

Stomach—The portion of the alimentary canal between the esophagus and small intestine. (5)

Stomatitis—An inflammation of the mouth. (14, 18)

Stress—The total biological reaction to a stimulus, whether physical, mental, or emotional, that threatens to disturb the body's equilibrium. (21)

Stress factor—A number used to predict how much a patient's kilocalorie need has increased as a result of a disease state. (21)

Subcutaneously—Beneath the skin. (16)

Submucosa—Structural layer of the alimentary canal below the mucosa; contains tissues and blood vessels. (5)

Sucrase—An enzyme in the intestinal mucosa that splits sucrose into glucose and fructose. (5)

Sucrose—A disaccharide; one unit of glucose and one unit of fructose joined together; ordinary white table sugar. (2)

Superior vena cava—One of the largest diameter veins in the human body; used to deliver total parenteral nutrition. (13)

System—An organized grouping of related structures or parts. (10)

Systemic circulation—Refers to the blood flow from the left part of the heart through the aorta and all branches (arteries) to the capillaries of the tissues. Systemic circulation also includes the blood's return to the heart through the veins. (18)

Systolic pressure—Pressure exerted against the arteries when the heart contracts; the upper number of the blood pressure reading. (17)

T-lymphocytes (T-cells)—White blood cells that recognize and fight foreign cells such as cancer; thymic lymphocytes. (20)

Tapeworm—A parasitic intestinal worm that is acquired by humans through the ingestion of raw seafood or undercooked beef and pork. (12)

Target heart rate—Seventy percent of maximum heart rate (number of heartbeats per minute); a person's target heart rate can be objectively determined by a stress test. Individuals can estimate their target heart rate by subtracting their age from 220 and multiplying the difference by 70 percent. A person's target heart rate is the rate at which the pulse should be maintained for at least 20 minutes during aerobic exercise. (8)

Teratogenic—Capable of causing abnormal development of the embryo; results in a malformed fetus. (10)

Term infant—Any newborn, regardless of birth weight, born between weeks 38 and 42 of gestation inclusive. (10)

Tetany—Muscle contractions, especially of the wrists and ankles, resulting from a disorder characterized by severe and painful low levels of ionized calcium in the blood; causes include parathyroid deficiency, vitamin D deficiency, and alkalosis. (6)

Thermic effect of exerise—The number of kilocalories used above resting energy expenditure as a result of physical activity.

Thermic effect of foods (diet-induced thermogenesis, specific-dynamic action)—The energy cost to extract and utilize the kilocalories and nutrients in foods; the heat produced after eating a meal. (8)

Thiamin—Coenzyme in the metabolism of carbohydrates and fats; vitamin B_1. (6)

Thiaminase—An enzyme in raw fish that destroys thiamin. (6)

Thoracic—Pertaining to the chest, or thorax. (5)

Threonine—Essential amino acid often lacking in grains. (5)

Thrombus—A blood clot that obstructs a blood vessel; obstruction of a vessel of the brain or heart are among the most serious effects. (17)

Thrush—An infection caused by the organism *Candida albicans;* characterized by the formation of white patches and ulcers in the mouth and throat. (22)

Thymus—Gland in the chest, above and in front of the heart, which contributes to the immune response, including the maturation of T-lymphocytes. (20)

Thyroid stimulating hormone (TSH)—A hormone secreted by the pituitary gland that stimulates the thyroid gland to secrete thyroxine and triiodothyronine; thyrotropin. (7)

Thyrotropin releasing factor (TRF)—Stimulates the secretion of thyroid-stimulating hormone; produced in the hypothalamus. (7)

Thyroxine—A hormone secreted by the thyroid gland; increases energy production. (7)

Tissue—A group or collection of similar cells and their similar intercellular substance that acts together in the performance of a particular function. (10)

Tolerance level—The highest dose at which a residue causes no ill effects in laboratory animals. (12)

Total parenteral nutrition (TPN)—An intravenous feeding that provides all nutrients known to be required. (7, 13)

Traction—The process of using weights to draw a part of the body into alignment. (13)

Transferrin—Protein in the blood that binds and transports iron. (7)

Trauma—A physical injury or wound caused by an external force; an emotional or psychological shock that usually results in disordered behavior. (21)

Trichinella spiralis—A worm-like parasite that becomes embedded in the muscle tissue of pork. (12)

Trichinosis—The infestation of *Trichinella spiralis;* a parasitic roundworm, transmitted by eating raw or insufficiently cooked pork. (12)

Triglyceride—Three fatty acids joined to a glycerol molecule. (3)

Triiodothyronine (T$_3$)—A hormone secreted by the thyroid gland that increases energy production. (7)

Trousseau's sign—Spasms of the forearm and hand upon inflation of the blood pressure cuff; sign of tetany or lack of ionized calcium in the blood. (7)

Trust—First stage of Erikson's theory of psychosocial development, in which the infant learns to rely on those caring for it. (10)

Trypsin—An enzyme formed in the intestine that assists in protein digestion. (5)

Tryptophan—An essential amino acid, often lacking in legumes. (4)

Tubular reabsorption—The movement of fluid back into the blood from the renal tubule. (18)

Tubule—A small tube or canal. (18)

Turgor—The resistance of the skin to being pinched; in a healthy young person the effect of pinch disappears rapidly; in a dehydrated or elderly person, the pinched skin remains elevated longer. (9)

Tyramine—A monoamine present in various foods that will provoke a hypertensive crisis in persons taking monoamine oxidase (MAO) inhibitors. (14)

Ulcer—An open sore or lesion of the skin or mucous membrane. (19)

Ulcerative colitis—Inflanmmatory disease of the large intestine that usually begins in the rectum and spreads upward in a continuous pattern.

Uncomplicated starvation—A food deprivation without an underlying stress state. (21)

Undernutrition—The state that results from a deficiency of one or more nutrients. (1)

Universal precautions—A list of procedures developed by the Centers for Disease Control for when blood and other certain body fluids should be considered contaminated and treated as such. (22)

Unsaturated fat—A fat in which the majority of fatty acids contain one or more carbon-to-carbon double bonds. (3)

Urea—The chief nitrogenous constituent of urine; the final product, along with CO_2, of protein metabolism. (5)

Uremia—A toxic condition produced by the retention of nitrogen-containing substances normally excreted by the kidneys. (18)

Ureter—The tube that carries urine from the kidney to the bladder. (18)

Urinary calculus—A kidney stone, or deposit of mineral salts. (18)

Urinary tract infection (UTI)—The condition in which disease-producing microorganisms invade a patient's bladder, ureter, or urethra. (18)

Usual food intake—A description of what a person habitually eats. (1)

Vaginitis—Inflammation of the vagina, most often caused by an infectious agent. (16)

Ventilation—Process by which gases are moved into and out of the lungs; two aspects of ventilation are inhalation and exhalation. (21)

Very low-calorie diet (VLCD)—Diet that contains less than 800 kilocalories per day. (15)

Very low-density lipoprotein (VLDL)—A plasma protein containing mostly triglycerides with small amounts of cholesterol, phospholipid, and protein; transports triglycerides from the liver to tissues. (17)

Villi—Multiple minute projections on the surface of the folds of the small intestine that absorb fluid and nutrients; plural of villus. (5)

Virus—Very small noncellular parasite that is entirely dependent on the nutrients inside host cells for its metabolic and reproductive needs. (12)

Visible fat—Dietary fat that can be easily seen, such as the fat on meat or in oil. (3)

Vitamin—Organic substance needed by the body in very small amounts; yields no energy and does not become part of the body's structure. (6)

Warfarin sodium—Anticoagulant that interferes with the liver's synthesis of vitamin K–dependent clotting factors II, VII, IX, and X. (6)

Weight cycling—The repeated gain and loss of body weight. (15)

Wernicke-Korsakoff syndrome—A disorder of the central nervous system seen in chronic alcoholism and resulting thiamin depletion; signs and symptoms include motor, sensory, and memory deficits. (6)

Wilson's disease—Rare genetic defect of copper metabolism. (14)

Xerophthalmia—Drying and thickening of the epithelial tissues of the eye; can be caused by vitamin A deficiency. (6)

Xerostomia—Dry mouth caused by decreased salivary secretions. (11)

Yo-yo dieting—The repeated loss and gain of body weight. (15)

Index

Numbers followed by an "f" indicate figures; numbers followed by a "t" indicate tabular material.